Geriatric Emergency Medicine

Principles and Practice

Geriatric Emergency Medicine

Principles and Practice

Edited by

Joseph H. Kahn, MD, FACEP
Associate Professor of Emergency Medicine, Boston University School of Medicine;
Director of Medical Student Education, Department of Emergency Medicine,
Boston Medical Center, Boston, MA, USA

Brendan G. Magauran Jr., MD, MBA
Assistant Professor of Emergency Medicine, Boston University School of Medicine, and Physician Advisor for
Utilization Management, Boston Medical Center, Boston, MA, USA

Jonathan S. Olshaker, MD, FACEP, FAAEM
Professor and Chair, Department of Emergency Medicine, Boston University School of Medicine;
Chief, Department of Emergency Medicine, Boston Medical Center, Boston, MA, USA

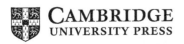

CAMBRIDGE UNIVERSITY PRESS

CAMBRIDGE
UNIVERSITY PRESS

University Printing House, Cambridge CB2 8BS, United Kingdom

One Liberty Plaza, 20th Floor, New York, NY 10006, USA

477 Williamstown Road, Port Melbourne, VIC 3207, Australia

314-321, 3rd Floor, Plot 3, Splendor Forum, Jasola District Centre, New Delhi - 110025, India

79 Anson Road, #06-04/06, Singapore 079906

Cambridge University Press is part of the University of Cambridge.

It furthers the University's mission by disseminating knowledge in the pursuit of
education, learning and research at the highest international levels of excellence.

www.cambridge.org
Information on this title: www.cambridge.org/9781107677647

© Cambridge University Press 2014

First published 2014

A catalogue record for this publication is available from the British Library

Library of Congress Cataloging in Publication data
Geriatric emergency medicine (2014)
Geriatric emergency medicine : principles and practice / edited by Joseph H. Kahn, Brendan
G. Magauran Jr., Jonathan S. Olshaker.
    p. ; cm.
Includes bibliographical references and index.
ISBN 978-1-107-67764-7 (pbk.)
I. Kahn, Joseph H., 1953– editor of compilation.   II. Magauran, Brendan G., Jr., editor of compilation.
III. Olshaker, Jonathan S., editor of compilation.   IV. Title.
[DNLM: 1. Geriatrics–methods.   2. Aged.   3. Emergencies.   4. Emergency
Medicine–methods. WT 100]
RC952.5
618.97′025–dc23
2013028335

ISBN 978-1-107-67764-7 Paperback

....

Contents

Contributors

Robert S. Anderson Jr., MD
Assistant Professor of Emergency Medicine and Internal Medicine, Tufts University School of Medicine, Boston, MA, USA, and Attending Physician, Departments of Emergency and Internal Medicine, Maine Medical Center, Portland, ME, USA

(Mary) Colleen Bhalla, MD
Emergency Medical Research Director, Summa Akron City Hospital, Akron, OH, and Assistant Professor of Emergency Medicine, Northeast Ohio Medical University, Rootstown, OH, USA

Michelle Blanda, MD, FACEP
Chair, Department of Emergency Medicine, Summa Health System, Akron, OH, and Professor, Department of Emergency Medicine, Northeast Ohio Medical University, Rootstown, OH, USA

Christopher Carpenter, MD, MSc, FACEP, FAAEM
Associate Professor of Emergency Medicine, and Director, Evidence Based Medicine, Division of Emergency Medicine, Washington University School of Medicine, St. Louis, MO, USA

Chris Chauhan, MD
Resident, Jacobi/Montefiore Residency in Emergency Medicine, Jacobi Medical Center, Bronx, NY, USA

Paul L. DeSandre, DO
Assistant Professor of Emergency Medicine and Associate Program Director, Fellowship in Hospice and Palliative Medicine, Emory University School of Medicine, and Assistant Chief, Section of Palliative Care, Department of Veterans Affairs Medical Center, Atlanta, GA, USA

Maura Dickinson, DO
Resident Physician, Department of Emergency Medicine, Boston Medical Center, Boston, MA, USA

Jonathan A. Edlow, MD, FACEP
Professor of Medicine, Harvard Medical School, and Vice-Chairman of Emergency Medicine, Beth Israel Deaconess Medical Center, Boston, MA, USA

Dany Elsayegh, MD
Division of Pulmonary/Critical Care/Sleep Medicine, Staten Island University Hospital, Staten Island, NY, USA

Kara Iskyan Geren, MD, MPH
Department of Emergency Medicine, Maricopa Integrated Health Systems, Assistant Professor of Emergency Medicine, University of Arizona, Phoenix Campus, Phoenix, AZ, USA

Peter J. Gruber, MD, FAAEM
Assistant Professor of Emergency Medicine, Albert Einstein College of Medicine, and Coordinator of Resident Education, Department of Emergency Medicine, Jacobi Medical Center, Bronx, NY, USA

Jin H. Han, MD, MSc
Assistant Professor of Emergency Medicine, Vanderbilt University School of Medicine, Department of Emergency Medicine, Nashville, TN, USA

Marianne Haughey, MD
Associate Professor of Emergency Medicine, Jacobi Medical Center, Albert Einstein College of Medicine, Bronx, NY, USA

Teresita M. Hogan, MD, FACEP
Director of Geriatric Emergency Medicine, University of Chicago, Chicago, IL, USA

Ula Hwang, MD, MPH
Department of Emergency Medicine, Brookdale Department of Geriatrics and Palliative Medicine, Mount Sinai School of Medicine, New York, and Geriatric Research, Education and Clinical Center, James J. Peters VAMC, Bronx, NY, USA

Lindsay Jin, MD
Attending, Department of Emergency Medicine, Resurrection Emergency Medicine Residency, Partner of Infinity Healthcare, Saint Francis Hospital, Evanston, IL, USA

Michael P. Jones, MD
Associate Residency Program Director, Department of Emergency Medicine, Jacobi Medical Center, and Assistant Professor, Department of Emergency Medicine, Albert Einstein College of Medicine, Bronx, NY, USA

Joseph H. Kahn, MD, FACEP
Associate Professor of Emergency Medicine, Boston
University School of Medicine, and Director of Medical
Student Education, Department of Emergency
Medicine, Boston Medical Center, Boston, MA, USA

Keli M. Kwok, MD
Department of Emergency Medicine, Boston Medical Center,
Boston, MA, USA

Denise Law, MD
Department of Emergency Medicine, Boston Medical Center,
Boston University School of Medicine, Boston, MA, USA

Megan M. Leo, MD, RDMS
Assistant Professor, Department of Emergency Medicine,
Boston University Medical Center, Boston, MA, USA

Stephen Y. Liang, MD
Instructor of Medicine, Divisions of Infectious Disease and
Emergency Medicine, Washington University School of
Medicine, Saint Louis, MO, USA

Judith A. Linden, MD, FACEP
Associate Professor of Emergency Medicine, Boston
University School of Medicine, Boston Medical Center,
Boston, MA, USA

Brendan G. Magauran Jr., MD, MBA
Assistant Professor of Emergency Medicine, Boston University
School of Medicine, and Physician Advisor for Utilization
Management, Boston Medical Center, Boston, MA, USA

Joseph P. Martinez, MD
Assistant Professor of Emergency Medicine, University of
Maryland School of Medicine, Baltimore, MD, USA

Amal Mattu, MD
Professor and Vice Chair of Emergency Medicine, University
of Maryland School of Medicine, Baltimore, MD, USA

Karen M. May, MD
Fellow, Hospice and Palliative Medicine, Emory University
School of Medicine, Atlanta, GA, USA

Aileen McCabe, MB, BCh, BAO, BMed Sci, DCH, MSc, MCEM
Emergency Care Research Unit (ECRU), Division of
Population Health Sciences, Royal College of Surgeons in
Ireland

Kerry K. McCabe, MD
Assistant Professor of Emergency Medicine, Boston Medical
Center, Boston University School of Medicine, Boston,
MA, USA

Jolion McGreevy, MD, MBE, MPH
Emergency Medicine Resident, Department of Emergency
Medicine, Boston Medical Center, Boston, MA, USA

Ron Medzon, MD
Associate Professor, Department of Emergency Medicine,
Boston Medical Center, Boston University School of
Medicine, Boston, MA, USA

Ravi K. Murthy, MD
Department of Emergency Medicine, Boston Medical Center,
Boston, MA, USA

Aneesh T. Narang, MD
Emergency Professional Services, Banner Good Samaritan
Medical Center/Banner Estrella Medical Center,
Phoenix, AZ, USA

Lauren M. Nentwich, MD
Attending, Department of Emergency Medicine, Boston
University Medical Center, Boston, MA, USA

David E. Newman-Toker, MD, PhD, FAAN
Assistant Professor of Neurology, Johns Hopkins School of
Medicine, Baltimore, MD, USA

Jonathan S. Olshaker, MD, FACEP, FAAEM
Professor and Chair, Department of Emergency Medicine,
Boston University School of Medicine, and Chief, Department
of Emergency Medicine, Boston Medical Center, Boston,
MA, USA

Joseph R. Pare, MD
Resident Physician, Department of Emergency Medicine,
Boston Medical Center, Boston, MA, USA

Thomas Perera, MD
Residency Program Director, Jacobi/Montefiore Medical
Centers, and Associate Professor, Department of Emergency
Medicine, Albert Einstein College of Medicine, Bronx,
NY, USA

Joanna Piechniczek-Buczek, MD
Vice-Chair, Clinical Services, Boston Medical Center, Division
of Psychiatry, Boston University School of Medicine, Boston,
MA, USA

Jesse M. Pines, MD, MBA, MSCE
Director, Office for Clinical Practice Innovation, Professor of
Emergency Medicine and Health Policy, George Washington
University, Washington, DC, USA

Timothy Platts-Mills, MD
Department of Emergency Medicine and Department of
Anesthesiology, University of North Carolina Chapel Hill,
Chapel Hill, NC, USA

Suzanne Michelle Rhodes, MD
Assistant Professor of Emergency Medicine,
University of Arizona College of Medicine, Tuscon,
AZ, USA

Lynne Rosenberg, PhD, MSN
President, Practical Aspects LLC, Denville, NJ, USA

Mark Rosenberg, DO, MBA
Chairman, Department of Emergency Medicine; Chief, Geriatric Emergency Medicine; and Chief, Palliative Medicine, Department of Emergency Medicine, St Joseph's Healthcare System, Paterson, NJ, USA

Todd C. Rothenhaus, MD
Chief Medical Officer, Athenahealth Inc., Watertown, MA, USA

Kristine Samson, MD
Assistant Professor, Department of Emergency Medicine, Jacobi/NCB Hospital Center and Albert Einstein College of Medicine, Bronx, NY, USA

Arthur B. Sanders, MD
Professor of Emergency Medicine, University of Arizona College of Medicine, Tuscon, AZ, USA

Jeffrey I. Schneider, MD, FACEP
Assistant Professor of Emergency Medicine and Residency Program Director, Boston University School of Medicine, Boston Medical Center, Boston, MA, USA

Rishi Sikka, MD
Vice President, Clinical Transformation, Advocate Health Care, and Clinical Associate Professor, University of Illinois Chicago School of Medicine, Chicago, IL, USA

Kirk A. Stiffler, MD, MPH
Associate Director, Emergency Medicine Research Center, Summa Akron City Hospital, Akron, and Associate Professor of Emergency Medicine, Northeast Ohio Medical University, Rootstown, OH, USA

Morsal R. Tahouni, MD
Assistant Professor of Emergency Medicine, Boston University School of Medicine, Department of Emergency Medicine, Boston Medical Center, Boston, MA, USA

Mary E. Tanski, MD
Department of Emergency Medicine and Health Policy, George Washington University, Washington, DC, USA

Abel Wakai, MD, FRCSI, FCEM
Emergency Care Research Unit (ECRU), Division of Population Health Sciences, Royal College of Surgeons in Ireland, and Department of Emergency Medicine, Beaumont Hospital, Dublin, Ireland

Scott T. Wilber, MD, MPH
Director, Emergency Medicine Research Center, Summa Akron City Hospital, Akron, OH, and Associate Professor of Emergency Medicine, Northeast Ohio Medical University, Rootstown, OH, USA

Deborah R. Wong, MD
Clinical Instructor of Emergency Medicine, Harvard Medical School, Cambridge, MA, USA

Preface

Geriatric emergency medicine has emerged rapidly as a subspecialty within emergency medicine. The emergence of this new subspecialty fills a growing need, which is the provision of high-quality emergency care to the elderly population in the United States and elsewhere in the world. Today, people 65 years of age and older account for 13% of the US population and 20% of emergency department (ED) visits. By 2030, elders will comprise 20% of the US population.

Elderly patients, in addition to often having multiple comorbidities, have a unique physiology which may mask the presentation of acute illnesses and injuries. The first section of this textbook presents chapters outlining some of the fundamental physiologic differences between the elderly and the general population. It includes an overview of geriatric emergency medicine, and chapters on the geriatric emergency department, the general approach to the geriatric patient, principles of resuscitation, pharmacology, generalized weakness in the elderly, management of trauma, and pain management in the elderly.

The second section focuses on the expedited evaluation and management of common high-risk chief complaints of elderly patients. This section includes chapters on chest pain, dyspnea, abdominal pain, altered mental status, syncope, dizziness and dysequilibrium, headache, and back pain.

The third section reviews the various systems in order to provide the reader with a comprehensive review of geriatric emergency medicine. Chapters include ophthalmologic and ear, nose and throat emergencies, neurologic emergencies, pulmonary emergencies, cardiovascular emergencies, gastrointestinal emergencies, genitourinary and gynecologic emergencies, rheumatologic and orthopedic emergencies, infectious diseases, hematologic and oncologic emergencies, psychiatric emergencies, and metabolic and endocrine emergencies.

The fourth and final section is devoted to special topics unique to geriatric emergency medicine, including alternative geriatric care and quality metrics, functional assessment, palliative and end-of-life care, social services and case management, falls and fall prevention, financial issues in geriatric emergency medicine, and elder mistreatment.

We want to thank the authors, many of whom are nationally recognized leaders in geriatric emergency medicine, for their well-referenced, excellently written, informative chapters. We would like to thank Jonathan Howland for his extremely helpful contributions. We also want to thank the editors at Cambridge University Press, especially Nicholas Dunton, Joanna Chamberlin, and Katrina Hulme-Cross for their expert guidance and patience. Most of all, we would like to thank those of you who read this text or use it as a reference; we sincerely hope you find it useful in your practice and pursuit of geriatric emergency medicine.

Joseph H. Kahn, MD, FACEP
Brendan G. Magauran Jr., MD, MBA
Jonathan S. Olshaker, MD, FACEP, FAAEM

Overview of geriatric emergency medicine

Jolion McGreevy and Joseph H. Kahn

Geriatric emergency medicine

The care of elderly emergency department (ED) patients often presents multiple clinical, social, ethical, and economic challenges. As a result, elders commonly influence flow and tax resources in EDs to a greater degree than more acutely ill younger adults. Consider a 75-year-old woman with diabetes, hypertension, and heart disease who presents with weakness after falling at home. The initial differential diagnosis for this elderly woman includes typical and atypical presentations of many life-threatening conditions. She will likely require extensive evaluation and treatment, and her disposition may depend on, in addition to her diagnosis, her ability to manage her multiple comorbidities, her personal financial resources, her family support, and the availability of home-care providers or rehabilitation facilities in the community. In addition, treatment and disposition decisions will need to take into account her baseline functional status and her beliefs about which clinical and social interventions align with her vision of a quality life.

Emergency departments vary in their ability to care for elderly patients [1]. Clinicians at a small community hospital with close ties to primary care providers can make collaborative decisions about care and disposition, reducing both unnecessary admissions and repeat ED visits. Clinicians at a large center are more likely to have immediate access to specialists who, for example, can definitively manage an expanding subdural hematoma sustained in a fall. Larger facilities also tend to have more extensive resources, including ED social workers and case managers, to connect elders with skilled nursing and rehabilitation facilities. Regardless of the size of a given hospital, recognition by clinicians and administrators that the care of elders in the ED does not end with addressing the chief complaint is an essential step toward improving the quality of care for the rapidly growing cohort of elders in the United States (US).

Research questions related to the emergency care of elders abound, as do opportunities to improve geriatric emergency medicine (EM) education in residency programs. In the US, the population of adults over 65 years of age is growing much faster than the population as a whole, with the fastest growth observed in the "oldest old," persons aged 85 years and above. In the US, approximately 30% of the annual Medicare budget is directed toward patients in the final year of life, with 80% of the expenditure paying for Intensive Care Unit (ICU) level care in the final month [2]. A study from two emergency departments in the United Kingdom found that half of elder patients who died in the ED had visited the ED or had been admitted to hospital within the previous year [3]. Elders should be given an early opportunity to express their end-of-life care preferences, particularly with regard to cardiopulmonary resuscitation. Yet do-not-resuscitate orders (DNR) are often written in the last days of life [4]. Earlier discussions with patients and families regarding prognoses also allow for introduction of palliative care options. Improving the quality and efficiency of care and the satisfaction of elders and their families is an exciting challenge in EM – one that will have a significant impact on the overall quality and cost of health care nationally.

Population aging

Elders are a heterogeneous group. Individuals over 65 years old vary greatly in terms of functional status, comorbidities, risk of adverse medication effects, financial resources, social support, and treatment goals. A health-conscious individual among the oldest old may be overall better off than a much younger person with multiple comorbidities. However, on average, elder patients are more likely to come to the ED by ambulance, spend more time in the ED, require more tests, and be admitted to higher levels of care. All of these increase the cost of care for the elderly.

Today patients over 65 years old account for 13% of the US population and 20% of ED visits [5]. By 2030, elders will comprise 20% of the US population [6]. Among elders, the fastest growth is seen among the oldest old who, by 2050, will account for double the population segment compared with that in the year 2000 [7]. Given that this group has the highest ED visit rate among elders, the expansion of this age cohort will likely have a substantial impact on ED utilization. By 2050, the ratio of working adults to elderly will be 2:1, compared with 4:1 today [8].

In countries with extensive health care safety nets, working taxpayers bear an enormous financial burden that will no doubt continue to increase. The economic impact of care for the elderly depends not only on the increase in the number of persons in this age cohort, but also on changes in family structure as a

---

whole. As nearly all developed countries shift toward a higher prevalence of one-child families, more individuals and couples will be the sole support for elderly parents.

Although elders are on average more financially secure today compared with a few decades ago, ED personnel increasingly find themselves talking to patients and families about the relative safety and cost of self-care at home versus alternatives, such as home health professionals and nursing homes [9]. Home health care is the second fastest-growing job category in the US [10]. The percentage of elders living in nursing homes has remained constant over the last two decades, but the population is trending toward older, more dependent patients, creating more competition for limited nursing home beds [9].

Emergency departments need to provide efficient, high-quality care to a rapidly increasing number of elderly patients and at the same time work with families, primary care physicians and other community care providers to improve out-of-hospital care for elders and decrease costly repeat ED visits and hospital admissions. Prevention of costly acute care visits will become increasingly important as the health care system shifts away from fee-for-service toward a global payment system.

Health system aim

High-quality care of geriatric ED patients contributes to the larger health system aim of maximizing active (disability-free) life expectancy. By identifying acute conditions in older patients, ED clinicians reduce death and disability. Older patients are more likely than younger patients to display atypical signs and symptoms of acute illness; yet clinical research that specifically addresses the diagnosis and treatment of emergent conditions in elderly patients is limited.

Emergency departments can further improve the health of elder patients by preventing adverse medication events and screening for cognitive and functional impairment that may lead to injury or limit older patients' ability to perform activities of daily living (ADL). However, just as elder-specific evidence for acute disease management is limited, there is a dearth of high-quality studies related to ED-based assessment of functional status and injury risk among elders [11].

Health systems are not limited to formal health care providers. Family members play an important role in promoting the health of geriatric patients. Elders who lack social support are at increased risk of repeat ED visits [12]. Interventions that reduce the burden on informal caregivers, such as arranging for home health services, may reduce ED and hospital utilization and ultimately be a cost-effective way to improve the health of elderly patients, especially given that such patients are at increased risk of functional decline following discharge from the ED [13].

While larger hospitals may have personnel in the ED who can set up home health services, smaller hospitals will likely need to work closely with primary care physicians to ensure that geriatric patients who are discharged from either the ED or inpatient wards receive appropriate evaluation for subsequent home health need. Geriatric patients who have been hospitalized within the previous six months or who suffer from depression are at increased risk of returning to the ED or having an adverse event, such as a significant decline in functional status, long-term hospitalization, or death [12]. Although there is no evidence-based standard of care regarding the prevention of adverse events among geriatric patients following discharge from the ED, some simple screening tools, including self-reporting questionnaires, have been studied. Limited evidence suggests that ED screening for abuse, depression, substance abuse, and decline in cognition, vision or hearing can effectively identify elders at risk for adverse events after discharge from the ED or hospital [13,14]. However, it is not clear to what extent a busy ED should accept responsibility for screening, given its primary aim to evaluate and treat for acute illness. One solution is to have social workers and case managers, rather than physicians, screen elders for conditions or home situations likely to reduce active life expectancy [15,16].

The extensive needs of elders during ED visits have prompted the development of separate EDs dedicated to this population. Geriatric EM physicians specialize in managing acute illness in the elderly. An "atypical presentation" in an elderly patient may be seen as fairly typical by a clinician who specializes in the emergency care of the elderly. A section of an ED devoted to elderly patients allows these clinicians, in collaboration with ED social workers, case managers, and pharmacists, to take the time necessary to consider the effects of multiple comorbidities and polypharmacy on clinical presentations and to employ geriatric-specific screening tools without slowing the care of other patients. A central aim of geriatric EM is to develop more fair, affordable, evidence-based interventions for the prevention and treatment of conditions that reduce the active life expectancy of older persons.

Clinical challenge

Complex patients

Geriatric patients are complex, and medical evaluations of elderly patients in the ED tend to be more costly and time-intensive than evaluations of younger patients. There is a higher percentage of emergent and urgent ED presentations among elders than among younger patients [17].

The American College of Emergency Physicians (ACEP) predicts that by 2030 the number of people over age 65 in the US will be 70 million, comprising 20% of the population. This is up from the year 2000 when there were 35 million people over age 65, comprising 13% of the population. By 2030, geriatric patients will account for at least one quarter of ED visits [18]. In addition, the oldest old population in the US continues to grow. In 2010, there were 1.9 million people aged 90 and above; by 2050, according to US Census Bureau predictions, there will be 9 million Americans in this age group [19]. Geriatric patients presenting to the ED tend to have multiple comorbidities, so their evaluations are frequently not straightforward. They also have a higher likelihood of serious illness than their younger counterparts [17]. Homebound elders have a higher rate of metabolic abnormalities, cardiovascular disease, cerebrovascular disease, musculoskeletal disorders, cognitive impairment, dementia, and depression compared with the general elderly population [20]. A recent study by Grossmann et al. in

Switzerland revealed that elderly patients presenting to the ED are under-triaged as frequently as 23% of the time, especially for the chief complaint of generalized weakness [21].

Polypharmacy is a common problem among elderly patients presenting to the ED. Elders may see multiple physicians, including their primary care physician (PCP) and specialists, and each may prescribe multiple medications. Comprehensive medication lists may not be available to ED providers, complicating the evaluation and treatment of elderly patients in the emergency setting. Transitions in care make patients particularly vulnerable to medication-related problems [22]. Medications that are potentially inappropriate for elders are frequently prescribed as first-line treatment [23]. Interestingly, the majority of hospitalizations for adverse drug events in the elderly are not due to inappropriate medications, but rather to commonly used medications such as warfarin, insulin, antiplatelet agents, and oral hypoglycemics [24].

Cognitive impairment may make the obtaining of a reliable history very difficult. Patients may not be able to express themselves well as a result of dysarthria, confusion, or dementia [17]. Acute medical conditions may cause delirium, making communication with elderly patients even more difficult than when they are at their baseline [17]. Elderly patients frequently do not remember why they were sent to the ED, highlighting the importance of communication with family members, emergency medical service (EMS) providers, and chronic care facilities [17]. After discharge from the ED, the incidence of worsening morbidity and mortality is higher for elders than for younger people. For this reason, communication with PCPs, family, and long-term care facilities is essential prior to discharge. This helps ensure that the intended treatment plan is carried out, timely follow-up care is arranged, and the patient will be returned to the ED immediately if he or she decompensates.

Elders who are discharged from the ED subsequently have a high risk of unplanned readmission. Screening tools such as the Identification of Seniors at Risk (ISAR) and the Triage Risk Stratification Tool (TRST) have been developed to predict which geriatric patients are at high risk for readmission [25]. Because Medicare may penalize hospitals with high readmission rates, some US hospitals now hold elderly patients for observation rather than admitting them [26].

In Europe, short-stay geriatric units allow ED geriatric patients to be admitted for brief periods, without increasing readmissions in the subsequent month [27]. The disposition of elderly patients living at home may depend on whether informal caregivers and home health care providers can help patients maintain safe environments and manage their chronic conditions. Even minor injuries may make it unsafe for marginally functioning patients to remain in their homes. The additional burden of acute illness or injury may be too much for family members caring for these patients. This is an important assessment for the emergency physician or case manager to carry out, as additional home care resources may be needed or patients may require temporary placement in skilled nursing facilities. Elderly ED patients should also be screened for elder abuse and neglect, which have mandated reporting requirements. With training, Emergency Medical Technicians (EMTs) can accurately identify elders at risk for abuse and neglect and notify staff at receiving hospitals [28].

Chest pain and dyspnea are the most common ED presentations among elder Americans, accounting for 11% of ED visits in this population. Elderly people often have atypical, subtle signs and symptoms of serious diseases such as myocardial infarction, surgical abdomen, and sepsis and, therefore, often require extensive work-up, even for seemingly minor complaints. Multiple trauma can be particularly devastating to elderly patients. Methodist Health System in Dallas, Texas has created a geriatric trauma unit to facilitate treatment of both acute injuries and chronic illnesses though a multidisciplinary approach [29]. Lancaster General Hospital in Pennsylvania has instituted a trauma protocol for the elderly, which attempts to promptly identify and aggressively treat occult shock. This protocol has significantly reduced mortality in geriatric trauma patients [30].

Important research questions related to the complexity of emergency care in the elderly include the following: whether medication management and functional assessment screening and intervention in the ED allow more geriatric patients to be safely discharged home; whether multidisciplinary geriatric units improve the safety and efficiency of ED disposition planning; and whether outpatient use of parenteral antibiotics can safely reduce and/or shorten hospital admissions among elderly patients [11,31].

Expensive care

Care of the geriatric emergency patient tends to be more expensive than that of their younger counterparts for a variety of reasons. Geriatric patients are more likely to arrive by ambulance than younger ED patients. The hospital admission rate is higher among elder patients, as is the proportion of these patients who require ICU-level care. More than 75% of geriatric patients who present to the ED in their final month of life are admitted to the hospital [32,33]. Many emergency medicine physicians feel less confident in the management of older patients and desire more training in the field of geriatric emergency medicine [34]. This has prompted efforts to increase exposure to geriatric topics in EM residency training, including through high-fidelity simulations of atypical presentations in the elderly. Because of the higher incidence of serious disease and increased likelihood of subtle presentations of life-threatening illness, more tests are ordered in elderly patients than in younger people. This expensive care is counter to the American push to decrease health care expenditures at all levels, including emergency care.

Research questions include whether more expensive care with more testing and higher rates of inpatient and ICU-level care translates into a decrease in morbidity and mortality for elderly patients. Another important research question is whether EMS can perform accurate home assessments prior to transferring patients to the hospital without delaying their medical care [35].

Chaotic environment

The ED environment per se can work against efficient care of the elderly patient. The noise and activity level may disorient and agitate even reasonably well-functioning elderly people. Staff in EDs may find it challenging to accommodate the needs of the geriatric patient [36]. Geriatric patients may not be able to tolerate lying on stretchers for extended periods of time and often have increased toilet needs compared with younger people [32]. Furthermore, trying to get down from the stretcher and walk to the bathroom unassisted is a frequent cause of falls in the ED. Patient falls have been targeted by the Centers for Medicare and Medicaid Services as an event which should never happen in the hospital [37]. Overtaxed nurses and nursing assistants may be unable to provide the care demanded by the geriatric patient in a busy ED. Similarly, emergency physicians, who are accustomed to performing a goal-directed history and physical exam focused on a single chief complaint, may not have the time to perform the comprehensive evaluation that many elder patients require. This may cause the emergency physician to miss important findings that signal a more serious clinical problem than originally suspected.

Since the creation of the first geriatric emergency department at Holy Cross Hospital in Silver Spring, Maryland in 2008, other hospitals have followed suit, including St. Joseph's Regional Medical Center in New Jersey, St. Joseph Mercy Ann Arbor Hospital in Michigan, Mt. Sinai Medical Center in New York, and Newark Beth Israel Medical Center in New Jersey [38]. There are currently at least 35 geriatric emergency departments in the US [39]. These geriatric EDs address the special needs of the geriatric patient, with a quieter environment, more comfortable stretchers, and a higher staff-to-patient ratio. They often have better access to social services and case management than the typical ED. The patient satisfaction ratings are very high in geriatric EDs, and many more geriatric EDs are in the planning stage across the US [40]. Geriatric EDs will be discussed in more detail in Chapter 2.

Chronically ill elders should be connected with palliative care services. Palliative care can be initiated in the ED for patients who do not desire aggressive resuscitation [41]. Many patients who would prefer to die at home with their loved ones are transferred to the ED when a near-terminal event occurs, and EDs should link these patients with palliative care providers [42]. It is important to note that palliative care is no longer administered only as a last resort; it also includes open communication with and support for patients and families and provision of pain management for patients who are being treated for any serious illness [43]. Unfortunately, pain in the elderly patient presenting to the ED is often undertreated. Further research is needed to determine the extent to which geriatric emergency departments and initiation of palliative care services in the ED improve patient and family satisfaction.

Families

A review of the literature by Luppa et al. identified six factors that predict nursing home placement in the elderly: increased age, low self-rated health status, functional and cognitive impairment, dementia, placement in a nursing home in the past, and multiple prescription medications. Predictors less strongly supported by evidence include male gender, depression, limited education, low economic status, and a history of stroke, hypertension, incontinence, or prior hospitalizations [44]. Nursing home care is often both expensive and impersonal, and in many cases sustainable home care is a better option for the elder patient and his or her family.

Home care requires additional resources for most families, including visiting nurses, visiting nursing assistants, lab collection at home, and nurse practitioner and physician home visits [45]. In order for elders to remain in their homes and continue to be active members of their communities, not only are additional medical and social services required, but these services must be integrated [46]. Education of the patient and family regarding safe home care should include instruction on accident and fall prevention. The importance of home assessments and fall prevention cannot be overestimated, as a fall may represent a sentinel event leading to rapid decline in function [47].

Maintaining continence may allow for continued home care in the elderly population, and programs promoting continence may delay long-term care facility placement [48]. Before an elderly person loses decision-making capacity, a health care proxy should be identified. The health care proxy is often the next of kin or closest family member, but this should be established prior to the occurrence of a catastrophic event. Also, advance directives should be discussed with the patient and family and health care proxy while the elder still has the ability to express his or her wishes. This makes it easier for the health care proxy to make a reasonable decision when a catastrophic event occurs. The decision to withhold medical care is very difficult for a loving family member, and establishing the patient's wishes in advance can be extremely helpful in a time of crisis.

Research questions related to the involvement of family members in the care of the elderly include what percentage of elder Americans have a health care proxy, what percentage have advance directives, and whether families and medical care providers make decisions in accordance with advance directives when serious medical illness strikes. It is also important to develop home care models that effectively reduce ED visits, hospitalizations, and long-term care placements [45,49].

Special challenges

Certain groups within the elder population are especially challenging. Low-income inner city and rural families often lack health insurance and additional resources needed to care for an elderly person at home. Racial disparities in health care in the US may affect access to adequate home care. Many immigrants are uninsured and unaware of available resources to enable home care of elders. Elderly people who do not receive medical care on a regular basis are unlikely to have a health care proxy or advance directive, often leaving their families in crisis when they sustain serious medical illnesses or injuries. Additional research is needed to identify patterns of home care versus placement in skilled nursing facility based on geography and demographics.

Palliative care in the ED

Palliative care for chronically ill older patients reduces pain, dyspnea, and depression [41,50]. It also reduces ED visits and hospital stays and increases patient and family satisfaction [41]. Most older people prefer to die at home [42]. However, many die in emergency rooms or intensive care units. Older patients who die in the ED often have recent visits to the same ED or admissions to the same hospital [3], yet few have advance directives or contact with palliative care services. ED services that link chronically ill older adults with palliative care, home care, and hospice services improve well-being and reduce ED visits and deaths in the hospital [42,51]. Research priorities related to ED palliative care include clinician education, ED-specific screening tools, outcomes for palliative care initiated in the ED, and appropriate, cost-effective alternatives to inpatient admission for geriatric patients who cannot safely return home [52].

Interfacing with PCPs and care facilities

Strong communication between EDs and PCPs can reduce hospital admissions. Primary care providers can see geriatric patients either in the clinic or the patients' homes and treat many acute illnesses and exacerbations of chronic diseases before they lead to costly ED visits and hospitalizations. When elder patients require hospital-level care, primary care providers can notify EDs in advance of the reason for the visit and, perhaps more importantly, note which aspects of the anticipated follow-up care they can provide upon discharge. In some instances, clinicians in the ED may be able to rule out a life-threatening condition and allow a patient to return home if they are able to arrange expedited follow-up with the primary care provider.

Collaboration between ED clinicians and hospital care providers is also essential. While ED clinicians may screen elders likely to be discharged for conditions that would increase their risk of repeat ED visits or adverse events at home, they may reasonably defer screening and prevention planning for elders who are being admitted to the hospital. Inpatient providers can reduce repeat ED visits and hospitalizations among elders by carefully reviewing patients' medication lists for undertreatment, potential adherence problems, and adverse medication events, as well as by screening for depression and malnutrition and by communicating with outpatient providers [53]. Additional research on ways to improve communication among ED clinicians, hospital providers, and community primary care clinics is needed to increase the likelihood that geriatric patients who are discharged from the ED or hospital are able to return home as active as or even more active than before the hospital visit.

Geriatric emergency medicine education

Emergency departments in the US need to continue to increase their ability to provide consistent, high-quality care for geriatric patients [54,55]. The dramatic increase in volume of ED visits by elder patients expected over the next decade threatens to strain clinician knowledge and department resources further, putting elders at increased risk for less than optimal outcomes. Emergency physicians should be comfortable evaluating and treating geriatric patients; yet many find it more difficult to care for elder patients than for younger adults and feel they received inadequate geriatric-specific training during residency [56,57]. Hogan et al. (2010) developed a set of competencies which residency programs, as well as geriatric EM fellowships, can use to develop curricula. Broadly, geriatric EM competencies include the ability to recognize atypical presentations, manage trauma and cognitive disorders, assess the risks and benefits of interventions in elderly patients, manage medications, participate in safe transitions of care, and contribute to the long-term management of comorbid conditions [54].

There are only a few geriatric emergency medicine fellowships in the US, compared with more than 100 geriatric subspecialty training programs for internists [58,59]. The vast majority of geriatric EM training occurs in residency programs. Given that both residents and attending physicians benefit from additional training in the care of the elderly, close teaching collaborations with geriatric medicine departments should be developed. Such collaborations would allow emergency physicians to learn from geriatricians, who have significant experience in the care of the elderly, but perhaps more importantly, they would lay the foundation for better continuity of care between emergency departments and primary care offices. Close collaboration between emergency physicians and geriatricians can facilitate safe transitions for elders with acute illnesses from their homes to acute care settings, rehabilitation facilities, and back to their homes. Such continuity of care is critical if the health system is to meet the needs of a dramatically increasing elderly population.

Summary

The aging US population will present numerous challenges to the health care system in the coming decades. EDs will need to prepare by improving education in geriatric emergency medicine for nurses and physicians and devoting additional resources to the care of elderly ED patients. Patients with atypical presentations of serious disease need to be identified rapidly and treated aggressively. Elders with chronic illnesses and functional decline need social services and case management, with input from families and primary care physicians, to determine appropriate disposition, establish advance directives, and connect with palliative care services. Measures that reduce costly hospital admissions and repeat ED visits will help hospitals continue to provide high-quality care to elder patients as the health care system shifts toward global payment. Innovation in response to these challenges may lead to a new paradigm of caring for the elderly emergency department patient in the US.

Pearls and pitfalls

Pearls

- Currently, elders comprise 13% of the population and 20% of ED visits in the US By 2030, 20% of the US population will be over age 65 and will account for over 25% of ED visits.

- There is a role for screening elderly patients for impaired functional status prior to discharge from the ED. Case managers and social workers can carry out many screening responsibilities.
- Emergency department visits provide an opportunity to discuss advance directives, establish health care proxies, and connect elder patients and their families with palliative care services.

Pitfalls

- Elderly patients frequently have atypical presentations of serious disease.
- Geriatric patients discharged from EDs or inpatient wards have high rates of repeat ED visits and subsequent readmission to the hospital.
- Polypharmacy is a common problem among elderly patients presenting to EDs.

References

1. McCusker J, Ionescu-Ittu R, Ciampi A, et al. Hospital characteristics and emergency department care of older patients are associated with return visits. *Acad Emerg Med.* 2007;14(5):426–33.

2. Hogan C, Lunney J, Gabel J, et al. Medicare beneficiaries' costs of care in the last year of life. *Health Affairs.* 2001;20(4):188–95.

3. Beynon T, Gomes B, Murtagh FE, et al. How common are palliative care needs among older people who die in the emergency department? *Emerg Med J.* 2011;28(6):491–5.

4. Bailey FA, Allen RS, Williams BR, et al. Do-Not-Resuscitate orders in the last days of life. *J Palliat Med.* 2012;20(4):751–9.

5. *Ambulatory Medical Care Utilization Estimates for 2007* (United States Department of Health and Human Services, Centers for Disease Control and Prevention, 2011, Series 13, Number 169).

6. *A Profile of Older Americans: 2011* (Department of Health and Human Services, Administration on Aging [online; cited July 19, 2012]), accessed from www.aoa.gov/aoaroot/aging_statistics/Profile/2011/4.aspx

7. Crescioni M, Gorina Y, Bilheimer L, Gillum R. *Trends in Health Status and Health Care Use among Older Men* (United States Department of Health and Human Services, Centers for Disease Control and Prevention, National Center for Health Statistics, 2010).

8. Hobbs F, Damon B. 65+ in the United States. In *Current Population Reports, Special Studies* (Washington, DC: United States Census Bureau, 1996), pp. 23–190.

9. *Geriatrics Review Syllabus: A Core Curriculum in Geriatric Medicine*, 5th edn (Malden, MA: Blackwell Publishing, 2002).

10. Boris E, Klein J. Home-care workers aren't just 'companions'. *The New York Times.* 2012, July 1.

11. Carpenter CR, Heard K, Wilber S, et al. Research priorities for high-quality geriatric emergency care: medication management, screening, and prevention and functional assessment. *Acad Emerg Med.* 2011;18(6):644–54.

12. McCusker J, Bellavance F, Cardin S, et al. Prediction of hospital utilization among elderly patients during the 6 months after an emergency department visit. *Ann Emerg Med.* 2000;36(5):438–45.

13. McCusker J, Verdon J, Tousignant P, et al. Rapid emergency department intervention for older people reduces risk of functional decline: results of a multicenter randomized trial. *J Am Geriatr Soc.* 2001;49(10):1272–81.

14. Carpenter CR, Bassett ER, Fischer GM, et al. Four sensitive screening tools to detect cognitive dysfunction in geriatric emergency department patients: brief Alzheimer's Screen, Short Blessed Test, Ottawa 3DY, and the caregiver-completed AD8. *Acad Emerg Med.* 2011;18(4):374–84.

15. Mion LC, Palmer RM, Anetzberger GJ, et al. Establishing a case-finding and referral system for at-risk older individuals in the emergency department setting: the SIGNET model. *J Am Geriatr Soc.* 2001;49(10):1379–86.

16. Sinha SK, Bessman ES, Flomenbaum N, et al. A systematic review and qualitative analysis to inform the development of a new emergency department-based geriatric case management model. *Ann Emerg Med.* 2011;57(6):672–82.

17. Kahn JH, Magauran B. Trends in geriatric emergency medicine. *Emerg Med Clin North Am.* 2006;24(2):243–60.

18. Fitzgerald R. *The Future of Geriatric Care in our Nation's Emergency Departments: Impact and Implications* (Irving, TX: American College of Emergency Physicians; 2008).

19. He W, Muenchrath M. *90+ in the United States: 2006–2008* (National Institutes of Health, National Institute on Aging; 2011).

20. Qiu WQ, Dean M, Liu T, et al. Physical and mental health of homebound older adults: an overlooked population. *J Am Geriatr Soc.* 2010;58(12):2423–8.

21. Grossmann FF, Zumbrunn T, Frauchiger A, et al. At risk of undertriage? Testing the performance and accuracy of the emergency severity index in older emergency department patients. *Ann Emerg Med.* 2012;60(3):317–25.

22. Garcia-Caballos M, Ramos-Diaz F, Jimenez-Moleon JJ, et al. Drug-related problems in older people after hospital discharge and interventions to reduce them. *Age Aging.* 2010;39(4):430–8.

23. American Geriatrics Society 2012 Beers Criteria Update Expert Panel. American Geriatrics Society updated Beers Criteria for potentially inappropriate medication use in older adults. *J Am Geriatr Soc.* 2012;60(4):616–31.

24. Budnitz DS, Lovegrove MC, Shehab N, et al. Emergency hospitalizations for adverse drug events in older Americans. *N Engl J Med.* 2011;365(21):2002–12.

25. Graf CE, Giannelli SV, Herrmann FR, et al. Identification of older patients at risk of unplanned readmission after discharge from the emergency department – comparison of two screening tools. *Swiss Med Wkly.* 2012; 141:w13327.

26. Bowman L. Hospitals hold off admitting Medicare patients. *The Republic.* 2012, June 20.

27. Traissac T, Videau MN, Bourdil MJ, et al. The short mean length of stay of post-emergency geriatric units is associated with the rate of early readmission in frail elderly. *Aging Clin Exp Res.* 2011;23(3):217–22.

28. Sanders AB. The training of emergency medical technicians in geriatric emergency medicine. *J Emerg Med.* 1996;14(4):499–500.

29. Mangram AJ, Shifflette VK, Mitchell CD, et al. The creation of a geriatric trauma unit "G-60." *Am Surg*. 2011;77(9):1144–6.

30. Wendling P. Team-based protocol cut geriatric trauma mortality. *ACEP News*. 2012.

31. Nguyen HH. Hospitalist to home: outpatient parenteral antimicrobial therapy at an academic center. *Clin Infect Dis*. 2010;51 Suppl. 2:S220–3.

32. Span P. At the end, a rush to the ER. *The New York Times*. 2012, June 5.

33. Sanders AB. Care of the elderly in emergency departments: conclusions and recommendations. *Ann Emerg Med*. 1992;21(7):830–4.

34. Schumacher JG, Deimling GT, Meldon S, et al. Older adults in the Emergency Department: predicting physicians' burden levels. *J Emerg Med*. 2006;30(4):455–60.

35. Wilber ST, Gerson LW. A research agenda for geriatric emergency medicine. *Acad Emerg Med*. 2003;10(3):251–60.

36. Singler K, Christ M, Sieber C, et al. [Geriatric patients in emergency and intensive care medicine]. *Internist (Berl)*. 2011;52(8):934–8.

37. Mattie AS, Webster BL. Centers for Medicare and Medicaid Services' "never events": an analysis and recommendations to hospitals. *Health Care Manag (Frederick)*. 2008;27(4):338–49.

38. Baker B. Serenity in emergencies: a Silver Spring ER aims to serve older patients. *The Washington Post*. 2009, January 27.

39. http://adgap.americangeriatrics.org/retreat/2013/biese_and_hwang.pdf. Accessed 19 August, 2013.

40. Hartocollis A. For the elderly, emergency rooms of their own. *The New York Times*. 2012, April 9.

41. Meier DE. Increased access to palliative care and hospice services: opportunities to improve value in health care. *Milbank Q*. 2011;89(3):343–80.

42. Bell CL, Somogyi-Zalud E, Masaki KH. Factors associated with congruence between preferred and actual place of death. *J Pain Symptom Manage*. 2010;39(3):591–604.

43. Morhaim D. Viewpoint: Palliative care belongs in the ED. *Emerg Med News*. 2012;34(6).

44. Luppa M, Luck T, Weyerer S, et al. Prediction of institutionalization in the elderly. A systematic review. *Age Aging*. 2010;39(1):31–8.

45. Tung TK, Kaufmann JA, Tanner E. The effect of nurse practitioner practice in home care on emergency department visits for homebound older adult patients: an exploratory pilot study. *Home Healthc Nurse*. 2012;30(6):366–72.

46. Bélacd F, Hollander MJ. Integrated models of care delivery for the frail elderly: international perspectives. *Gac Sanit*. 2011;25 Suppl. 2:138–46.

47. Sanders AB. Changing clinical practice in geriatric emergency medicine. *Acad Emerg Med*. 1999;6(12):1189–93.

48. Roe B, Flanagan L, Jack B, et al. Systematic review of the management of incontinence and promotion of continence in older people in care homes: descriptive studies with urinary incontinence as primary focus. *J Adv Nurs*. 2011;67(2):228–50.

49. Genet N, Boerma WG, Kringos DS, et al. Home care in Europe: a systematic literature review. *BMC Health Serv Res*. 2011;11:207.

50. Seah ST, Low JA, Chan YH. Symptoms and care of dying elderly patients in an acute hospital. *Singapore Med J*. 2005;46(5):210–14.

51. Mahony SO, Blank A, Simpson J, et al. Preliminary report of a palliative care and case management project in an emergency department for chronically ill elderly patients. *J Urban Health*. 2008;85(3):443–51.

52. Quest TE, Asplin BR, Cairns CB, et al. Research priorities for palliative and end-of-life care in the emergency setting. *Acad Emerg Med*. 2011;18(6):e70–6.

53. Legrain S, Tubach F, Bonnet-Zamponi D, et al. A new multimodal geriatric discharge-planning intervention to prevent emergency visits and rehospitalizations of older adults: the optimization of medication in AGEd multicenter randomized controlled trial. *J Am Geriatr Soc*. 2011;59(11):2017–28.

54. Hogan TM, Losman ED, Carpenter CR, et al. Development of geriatric competencies for emergency medicine residents using an expert consensus process. *Acad Emerg Med*. 2010;17(3):316–24.

55. *Emergency Medical Services at the Crossroads* (Washington, DC: National Academies Press, Institute of Medicine Committee on the Future of Emergency Care in the US Health System, 2006).

56. McNamara RM, Rousseau E, Sanders AB. Geriatric emergency medicine: a survey of practicing emergency physicians. *Ann Emerg Med*. 1992;21(7):796–801.

57. Carpenter CR, Lewis LM, Caterino JM, et al. Emergency physician geriatric education: An update of the 1992 Geriatric Task Force Survey. Has anything changed? *Ann Emerg Med*. 2008;52(4):554–6.

58. *Fellowship Directory* (Society for Academic Emergency Medicine [online; cited July 18, 2012]), accessed from www.saem.org/fellowship-directory

59. *Subspecialty Careers: Geriatric Medicine* (American College of Physicians [online; cited July 18, 2012]), accessed from www.acponline.org/medical_students/career_paths/subspecialist/geriatric_medicine.htm

Chapter

2

The geriatric emergency department

Mark Rosenberg and Lynne Rosenberg

Introduction

Populations have been experiencing longevity and improved health in recent decades, forcing professions around the globe to struggle to keep up with the effects of this demographic tsunami. Health care in particular has had to grapple with shifting paradigms of aging, replacing the outdated notion of 65 and older as "old age." Once viewed as a homogenous cohort, it is now recognized that people 65 years of age and older are a heterogeneous population that can be further divided into at least three categories: young-old (65–74), the old (75–84), and the oldest old (85+).

The emergency medicine (EM) literature reflects the discussion and strategies to embrace this segment of the population while recognizing that resources are limited [1–5]. Interestingly, this discussion has been consistent for the past 30 years. In 1982, Gerson noted the potential impact the shift in demographics would have on the emergency medical system and urged a national data reporting system to prepare for the increased demands on emergency medical and advanced life support services [6]. Lowenstein et al. noted trends related to health and demographics that stimulated public interest in the aging population which remain applicable today: the increasing size of the population, the additional financial and personal support required as the population ages, and that they are the largest consumers of health care and account for a disproportionate share of expenditures for health care [4]. Thirty years ago, 19% of emergency patients were 65 years of age and older [4], had a longer length of stay in the emergency department (ED) [5], higher ED charges [5], more diagnostic tests [5], higher rates of hospitalization [3,5], and high rates of recidivism [1,2,4]. Researchers concluded that the health community needed to "prepare now to meet the growing needs of the frail, chronically impaired elderly" [4] since EDs were already facing overcrowding and limited resources on a daily basis [2]. Past recommendations included evaluating how emergency care is delivered to the elderly and possibly considering a "geriatric emergency health center" similar to trauma centers or pediatric emergency departments [1].

Where are we today?

As predicted, the appropriateness, effectiveness, cost, and outcome of emergency care provided to this cohort are of special concern [4]. Emergency departments continue to be the gateway to the acute health care system as well as long-term health care, and provide emergency treatment and primary care as needed [4]. In recent years, the ED has been utilized as a safety net to provide medical care or as a point of transition between levels of medical care [7].

Older patients continue to use the ED more frequently than younger patients, representing up to 24% of the general ED population [8]. Similar to 30 years ago, older patients continue to have longer lengths of stay in the ED [8–10], require more diagnostic tests [8,9], have higher rates of admission [8], and a higher ICU admission rate [7–9].

Advances in education have resulted in geriatric fellowships and core geriatric modules in most EM curriculums of health professionals. However, the geriatric patient as a whole experiences poorer clinical outcomes [9] due to misdiagnosis [7] and lack of appropriate outpatient resources [8]. Other contributing factors include the current paradigm of the ED with a focus toward rapid assessments and dispositions versus the complexities and needs of the geriatric patient (Table 2.1).

Barriers

Barriers to emergency medical care for older populations are significant. Stereotypes of confused, dependent elderly may contribute to the reluctance to engage these patients when they present for treatment in the ED. Health professionals, in general, are often not comfortable with older patients [1,8] regardless of abundant educational programs and research studies focused on the geriatric population and their specific need.

Many obstacles to emergency care are intrinsic within the ED model of care. The ED is not an environment conducive to eliciting a comprehensive history and work-up for these patients. The complexity of an older patient presenting for emergency treatment may not be taken into consideration as

Geriatric Emergency Medicine, ed. Joseph H. Kahn, Brendan G. Magauran Jr., and Jonathan S. Olshaker. Published by Cambridge University Press.
© Cambridge University Press 2014.

Table 2.1. Two paradigms of emergency care

General ED population	Geriatric ED population
☐ Single complaint	☐ Multiple problems: medical, functional, social
☐ Acute	☐ Acute on chronic, sub-acute
☐ Diagnose and treat	☐ Control symptoms
	☐ Maximize function
	☐ Enhance quality of life
☐ Rapid disposition	☐ Continuity of care

patients are often referred to as a "bed number" or presenting complaint. Older patients spend more time in the ED [9,11], necessitating additional use of valuable personnel resources as well as preventing the use of an ED bed for an extended period of time. The current ED model is not optimal for older patients because it does not allow the ED staff the time to recognize the presentation of older patients nor the support to provide optimal care [9].

Defining the goal

When considering a change in the delivery of emergency care it is essential to define the goals of the program. Will hospital administration support the design of a physical space within the ED for geriatric patients? Or do space limitations and budget require shifts in policy to accommodate the geriatric emergency population? When considering how to deliver emergency care to this population it is essential to know the characteristics of the older people living in the community as well as the medical resources available. What is the current percentage of the community population aged 65 and older? Are they living independently in the community or residing in a residential facility? What is the overall goal of this project: to increase or decrease admissions, maintain independence, or to provide better emergency care for seniors? What is the marketing strategy? Is this for marketing, quality care, or both?

Discussions surrounding these questions and topics will provide the framework for improving emergency care for the geriatric population. Maintaining focus and perspective may be difficult when collaborating with architects, consultants, and other vendors. It is not always prudent to build bigger and better rather than evaluate existing resources and current utilization of space and personnel. Ultimately, the primary function, regardless of infrastructure, is to deliver quality emergency care to the surrounding community.

Considering a geriatric emergency department

Reasons to consider a geriatric ED include the impact of global demographic changes, the influence of contributing factors from changing health care regulations, and clinical

outcomes for older ED patients. The aging of the population is a global experience in terms of increasing longevity and percentages of total population. More importantly, the demographics of the specific community each ED serves need to be discussed in terms of age group percentages, available resources, and clinical outcomes. Contributing factors, unrelated to demographics, focus on changes within the practice of medicine. There is a shrinking primary care pool in terms of the population as a whole, compounded by a 50% reduction in Family Practice (FP) residents, a deficit of 25,000 gerontologists by 2030, and a decrease in the number of Internal Medicine (IM) residents moving into primary care [8]. Many physician practices are no longer accepting new Medicare patients. Medicare, as the primary insurance of many older patients, emphasizes a lack of financial incentive to care for this particular population by paying 25–31% less than private insurers [9,12,13].

Research has demonstrated that older people have increased health care needs [1] and represent 15–20% of all ED patients [8]. Older people use seven times more ED services and account for 43% of all admissions including 48% of critical care admissions [2,9]. This group also has a 20% longer length of stay as acute care inpatients [9].

The American College of Emergency Physicians (ACEP) report on geriatric care in the ED depicted poorer clinical outcomes for the geriatric patient [9]. Poor outcomes were evidenced by delayed or missed diagnosis; unsuspected diagnoses such as depression; overtreatment with high rates of urinary catheterization and administration of medications; and undertreatment for pain management [14]. Furthermore, older patients usually have a complex presentation due to multiple chronic diseases often compounded by social issues [8]. This group utilizes 400% more social service interventions and 50% more diagnostic studies [9]. Medical management concerning cognition, mobility, transportation, and subspecialist availability needs to be taken into consideration for each geriatric patient [1,9,12], and may be impossible to manage on an outpatient basis. By contrast, during an ED visit the work-up can be completed to include labs, X-rays, and consultations providing a diagnosis and plan of care.

Contrary to popular belief, the ED may not be more expensive if comparisons are made between a FP work-up as an outpatient versus an ED work-up. The benefit to everyone is time invested in assessing and diagnosing the patient. The treatment plan that can take days or weeks as an outpatient can be done in a matter of hours through the ED. A geriatric ED can provide a safety net for this vulnerable population. According to Hwang and Morrison [15]:

> The ED sits at a unique junction in the continuum of patient care, overlapping with outpatient, inpatient, prehospital, home and extended care settings. By addressing how care is delivered not only within the ED itself but also at transitions of care to and from the ED – to and from nursing homes, outpatient clinics and offices, hospital inpatient services – it is hoped that overall geriatric patient care would be improved on all fronts.

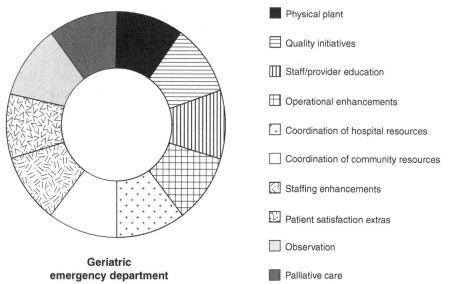

Physical plant

Quality initiatives

Staff/provider education

Operational enhancements

Coordination of hospital resources

Coordination of community resources

Staffing enhancements

Patient satisfaction extras

Observation

Palliative care

Geriatric emergency department

Figure 2.1. Components of a geriatric ED.

For these reasons and more, geriatric EDs are increasing in number and likely to become the standard within the practice of EM. The specialty of EM has responded before when a segment of the population required a different approach to the standard delivery of care, illustrated by Pediatric EDs, Trauma Care, or Chest Pain Centers to name but a few. This has led to a paradigm shift in EM and a new model of ED care – namely geriatric EM and the geriatric ED.

The geriatric emergency department

Key points for discussion when considering a geriatric ED include: administrative support; identification of local champions to attain and sustain the initiatives; delineating the appropriate patient population; the actual physical location for services; the financial and logistic feasibility of structural modifications; and the education of all staff members in the department.

EDs must meet the needs and demands of a diverse population. Hospital communities must consider this when discussing how to deliver geriatric emergency services. Geriatric EDs use specific interventions to improve patient satisfaction, comfort, and outcomes [11]. Some hospitals support separate units similar to pediatric units while others embrace this population within the existing ED structure. Data from the Emergency Department Benchmarking Alliance (EDBA) indicate that EDs can see approximately 1500 visits/exam area [16]. If an ED sees 9000 geriatric visits, the department would benefit from the use of six (6) senior beds. If the decision is made not to build a separate geriatric ED, geriatric protocols and processes can guide the care for older patients while providing emergency services for everyone.

Factors such as existing space and financial constraints impact the decision of how to operationalize a geriatric emergency department. Contrary to the traditional image of physical infrastructure, the geriatric ED does not necessarily need

to include bricks and mortar. A physical entity is just one of the ten parts of a geriatric ED (Figure 2.1), yet not necessarily essential to the success of the department.

Physical plant

Each hospital or institution needs to consider its specific ED population and surrounding community to determine how best to meet the needs of the aging population. In addition, the hospital mission as well as financial capacity needs to be kept in mind when determining whether the geriatric ED should be a physical structure or space. The "space" may range from dedicated beds in the ED to a separate unit, with attention to the needs of older patients incorporated in the design. Features to be considered include location of diagnostic and treatment services, consultant and caregiver workspace, and additional accommodations for family members [9]. It may be considered a luxury to appropriate dollars and space for the specific needs of the geriatric ED population; however, it is important to keep in mind that the physical plant design (new or existing) does not hinder the development of a geriatric ED.

Existing EDs can be modified using principles of universal design in which the entire ED would be geriatric friendly. universal design is a form of design that allows disabled people the same access as able-bodied people. From the architectural literature, the concept of universal design was defined by Ron Mace as "an approach to design that incorporates products as well as building features which, to the greatest extent possible, can be used by everyone" [17]. A common example would be cutouts on sidewalks at street corners. Originally mandated for ease of use when in a wheelchair, they are of benefit to people on bicycles, or those pushing strollers or carts. Or consider the unobtrusive experience of walking through automatic doors. Automatic doors are an excellent example of universal design already in place in most ED entrances and exits which can be used by everyone whether arriving by stretcher, wheelchair, or ambulating independently. Other areas to consider Universal

Design include protective shelters over entranceways, a clearly marked ED entrance, and patient-waiting areas allowing eye contact with staff, and large clear lettering on signs. Creating an environment for emergency care that meets the physical and psychological needs of the geriatric patient will also benefit the greater ED population [12].

Whether building a separate unit or modifying the current ED, key modifications can be made based on the geriatric literature. There is growing recognition that the physical environment can enhance or deter the mobility and independence of older patients [18]. Lengthy ED visits can contribute to mental status changes such as confusion in this population [11]. Specific interventions in the geriatric ED can improve patient satisfaction, comfort, and outcomes [12] as well as promote an overall supportive and safer environment. A visual inventory needs to be taken from the view of the patient to identify areas of potential injury such as slippery tile floors and poor lighting. Intravenous lines, catheters, and tubes can restrict movement or become tangled in the patient's gown. Strategically placed handrails and natural lighting can improve patient safety in corridors. Non-slip, non-glare flooring improves safe ambulation and can also be useful in absorbing sound.

The impact of noise on both the patient and the care provider has been studied extensively and the ED routinely has excessive noise [19]. Therefore the actual physical location of the geriatric ED becomes another factor for consideration. Research suggests that a quieter examination area yields better outcomes because of decreased mental stress for staff and a more comfortable environment for patients [12]. A quieter atmosphere may be more conducive to eliciting an accurate history of the older patient's current illness without the distraction of trauma alerts and intoxicated patients in a busy tertiary care center.

The elderly typically spend more time in the ED due to their complex presentation and frequently experience back pain as a result of hard mattresses [12]. The ED bed is usually a narrow stretcher that restricts mobility and repositioning. Potential solutions include replacing ED stretchers with hospital beds or using thicker mattresses on the stretchers to improve patient comfort, as well as providing supportive surfaces to prevent skin breakdown while in the ED [10,12]. In the case of the ED patient rooms, the use of a variety of lighting solutions in one treatment room can accommodate both the medical staff in terms of exams and procedures as well as the patients, whether for light-sensitivity or difficulty seeing in low-light conditions.

Quality initiatives

It is easy for hospitals that are developing a geriatric ED process to get so involved in the physical plant that the purpose for the changes can be forgotten. The goal of the geriatric ED is to improve emergency health care for functioning independent seniors. Therefore, quality care and ongoing quality initiatives are critical and are an essential part of any geriatric ED program.

Ideally quality initiatives or metrics should be guided by the quality improvement activities within the existing ED and focus on areas of high risk such as potential for medication interactions or risk for falls. This process helps identify areas for operational improvement and functions as a needs assessment for ongoing staff education programs.

The ED quality committee performs chart reviews and monitors clinical outcomes associated with the metrics identified for inclusion in the quality program. The committee may be a subcommittee of the existing ED quality committee or report as a separate entity. The composition of the committee typically includes the program coordinator, geriatric physician, nurse manager, geriatric nurse, case manager, social worker, and pharmacist. Sample quality metrics include: falls, Foley catheter usage, restraint use, returns within 72 hours and 30 days, medication usage, delays in ST segment elevation myocardial infarction (STEMI) identification, all deaths, quality referrals from other hospital departments, and patient complaints (Figure 2.2). It is important that the quality program reflect the specific needs of the community's geriatric ED population in terms of metrics, committee composition, and frequency of meetings.

Falls and fall assessment

A fall-risk assessment is an integral part of any hospital geriatric ED program. It is important to perform this assessment early in the ED visit during intake or triage. Any patient that presents with a fractured wrist, for example, is not "just" a fractured wrist but is a fall. The program needs to identify and protect individuals at risk. A patient who just received a medication treatment with a sedating medication, such as an antihistamine, benzodiazepines, or pain medication should be screened for falls potential *prior* to allowing independent ambulation to ensure patient safety.

Many fall assessment screens are available for this population. One possible tool is the "Get-up and Go Test" [20]. This testing is simple and can be completed by most members of the patient care team. Regardless of the tool selected, the fall assessment should be standardized throughout the department.

Medications

An integral part of quality and patient safety in the geriatric ED is a medications program that addresses two main areas: Drug interactions and limiting the use of potentially inappropriate medications in older adults. Increasing frailty, comorbid conditions, age-related physiologic changes, and polypharmacy are associated with adverse drug reactions (ADR) in this population [21].

The geriatric population typically has multiple prescriptions from multiple physicians. And as people age, the tendency may be to take more and more medications. Forty percent of people 65 years of age and older take five to nine medications [21]. Included in this list are prescription medications, over-the-counter medications, vitamins, and supplements. Alcohol consumption should also be taken into consideration. Research has shown that the greater the number of medications, the greater the risk of drug–drug interactions [21]. This is significant for this population as there is a

Geriatric ER PI Review Matrix	Jan	Feb	Mar	Apr	May	Jun	Jul	Aug	Sep	Oct	Nov	Dec
Global Measures												
Geriatric volume age > 65												
Admissions and % of total admits												
Readmissions												
RTED within 72 hours												
Geriatric transfers for HLOC												
Admission upgrade within 24 hours												
Geriatric Abuse or neglect												
Cardiopulmonary arrests												
Deaths												
Disease Specific Measures												
Falls												
Hip fractures												
Traumatic ICH												
Blunt abdominal injuries												
Death												
Polyphamacy screen												
Fall screens												
Urinary Catheters												
#Indwelling catheter POA												
Foley insertion												
Check list used												
Catheter days												
Automated discontinuation used												
LOS w and wo CAUTI												
Medication Management												
Documentation high risk meds												
ED use of high risk meds												
Revisits for adverse reaction												
Revisits for non-compliance												
Delirium and Restraint review												
Indications documented												
Chemical restraint attempted												
Behavioral physical restraint used												

Figure 2.2. Quality metrics. Used with permission. Jason Greenspan MD FACEP, James De La Torre MD. "Emergent Medical Associates Geriatric Emergency Room Initiative – Working Draft."

100% chance of an ADR during the time a patient is taking five or more medications [22].

Not all reactions are serious but all need to be considered. Presenting symptoms such as constipation, depression, confusion, falls, fractures, and immobility may be due to an ADR rather than a disease [22]. It is believed that 80% of ADR are due to prescription medications including warfarin, insulin, and digoxin [22]. Warfarin in particular is associated with one-third of the emergency hospitalizations for ADR in older adults [22].

Every geriatric ED needs a mechanism to evaluate a patient's current medications with those being prescribed in the ED for drug–drug interactions. There are a variety of options and combinations to consider depending on the

specific needs and resources of the ED. Basically there are three considerations: A pharmacist-screening program in which an ED pharmacist would review medications concurrently with the patient's ED visit or within a defined timeline; applications such as Epocrates [23] or Medscape [24] designed for the ED physician's smartphone; and electronic medical records with computerized programs for detecting ADRs. Other tools to identify high-risk medications include Beers [25] criteria, START [26] criteria, and STOPP [27] criteria. The Beers criteria, used to identify potentially inappropriate medication use in older adults, are the most widely used criteria while also being the most controversial [25]. It has been suggested that the START/STOPP criteria, organized according to physiological systems, should be used in a "complementary manner" with Beers criteria for a comprehensive medication program [25].

Staff education

Physicians, nurses, and most staff associated with emergency care consider themselves capable of caring for patients of all ages. One of the largest hurdles in gaining support is having staff recognize that geriatric patients present differently than other age groups. Elderly patients often present with vague complaints, comorbid conditions, co-existing chronic medical problems, and polypharmacy, necessitating staff education related to their unique presentation [12]. This cohort has more complex medical needs and is labor-intensive; meaning they require more time devoted to unraveling vague medical histories and complaints.

The most important component of a geriatric ED is staff awareness and education. Both are fundamental to improving care for geriatric ED patients and the success of the geriatric ED. A department's quality program can identify and focus on areas of risk thereby guiding staff education programs. The staff needs to demonstrate competencies specific to the needs of geriatric patients. General information concerning demographics, attitudes towards older adults, and normal changes associated with aging provide a foundation for all staff with other specific modules identified via a needs assessment. The Emergency Nurses Association (ENA) provides specific education modules for nurses via Geriatric Emergency Nursing Education (GENE) [28].

The ED medical staff needs to be cognizant of the physiological changes that occur with aging resulting in decreased functional reserve. Certain complaints, such as abdominal pain, should be red flags that caution the practitioner to "prepare for the worst" and "hope for the best." If a geriatric patient presents to the ED with a fractured wrist, a comprehensive work-up is needed with a detailed history to determine the etiology of the fall and potential complications.

ACEP and the Society for Academic Emergency Medicine (SAEM) have developed a geriatric curriculum and a series of videos [29] that include:

- general assessment of the elder patient;
- physiology of aging;
- delirium, altered mental status;
- abdominal pain;
- falls and trauma;
- infectious disease;
- the dizzy patient;
- pharmacology;
- chest pain and dyspnea;
- end of life;
- polypharmacy/medication/drug interactions.

Geriatric competences for EM resident programs cover the domains of core geriatric concepts, EM trauma and interventions, and fundamental geriatric principles adapted to the emergency patient [30]. Geriatric EM fellowships further promote understanding of the complexities of the geriatric population presenting for emergency care.

Operations

Advancing emergency severity index criteria for elderly

Triage, staffed by ED physicians or ED nurses, is usually the entry point into the ED system (Figure 2.3). Triage becomes an opportunity to identify high-risk patients through specific policies and education. "Practice patterns would be modified for the screening and assessment of conditions specific to the geriatric patient population" [31]. Brief validated screening tools, such as the Identification of Seniors at Risk [31], are essential in identifying geriatric patients at risk for hospitalization or having a return ED visit. Patients would also be triaged to the geriatric ED depending upon time of day and hours of operation.

The Emergency Severity Index (ESI) [32] is a triage algorithm that provides five levels from least to most urgent, based on patient acuity and resource need. In elderly ED patients, vague complaints and presentations may warrant modifying the ESI (Figure 2.4).

Staff should be aware of vague complaints from geriatric patients such as "I just don't feel well." Awareness that normal vital signs, such as 120/80 blood pressure, may actually be abnormal for this cohort or that chest pain is not a common complaint when geriatric patients present with ischemic heart disease allow the staff to triage appropriately and initiate diagnostics and treatment sooner.

The complexities of the geriatric patient necessitate this strategic approach and for practitioners to be hyper-vigilant, always "prepared for the worst ..." In some institutions there "is no such thing" as a Level 3 geriatric patient. In this case, geriatric EDs make seniors a higher priority as dictated by the hospital's specific policies and procedures [33]. Elderly patients can be triaged according to either standard ESI levels or modified ESI levels in which Level 3 is bumped to Level 2 [33]. A patient example best describes uptriaging. Mrs. S. is an 82-year-old who presents to triage with vague abdominal pain and thinks she is constipated. She is awake, aware, and crocheting when you see her. Triage level could be a 3 but with uptriaging, she is a 2. Mrs. S. was diagnosed with a ruptured appendix with abscess formation requiring a large amount of resources. Another example is the 75-year-old female with a chief complaint of weakness that turns out to be a myocardial infarction (MI), or the lethargic 80-year-old who in reality is septic. Without moving the 3's to a higher triage level, the vagueness of many seniors' complaints results in undertriaging. In a busy ED where resources are already stretched and timeliness of care is based on the ESI, uptriaging helps provide more timely care and possibly improved outcomes for the geriatric population.

Two-step geriatric program

A large percentage of geriatric ED patients have functional decline within 30 days of ED discharge. The literature [34,35] suggests that this decline is related to a continuation or exacerbation of the original problem that brought the patient to the ED for treatment. Occasionally the decline can be attributed to

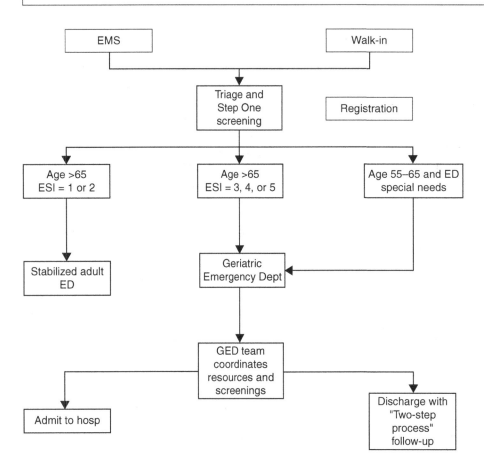

Figure 2.3. Geriatric ED triage.

Standard ESI	Geriatric modified ESI	
If patient presents as:	Modification I	Modification II
1	1	1
2	1	2
3	2	2
4	4	4
5	5	5

Figure 2.4. Geriatric triage using Modified ESI criteria.

a new problem or condition. Therefore, an ED visit by an elderly person becomes an opportunity to identify high-risk seniors and initiate valuable community support services.

The Two-step Geriatric Program in the ED is a process to identify older patients with potential problems and prevent functional decline after the ED visit. This program operates 24 hours a day, seven days a week. During Step One a screening tool [34] identifies patients at risk using criteria specific to the individual hospital population. Screening tools such as the identification of "Seniors at Risk" [31] predict possible decrease in functional status, the need for community services, revisits to the ED, admissions to long-term care, and mortality [36]. A further more detailed evaluation is performed for at-risk patients to develop a plan of care, identifying the full complement of hospital and community resources. Essentially Step One occurs during the ED visit and establishes the transition of care.

The most important element of follow-up is the transition of care, which occurs in Step Two. A member of the geriatric team calls the patient within 24 hours of discharge from the ED to determine whether the patient was able to comply with discharge instructions. Further needs are identified during the phone interview with a call-back algorithm (Figure 2.5). If appropriate, a pharmacologist and toxicologist review current medications and hospital and community resources are coordinated and mobilized. The communication between the discharged ED patient and member of the geriatric team is not for patient satisfaction: it is an essential part of the ED visit. The Two-step Geriatric Program [33] is an example of one hospital's approach to improving emergency care for their senior population. The program is promising in its potential and requires further study and validation.

Notification of the Primary Medical Doctor (PMD) is paramount in the effort to provide a safety net and continuum of care for geriatric patients. If the patient does not have his or her own PMD, one will need to be assigned. It is best to provide the names of a few practitioners in the patient's neighborhood and allow them to select someone based on their own preferences (gender, age, spoken language) and comfort. If a patient's symptoms become worse or if some new information

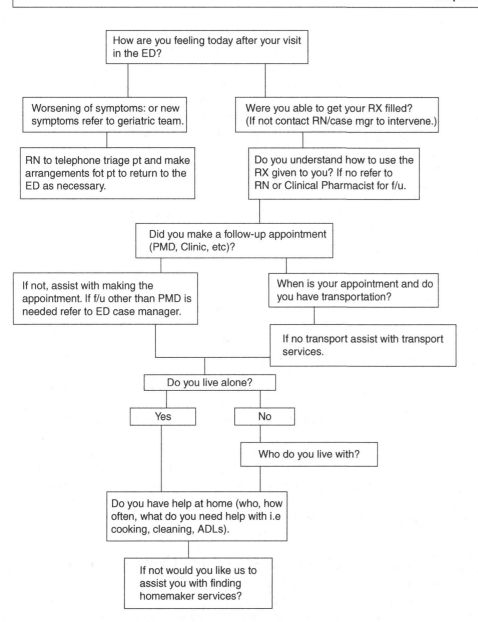

Figure 2.5. Call-back algorithm. Used with permission from St. Joseph's Regional Medical Center, Paterson, NJ.

is available (e.g., "I forgot to tell you …"), the patient can be brought back to the ED. In this case the revisit is streamlined.

Coordination of hospital resources

In operationalizing a geriatric ED, it is essential to identify and structure the available resources within the hospital itself as well as within the community. Staff resources within the ED and extending to the hospital system need to be evaluated and considered for their role in the geriatric ED. In most hospitals there are resources that are available beyond the emergency department. Many acute care hospitals have social workers, case managers, access to physical therapists, occupational therapists, mental health staff, translation services, speech pathology, spiritual care, palliative care, and pharmacists for consultations for medications and drug interactions. Toxicologists are available, if not within the hospital then at the local poison control center. Some hospitals may have telemedicine capabilities available to access other resources or consultants. For a geriatric process to

be successful there must be a working relationship with these departments and others to provide these services to the geriatric patients in the ED. In a large geriatric ED, it may be necessary to have these services function only for the ED itself and the patients that it serves. For instance, the geriatric population may require the services of a full-time social worker.

Coordination of community resources

The level of care in the community depends upon the discharge diagnosis as well as the assessment from the Two-step Geriatric Program. Most communities and hospitals can provide visiting nurses, home care, skilled nursing facilities (SNF), long-term care facilities, acute rehabilitation, long-term acute care (LTAC), hospice, and emergency medical services (EMS). Additional county resources may include meals on wheels or dial-a-ride for transport to doctor appointments or errands. Again, in operationalizing a geriatric ED, it is essential to identify key individuals in the community and structure those community resources that are available to and can support the discharged geriatric ED patient.

Staffing enhancements

Operations or operational enhancements will depend upon the individual goals of the geriatric ED. A hospital program can choose to have numerous staffing enhancements or none depending on the needs of the program and the community. Ideally an advocate for the geriatric ED can be instrumental in championing the culture change needed to embrace the new model of care for seniors. This role can be assumed by anyone knowledgeable and passionate about the program.

For day-to-day operations, key participants integral to the success of the program need to be identified early in the discussion. It is recommended that physicians interested in geriatric EM be board certified in EM. ED physicians may also have a geriatric fellowship or be double boarded in EM and internal medicine or EM and FP.

At a minimum, a program coordinator is a benefit in terms of overall responsibility and follow-through and best suited to administrative personnel. However, the program coordinator may be a physician, nurse, or administrator with overall responsibility for the program. This individual needs excellent communication and organization skills with meticulous attention to detail for follow-up.

Other enhancements may include: a nurse coordinator, geriatric fellowship trained EM, geriatric ED medical director, pharmacist, and physical therapist. Some geriatric EDs choose to consult with toxicologists for serious drug interactions while pharmacists provide routine medication reviews. Toxicologists are an important resource for this population due to the frequency of polypharmacy and the potential for severe drug–drug interactions. The support staff is most important and includes the services of social workers, case managers, and administrative staff. The geriatric population utilizes 400% more services [9], necessitating access to physical therapy, occupational therapy, and home care. The staffing composition and staffing patterns of the geriatric ED must reflect the needs of the community's senior population.

ACEP suggests the geriatric ED team consist of a MD, RN, social worker/case manager, and geriatric mid-level provider (MLP). A pharmacist, pastoral care, and occupational/physical therapist would supplement this team. According to ACEP:

> The ED physician and nurse need to address acute medical problems but the rest of the team will often be necessary to gather all relevant clinical information, address important but not acute medical issues, to evaluate all disposition options and to screen for other conditions that may affect outcomes [9].

Patient satisfaction

"Why is patient satisfaction important? Because it makes your job delivering quality care easier" [34]. Some very simple patient satisfaction extras should be considered as part of a geriatric ED. These include having pillows and blankets, as elderly patients tend to be cold. Televisions with or without educational programs, reading glasses, and hearing assist devices are other considerations. Basic manners such as introducing staff and refraining from calling patients by their first names unless asked to do otherwise are important.

Of primary importance is taking the time to set an environment conducive to making a connection and establishing trust – which is easier said than done in an ED. Establishing a relationship with geriatric patients may result in better history of the presenting complaint and a better outcome.

Patient satisfaction goes beyond non-glare lighting and large print signs. *A paradigm shift is required to improve patient satisfaction and quality of care for the geriatric ED patient. This shift requires changes in thought and action through leadership and training.*

The patient cannot measure the quality of emergency care they receive; yet they expect quality care. Tools to measure satisfaction usually do not measure medical care and outcomes. Subjective assessments are often the basis of patient satisfaction surveys and illustrate their perceptions of care based on the attentiveness of staff or the cleanliness of the department.

Patient satisfaction is also reflected in reimbursements. Value-based purchasing (VBP) is related to quality metrics and patients' perception of their care. In the era of health care reform, it becomes important to understand VBP for both financial reasons and patient care. VBP consists of quality metrics and patient experiences of care. These scores focus on how nurses and doctors interact with patients and their families concerning overall communication, management of pain, and explanations of medications, procedures, and discharge instructions. Hospital and department cleanliness and noise levels are also surveyed.

Observation and extended home observation

The ED may be a gatekeeper for admissions as insurance regulations change. Patients arrive at the ED from different pre-hospital locations, which may include home, assisted living, and long-term care among others. The ED establishes the plan of care, the transition of care whether it is admission or discharge or observation. If observation is not available or not appropriate, extended home observation may be an option.

A coordinated approach of the geriatric team is essential to maximize efficiency to expedite the ED stay. The staff may be expected to do more extensive evaluations, observe patients longer, seek more consultations, and explore outpatient alternatives. The timeframe of most ED visits is frequently inadequate for assessments of geriatric patients. Consequently older patients may be discharged or admitted based on available information at the time of disposition. Every effort should be made "not" to admit geriatric patients to the hospital when they can be managed at a lesser level of care; therefore appropriate level of care is important. However, if acute care hospitalization is required then it should be expedited and the geriatric patient transferred to an in-house bed as quickly as possible.

The ED may utilize observation units largely to prevent questionable hospital admissions [9] for geriatric patients. Observation, or stays 23 hours or less, provides an opportunity for a more comprehensive assessment of the geriatric patient and presenting complaint. If the patient is subsequently admitted, the inpatient unit is provided with a working diagnosis along with results from any consults, lab studies, and other diagnostics.

The concept of an observation unit available to the ED is best illustrated through an example of a 70-year-old female patient presenting with abdominal pain. A complete work-up reveals diverticulitis. A conservative plan of treatment is established yet it is unclear how this patient will tolerate the therapy. Keeping this patient in the geriatric observation unit allows a therapeutic trial of oral medications and repeat examinations until stable. The patient can be safely discharged with a transition of care to her geriatrician if complete resolution is not achieved.

Another tool to consider using is extended home observation. This model is undergoing significant research and study. Using extended home observation the same 70-year-old patient can be discharged from the ED or observation area. The patient receives written instructions to continue their therapy at home and an appointment is made to return to the ED at a time convenient for the patient and her family. Upon return, a member of the geriatric team brings the patient directly to a bed, bypassing the triage and registration desks. A re-examination is performed with repeated studies such as a computed tomography scan or laboratory tests.

Extended home observation with a scheduled ED return has several advantages. This model provides seamless continuity of care and at the same time allows the patient to be in the comfort of her own surroundings. The Two-step Geriatric Program coordinates support services at home and the follow-up ED appointment. The disadvantages of this model are clear: billing issues; transportation; location of the re-evaluation; living conditions; family concerns. The extended home observation model is an option to consider but will not work in all situations. It may be possible to request that the patient return to the ED during "downtime." Already overburdened EDs may not welcome "scheduling" patients for return visits. If this cannot be accomplished, arranging for follow-up with the primary doctor will suffice.

Geriatric palliative care

Older adults with chronic illnesses represent a complex, vulnerable population and often present to the ED multiple times in their last year of life. Providers of emergency care have a unique opportunity to support palliative care interventions early in this patient's disease trajectory, promoting quality of life as well as reducing cost associated with treatments [37–41].

The ED offers a solution to the large gap in outpatient services for these patients by providing access to multidisciplinary teams for interventions 24 hours a day, seven days a week [42]. However, the typical response of emergency clinicians to offer life-prolonging interventions may not be in alignment with the goals of this particular cohort. Therefore, clinical protocols may be instrumental in providing palliative medicine in response to the various presenting complaints of

these patients [43]. Palliative interventions in the ED provide ample benefits which include timely provision of care [40,44], improved outcomes [44,45], direct referrals to hospice [40], reduced length of stay [40,44,45], improved patient and family satisfaction [45], less utilization of intensive care compared with similar patients receiving usual care [39,46], and cost savings [39,40,44–47].

Summary

The geriatric population and its medical needs are increasing rapidly. The need for a better model of care is apparent. A geriatric ED can meet the needs of this vulnerable population by providing quality care, transitioning care, and preventing functional decline. The goal of the geriatric ED program is to improve emergency care for functioning, independent seniors in an efficient safe model of care.

This chapter reviewed the need for geriatric EDs and helped define this through ten key areas. This is an international problem and geriatric EDs may provide the solution. Many countries including Canada, China, Singapore, and South Korea have been working with geriatric ED initiatives. This may be the biggest change of emergency care since the development of pediatric EDs.

Lastly, a word of caution when considering geriatric emergency services. The infrastructure and design planning may demand significant attention from the hospital committee considering a geriatric ED. However, a paradigm shift is required to improve patient satisfaction and quality of care for the geriatric ED patient. This shift requires changes in thought and action through leadership and training. Ultimately, the success of the geriatric ED program rests with every staff member.

Pearls and pitfalls

Pearls

- Develop a geriatric-specific quality program. This will identify education need.
- Staff education is the key to success.
- Make a list of all hospital and community resources. Then set up a meeting with all on the list and invite them to be part of your team.
- Call back all seniors that have been discharged from the ED to evaluate their treatment and follow-up.
- Every fracture needs a fall assessment.

Pitfalls

- A physical plant alone will not improve outcomes.
- Beware of polypharmacy and drug–drug interactions.
- Vague complaints are frequently the biggest challenge.

References

1. Sanders A. Care of the elderly in emergency departments: Conclusions and recommendations. *Ann Emerg Med.* 1992;21:830–4.

2. Sanders A. Care of the elderly in emergency departments: Where do we stand? *Ann Emerg Med*. 1992;21:792–4.

3. Strange G, Chen E, Sanders A. Use of emergency departments by elderly patients: Projections from a multicenter database. *Ann Emerg Med*. 1992;21:819–24.

4. Lowenstein S, Crescenzi C, Kern D, Steel K. Care of the elderly in the emergency department. *Ann Emerg Med*. 1986;15:528–34.

5. Singal B, Hedges J, Rousseau E, et al. Geriatric patient emergency visits Part I: Comparison of visits by geriatric and younger patients. *Ann Emerg Med*. 1992;21:802–7.

6. Gerson LW. Emergency medical service utilization by the elderly. *Ann Emerg Med*. 1982;11:610–12.

7. Aminzadeh F, Dalziel W. Older adults in the Emergency Department: A systematic review of patterns of use, adverse outcomes and effectiveness of interventions. *Ann Emerg Med*. 2002;39:238–46.

8. Samaras N, Chevalley T, Samaras D, Gold G. Older patients in the emergency department: A review. *Ann Emerg Med*. 2010;56:261–9.

9. Fitzgerald R. *The Future of Geriatric Care in Our Nation's Emergency Departments: Impacts and Implications* (Irving, TX: American College of Emergency Physicians, 2008), accessed October 1, 2011 from http://apps.acep.org/WorkArea/DownloadAsset.aspx?id=43376

10. Naccarato MK, Kelechi T. Pressure ulcer prevention in the emergency department. *Adv Emerg Nurs J*. 2011;33:155–62.

11. Kihlgren A, Nilsson M, Skovdahl K, Palmblad B, Wimo A. Older patients awaiting emergency department treatment. *Scand J Caring Sci*. 2004;18:169–76.

12. Rosenberg M, Rosenberg L. Improving outcomes of elderly patients presenting to the emergency department. *Ann Emerg Med*. 2011;58:479–81.

13. *Profile of Older Americans: 2011* (Administration on Aging (AoA), US Department of Health and Human Services), accessed from www.aoa.gov/aoaroot/aging_statistics/Profile/2011/docs/2011profile.pdf.

14. Iyer R. Pain documentation and predictors of analgesic prescribing for elderly patients during emergency department visits. *J Pain Symptom Manage*. 2011;41:367–73.

15. Hwang U, Morrison S. The geriatric emergency department. *J Am Geriatr Soc*. 2007;55:1873–6.

16. Emergency Department Benchmarking Alliance (www.EDBA.org).

17. Connell BR, Jones M, Mace R, et al. The Center for Universal Design. *The Principles of Universal Design*. Accessed February 15, 2005 from www.design.ncsu.ed/cud/univ_design/principles/udprinciples.htm.

18. Demirbilek O, Demirkan H. Universal product design involving elderly users: a participatory design model. *Appl Ergon*. 2004;35;361–70.

19. Tijunelis MA, Fitzsullivan E, Henderson SO. Noise in the ED. *Am J Emerg Med*. 2005;23:332–5.

20. Mathias S, Nayak USL, Isaacs B. Balance in elderly patients: the "get-up and go" test. *Arch Phys Med Rehab*. 1986;67:387–9.

21. Budnitz DS, Lovegrove MC, Shehab N, Richards CL. Emergency hospitalizations for adverse drug events in older Americans. *N Engl J Med*. 2011;365:2002–12.

22. Winbery S. Medication management, simplification & the older adult: Putting the problem into perspective. In *Quality Insights of Pennsylvania*, accessed October 20, 2011 from www.qualitynet.org/dcs/BlobServer?blobkey

23. Epocrates Inc. 2012 (www.Epocrates.com).

24. WebMD LLC. Medscape Reference (www.reference.medscape.com).

25. Fick D, Semla TP. American Geriatrics Society Beers Criteria: New year, new criteria, new perspective. *J Am Geriatr Soc*. 2012;60:614–15.

26. Barry PJ, Gallagher P, Ryan C, O'Mahony D. START (screening tool to alert doctors to the right treatment) – an evidence-based screening tool to detect prescribing omissions in elderly patients. *Age Aging*. 2007;36:632–8.

27. Hamilton H, Gallagher P, Ryan C, Byrne S, O'Mahony D. Potentially inappropriate medications defined by STOPP criteria and the risk of adverse drug events in older hospitalized patients. *Arch Intern Med*. 2011;171:1013–19.

28. *Geriatric Emergency Nursing Education*. (Emergency Nurses Association), accessed from www.ena.org/coursesandeducation/education/GENE/Pages/CourseOutlin.aspx

29. ACEP. Clinical Resources-Geriatric Videos, accessed from www.acep.org/Clinical – Practice-Management/Geriatric-Videos/

30. Hogan T, Losman E, Carpenter C, et al. Development of geriatric competencies for emergency medicine residents using an expert consensus process. *Acad Emerg Med*. 2010;17:316–24.

31. Hwang U, Morrison RS. The geriatric emergency department. *J Am Geriatr Soc*. 2007;55:1873–6.

32. Gilboy N, Tanabe T, Travers D, et al. *Emergency Severity Index (ESI): A Triage Tool for Emergency Department Care, Version 4*. Implementation Handbook, 2012 edn (Rockville, MD, AHRQ Publication No. 12–0014), Agency for Health Care Research and Quality, November 2011.

33. Rosenberg M. *The Geriatric Emergency Department* (April 28, 2011), accessed from www.urgentmatters.org/webinars.

34. Dendukuri N, McCusker J, Belzile E. The identification of seniors at risk screening tool: further evidence of concurrent and predictive validity. *J Am Geriatr Soc*. 2004;52:290–6.

35. Caplan GA, Brown A, Croker WD, Doolan J. Risk of admission within 4 weeks of discharge of elderly patients from the emergency department – the DEED study. *Age Aging*. 1998;27:697–702.

36. David J. The life cycle of the banana: Rethinking geriatric falls in the ED. *Emergency Physicians Monthly*. 2011; August 10.

37. Mayer TA, Cates RJ. *Leadership for Great Customer Service*, ACHE Management Series (Chicago, IL: Health Administration Press, 2004).

38. Quest T, Asplin B, Cairns C, Hwang U, Pine J. Research priorities for palliative and end-of-life care in the emergency setting. *Acad Emerg Med*. 2011;18:e70–6.

39. Lamba S. Early goal-directed palliative therapy in the emergency department: A step to move palliative care upstream. *J Palliat Med*. 2009;12:767.

40. Penrod J, Deb P, Dellenbaugh C, et al. Hospital-based palliative care consultation: Effects on hospital cost. *J Palliat Med*. 2010;13:973–7.

41. Stone S. Emergency department research in palliative care: Challenges in recruitment. *J Palliat Med*. 2009;12:867–8.

42. O'Mahony S, Blank A, Simpson J, et al. Preliminary report of a palliative care and case management project in an emergency department for chronically ill elderly patients. *J Urban Health*. 2008;85:443–51.

43. Grudzen CR, Stone S, Morrison S. The palliative care model for emergency department patients with advanced illness. *J Palliat Med*. 2011;14:945–50.

44. *Improving Palliative Care in Emergency Medicine*. Retrieved March 11, 2012 from www.capc.org/ipal/ipal-em

45. Meier D, Beresford L. Fast response is key to partnering with the emergency department. *J Palliat Med*. 2007;10:641–5.

46. Beemath A, Zalenski R. Palliative emergency medicine: Resuscitating comfort care? *Ann Emerg Med*. 2009;54:103–4.

47. Penrod J, Deb P, Luhrs C, et al. Cost and utilization outcomes of patients receiving hospital-based palliative care consultation. *J Palliat Med*. 2006;9:855–60.

Chapter 3

General approach to the geriatric patient

Suzanne Michelle Rhodes and Arthur B. Sanders

Introduction

The emergency department approach to the geriatric patient is different than the traditional approach to younger emergency patients, and requires an evaluation combining medical, functional, and psychosocial issues. This chapter will also review the processes which make the geriatric patient susceptible to disease yet lack the typical symptoms and signs of life-threatening illnesses.

Principles of geriatric emergency medicine

Emergency medicine (EM) is a specialty focused on chief complaints to identify life- or limb-threatening problems as well as urgent disease processes that require immediate attention. A focused history and physical exam, as is the norm for most emergency department (ED) visits, may not be adequate for many elders. Generally, the aging population presents with less specific and localized complaints. Adding to this difficulty is that of obtaining a history in some elder patients who may have cognitive or hearing impairment [1]. Geriatric patients are at increased risk for return visits, misdiagnosis, hospitalization, morbidity, and death [2]. Mortality due to acute coronary syndrome (ACS), appendicitis, sepsis, and trauma, as well as many other conditions, is significantly increased in elders compared with that of the younger population [3]. An appreciation of the importance of the multiple factors, related acute exacerbations of chronic disease, and social and functional issues is required to address the elder in the ED in a meaningful way [4].

Geriatric patients are unique and similarly to pediatric, obstetric, and trauma patients, require an alternative model to the traditional EM approach [3,5,6]. Altered physiology, response to medications, differences in disease presentation, and response to therapy differentiate the geriatric population from that of younger adults. Care is particularly difficult for the emergency physician (EP) who is typically meeting the patient for the first time without prior knowledge of medical history, comorbidities, and social support [6]. As with pediatric patients, EPs feel less confident treating geriatric patients compared with younger adults [7]. Elders, much like pregnant women and pediatric patients, are excluded from most clinical trials, making extrapolation of the findings difficult for

practitioners [8,9]. Vaccine coverage is an important consideration and has been shown to be effective in the aged population [10]. Abuse is another similarity to pediatrics, with rates of elder abuse (estimated at 1–2.5 million per year in the US) just below that of pediatrics [11,12]. The pediatric approach to EM evaluation includes the social environment, caretakers and special needs, feeding and immunizations, as well as consideration for non-accidental trauma [5]. Table 3.1 lists special needs and concerns in the model for the emergency care of elder patients.

Healthy aging

Aging can be viewed as another stage of life that comes with different experiences of joy and pain [5]. Elders are valued in many cultures for being wise and having more time to devote to important parts of their lives, such as family. Wealth of knowledge and experience accompany aging. Elders are a diverse population, and it is important to avoid negative attitudes and stereotypes. Emergency health care professionals often treat the sickest of the elders with many chronic medical conditions. It is important to realize that this population is only a subset of elders, many of whom are extremely active and productive in their lives.

Physiologic changes can be difficult to classify as part of normal aging versus disease process due to the ubiquitous nature of some disease states such as atherosclerosis and benign prostatic hypertrophy [13]. Frequently associated conditions such as incontinence, confusion, and frailty are not normal processes of aging and require identification and aggressive treatment [5]. While loss of loved ones and physical changes are prevalent in the elder population and sadness can be a normal response, depression is not normal and should be assessed and treated appropriately [14]. Similarly, falls should not be considered normal aging and need to be investigated and treated.

Physiologic changes with age

There is a marked variability in biologic and physical function with aging from one individual to another of the same age, representing the difference between chronologic and biologic age. This is most likely due to variability in genetics, environmental

Geriatric Emergency Medicine, ed. Joseph H. Kahn, Brendan G. Magauran Jr., and Jonathan S. Olshaker. Published by Cambridge University Press.
© Cambridge University Press 2014.

Table 3.1. Principles of geriatric emergency medicine

- Complex presentation
- Atypical presentations of common disease
- Confounding effects of comorbid illness
- Polypharmacy as a factor in presentation, diagnosis, and management
- Role of cognitive impairment
- Different normal values for diagnostic tests
- Decreased functional reserve
- Adequacy of social support and reliance on caregivers
- Importance of baseline functional status
- Psychosocial adjustments to health problems
- Assessment of living conditions

Sanders AB, Witzke DB, Jones JS, Richmond K, Kidd P. Principles and models of care. In: Sanders AB, ed. *Emergency Care of the Elder Person*. St. Louis, MO: Beverly Cracom; 1996. p. 62. Adapted with permission from the Society for Academic Emergency Medicine.

exposures, disease states, healthy and unhealthy behaviors, and many other factors. It is important to consider the patient before you as to where they may fall in the spectrum of aging. An 80-year-old patient with no diseases or medications may be physiologically better off than a 40-year-old patient with multiple disease processes, medications, and cardiovascular risk factors. Table 3.2 summarizes the common physiologic changes with age.

Body composition

While body weight should not vary greatly with aging, there is a significant change in composition. There is a proportional decrease in lean body weight and bone mass with an increase in adiposity [5]. This leads to a decrease in percentage of total body water [5]. Resultant changes in distribution of drugs include potential for accumulation of lipophilic drugs, and a decrease in volume for drugs that distribute in lean tissue with increased potential for toxicity [5]. Decreased total body water makes elders more prone to dehydration and electrolyte and osmolarity abnormalities in times of stress [5]. Adipose is redistributed from peripheral and subcutaneous areas to central sites. With redistribution, there is a loss of subcutaneous fat that increases risk of skin breakdown at bony prominences [5].

Vital signs

With aging there is an overall decreased variability in vital signs and a reduction in the ability to appropriately compensate in times of stress [13]. While respiratory rate and pulse oximetry do not vary markedly with aging, there are changes in temperature, blood pressure, and pulse. Normal vital signs do not rule out significant illness in the geriatric population. Age-related decrease in maximum heart rate and decreased responsiveness to catecholamines will blunt the initial tachycardic response to stress [13]. In the setting of trauma, elder patient vital signs may not respond according to teaching by Advanced Trauma Life Support (ATLS) as an early guide to shock [3]. Due to increased arterial stiffness from a variety of molecular changes

and insults throughout life, there is a requirement for increased systolic pressure to achieve forward flow [13]. Hypertension is very common in the elder population [5]. Geriatric patients are also at increased risk for orthostatic hypotension due to decreased sensitivity of the baroreflex, decreased atrial compliance, decreased plasma volume, and other factors [5]. Aging also results in a lower basal body temperature, change in response to pyogenic molecules, and temperature regulation [13,15]. Elder adults are less able to mount a febrile response, and small changes in temperature from baseline may represent underlying infection [13]. Knowing a patient's baseline temperature can be helpful, and an increase of 1.0–1.3°C should be considered a febrile response in an elder patient, though this information may not always be available in the ED [13,16,17]. A reduced threshold for fever, such as 37.8°C, should be used in this population [13,16,18].

Skin/mucosa

Reduced elasticity and atrophy combined with decreased blood flow result in an increased number of skin wounds and breakdown even from minor trauma [18]. Decreased blood flow is further exacerbated in many by diabetes mellitus and peripheral vascular disease with a resultant increased risk of skin infections [18]. Healing is further slowed by decreased epithelial proliferation [3]. Mucous membranes are another important barrier to infection. Elders are prone to xerostomia through age-related and medication changes; this also negatively impacts defense against infection, promotes dental carries, and changes the normal oral flora (increases colonization of Gram-negative enteric organisms) [5,18]. Decreased number of sweat glands results in increased risk of hyperthermia [19].

Cardiovascular

Cardiac output at rest declines at a rate of 1% per year after age 30, decreasing perfusion to all organ systems [5,13]. With increasing age, there is an increase in the amount of collagenous and elastic tissue in the conduction tissues of the heart [20]. This contributes to decreased maximal rate of the sinus node which may lead to sinus bradycardia or, in severe cases, sick sinus syndrome [20]. Elders are more dependent on circulating catecholamines for inotropy [5]. Other age-related changes include reduced arterial compliance, increase in afterload (due to increases in systolic pressure), and left ventricular diastolic dysfunction [21]. Changes within the ventricle including decreased number of myocytes as well as accumulation of collagen lead to increase in left ventricular size and result in diastolic dysfunction [13]. Aforementioned changes as well as increased adiposity, kyphoscoliosis, and change in makeup of the chest wall lead to changes over time in the electrocardiogram (ECG) with many aged patients [20]. For example, left ventricular hypertrophy with associated ECG changes has been estimated to be present in up to 40% of elderly [20]. Bundle branch blocks are also more frequently found and may be due to ischemia or fibrosis [20]. Other changes include left axis deviation, prolonged PR and QT intervals, and low wave amplitudes [20].

Table 3.2. Physiologic changes of aging and potential effects

Physiologic change	Potential effect
Nervous system	
Decreased efficiency of blood–brain barrier	Increased risk of meningitis
	Potential of exaggerated medication responses
Decreased response to changes in temperature	Impaired thermoregulation
Alteration of autonomic system function	Variations in blood pressure; risk of orthostatic hypotension
	Reduced erectile function
	Urinary incontinence
Alterations in neurotransmitters	Slowing of complex mental functioning
Skin/mucosa	
Atrophy of all skin layers	Decreased insulation
	Increased risk of skin injury
	Increased risk of infection
Sweat glands decrease in number or activity	Potential for hyperthermia
Musculoskeletal system	
Progressive bone loss	Increased risk of fractures
Atrophy of fibrocartilaginous & synovial tissues	Joint instability and pain
	Impaired balance and mobility
Decrease in lean body mass	Alteration in pharmacokinetics
Increase in proportion of adipose tissue	Alteration in pharmacokinetics
Immune system	
Decrease in cell-mediated immunity	Increased susceptibility to neoplasms
	Tendency to reactivate latent disease
Decreased antibody titers	Increased risk of infection
Cardiovascular system	
Decreased inotropic response	Less efficient response to myocardial wall stress
Decreased chronotropic response	Decreased maximal heart rate
Increased peripheral vascular resistance	Increased blood pressure
Decreased ventricular filling	Changes in organ perfusion
Pulmonary system	
Decreased vital capacity	
Decreased lung/airway compliance	Increased airway resistance
Decreased chemoreceptor response to hypercapnia/hypoxemia	Potential for rapid decompensation
Decreased ventilatory drive	Decreased PaO_2 and increased $PaCO_2$
Decreased diffusion capacity	Decreased PaO_2
Hepatic function	

Physiologic change	Potential effect
Decrease in hepatic cell mass	Reduced ability to regenerate
Decrease in hepatic blood flow	Alteration in pharmacokinetics
Alterations in microsomal enzyme activity	Alteration in pharmacokinetics
Renal system	
Decrease in renal cell mass	Decreased drug elimination
Thickening of basement membrane	Decreased drug elimination
Reduced hydroxylation of vitamin D	Risk of hypocalcemia, osteoporosis
Decrease in total body water	Alteration in pharmacokinetics
Decreased thirst response	Risk of dehydration/electrolyte abnormalities
Decreased renal vasopressin response	Risk of dehydration/electrolyte abnormalities
Gastrointestinal system	
Decrease in gastric mucosa	Increased risk of gastric ulcer
Decrease in bicarbonate secretion	Increased risk of gastric ulcer
Decrease in blood flow to gastrointestinal system	Increased risk of perforation
Decreased epithelial cell regeneration	Longer healing times

Birnbaumer DM. The elder patient. In: Marx JA, Hockberger RS, Walls RM, Adams J, Rosen P, eds. *Rosen's Emergency Medicine: Concepts and Clinical Practice*. Philadelphia: Mosby/Elsevier; 2010. p. 2349. Reproduced with permission from Mosby/Elsevier.

Respiratory

Changes in the shape of the thorax including kyphosis, calcification of costal cartilage, and muscle stiffness reduce the efficiency of the diaphragm resulting in increased work of breathing and decreased physiologic reserve [5,13]. Additionally the movement of cilia decreases with age, allowing more bacteria from the oral pharynx into the lower airways [18]. This is further exacerbated by smoking [18]. Osteoporosis also predisposes to fractures of the ribs and sternum and pulmonary contusion with relatively minor trauma [3]. While total lung capacity changes little, there is an increase in residual volume and decrease in vital capacity [5]. There is a predictable decline in PaO_2 primarily due to ventilation–perfusion mismatch [3,5]. There is a decrease in ventilatory drive due to decreased chemoreceptor sensitivity to hypercapnia and hypoxia [5].

Gastrointestinal

Decreased amplitude of peristaltic waves of the esophagus and incomplete relaxation of the lower esophageal sphincter make elders prone to gastro-esophageal reflux [22]. Elevated gastric pH means less efficient elimination of *Listeria* and *Salmonella* [5]. The presence of *Helicobacter pylori* increases with age and has been isolated in 80% of patients [23]. Coupled with decreased mucosal thickness and bicarbonate secretion, there is increased risk for ulcers [19]. Changes in the appendix itself, including decreasing amounts of lymphoid tissue and thinning of the wall as well as diminished blood supply, have been hypothesized to increase the risk of perforation in this patient population [24]. Decreased number of neurons in the mesenteric plexus result in slowed fecal transit through the colon, partially accounting for increased frequency of constipation [22]. Autopsy studies have found 50% of adults over 75 have diverticulosis [15]. Cholelithiasis is present in more than 50% of patients aged over 70 [1]. Decreases in hepatic cell mass and function result in changes in pharmacokinetics [19].

Genitourinary

Renal function is reduced as a result of decrease in the number and function of glomeruli, affecting drug elimination [15]. Kidneys are also less able to concentrate urine, making geriatric patients prone to dehydration [15,25]. The frequency of volume contraction and reduced glomerular filtration rate (GFR) make elders prone to the adverse effects of intravenous contrast agents [3]. Diminished thirst response and decreased renal responsiveness to antidiuretic hormone, particularly if combined with decreased access to water due to immobility, lead to increased risk of dehydration [5]. An increased risk of hyperkalemia results from decreased GFR, decreased responsiveness to the renin–aldosterone system, and myriad pharmacologic causes and disease states [5]. On the other hand, dietary changes and diuretic use predispose to hypokalemia [5]. There is also development of diverticula in the basement membranes, which results in urinary stasis and predilection for urinary tract infection (UTI) [15]. In women, the periurethral area is less protected due to decreased estrogen exposure. There is incomplete bladder emptying due to pelvic floor abnormalities, and in men, increased rates of benign prostatic hypertrophy lead to increased urine stasis [18,19].

Musculoskeletal

There is a decline in skeletal muscle mass resulting in decreased strength [26]. Drying and deterioration of cartilage results in high rates of arthritis, which may negatively affect quality of life [19,26]. Osteoporosis, as well as increased rates of Paget's disease, malignancy, and metabolic derangements mean increased risk of fracture with relatively minor trauma such as falls [26].

Neurologic

The mature brain loses 10% of its weight by age 65, leaving increased space and stretching of bridging veins with increased risk of subdural hematoma [3]. The increased space within the skull also means smaller bleeds can have a more subtle presentation [3]. Adherence of the dura to the calvarium makes epidural hematomas less likely [19]. The circulating concentration of norepinephrine increases by 10–15% per decade, suggesting increase in sympathetic nervous system output particularly to skeletal muscle and the heart [27]. Changes in the type of nerve fiber (from fast delta A to C fibers) decrease the speed of pain perception and may contribute to lack of peritoneal signs [15]. While cognitive impairment is not part of healthy aging, it is very prevalent in the elder community, particularly

in those visiting the ED [28]. There is an increase with age to 50% of patients aged over 85 years having some form of cognitive impairment [29]. As many as two-thirds of nursing home residents are cognitively impaired [30].

Psychological

Elder adults have the highest risk of death by suicide of any age group [14]. In patients 85 years and older the rate is even higher at 18/100,000 compared with an overall average of 11/100,000 [14]. Depressed elders are also at higher risk of death by any cause (aside from suicide) at four times that of matched non-depressed elders [14]. Depressed elder patients are also twice as likely to use emergency services [14].

Endocrine

There is a decrease in secretion of epinephrine by the adrenal medulla, though the heart does secrete epinephrine in aged individuals, unlike in the young [27]. Epinephrine release in the setting of stress is also reduced in healthy aged adults [27]. Secretion of estrogen, testosterone, growth hormone, and many other hormones is decreased, while secretion of norepinephrine, insulin, and cortisol is increased [31]. Thyroid hormone is unchanged, except in disease states [31].

Immunologic

Changes with aging are multiple and occur at both the cellular and system level. Immunosenescence is one of these changes and leads to increased risk of reactivation of latent infections such as tuberculosis and varicella (zoster) and increased risk for malignancy [15,16,18]. There is a decrease in the quality and quantity of T cells, which results in both deficient cell-mediated immunity and reduced humoral immunity partially through less robust helper T-cell response [5]. There are reduced circulating antibodies [19]. Rates of seroprotection against tetanus are lower (60%) in adults 70 and older versus greater than 90% coverage in patients aged 18–49 [32]. Environmental factors, such as residing in a long-term care facility, expose elder patients to multidrug-resistant organisms [16].

Hematologic

While hemoglobin should remain constant, there is a decrease in 2,3-diphosphoglycerate that shifts the hemoglobin dissociation curve leftward [5]. Although anemia is not a natural consequence of aging, decreased quantity of hematopoietic tissue may contribute to decreased ability to respond to blood loss [5]. Decreased production of erythropoietin also contributes to anemia [15,25].

Polypharmacy and elders

Chief complaints of elder patients in the ED may be effects of medications, interactions of medications, or adverse effects of medications. Polypharmacy is much more common in the elderly and further complicates the presentation and evaluation of patients in this age group [23]. The average elder takes 4.5 prescription medications and 2.1 over-the-counter drugs [5].

Most elder patients receive new medications during the ED visit. The recently revised Beer's List is a good resource to take into account when assessing new or old medication effects on older ED patients [33]. Chapter 5 reviews pharmacology in older patients in more depth.

Diagnostic testing and age

While some laboratory changes are attributable to aging, such as increase in alkaline phosphatase, decreases in albumin are slight and should not be attributed to aging [23]. In one study of 200 patients aged 65 and above using urine dip, there was poor performance with 30% of positive cultures having a negative nitrite and leukocyte esterase [16]. On the other hand, those with positive nitrite or leukocyte esterase had negative cultures over 50% of the time [16]. In addition to the vague symptoms of UTI, and difficulty with diagnosis based on testing, many elder patients will have asymptomatic bacteriuria, including 15 to 50% of people in long-term care facilities (LTCF) and 5 to 20% of community-dwelling elders [16]. In the setting of a positive urinalysis, physicians must still consider other sources as causes of potential infection [15,16], and 20 to 45% of bacteremic elder patients will have a normal white blood cell (WBC) count [16]. Table 3.3 lists the common diagnostic tests that do and do not vary with age.

Atypical disease presentation

Infections

Elder patients have increased susceptibility to infections due to previously listed changes associated with aging, comorbid conditions, and in some cases, living environment [16]. Blunted febrile response and atypical signs of infection may lead to more difficulty with diagnosis and may partially account for increased morbidity and mortality in the elder population [18]. Urinary tract infection has five to ten times the mortality of younger adults while pneumonia (PNA) has three times the mortality [16]. Ninety percent of influenza deaths occur in patients older than 65 years of age (prior to the H1N1 strain) [16]. Sepsis, another major cause of morbidity and mortality in elders, is both more common in this population and is associated with higher rates of death and morbidity [16].

Atypical and subtle presentations of infectious etiologies of illness are common in the geriatric population. In elder patients with serious bacterial or viral infection, 20 to 30% will have no elevation in body temperature [34]. The oldest patients tend to have the lowest temperatures, and studies among nursing home residents have found temperature of 38.3°C to be only 40% sensitive for presence of bacterial illness [13,16,18]. When an elder patient does have a fever, it is due to an infectious etiology 90% of the time and is most likely bacterial in nature [16]. UTI may present as incontinence, altered mental status (AMS), or change in functional status [18]. Patients with PNA may present without fever or elevated WBC count and frequently will have a cough with lack of sputum production [18]. Elder patients may be completely asymptomatic 10% of the time with PNA [16]. Bacteremia is more common in elder

patients than in their younger counterparts [16]. Many of the common signs, symptoms, and objective measures relied upon in searching for bacteremia may be absent in the aged [16]. Fontanarosa et al. found only bands greater than 6%, altered mental status, and vomiting to correlate with bacteremia [16]. Those factors that failed to predict bacteremia included WBC count, temperature, respiratory or urinary symptoms, hemoglobin, vital signs, blood urea nitrogen, and creatinine levels [16]. Other common symptoms of infection include weakness, decrease in functional status, falls, and confusion, and should prompt a search for an infectious etiology [16]. Physical exam findings such as relative hypotension, tachypnea, and hypothermia may also be subtle clues to an infectious etiology [16].

Another consideration in the elder with an infection is that different organisms may cause disease. For example, while UTI in adults (usually women) is typically due to *Escherichia coli*, elders have more diverse causes including *Proteus*, *Klebsiella*, *Pseudomonas*, and *Enterobacter*, and this must be considered when choosing treatment [17]. Similarly, with meningitis, *Listeria* must be a consideration in geriatric patients, in addition to the more common pathogens [17]. Elder patients with prolonged recent hospitalizations or residing in long-term care facilities may be infected with multidrug-resistant bacteria [16].

Acute coronary syndrome

Heart disease is the leading cause of death in the elderly population [35]. The prevalence of atherosclerosis in the elderly at autopsy is very high (50–70%) while the rates of angina are much lower (10–23%) [8]. This, combined with rates of arrhythmia and sudden cardiac death as initial manifestation of cardiac disease in the aged population, has led many to believe there are high rates of asymptomatic acute coronary syndrome (ACS) in the elderly [8]. Silent myocardial ischemia (evidence of Q-wave myocardial infarction (MI) on ECG with no symptoms attributed to ACS) affects 21 to 68% of older adults [36]. In addition to autonomic dysfunction, collateral circulation and cognitive impairment are suspected reasons for increased rates of silent MI with age [36]. Atypical manifestations of myocardial ischemia, rather than typical chest pain, may be a decrease in physical function, dyspnea, neurologic symptoms, or gastrointestinal symptoms [8,9,36]. Elders may present with the results of ischemia such as poor cardiac output or congestive heart failure (CHF) rather than pain from the ischemic event. With atypical presentations of ACS, the symptoms may be attributed to other comorbid illnesses such as chronic obstructive pulmonary disease (COPD) [20]. ACS can also be precipitated in the elderly population by dehydration or infection [9].

Morbidity and mortality due to ACS are higher in elder patients. A study by Aronow found that among patients with silent ACS, rates of MI and sudden cardiac death were twice that of a population with no history of silent MI in a 45-month follow-up study [36]. This may be secondary to higher rates of non-ST elevation MI (NSTEMI), with ST-elevation myocardial infarction (STEMI) accounting for a smaller percentage of ACS in older patients [37]. The Global Registry of Acute Coronary

Table 3.3. Laboratory assessment of the geriatric patient

Laboratory parameters unchanged[1]

Hemoglobin & hematocrit
White blood cell count
Platelet count
Electrolytes (sodium, potassium, chloride, bicarbonate)
Blood urea nitrogen
Liver function tests (transaminases, bilirubin, prothrombin time)
Free thyroxine index
Thyroid-stimulating hormone
Calcium
Phosphorus

Common abnormal laboratory parameters[2]

Parameter	Clinical significance
Sedimentation rate	Mild elevations (10–20 mm) may be an age-related change
Glucose	Glucose tolerance decreases; elevations during acute illness are common
Creatinine	Because lean body mass and daily endogenous creatinine production decline, high–normal and minimally elevated values may indicate substantially reduced renal function
Albumin	Average values decline (<0.5 g/ml) with age, especially in the acutely ill, but generally indicate undernutrition
Alkaline phosphatase	Mild asymptomatic elevations common; liver and Paget's disease should be considered if moderately elevated
Serum iron, iron-binding capacity, ferritin	Decreased values are not an aging change and usually indicate undernutrition and/or gastrointestinal blood loss
Prostate-specific antigen	May be elevated in patients with benign prostatic hyperplasia. Marked elevated or increasing values when followed over time should prompt consideration of further evaluation in patients for whom specific therapy for prostate cancer would be undertaken if cancer were diagnosed
Urinalysis	Asymptomatic pyuria and bacteriuria are common and rarely warrant treatment; hematuria is abnormal and needs further evaluation
Chest radiographs	Interstitial changes are a common age-related finding; diffusely diminished bone density generally indicates advanced osteoporosis
Electrocardiogram	ST-segment and T-wave changes, atrial and ventricular arrhythmias, and various blocks are common in asymptomatic elderly and may not need specific evaluation or treatment.

Evaluating the geriatric patient. In: Kane RL, Ouslander JG, Abrass IB, Resnick B. *Essentials of Clinical Geriatrics*, 6th edn. New York: McGraw-Hill; 2009. p. 56–7. Adapted with permission from McGraw-Hill.

1 Aging changes do not occur in these parameters; abnormal values should prompt further evaluation.

2 Includes normal aging and other age-related changes.

Events (GRACE) Trial found NSTEMI to be 11% more common among patients over 85 than among those under 65 [38]. Other contributing factors are likely history of prior MI, multivessel disease, hypertension (HTN), ventricular hypertrophy, and delay in seeking medical attention for symptoms that may be attributed to ACS [36,38].

A high index of suspicion is needed to diagnose ACS in the elderly [9]. In elders, symptomatic ACS may present as confusion, behavioral changes, abdominal pain, syncope, dyspnea, or vertigo [39]. In the National Registry of Myocardial Infarction (NRMI) trial, atypical symptoms (lack of pain) were found in many aged patients with only 40% of those 85 years or older having chest pain [21]. Patients in one large observational study were found to present without chest pain 33% of the time [40]. Patients without chest pain presented with dyspnea (49%), diaphoresis (26%), nausea and vomiting (24%),

and syncope (19%) [21,41]. These patients tend to be older (74.2 versus 69.9), women (49 versus 38%), and diabetic (36.2 versus 25.4%) [40]. Older patients are more likely to have non-diagnostic ECGs [21]. In the NRMI trial, NSTEMI patients with a non-diagnostic ECG increased from 23% in those older than 65 to 43% in those 85 and older [21]. Left bundle branch block has been found in up to one-third of ECGs in patients older than 85 [37].

Secondary ACS is also more likely to occur in aged individuals who are stressed by other conditions such as pneumonia, fall with injury, COPD exacerbation, or other stressors, and is due to increased myocardial oxygen demand in the setting of coronary artery disease [21]. Due to secondary causes, atypical presentations, potential cognitive limitations, and more, it is important to maintain a high index of suspicion to make the diagnosis in a timely fashion [21].

Evidence-based treatments are often underutilized in the aged population [9,38]. Elder patients presenting with ACS who previously had an advance directive indicating "allow natural death" (AND) or resided in an extended care facility were less likely to undergo cardiac catheterization [42]. These patients also tended to present to the hospital later, were less likely to receive evidence-based treatments including aspirin, cardiac catheterization, and lytics, and had higher mortality [40]. While advance directives that limit health care treatment do not prohibit aggressive therapies, they should prompt a conversation regarding desired therapies and treatment plans.

Acute abdomen

Abdominal pain is the fourth most common cause of older adults presenting to the ED [15]. Up to 60% of complaints are surgical in nature [19]. EPs consider this to be the most difficult complaint to evaluate in the aged patient [43]. Atypical presentations of abdominal emergencies are myriad and differ from younger patients in presentation, etiology, and potential mortality [19]. One review of patients with perforated peptic ulcer found only 21% presented with peritoneal signs [15]. Previous surgeries may decrease older patients' perception of pain [15]. There are many hypotheses for reasons, including differences in pain perception of intra-abdominal pathology [44].

Aged adults are also at increased risk of vascular causes of abdominal pain due to increased prevalence of atrial fibrillation, atherosclerosis, HTN, and peripheral arterial disease [15]. Mesenteric ischemia is rare, but potentially fatal (mortality 60–90% depending on cause) and difficult to diagnose [15]. Peptic ulcer disease is more common in the elderly due to medications and increased incidence of *H. pylori* [15]. Obstruction is the cause of abdominal pain in elderly presenting to the ED in 10 to 12% of cases [15,45]. Disorders and diseases less common in younger populations, including diverticulitis, volvulus, large bowel obstruction, and acalculous cholecystitis, are more common and are included in the differential of the elder with abdominal pain [23,46].

Estimates of misdiagnosis in elders presenting to the ED with abdominal pain are as high as 40%, contributing to a 10% mortality rate [1]. Aged adults tend to present later, with non-specific complaints, and have higher mortality than younger patients for many common conditions including biliary disease, pancreatitis, and appendicitis [23,47]. In one study, a mortality difference among those elderly patients presenting with abdominal pain with a diagnosis made in the ED versus that post-admission was 8 versus 19% [1]. Because of the difficulty of diagnosis, many aged patients with abdominal pain have a computed tomography (CT) scan to further evaluate the cause of their pain. In a recent prospective, multi-center study, abdominal CT scans were obtained in 37% of patients ≥60 years old and 57% were diagnostic [48]. Difficulty with diagnosis, increased morbidity and mortality, and high positive rates of CT support a low threshold for CT imaging of elders with this complaint.

Appendicitis

In older adults with abdominal pain, 3 to 4% will have appendicitis [15]. In one retrospective study from a single institution, only 10% of patients aged 60 or older had a typical presentation of appendicitis (right lower quadrant abdominal pain, fever, elevated WBC count, nausea, or vomiting) [49]. The rate of perforation in the elderly population is about 50%, which is much higher than that in younger adults [1]. Complications from appendicitis in elders have been documented in as many as 70% of patients versus a 1% complication rate in younger patients [50]. In a study comparing characteristics of appendicitis in the aged in the pre- and post-CT eras at a single institution, the elderly population continued to have delayed presentation [50]. Incorrect diagnosis was the factor that placed patients at increased risk of perforation (as well as delayed presentation), which has continued to occur in the era of CT [50]. There was a reduction in perforation rates (72 to 51%) though mortality remained constant [50]. Another study that evaluated patients ≥70 years of age before and after the era of increased use of CT and laparoscopic appendectomy found that perforation rates, morbidity, and mortality have remained constant in this population [51]. While many have argued that atypical presentation is the cause of increased morbidity, others have argued that delayed presentation, comorbidities, and faster progression of the disease due to changes in the appendix associated with aging are the cause [23].

Geriatric emergency care model

Approach

A separate chart used for the elder, much like pediatric patients, may help to remind emergency physicians of the importance of history and exam findings particular to the aging patient such as support at home, mental status screening, vaccinations, activities of daily living (ADL), and screening for elder abuse [52].

Pre-hospital care

The importance of the emergency medical system (EMS) assessment of the home environment and living conditions cannot be overstated. Approximately 30% of geriatric patients will arrive at the ED by EMS [5]. Any information available from EMS such as contact information from family members, risk for elder abuse, environmental factors contributing to a fall, general state of the residence, medication list, and recent adjustments is extremely useful [3]. Pre-injury or illness function and mental status are also very helpful [3]. EMS has been used for case finding for unmet needs (falls, medications, depression) among elder patients who accessed EMS in a rural community with success [53]. EMS providers can also facilitate communication by ensuring elders bring hearing aids, glasses, or other necessary assistive devices [5]. They should also be encouraged to bring all medications to the hospital [5].

When treating and transferring elders, EMS must also consider poor thermoregulation and treat and prevent hypothermia aggressively [3]. If an elder patient does require spinal immobilization, it is important to pad pressure points and limit the time of immobilization because relatively short periods on a hard board can result in skin breakdown due to physiologic changes [19]. Some have suggested a lower threshold for geriatric trauma patients (>70 years) to be transported to dedicated trauma centers due to a markedly increased mortality compared with patients aged 16–70 years [54]. A Glasgow Coma Scale (GCS) score of ≤14 has been proposed specifically for transfer to a trauma center because elders, unlike younger adults, have a significant increase in mortality with GSC 14 or 13 [54].

EMS commonly transports elders from LTCF to and from the ED. Up to 25% of nursing home residents will visit the ED yearly [30]. It has been reported that 10% of nursing home residents arrive without any documentation and much important information is missing for the other 90% [30]. Nursing home staff also report frustration with the ED in that patients return unexpectedly, without the results of studies and missing other important information [30]. The Society for Academic Emergency Medicine (SAEM) geriatric EM Task Force has recommended as a quality indicator that nursing homes, when transferring patients to the ED, provide clearly documented: reason for transfer, code status, medication allergies, medication list, and contact information (for power of attorney, next of kin, nursing home, and primary care provider) [55]. In the age of multidrug-resistant bacteria, it is also important to know whether the patient is infected with any of these for contact precautions. Basic information that should accompany a patient transferred from a nursing home includes: demographics, current medications, medical and surgical history, allergies, baseline physical and mental status, code status and advance directives, recent vital signs, most recent lab results, name of nursing home with contact information, name of primary doctor, and family members with contact information [30].

ED assessment

Triage

The Emergency Severity Index (ESI) has been validated in the geriatric population and found to be predictive of hospitalization, resource utilization, length of stay, and survival [56]. Of note, 81.8% of patients aged ≥65 years were in the first three triage categories [56]. The hospitalization rate was 41.2% overall [56]. As much as possible, elders should not be left waiting on hard chairs without access to food, water, or their medications, and should be re-evaluated frequently if there are long wait times or they are triaged to lower acuity levels.

History

Reasons for difficulty with obtaining a complete and accurate history include hearing issues, cognitive deficits, acute or chronic altered mental status (AMS), stoicism, fear of being hospitalized, and memory problems [44]. Interactions with elder patients are best if the EP allows plenty of time for answering questions and gives reassurance. This will reduce fear on the part of the elderly patient [57]. Lowering the pitch of the

voice, minimizing background noise, and speaking slowly and clearly can help overcome difficulties in conversing due to age-related hearing changes. In patients with cognitive difficulties, a family member, primary care provider, or past records can be used to supplement the history.

The history should include the presenting symptom, baseline functional status, and questions regarding treatment preferences and advance directives, in addition to the usual medications, allergies, past medical history, and review of systems [5]. It is vital to have an accurate medication list with knowledge of which medications are new and any recent changes in doses. This is of particular importance in many common presentations including falls, weakness, and AMS. A history of baseline cognitive and functional status is important. Elders should be screened for possible abuse.

Physical exam

Taking into account general appearance and grooming is helpful to evaluate self-care or signs of neglect [26]. The skin of an elder may be thin and dry with loss of elasticity [5]. Mucous membranes or the lateral cheek may be more accurate than skin turgor for assessment of hydration status [5]. Senile purpura may be normal in the geriatric population, but bruising should be evaluated for coagulopathy, neglect, stigmata of falls, or abuse [5]. Aging results in a loss of orbital fat and enophthalmos, which again is not a reliable indicator of hydration status [5]. Hearing loss may be caused or compounded by cerumen impaction and should be evaluated [5]. Rales are commonly auscultated in the lung bases of elders [5]. Subtle systolic ejection murmurs are common and typically due to aortic valve sclerosis, though diastolic murmurs, louder systolic murmurs, and those in the setting of syncope or angina symptoms require further evaluation [5].

Thinning of the abdominal wall can make it easier to palpate for an abdominal aortic aneurysm, but this can be difficult to distinguish from a tortuous aorta [5]. Loss of abdominal wall musculature results in fewer or absent peritoneal signs, even in the setting of severe peritonitis [5]. The SAEM geriatric EM Task Force recommends a mental status screening exam be done on all geriatric patients [2]. As many as 25% of elder patients presenting may have AMS on presentation to the ED [2]. Approximately 10% will have delirium [52]. This cognitive impairment is recognized only 28 to 38% of the time by EPs [55]. Patients discharged with delirium have a threefold increased risk of death [55,58]. In addition to the importance of diagnosing delirium, it is important to recognize cognitive impairment as this will affect the reliability of history as well as the ability to follow discharge instructions and take medications as prescribed [55]. There are many screening tools that have been developed in the ED for this purpose, and these will be discussed in more detail in later chapters [58]. Regardless of the tool used, a systematic approach is recommended with attention to level of consciousness (LOC), level of confusion, and, for high-risk patients, a test such as the Mini-Mental State Exam (MMSE) [58]. The patient's gait should also be observed, particularly in patients with falls. The "get up and go test," which is simply the patient's ability to get up from the chair or gurney and walk, is vital in the community-dwelling elder with a fall [46,59].

Preventive care

Preventative care, including immunizations and fall prevention, is important in the elder population, with the potential to reduce morbidity and mortality. Vaccination rates for pneumococcus and influenza are significantly below the Centers for Disease Control and Prevention (CDC) goal of 80% in the elder population (62 and 66%, respectively) [19]. Given that pneumonia and influenza are the fifth leading cause of death in elders, vaccination has the potential to reduce mortality in this population [60]. The CDC has recommended that vaccination sites be expanded to the ED and other acute care sites for improved vaccination rates. Aged patients at risk are those without a complete tetanus vaccine series (3 or more vaccines), and it is important to identify these patients in wound management as they will require tetanus immune globulin in addition to tetanus vaccine [32]. Studies have shown poor compliance with recommendations for this age group by EPs [32].

Disposition

Currently, about half of elder patients evaluated in the ED are admitted to the hospital [5]. In the future, the "hospital at home model" or direct LTCF admission may divert some inpatient admissions [6]. There is some evidence that admission to a geriatric ward, if available, rather than an internal medicine ward may have a mortality benefit [61].

For patients that are discharged back to a nursing home, the EP should contact the nursing home, primary care physician (PCP), or on-call physician and should provide the diagnosis as well as test results [55]. It is important that for patients returning to a nursing home, they arrive with important discharge information including: diagnosis, treatments rendered, test results, treatment recommendations, and information for follow-up [30].

Discharge planning is vital for a successful experience for the elder patient. Geriatric patients are at increased risk for return visits to the ED, with rates from 12 to 24% at 1 month and 19 to 24% at 3 months [62]. There are several screening tools developed to predict which patients may be at increased risk and who therefore need more intensive resources [62].

Up to 13% of patients had significant functional decline following an ED visit [63]. Clarification of discharge instructions was required for 40% of patients [63]. Elder patients may suffer inability to care for themselves at home after discharge from the ED. Studies have found rates of 27 to 52% with resultant unplanned admission to the hospital in 6 to 18% over subsequent weeks [64]. Case management and social services can help with a smooth transition to home or with community support in the outpatient setting. Chapter 31 will discuss this in more detail.

New medications are prescribed with careful consideration. When a new medication is added, it is important to ensure there will not be interactions with the current medications and elders understand how to properly take the new medication. The Beers list of medications to avoid in this population should be considered prior to addition of medications [33]. Geriatric patients are the most likely to receive inadequate pain control [55]. When an opioid analgesic is prescribed, a bowel regimen should also be prescribed [55]. Medication issues in the elderly are further discussed in Chapter 5.

If a patient with new cognitive impairments is sent home, it is important to arrange and document adequate home support and specific follow-up plans [55]. Identification of potentially reversible causes of cognitive impairment, if not found in the ED, should continue as an outpatient with a specific referral [55]. With few exceptions, delirious patients should be admitted to the hospital to further identify and treat the cause as such patients have high mortality and require constant observation to prevent injury [29]. (Figure 3.1).

Patient satisfaction

Increased importance of patient satisfaction metrics, combined with the increasing proportion of visits by elders, should result in focusing on improving the experience for this patient population. Elders cite significant anxiety associated with an ED visit [65]. The ED is perceived as uncomfortable and confusing. Elders have voiced fear associated with ED visits in which they are left on hard gurneys for extended periods of time without their medications, access to food or water, and some even cited fears of being unable to call for help [66]. Updates on delays and what to expect can alleviate some of this anxiety [65]. Elder

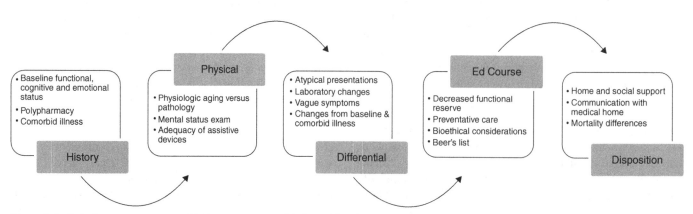

Figure 3.1. Geriatric emergency care model. The emergency model of care differs from that of traditional medical care. This model of emergency care contains important considerations and differences for the elder patient.

patient satisfaction in an urban academic ED was tied to not feeling as though the ED visit was too lengthy, having adequate pain control, being informed about testing and results, having a relationship of trust, as well as patient factors of having fewer comorbid illnesses and perception of greater health status [67].

Pearls and pitfalls

- Knowledge of the physiologic changes associated with aging is important to distinguish normal aging from pathologic changes.
- Emergency health care professionals should use a geriatric ED care model in assessing elder adults' complaints. This involves a more comprehensive approach to the elder patient, taking into account atypical disease presentations, comorbid conditions, and polypharmacy.
- Mental status evaluation is a key element in the ED given the effects on reliability of history and physical, discharge planning, and screening for delirium.
- Diagnostic testing may be misleading and must account for differences with age.
- Baseline functional status and social support systems, including the role of caregivers, need to be considered in evaluating and treating elder ED patients.

Summary

Aging is associated with differences in physiology, response to therapy, morbidity from common illness, and disease presentation. A specialized approach to the elder patient, similar to pediatric patients, is required to optimally care for this rapidly expanding ED population.

References

1. Chang CC, Wang SS. Acute abdominal pain in the elderly. *Int J Gerontology*. 2007;1:77–82.

2. Samaras N, Chevalley T, Samaras D, Gold G. Older patients in the Emergency Department: A review. *Ann Emerg Med*. 2010;56:261–9.

3. Mandavia D, Newton K. Geriatric trauma. *Emerg Med Clin North Am*. 1998;16:257.

4. Aminzadeh F, Dalziel WB. Older adults in the emergency department: a systematic review of patterns of use, adverse outcomes, and effectiveness of interventions. *Ann Emerg Med*. 2002;39:238–47.

5. Sanders AB. Emergency care of the elder person. In *Geriatric Emergency Medicine Task Force* (St. Louis, MO: Beverly Cracom Publications, 1996:53–83).

6. Wilber ST, Gerson LW, Terrell KM, et al. Geriatric emergency medicine and the 2006 Institute of Medicine reports from the committee on the future of emergency care in the US health system. *Acad Emerg Med*. 2006;13:1345–51.

7. Schumacher JG, Deimling GT, Meldon S, Woolard B. Older adults in the emergency department: Predicting physicians' burden levels. *J Emerg Med*. 2006;30:455–60.

8. Ambepitiya GB, Iyengar EN, Roberts ME. Silent exertional myocardial ischemia and perception of angina in elderly people – review. *Age Aging*. 1993;22:302–7.

9. Jokhadar M, Wenger NK. Review of the treatment of acute coronary syndrome in elderly patients. *Clin Interv Aging*. 2009;4:435–44.

10. Wilber ST, Gerson LW. A research agenda for geriatric emergency medicine. *Acad Emerg Med*. 2003;10:251–60.

11. Clarke ME, Pierson W. Management of elder abuse in the emergency department. *Emerg Med Clin North Am*. 1999;17:631.

12. Geroff AJ, Olshaker JS. Elder abuse. *Emerg Med Clin North Am*. 2006;24:491.

13. Chester JG, Rudolph JL. Vital signs in older patients: Age-related changes. *J Am Med Directors Assoc*. 2011;12:337–43.

14. Piechniczek-Buczek J. Psychiatric emergencies in the elderly population. *Emerg Med Clin North Am*. 2006;24:467.

15. Ragsdale L, Southerland L. Acute abdominal pain in the older adult. *Emerg Med Clin North Am*. 2011;29:429.

16. Fontanarosa PB, Kaeberlein FJ, Gerson LW, Thomson RB. Difficulty in predicting bacteremia in elderly emergency patients. *Ann Emerg Med*. 1992;21:842–8.

17. Yoshikawa TT. Epidemiology and unique aspects of aging and infectious diseases. *Clin Infect Dis*. 2000;30:931–3.

18. Bender BS. Infectious disease risk in the elderly. *Immunology Allergy Clin North Am*. 2003;23:57.

19. Marx JA, Hockberger RS, Walls RM, Adams J, Rosen P. *Rosen's Emergency Medicine: Concepts and Clinical Practice*, 7th edn (Philadelphia, PA: Mosby/Elsevier, 2010).

20. Jones J, Srodulski ZM, Romisher S. The aging electrocardiogram. *Am J Emerg Med*. 1990;8:240–5.

21. Alexander KP, Newby K, Cannon CP, et al. Acute coronary care in the elderly, Part I Non-ST-segment-elevation acute coronary syndromes – A scientific statement for health care professionals from the American Heart Association Council on Clinical Cardiology – in collaboration with the Society of Geriatric Cardiology. *Circulation*. 2007;115:2549–69.

22. Grassi M, Petraccia L, Mennuni G, et al. Changes, functional disorders, and diseases in the gastrointestinal tract of elderly. *Nutricion Hospitalaria*. 2011;26:659–68.

23. Shamburek RD, Farrar JT. Disorders of the digestive system in the elderly. *N Engl J Med*. 1990;322:438–43.

24. Podnos YD, Jimenez JC, Wilson SE. Intra-abdominal sepsis in elderly persons. *Clin Infect Dis*. 2002;35:62–8.

25. Zhou XJ, Saxena R, Liu ZH, Vaziri ND, Silva FG. Renal senescence in 2008: progress and challenges. *Int Urol Nephrol*. 2008;40:823–39.

26. Kane RL, Kane RL. *Essentials of Clinical Geriatrics*, 6th edn (New York: McGraw-Hill Medical; 2009).

27. Seals DR, Esler MD. Human aging and the sympathoadrenal system. *J Physiol London*. 2000;528:407–17.

28. Gerson LW, Counsell SR, Fontanarosa PB, Smucker WD. Case-finding for cognitive impairment in elderly emergency medicine department patients. *Ann Emerg Med*. 1994;23:813–17.

29. Wilber ST. Altered mental status in older emergency department patients. *Emerg Med Clin North Am*. 2006;24:299.

30. Terrell KM, Miller DK. Challenges in transitional care between nursing homes and emergency departments. *J Am Med Dir Assoc*. 2006;7:499–505.

31. Banks WA, Morley JE. Endocrine and metabolic changes in human aging. *J Am Aging Assoc*. 2000;23:103–15.

32. Talan DA, Abrahamian FM, Moran GJ, et al. Tetanus immunity and physician compliance with tetanus prophylaxis practices among emergency department patients presenting with wounds. *Ann Emerg Med.* 2004;43:305–14.

33. American Geriatrics Society Beers Criteria Update Expert P. American Geriatrics Society updated Beers Criteria for potentially inappropriate medication use in older adults. *J Am Geriatr Soc.* 2012;60:616–31.

34. Norman DC. Fever and aging. *Infect Dis Clin Pract.* 1998;7:387–90.

35. Skolnick AH, Alexander KP, Chen AY, et al. Characteristics, management, and outcomes of 5,557 patients age >= 90 years with acute coronary syndromes – Results from the CRUSADE initiative. *J Am Coll Cardiol.* 2007;49:1790–7.

36. Aronow WS. Silent MI – Prevalence and prognosis in older patients diagnosed by routine electrocardiograms. *Geriatrics.* 2003;58:24.

37. Alexander KP, Newby LK, Armstrong PW, et al. Acute coronary care in the elderly, Part II – ST-segment-elevation myocardial infarction – A scientific statement for health care professionals from the American Heart Association council on clinical cardiology – In collaboration with the Society of Geriatric Cardiology. *Circulation.* 2007;115:2570–89.

38. Avezum A, Makdisse M, Spencer F, et al. Impact of age on management and outcome of acute coronary syndrome: Observations from the Global Registry of Acute Coronary Events (GRACE). *Am Heart J.* 2005;149:67–73.

39. Tresch DD. Management of the older patient with acute myocardial infarction: Difference in clinical presentations between older and younger patients. *J Am Geriatr Soc.* 1998;46:1157–62.

40. Canto JG, Shlipak MG, Rogers WJ, et al. Prevalence, clinical characteristics, and mortality among patients with myocardial infarction presenting without chest pain. *JAMA.* 2000;283:3223–9.

41. Brieger D, Eagle KA, Goodman SG, et al. Acute coronary syndromes without chest pain, an underdiagnosed and undertreated high-risk group – Insights from the Global Registry of Acute Coronary Events. *Chest.* 2004;126:461–9.

42. Han JH, Miller KF, Storrow AB. Factors affecting cardiac catheterization rates in elders with acute coronary syndromes. *Acad Emerg Med.* 2007;14:228–33.

43. McNamara RM, Rousseau E, Sanders AB. Geriatric emergency medicine – a survey of practicing emergency physicians. *Ann Emerg Med.* 1992;21:796–801.

44. Martinez JP, Mattu A. Abdominal pain in the elderly. *Emerg Med Clin North Am.* 2006;24:371–88.

45. Kizer KW, Vassar MJ. Emergency department diagnosis of abdominal disorders in the elderly. *Am J Emerg Med.* 1998;16:357–62.

46. Baraff LJ, DellaPenna R, Williams N, Sanders A. Practice guideline for the ED management of falls in community-dwelling elderly persons. *Ann Emerg Med.* 1997;30:480–92.

47. Tong K, Merchant R. Nonacute acute abdomen in older adults. *J Am Geriatr Soc.* 2012;60:370–1.

48. Hustey FM, Meldon SW, Banet GA, et al. The use of abdominal computed tomography in older ED patients with acute abdominal pain. *Am J Emerg Med.* 2005;23:259–65.

49. Paranjape C, Dalia S, Pan J, Horattas M. Appendicitis in the elderly: a change in the laparoscopic era. *Surg Endosc.* 2007;21:777–81.

50. Storm-Dickerson TL, Horattas MC. What have we learned over the past 20 years about appendicitis in the elderly? *Am J Surg.* 2003;185:198–201.

51. Hui TT, Major KM, Avital I, Hiatt JR, Margulies DR. Outcome of elderly patients with appendicitis – Effect of computed tomography and laparoscopy. *Arch Surg.* 2002;137:995–8.

52. Sanders AB. Missed delirium in older emergency department patients: A quality-of-care problem. *Ann Emerg Med.* 2002;39:338–41.

53. Shah MN, Caprio TV, Swanson P, et al. A novel emergency medical services-based program to identify and assist older adults in a rural community. *J Am Geriatr Soc.* 2010;58:2205–11.

54. Caterino JM, Raubenolt A, Cudnik MT. Modification of Glasgow Coma Scale criteria for injured elders. *Acad Emerg Med.* 2011;18:1014–21.

55. Terrell KM, Hustey FM, Hwang U, et al. Quality indicators for geriatric emergency care. *Acad Emerg Med.* 2009;16:441–9.

56. Baumann MR, Strout TD. Triage of geriatric patients in the emergency department: Validity and survival with the Emergency Severity Index. *Ann Emerg Med.* 2007;49:234–40.

57. Hendrickson M, Naparst TR. Abdominal surgical emergencies in the elderly. *Emerg Med Clin North Am.* 2003;21:937.

58. Sanders AB. Mental status assessment in emergency medicine. *Int Emerg Med.* 2007;2:116–18.

59. Mathias S, Nayak USL, Isaacs B. Balance in the elderly – the get-up and go test. *Arch Phys Med Rehabil.* 1986;67:387–9.

60. Kahn JH, Magauran B. Trends in geriatric emergency medicine. *Emerg Med Clin North Am.* 2006;24:243–60.

61. Di Bari M, Balzi D, Roberts AT, et al. Prognostic stratification of older persons based on simple administrative data: Development and validation of the "Silver Code," to be used in emergency department triage. *J Gerontol A Biol Sci Med Sci.* 2010;65:159–64.

62. Moons P, De Ridder K, Geyskens K, et al. Screening for risk of readmission of patients aged 65 years and above after discharge from the emergency department: predictive value of four instruments. *Eur J Emerg Med.* 2007;14:315–23.

63. Jones JS, Young MS, LaFleur RA, Brown MD. Effectiveness of an organized follow-up system for elder patients released from the emergency department. *Acad Emerg Med.* 1997;4:1147–52.

64. Burns E. Older people in accident and emergency departments. *Age Aging.* 2001;30:3–6.

65. Baraff LJ, Bernstein E, Bradley K, et al. Perceptions of emergency care by the elderly – results of multicenter focus group interviews. *Ann Emerg Med.* 1992;21:814–18.

66. Nyden K, Petersson M, Nystrom M. Unsatisfied basic needs of older patients in emergency care environments – obstacles to an active role in decision making. *J Clin Nursing.* 2003;12:268–74.

67. Nerney MP, Chin MH, Jin L, et al. Factors associated with older patients' satisfaction with care in an inner-city emergency department. *Ann Emerg Med.* 2001;38:140–5.

Chapter

4

Resuscitation of the elderly

Aneesh T. Narang and Rishi Sikka

Introduction

The increasing proportion of elderly within the population has altered America's socioeconomic landscape and gradually transformed the practice of health care. Compared with the general population, the elderly are more acutely ill on presentation, consume more emergency department (ED) resources, are admitted more frequently to the hospital, and account for a greater proportion of intensive care unit admissions [1].

Given the current trends, EDs can anticipate an increase in the presentation of critically ill, elderly patients. Unfortunately, these patients remain a challenge to diagnose and to resuscitate. The normal physiologic changes associated with aging may masquerade a critical illness, and may impact the effectiveness of resuscitation. In many instances, physicians also must take into account issues of advance directives and medical futility when formulating their clinical decisions.

This chapter outlines the basic science and practical decision making involved in the resuscitation of the elderly patient. It will also review the challenges of managing common geriatric emergencies such as sepsis, respiratory failure, cardiac arrest, shock, seizures, and stroke. It is intended as a guide to assist in evidence-based, compassionate ED care for the critically ill geriatric patient.

Epidemiology and outcomes

Elderly individuals who are ill are at high risk for hospitalization and death. On average, an elderly person has three to four chronic illnesses and nearly a 20% annual risk of hospitalization [2]. Once admitted, up to two-thirds of elderly patients may be readmitted to the hospital within 6 months [3]. Unfortunately, the majority of elderly die in the hospital setting [4].

The first step in improving the resuscitation of the elderly in the ED is to better understand the outcomes and prognosis of resuscitation in this age group. The literature on the success of in-hospital and out-of-hospital cardiopulmonary resuscitation (CPR) provides some valuable guidance. The success of CPR in hospitalized patients has been well studied. Some earlier studies have demonstrated poor survival rates among hospitalized elderly patients after CPR, prompting some to question its utility in the geriatric population [5,6]. Contrary to older studies,

more recent studies have reported more favorable results. Most studies have shown a hospital discharge survival rate ranging from 10 to 29%, and shown age not to be a significant determinant of survival [7–16]. The presence of ventricular tachycardia/ventricular fibrillation (VT/VF) substantially improves these rates, while relatively few patients who demonstrate asystole survive. Duration of CPR as well as the patient's pre-arrest comorbidities also significantly affect survival to hospital discharge [14]. Follow-up data in many of these studies have shown that more than half of the patients were alive, and most were living independently at home without any compromise in daily activities [12,16]. In general, patients who are highly functional with fewer chronic illnesses, hospitalized for a cardiac etiology, and closely monitored before the arrest are more likely to benefit from CPR. In these circumstances, CPR can be very successful, and elderly patients will benefit as much as younger patients [17].

The results of studies examining the effectiveness of out-of-hospital resuscitation are conflicting. Survival rates following an out-of-hospital arrest for elderly patients with VF as a presenting rhythm are between 14 and 24% in most studies [18–23], but much lower in patients presenting with asystole or electromechanical dissociation. This wide range can be partially attributed to differences in study methodologies, downtime before CPR, the availability of advanced cardiac life support in the field, and the training level of the paramedics. In general, the majority of analyses indicate favorable resuscitation outcomes in the elderly, particularly if the inciting event is a ventricular arrhythmia [17]. In contrast to studies of in-hospital and out-of-hospital cardiac arrests, there are few data regarding the effectiveness of resuscitation in nursing home residents. CPR is rarely, if ever, performed in this setting. Most analyses report poor rates of survival in the majority of patients who receive CPR [24–26]. However, some data suggest that CPR can be effective if an arrest is witnessed and the initial rhythm is VT or VF [27,28].

The conclusions from these various studies show that age alone does not appear to be a significant determinant of survival in patients who receive CPR following cardiac arrest. Instead, those elderly patients with acute cardiac illnesses with fewer diseases and better baseline functional status have better resuscitation outcomes. Therefore, determining the potential success of resuscitation on the basis of age is shortsighted and not evidence-based. The potential response to CPR in an elderly patient with chronic, debilitating illnesses is not equivalent to that of an active, vigorous elderly patient with few comorbidities.

Pathophysiology

The difficulty in resuscitating elderly patients often can be attributed to significant pathophysiologic changes associated with aging, particularly within the cardiovascular system. Over time, there is a progressive decrease in the number of myocytes as well as an increase in collagen content, connective tissue, and fat. This results in a decline in ventricular compliance and in an increase in the incidence of sick sinus syndrome, atrial arrhythmia, and bundle branch block. There is also a substantial hardening of the major vessels, resulting in elevated systolic blood pressure, increased resistance to ventricular emptying, and ventricular hypertrophy. These physiologic changes lead to decreases in maximal heart rate, maximal aerobic capacity, peak exercise cardiac output, and peak ejection fraction. The elderly often are unable to compensate for decreased cardiac output by increasing their heart rate. Instead, they rely on augmenting ventricular filling and stroke volume to increase cardiac output. As a consequence, minor hypovolemia may precipitate a significant deterioration in cardiac function [29].

Pulmonary function is also affected by aging. As individuals age, there is a substantial decrease in the strength of respiratory muscles, chest wall compliance, and rib mobility. This results in a decline in maximum inspiratory and expiratory force by as much as 50%. Ventilatory responses to hypoxia and hypercapnia also fall by 50 and 40%, respectively. The respiratory system's ability to guard against environmental injury and infection also declines. A decline in T-cell function, mucociliary clearance, swallowing function, and the cough reflex all predispose the elderly to aspiration, with an increase in the incidence of respiratory infections and failure. All of these changes within the respiratory system combine to increase the incidence and severity of pneumonia, other respiratory infections, and respiratory failure [29].

Renal function is also not spared from the effects of the aging process. Along with a decline in glomerular filtration rate (GFR) of approximately 45% by age 80 years, renal tubular function also declines. As a result, assessing renal function and calculating creatinine clearance becomes important when determining the type and dosage of drugs used in the elderly. In addition, regulation of volume status becomes more problematic in the elderly. The ability to conserve sodium and excrete hydrogen ions falls, and therefore the aging kidney is not able to regulate fluid and acid–base balance as well. Dehydration may become exacerbated because the kidney does not compensate well for nonrenal losses of sodium and water, which is thought to be due to a decline in the renin–angiotensin system and decreased end-organ responsiveness to antidiuretic hormone. Volume overload also can be a problem due to the decline in GFR and functional impairment of the diluting segment of the nephron [29].

Other significant changes that occur with aging involve the central nervous system. Components of sensory perception such as visual acuity, proprioception, balance, and tactile sensation all decline with age and make it difficult for patients to adjust to new environments. When placed in this situation, they are more likely to become confused and depressed, and suffer a serious fall. Decline in hypothalamic function, along with decreased basal metabolic rates and changes in threshold for peripheral vasoconstriction and shivering causes a decrease in the ability to generate and conserve heat. In the postoperative or post-injury period, fever responses may be blunted as well. Changes in acute pain perception with aging are also problematic, and can lead to misdiagnosis and undertreatment. Several clinical observations have confirmed this, such as in the incidence of silent myocardial infarction and asymptomatic duodenal ulcer disease in this population [29].

Management of resuscitation

The elderly undergo many changes that pose challenges for emergency medicine (EM) physicians in recognizing a critically ill patient and impact the efficacy of various interventions during all stages of CPR. The initial steps in basic life support are aimed at establishing an airway and providing adequate oxygenation and ventilation. Unfortunately, the aging process renders the management of the geriatric airway slightly different from typical airway management. In the elderly, mouth opening may be limited by temporomandibular joint disease. Because there is often poor dentition and teeth can be dislodged into the oropharynx, special care must be taken during direct laryngoscopy. Dentures and bridges should be removed, although ventilation can be more difficult in an edentulous airway because the seal may be hard to establish in mouth-to-mouth or mouth-to-mask procedures. There may also be a decrease in the range of motion of the cervical spine, especially at the atlanto-occipital joint, sometimes making positioning of the head and visualization of the glottis difficult. Forced extension of the neck can result in atlanto-occipital subluxation and spinal cord injury [30].

Due to these numerous anatomic changes, the emergency physician (EP) often must use alternative strategies and techniques in securing an airway. Intubation and mechanical ventilation of the elderly often become necessary, due to respiratory insufficiency, depressed mental status, and poor tolerance to hypoxia. It should not be withheld because of the patient's age. However, intubation should not be undertaken lightly. The risk of barotrauma and nosocomial pneumonia increases substantially, and weaning an elderly patient from the ventilator often becomes very difficult.

If intubation is necessary, it is important to be wary of anatomical features in the elderly that can assist in predicting a difficult airway. Preoxygenation becomes an even more critical component in the elderly due to the fact they desaturate relatively quickly after paralytics. Pretreatment agents should be strongly considered in elderly patients, who have a disproportionately higher incidence of cardiovascular and cerebrovascular disease. Lidocaine can help in patients with suspected increased intracranial pressure or reactive airway disease, while fentanyl blunts the catecholamine response to laryngeal manipulation. Use caution as older patients are more sensitive to opioids, and if fentanyl is used it should be given more slowly [31]. It is recommended to avoid the small priming dose of a non-depolarizing neuromuscular blocker, which is often administered before succinylcholine in younger patients. In the elderly, even a small priming dose of non-depolarizing neuromuscular blockers can abolish ventilation and airway reflexes completely. Furthermore, doses of induction agents, including barbiturates, benzodiazepines, and etomidate, should be reduced by 20 to 40% to minimize cardiac depression and hypotension in this population. On the other hand, doses of neuromuscular blocking agents should not be reduced. A Miller blade can be useful because it has a smaller flange than a Macintosh and allows easier visualization of landmarks and passage of the endotracheal tube [1]. It is also important to consider adjunctive airway devices such as laryngeal mask airways, videolaryngoscopy, gum elastic bougie, and fiberoptic laryngoscopy in elderly patients with difficult airways [30,31].

Since elderly patients develop greater complications from intubation, the use of noninvasive positive pressure ventilation (NIPPV) such as continuous positive airway pressure or bilevel positive airway pressure should be strongly considered in the appropriate setting. It has especially proven to be advantageous in managing congestive heart failure (CHF) and chronic obstructive pulmonary disease (COPD) exacerbations, which are very common causes of respiratory failure in this population. Patients with respiratory insufficiency from easily reversible causes would also benefit from NIPPV. In acute COPD exacerbations, NIPPV decreases the work of breathing and improves alveolar ventilation. Several trials and meta-analyses support the use of NIPPV by reducing ventilator-associated pneumonia, intubation, duration of stay in the intensive care unit (ICU), and mortality. In CHF, NIPPV also improves oxygenation, reduces the work of breathing, and may prevent intubation and decrease mortality. NIPPV should be considered in patients hospitalized with acidotic COPD exacerbation or CHF not responding to medical intervention [32].

The assessment of breathing in the elderly also becomes problematic, as there are wide arrays of changes in respiratory physiology that occur in this group. Decreasing baseline arterial oxygen tension with advancing age is due to an age-related decrease in diffusion capacity and an age-related ventilation-perfusion mismatch. The increased work of breathing along with frequent underlying nutritional deficiency puts the elderly at increased risk of respiratory failure. Because both ventilatory and heart rate responses to hypoxia and hypercapnia are reduced, diagnosing occult respiratory insufficiency is very difficult and requires careful and frequent monitoring. A chest radiograph is important to perform in assessing respiratory distress. An electrocardiogram (ECG) in the elderly is also critical, as silent myocardial ischemia is common among acute illnesses. If concern for carbon dioxide retention exists, a Venturi mask is favorable over a nasal cannula because it provides a more precise method of oxygen delivery and does not vary depending on whether the patient is primarily mouth or nose

breathing. For chronic obstructive pulmonary disease patients requiring intubation, ventilatory therapy should avoid respiratory alkalosis, which is a significant hurdle in attempts at subsequent weaning and extubation. It is generally agreed that using lower respiratory rates in conjunction with tidal volumes from 6 to 8 ml/kg is more physiologic and reduces the patient's work of breathing, as well as minimizing peak pressures and chances of barotrauma. Pulmonary oxygen toxicity is minimized by using the lowest amount of oxygen necessary to keep PO_2 at least 60 mmHg [1].

After ventilation, the next step is the assessment of the circulation. Although the usual recommendation is to palpate a carotid pulse, this is often difficult in the elderly, secondary to carotid artery lesions and severe vascular narrowing. Potential complications include carotid flow occlusion or disruption of a plaque with subsequent distal embolization. Using the femoral pulse is a reasonable alternative in this population [30]. It is important to note that the elderly often do not have enough cardiac reserve to mount a significant response to stresses such as hypovolemia, sepsis, trauma, acute coronary ischemia, or respiratory failure. The initial approach to shock after addressing the airway begins with intravenous access and use of intravenous resuscitative fluids. Multiple small (250 ml) fluid boluses with repeated reassessment will often prevent significant volume overload and cardiogenic pulmonary edema [1].

Determination of intravascular volume status can be very difficult in the critically ill geriatric patient. Many patients in hypovolemic or septic shock may still be intravascularly depleted despite having received multiple liters of intravenous fluids. The use of vasopressors would be premature in this scenario and could worsen end-organ perfusion. On the other hand, some volume-depleted elderly patients in septic shock may also have pre-existing cardiomyopathy where excessive fluid administration can lead to flash pulmonary edema and respiratory failure [33]. If time permits, using a central venous or pulmonary artery catheter will help improve outcome and guide therapy. By measuring filling pressures, it will be easier to assess whether the patient may need inotropic support to maintain an adequate blood pressure [1].

The use of ultrasound to estimate filling pressures or overall cardiac function has also been shown to be valuable in guiding resuscitation. While absolute inferior vena cava (IVC) diameter has been shown to decrease in size in response to decreasing intravascular volume, respiratory variation in IVC size has better predictive value for estimation of right-sided filling pressures than static measurements. Testing for IVC collapse can be enhanced by having the patient sniff or forcefully inspire when able to follow commands. Greater than 50% IVC collapse with inspiration predicts central venous pressure (CVP) less than 10 mmHg, while less than 50% IVC collapse predicts CVP greater than 10 mmHg. A small (<1.5 cm) IVC that shows complete (or near complete) collapse with inspiration indicates that the hypotensive patient in shock is volume depleted. Aggressive volume loading is warranted in such cases. A large (>2.5 cm) IVC that shows no (or minimal) change with inspiration, referred to as a plethoric IVC, can be seen in patients who are volume overloaded but may also be observed in a number of other conditions, such as isolated right-sided heart failure and chronic pulmonary hypertension [33].

Bedside ultrasound can also be used to estimate global systolic function and help guide the EP in decisions regarding how aggressively to volume resuscitate and when inotropic support may be needed. Moreover, ultrasound can also be helpful in undifferentiated hypotensive elderly patients to assess for conditions such as aortic aneurysm, pericardial effusion, pneumothorax, and massive pulmonary embolism (PE) [33]. As EPs continue to become more adept with using ultrasonography in their practice, this will play a greater role in helping guide management decisions in the resuscitation of elderly people, as well as help in determining the etiologies of undifferentiated shock states.

Another predicament for the EP lies in determining which patients with normal vital signs may still have significant tissue hypoperfusion. Capillary refill and extremity temperature are late signs of shock in the elderly. An arterial or venous lactate level can be helpful, and has been shown to be a sensitive marker for intensive care unit admission and death. Unexplained metabolic acidosis on an arterial blood gas also suggests lactate production, although it is not as sensitive. Causes of shock in the elderly are numerous and include sepsis, dehydration, cardiac failure, and blood loss. A full laboratory work-up is essential, as well as a chest radiograph. It is important to note that fever may be absent in elderly patients with focal infections, bacteremia, or sepsis, and hypothermia can occur in the setting of sepsis because of significant hypoperfusion. An ECG is mandatory to determine whether acute coronary ischemia or an arrhythmia is playing a role [1].

Sepsis is a very common and important cause of morbidity and mortality in the older population and its incidence has increased in the last 10 years. Diagnosis and early management in older patients pose a myriad of challenges. Elderly patients may be less likely to mount a fever or leukocytosis response in the setting of infection than younger adults. Their heart rate is also often blunted due to AV nodal agents they may be taking. Therefore, systemic inflammatory response syndrome (SIRS) criteria are often absent in this population. The clinical manifestations of sepsis may be minimally present, unusual, nonspecific, or absent altogether. Presentations can include weakness, malaise, delirium, confusion, anorexia, falls, or urinary incontinence [34].

Early goal-directed therapy remains the mainstay of resuscitation in the management of severe sepsis and septic shock in the elderly population. Improving cardiac output in the elderly should focus on systolic function rather than heart rate, since heart rate response is blunted in the elderly. Therefore, it is imperative to maintain adequate preload to increase cardiac output. However, overaggressive fluid administration can also be precarious in light of worsening diastolic dysfunction that occurs with age. If physical exam findings are equivocal, the use of ultrasound can be helpful in ascertaining volume status and cardiac function. Otherwise, CVP monitoring is necessary to further guide management in these septic patients. Vasopressors such as dopamine or norepinephrine can be used to maintain perfusion if hypotension is not responsive to fluid resuscitation.

The early institution of broad-spectrum antimicrobial therapy has been shown to decrease mortality and should be initiated within 1 hour of the recognition of sepsis. The use of corticosteroids remains controversial and should only be considered in elderly patients not responding to intravenous fluids (IVF) or vasopressor therapy. Elderly patients with severe sepsis and septic shock will often require mechanical ventilation due to respiratory distress. The need for intubation has been shown to be independently associated with increased mortality in this population. A study by the Acute Respiratory Distress Syndrome (ARDS) Network demonstrated absolute risk reduction in mortality of 9% with relative risk reduction of 22% in the low-tidal volume (TV) (6 ml/kg) group compared with the conventional-TV (12 ml/kg) group. Thus, a tidal volume of 6 ml/kg predicted body weight in patients with acute lung injury (ALI) or ARDS is recommended even in elderly patients with upper limit goal for plateau pressure less than 30 cmH$_2$O [35].

Several studies have found age to be an independent predictor of mortality in sepsis [35]. It is important to note that while older people do have a higher mortality associated with severe sepsis, the prognosis of any given individual cannot be generalized to a population. While age is an important factor, the higher mortality rate observed is thought to be due to increased comorbidities, most important of which are metastatic neoplasm, chronic liver disease, non-metastatic neoplasm, chronic renal disease, and COPD [34]. Other factors have also been cited as independent predictors of outcome including preinfectious immune or genetic status, nosocomial events, comorbidities, severity of illness, age >75 years, and altered mental status. Other poor prognostic factors include presence of shock, elevated lactate level, and the presence of organ failure, especially respiratory or cardiac failure. The long-term prognosis of the elderly septic patient is chiefly dependent on functional status rather on severity of illness at admission [35]. Therefore, aggressive resuscitation is not futile in this population and prognosis is still very good in patients with few pre-existing comorbid illnesses and good functional status [34].

Managing shock in the elderly is problematic for other reasons as well. Although chest compressions are to be instituted to maintain cardiac output when the patient does not have evidence of adequate circulation, this may be even less effective in the elderly who have a higher incidence of underlying valvular dysfunction. It also produces significant injuries in the elderly, including trauma to the ribs, sternum, heart, lungs, great vessels, liver, and upper gastrointestinal tract. In patients with osteopenia and dorsal kyphosis, there have been case reports of chest compression-induced thoracolumbar transvertebral fractures. Several studies have addressed the use of manual and mechanical compression devices to standardize the force and depth of compression and minimize injuries and complications [30].

The aging process also may impact the standard dosages of medications used during resuscitation. Changes in body composition during aging result in an increase in the volume of distribution of lipophilic drugs, and a decrease in the volume of distribution of hydrophilic drugs. The degree of drug binding to plasma proteins is also affected because of the decrease in albumin often seen in aging. In addition, there is evidence of decreased beta-adrenergic responsiveness in the elderly. Despite all of these physiologic changes, the current recommended Advanced Cardiac Life Support (ACLS) guidelines on the use of drugs during resuscitation do not require modification in the elderly because there is no compelling evidence to suggest that they are not effective in this population. However, one ACLS medication of particular importance in the elderly may be magnesium. The elderly are susceptible to hypomagnesemia due to poor daily intake, diuretic therapy, as well as malabsorption and diabetes mellitus. Magnesium deficiency is often associated with cardiac arrhythmias, cardiac insufficiency, and sudden cardiac death. There have been no reports regarding the use of magnesium or incidence of torsades de pointes in the elderly, but some studies reported decreased in-hospital mortality in patients 70 years or older who received magnesium versus placebo following an acute myocardial infarction [30].

Another area of geriatric resuscitation that emergency physicians can expect to increasingly manage is acute stroke. While the assessment and management of airway, breathing, and circulation still take priority, an elderly patient presenting with stroke poses many other challenges that physicians should be attuned to. Older patients with stroke have more severe deficits at presentation and recover more slowly than younger patients. Elderly patients with ischemic stroke often receive less effective treatment and have poorer outcomes than younger individuals with this condition. The fundamental treatment of patients presenting with ischemic stroke is reperfusion and neuroprotection. Early clot lysis with recombinant tissue plasminogen activator (rtPA) up to 3 to 4.5 hours after ischemic stroke improves patient outcomes. However, elderly patients are unfortunately underrepresented or excluded in many of the largest studies on thrombolytics and therefore it is unclear how well they respond to this treatment and whether bleeding complications are more frequent or more severe. Some studies including the NINDS rtPA study, which only included 42 patients aged over 80, showed a beneficial effect of rtPA across all age groups and did not support the exclusion of candidates based on age alone. Other studies excluded these patients due to concerns regarding the risk of intracerebral hemorrhage (ICH), as some elderly patients are more predisposed to this after thrombolysis. A systematic review of patients aged over 80 years who were treated with rtPA had a threefold higher mortality and less favorable outcomes at 3 months than younger patients; the risk of symptomatic ICH, however, was similar in both groups. It is important to realize that advanced age is not a contraindication to administering rtPA; however, careful consideration should be given prior to doing so if the risks of ICH are considered high. More elderly patients need to be included in randomized controlled trials to better clarify whether the benefits of thrombolysis outweigh the potential risk of bleeding complications [36].

Another important principle in stroke treatment is management of glucose levels, as patients with hyperglycemia have higher rates of morbidity and mortality. The combination of advanced age and elevated glucose levels after stroke appears to be a more significant risk factor and therefore patients older than 75 years should be treated aggressively for their hyperglycemia within the first 48 hours. Fever control, blood pressure management, and use of aspirin are all also important factors in the early management of stroke for the ED physician [37].

Status epilepticus is another common condition among the elderly that physicians should be comfortable recognizing and managing. Acute seizures, epilepsy, and status have the highest incidence in those over the age of 60 as compared with any other age group [38]. Status epilepticus is also two to five times more common in the elderly than in young adults [39]. The increasing prevalence of age-related neurologic disorders such as cerebrovascular and neurodegenerative disorders is a likely contributing factor. The most common condition leading to epilepsy in older adults is cerebrovascular disease, particularly ischemic stroke. Overall, short-term mortality with status epilepticus is independently related not only to seizure duration but also to the etiology of the event and the age of the patient [39]. Therefore, early, prompt intervention of elderly patients presenting in status epilepticus is of paramount importance.

Diagnosing epilepsy is difficult because of the subtle manifestation of partial seizures as well as the presence of age-related cognitive dysfunction, comorbid illnesses, and medication. Many are initially misdiagnosed as change in mental status, confusion, and syncope [38]. There are also often serious, debilitating, and life-threatening problems arising from seizures including fractures, dislocations, aspiration pneumonia, and significant head injuries that ED physicians should recognize and treat [40].

Initial assessment as always should focus on the airway, breathing, and circulation. It is important to pay particularly close attention to evidence of trauma, especially to the head and face. Levels of consciousness and observation of motor and eye movements can all be useful in determining the nature of the seizures. Initial treatment of status epilepticus should be initiated with a benzodiazepine, preferably intravenous lorazepam. If seizures persist, the next best choice would be fosphenytoin, which has fewer cardiac side effects than phenytoin and can be infused more quickly. Other common agents such as levetriacetam, valproic acid, and lacosamide may prove to be beneficial in aborting seizures, but no randomized controlled trials have been reported to support their use as first- or second-line treatment options. Refractory status epilepticus generally warrants intubation and continuous infusions of medications such as phenobarbital, pentobarbital, propofol, midazolam, or ketamine, any of which can be given and titrated to desired levels. Choice of agent should be primarily based on medical comorbidities and on minimization of drug–drug interactions. Prolonged neuromuscular blockade should be avoided so that reliable neurological exams can be performed [39].

A non-contrast head computed tomography (CT) should be performed once the seizures are controlled and the patient is relatively stable. If infection is a possibility, empirical antibiotic and antiviral treatment should not be delayed prior to performing a lumbar puncture. Metabolic abnormalities or hyperthermia should also be aggressively corrected in these cases. If the mental status does not improve within 20 to 30 minutes after cessation of seizure activity, it is important to rule out the presence of non-convulsive status. Neurologic consultation is advised when status epilepticus is not responding to first- or second-line therapies, or when electroencephalography (EEG) may be indicated [39].

Ethics of resuscitation and end-of-life care

In addition to facing complex dilemmas regarding resuscitating elderly patients, EM physicians increasingly will also confront a myriad of other issues associated with end-of-life care. Unfortunately, some aspects of the care of the dying may be at odds with the professional mission of EM physicians and the environment of the ED [4]. EM physicians possess a reflexive instinct toward saving the dying and averting death. Expertise in difficult resuscitation is a hallmark of the specialty. However, the impulse to save life at all costs must be relinquished by the EM physician when approaching the terminal patient. Although the rapid pace and lack of privacy of the ED may conspire against optimal end-of-life care, EM physicians should attempt to embrace a more patient-centric, humane approach. EM physicians should acknowledge and respect an individual patient's needs for end-of-life care. This requires a working knowledge of advance directives and the concepts underlying medical futility.

Advance directives

An advance directive (AD) is a document providing guidance for a patient's wishes when they are unable to do so themselves. ADs may take the form of either a living will or a durable power of attorney. A living will outlines the interventions that should or should not be performed under certain clinical scenarios, particularly when the patient is terminally ill [2]. Living wills may vary in substance from highly detailed documents to vague instructions with dubious interpretation [41]. In contrast, a power of attorney identifies a surrogate decision maker in the event that a patient no longer has the capacity to make decisions [2].

ADs secure the autonomy of an individual who currently lacks, but once possessed, an appropriate decision-making ability [42]. This extension of patient autonomy has been protected and encouraged through legislation. All 50 states recognize the patient autonomy embodied within an AD [43]. The federal Patient Self-Determination Act of 1991 requires that patients admitted to the hospital have the opportunity to complete and incorporate an AD within their medical record [44].

Although professional organizations and the general patient community have embraced ADs, their use remains sporadic and their implementation is problematic [45–47]. In one study of approximately 700 nursing home residents, only 8% possessed an AD [48]. A second analysis of over 13,000 US deaths found that less than 10% of the deceased had an AD [49]. However, the mere creation of an AD far from guarantees its application. It is not uncommon for individuals at the end of life to arrive in the ED without their AD. The AD may have been lost, placed in an outpatient chart, or simply forgotten at the place of residence [41,42,50]. Patients also may fail to inform the treating physician of the presence of an AD [51].

Equally concerning is the reticence of EM physicians to engage their patients about ADs and resuscitation options [4]. EM physicians may feel inappropriate in initiating this process, and may wish to defer to a primary care provider who has an ongoing, established relationship with the patient. EM physicians may also feel that the process is difficult and too time-consuming. However, neither of these concerns is supported by the available evidence. Most patients welcome the opportunity to discuss their end-of-life care with a physician, and a do not resuscitate order may be established in as little as 16 minutes in an ambulatory care setting [52–54].

EM physicians require a strategy to cope with the implementation problems associated with ADs and the moral ambiguities associated with end-of-life care. If an AD exists but cannot be produced in the ED, the EM physician should evaluate the reliability of the information available and attempt to make a series of clinical decisions adhering to the patient's previously stated wishes [55]. Physicians should resist the temptation to infer a patient's preferences for life-sustaining treatment. In general, physicians are unable to accurately predict an individual patient's preferences for resuscitation at the end of life [56].

If an AD can be produced in the ED, then the EM physician should not overrule it. Overriding an AD has been described as immoral and an act of disrespect toward patient autonomy [4]. Physicians should adhere to the instructions of an AD, although this may be difficult when the patient is comatose and their next of kin or health care proxy wants them fully resuscitated [57]. If there is doubt about the validity of the AD, or the next of kin or health care proxy insist on resuscitation, it is reasonable to resuscitate the patient and then discuss these issues in more detail. Emergency physicians should also resuscitate when the wishes of the patient or family are ambiguous or unclear, and clarify preferences when the timing is appropriate. Physicians may also override an AD if there is clear evidence that the patient's preferences have changed since the drafting of the original document [4].

If an AD does not exist and the timing and moment are appropriate, EM physicians should embrace the opportunity to discuss ADs with the appropriate patients. It is a component of the process to facilitate the follow-up of inpatient and outpatient care for the terminally ill. This is a proactive stance that promotes the cooperation and accountability of the entire health care team that serves patients at the end of their life [4].

Medical futility

Often, an unknown elderly patient may present to the ED on the verge of death. In such a situation, there may be neither the time nor the means to engage in meditative reflection regarding the patient's wishes. A delay in action may significantly hinder the effectiveness of a resuscitation. Although the impulse may be to resuscitate, a physician is not under an overriding legal or ethical obligation to treat if they believe an intervention may be futile.

A futile intervention may encompass a variety of potential outcomes. It may be used to refer to an intervention with a low likelihood of success, or an intervention with a low probability of survival, or an intervention with an unlikely restoration of an adequate quality of life [58]. Physicians lack a consensus definition of the meaning of futility [59,60]. As a result of these ambiguities, any discussion with families and other professionals requires an exact specification of the interpretation of a potentially futile intervention [58].

Both professional organizations and the judicial system have made meaningful contributions to the debate on withholding ineffective interventions. The American College of Emergency Physicians (ACEP) has issued a policy statement stating that EM physicians may withhold a treatment that has no realistic chance of medical benefit toward the patient [61]. Although this recommendation provides some guidance, the legal ramifications also need to be considered. In the majority of jurisdictions, there is no state or federal law addressing the withholding of non-beneficial treatments. Instead, case law provides some guidance regarding the legal implications of withholding care. In general, courts and juries are reluctant to override a family's desire for continuing care. Similarly, they are reticent about holding a physician liable for their judgment regarding the ineffectiveness of an intervention. Nonetheless, EM physicians must bear in mind that their determination of a treatment's effectiveness may be subject to legal scrutiny [58]. Any decision regarding a treatment's effectiveness should have a solid grounding in the evidence for the outcomes of resuscitation.

Despite the endorsement of ACEP and recent legal precedent, EM physicians still remain reluctant to withhold care. Legal concerns and the fear of liability continue to dominate EM physicians' decisions regarding resuscitation [62]. The best strategy to deal with these concerns and to promote ethical, humane care relies on open communication and knowledge of scientific data. The key is to engage the patient, their family, and their surrogates as early as possible regarding their preferences. These preferences should be weighed in the context of the available evidence regarding the benefits and risks of various alternative interventions [58].

Family-witnessed resuscitation

One issue that has stirred considerable debate in the medical community worldwide is whether to allow family members to be present during resuscitation. As the number of elderly patients continues to increase, physicians and staff members will likely have to address this question more frequently. While traditional practice entails keeping family outside of the resuscitation room, some members may prefer to be present, rather than waiting to see their loved one after she/he has been pronounced dead [63]. In fact, a number of health organizations including the American Heart Association (2000, 2005), the Canadian Association of Critical Care Nurses (2006), the European Federation of Critical Care Nursing Associations, the European Society of Pediatric and Neonatal Intensive Care, and the European Society of Cardiology Council on Cardiovascular Nursing and Allied Professions have all advocated for family-witnessed resuscitation (FWR) [64].

Many advantages have been cited in allowing family members to witness the resuscitation. In cases where it was unsuccessful, most family members felt that witnessing the event was instrumental in them coming to terms with the loss of their loved one. Families were also reassured knowing that all attempts to resuscitate were performed, and they also appreciated building rapport with the staff and having questions answered immediately on the status of their loved one. It has also been shown that post-traumatic stress disorder (PTSD) is actually lower in family members witnessing than those not attending [65].

However, many physicians and medical staff express concern that family members may interfere with the resuscitation process, inhibit staff performance, increase anxiety, and contribute to unnecessary prolongation of resuscitation. There is also fear of increased litigation risk and the psychological effect on family members. There are also health and safety issues to consider as some family members have fainted during the resuscitation, requiring medical attention themselves. Staff needs to be more vigilant when resuscitations involving defibrillators and sharp instruments are present so family members are not inadvertently injured [65,66].

Some studies have shown that previous work experience in the ED, doctor's gender, and previous participation in EM Continuing Medical Education (CME) courses were found to influence doctors' attitudes towards FWR [66]. One study demonstrated that visible bleeding and resuscitation failure exert significant negative effects on attitudes to FWR among both staff members and families. Female staff physicians and nurses in general reacted more negatively to family presence than did male physicians and nurses [67]. Overall, with more experience, doctors felt more comfortable about including family members during resuscitation of patients [66].

To better ensure the success of FWR, it is important for an individual not participating in the resuscitation to be present for family support. Preparing the family member prior to entering the room is crucial, as is the establishment of clear ground rules explaining what they are likely to witness (e.g., invasive interventions) and encouraging families to make contact with and talk to the patient. This family support person should be present at all times with the family members and also be able to escort them out of the resuscitation room if they are feeling faint or unwell. Decisions to end resuscitation need to be dealt with in a sensitive manner. The family support person plays a role in helping them deal with decisions. It is always ideal to involve family members who are present in this decision. Most literature recommends a nurse undertake the role of the family support person, since they have clinical knowledge and experience with resuscitation as well as being available 24 hours a day. On the other hand, there may be insufficient staff members to serve in this role and the emotional impact on the nurses should not be underestimated. One study stated that 70% of nurses felt unable to deal with the needs of family members while witnessing a resuscitation. Others have advocated for chaplains to serve this role as the family support person, since they are very adept at providing emotional and spiritual support. However, they may not be available during all hours and some families may feel uncomfortable with a chaplain as the support person [65].

In summary, FWR should be strongly considered in circumstances when family members have been adequately prepared for the experience and a support person is available to assist. Other factors relevant to this decision include the emotional state of the family member(s) and the age and number of family members present [63]. With more training, professional development, and increased work experience, it is likely that physicians will feel more comfortable about allowing families to be present for resuscitations.

Summary

In the future, EM physicians can anticipate increasing ED visits from critically ill elderly patients. These individuals require prompt identification and early, aggressive intervention. Unfortunately, the effects of aging on normal physiology conspire to make the recognition of the critically ill geriatric patient a challenge. These same physiologic effects may also impact the effectiveness of standard life-saving interventions. EM physicians should redouble their efforts toward understanding the pathophysiology and effective treatment of these patients.

A more thorough knowledge of this information will also assist in the ethical treatment of critically ill elderly patients toward the end of their life. An evidence-based comprehension of patient prognosis is a key component of an elderly individual's treatment toward the end of life. This information assists in the interpretation of ADs and patient and family preferences.

Ultimately, improving the care of the critically ill geriatric patient hinges on improved communication. EM physicians should actively engage primary care providers, specialists, prehospital providers, patients, and families in this process. When feasible and with appropriate support, physicians should also strongly consider allowing family members to witness resuscitation. Hopefully, initiating this process will further the goal of more humane, patient-centric care of all geriatric patients.

Pearls and pitfalls

Pearls

- Be wary of anatomical features that can make ventilating and intubating the geriatric patient difficult.
- The use of ultrasonography can be very beneficial in assessing the volume status of the elderly patient in shock and help guide resuscitation.
- Advanced age by itself is not a contraindication for the use of thrombolysis in acute CVA.
- Be proficient in handling end-of-life care issues; if advanced directives are not available or wishes of patients are unclear, it is generally safer to resuscitate the patient.

Pitfalls

- Failure to appreciate the unique pathophysiological changes that occur in the geriatric population.
- Not aggressively resuscitating the geriatric patient due to the misconception that efforts will always be futile; many of these patients still have favorable prognosis with timely treatment.

- Overreliance on classical signs and findings such as fever, leukocytosis, and tachycardia in the clinical assessment of elderly patients can be misleading and delay appropriate care.
- Not recognizing that elderly patients with sepsis often present with vague and atypical symptoms.

References

1. Milzman D, Rothenhaus T. Resuscitation of the geriatric patient. *Emerg Med Clin North Am*. 1996;14:233–44.

2. Mueller PS, Hook CC, Fleming KC. Ethical issues in geriatrics: a guide for clinicians. *Mayo Clin Proc*. 2004;79:554–62.

3. Callahan E, Thomas D, Goldhirsch S, et al. Geriatric hospital medicine. *Med Clin North Am*. 2002;86:707–29.

4. Schears RM. Emergency physicians' role in end-of-life care. *Emerg Med Clin North Am*. 1999;17:539–59.

5. Murphy DI, Murry AM, Robinson BE, et al. Outcomes of cardiopulmonary resuscitation in the elderly. *Ann Intern Med*. 1989;111:199–205.

6. Tafet GI, Teasdale TA, Luchi RJ. In-hospital cardiopulmonary resuscitation. *JAMA*. 1988; 260:2069–72.

7. Gulati RS, Bhan GL, Horan MA. Cardiopulmonary resuscitation of old people. *Lancet*. 1983;2:267–9.

8. Bedell SE, Delbanco TL, Cook EF, et al. Survival after cardiopulmonary resuscitation in the hospital. *N Engl J Med*. 1983;309:569–75.

9. Woog RH, Torzillo PJ. In-hospital cardiopulmonary resuscitation: prospective survey of management and outcome. *Anaesth Intensive Care*. 1987;15:193–8.

10. George AL Jr, Folk BP III, Crecelius PL, et al. Pre-arrest morbidity and other correlates of survival after in-hospital cardiopulmonary arrest. *Am J Med*. 1989;97:28–34.

11. Tortolani AJ, Risucci DA, Rosati RJ, et al. In-hospital cardiopulmonary resuscitation: patient arrest and resuscitation factors associated with survival. *Resuscitation*. 1990;20:115–28.

12. Robinson GR II, Hess D. Postdischarge survival and functional status following in-hospital cardiopulmonary resuscitation. *Chest*. 1994;105:991–6.

13. Roberts D, Landolfo K, Light RB, et al. Early predictors of mortality for hospitalized patients suffering cardiopulmonary arrest. *Chest*. 1990;97:413–19.

14. Rosenberg M, Wang C, Hofman-Wilde S, et al. Results of cardiopulmonary resuscitation. *Arch Intern Med*. 1993;153:1370–5.

15. Berger R, Kelley M. Survival after in-hospital cardiopulmonary arrest of noncritically ill patients. *Chest*. 1994;106:872–9.

16. Tresch DD, Heudebert G, Kutty K, et al. Cardiopulmonary resuscitation in elderly patients hospitalized in the 1990s: a favorable outcome. *J Am Geriatr Soc*. 1994;42:137–41.

17. Tresch DD, Thakur RK. Cardiopulmonary resuscitation in the elderly. Beneficial or an exercise in futility? *Emerg Med Clin North Am*. 1998;16:649–63.

18. Tresch DD, Thakur RK, Hofmann RG, et al. Comparison of outcome of paramedic-witnessed cardiac arrest in patients younger and older than 70 years. *Am J Cardiol*. 1990;65:453–7.

19. Tresch DD, Thakur RK, Hofmann RG, et al. Should the elderly be resuscitated following out-of-hospital cardiac arrest? *Am J Med*. 1989;86:145–50.

20. Bonnin MJ, Pepe PE, Clark PS. Survival in the elderly after out-of-hospital cardiac arrest. *Crit Care Med.* 1993;21:1645–51.

21. Denes P, Long L, Madison C, et al. Resuscitation from out-of-hospital ventricular tachycardia/fibrillation (VT/VF): the effect of age on outcome. *Circulation.* 1990;82(Suppl.):III-81.

22. Eisenberg MS, Horwood BT, Larson MP. Cardiopulmonary resuscitation in the elderly. *Ann Intern Med.* 1990;113:408–9.

23. Longstreth WT Jr, Cobb LA, Fahrenbruch CE, et al. Does age affect outcomes of out-of-hospital cardiopulmonary resuscitation? *JAMA.* 1990;264:2109–10.

24. Applebaum GE, King JE, Finucane TE. The outcome of CPR initiated in nursing homes. *J Emerg Geriatr Soc.* 1990;38:197–200.

25. Awoke S, Mouton CP, Parrott M. Outcomes of skilled cardiopulmonary resuscitation in a long-term care facility: futile therapy? *J Am Geriatr Soc.* 1992;40:593–5.

26. Gordon M, Cheung M. Poor outcome of on-site CPR in a multilevel geriatric facility: three and a half years experience at the Baycrest Center for Geriatric Care. *J Am Geriatr Soc.* 1993;41:163–6.

27. Tresch DD, Neahring JM, Duthie EH, et al. Outcomes of cardiopulmonary resuscitation in nursing homes: can we predict who will benefit? *Am J Med.* 1993;95:123–30.

28. Ghusn HF, Teasdale TA, Pepe PE, et al. Older nursing home residents have a cardiac arrest survival rate similar to that of older persons living in the community. *J Am Geriatr Soc.* 1995;43:520–7.

29. Rosenthal R, Kavic S. Assessment and management of the geriatric patient. *Crit Care Med.* 2004;32:S92–105.

30. Liu L, Carlisle A. Management of cardiopulmonary resuscitation. *Anesthesiol Clin North Am.* 2000;18:143–58.

31. Walls RM, Murphy MF. *Manual of Emergency Airway Management* (Philadelphia, PA: Lippincott, Williams and Wilkins, 2008).

32. Delerme, S, Ray, P. Acute respiratory failure in the elderly: diagnosis and prognosis. *Age Aging.* 2008;37:251–7.

33. Byrne MW, Hwang JQ. Ultrasound in the critically ill. *Ultrasound Clinics.* 2011;6:235–59.

34. Destarac LA, Ely EW. Sepsis in older patients: An emerging concern in critical care. *Advances Sepsis.* 2002;2:15–22.

35. Nasa P, Juneja D, Singh O. Severe sepsis and septic shock in the elderly: An overview. *World J Crit Care Med.* 2012;1:23–20.

36. Chen RL, Balami JS, Esiri MM, et al. Ischemic stroke in the elderly: an overview of evidence. *Nat Rev Neurol.* 2010;6:256–65.

37. Llinas R. Acute stroke treatment and prevention in the elderly. *US Special Populations.* 2006;24–6 (accessed from www.touchbriefings.com/pdf/2032/Llinas.pdf July 15, 2012).

38. Verellen RM, Cavazos JE. Pathophysiological considerations of seizures, epilepsy, and status epilepticus in the elderly. *Aging Dis.* 2011;2:278–86.

39. Mauricio, EA, Freeman WD. Status epilepticus in the elderly: differential diagnosis and treatment. *Neuropsychiatr Dis Treat.* 2011;7:161–6.

40. Rowan, JA. Epilepsy in older adults: common morbidities influence development, treatment strategies, and expected outcomes. *Geriatrics.* 2005;60:30–4.

41. Walker RM, Schonwetter RS, Kramer DR, et al. Living wills and resuscitation preferences in the elderly population. *Arch Intern Med.* 1995;155:171–5.

42. Danis M, Southerland LI, Garrett JM, et al. A prospective study of advance directives for life-sustaining care. *N Engl J Med.* 1991;324:882–8.

43. Prendergast TJ. Advance care planning: pitfalls, progress, promise. *Crit Care Med.* 2001;29:N34–9.

44. Wolf SM, Boyle P, Callahan D, et al. Sources of concern about the Patient Self-Determination Act. *N Engl J Med.* 1991;325:1666–71.

45. American College of Physicians. Ethics manual, 4th edn. *Ann Intern Med.* 1998;128:576–94.

46. Orentlicher D. Advanced medical directives. *JAMA.* 1990;263:2365–7.

47. Emmanuel LL, Barry MJ, Stoeckle JD, et al. Advance directives for medical care – a case for greater use. *N Engl J Med.* 1991;324:889–95.

48. Jones JS, Dwyer PR, White LJ, et al. Patient transfer from nursing home to emergency department: outcomes and policy implications. *Acad Emerg Med.* 1997;4:908–15.

49. Hanson LC, Rodgman E. The use of living wills at the end of life: a national study. *Arch Intern Med.* 1996;156:1018–22.

50. Miles SH, Koepp R, Weber EP. Advanced end-of-life treatment planning: a research review. *Arch Intern Med.* 1996;156:1062–8.

51. Teno JM, Licks S, Lynn J, et al. SUPPORT Investigators. Do advance directives provide instructions that direct care? *J Am Geriatr Soc.* 1997;45:508–12.

52. Hakim RB, Teno JM, Harrell FE, et al. Factors associated with do-not-resuscitate orders: patients' preferences, prognoses, and physicians' judgments. *Ann Intern Med.* 1996;125:284–93.

53. Schonwetter RS, Walker RM, Solomon M, et al. Life values, resuscitation preferences and the applicability of living wills in an older population. *J Am Geriatr Soc.* 1996;44:954–8.

54. Smith TJ, Desch CE, Hackney MK, et al. How long does it take to get a "do not resuscitate" order? *J Palliat Care.* 1997;13:5–8.

55. Marco CA. Ethical issues of resuscitation. *Emerg Med Clin North Am.* 1999;17:527–38.

56. Hamel MB, Lynn J, Teno JM, et al. Age-related differences in care preferences, treatment decisions, and clinical outcomes of seriously ill hospitalized adults: lessons from SUPPORT. *J Am Geriatr Soc.* 2000;48:S176–82.

57. Ramos T, Reagan JE. "No" when the family says "go": resisting families' requests for futile CPR. *Ann Emerg Med.* 1989;18:898–9.

58. Marco CA, Larkin GL, Moskop JC, et al. Determination of "futility" in emergency medicine. *Ann Emerg Med.* 2000;35:604–12.

59. Solomon MZ. How physicians talk about futility: making words mean too many things. *J Law Med Ethics.* 1993;21:231–7.

60. McCrary SV, Swanson JW, Youngner SJ, et al. Physicians' quantitative assessments of medical futility. *J Clin Ethics.* 1994;5:100–5.

61. *Nonbeneficial ("Futile") Emergency Medical Interventions (Policy Statement)* (Dallas, TX: American College of Emergency Physicians, 1998, accessed from www.acep.org/policy/PO400198.HTM).

62. Marco CA, Bessman ES, Schoenfeld CN, et al. Ethical issues of cardiopulmonary resuscitation: current practice among emergency physicians. *Acad Emerg Med.* 1997;4:898–904.

63. Wagner JM. Lived experience of critically ill patients' family members during cardiopulmonary resuscitation. *Am J Crit Care.* 2004;13:416–20.

64. Al-Mutair AS, Plummer V, Copnell B. Family presence during resuscitation: a descriptive study of nurses' attitudes from two Saudi hospitals. *Nurs Crit Care.* 2012;17:90–8.

65. Cottle EM, James JE. Role of the family support person during resuscitation. *Nursing Standard.* 2008;23:43–7.

66. Gordon ED, Kramer E, Couper, I, et al. Family-witnessed resuscitation in emergency departments: Doctors' attitudes and practices. *S Afr Med J.* 2011;101:765–7.

67. Itzhaki M, Bar-Tal Y, Barnoy S. Reactions of staff members and lay people to family presence during resuscitation: the effect of visible bleeding, resuscitation outcome and gender. *J Adv Nurs.* 2012;68:1967–77.

Pharmacology in the elderly

Michelle Blanda

Introduction

Significant emphasis has been given to the needs of seniors in emergency medicine due to their significant impact on resources and utilization of emergency services. In fact, it is recommended there be a geriatric emergency care model emphasizing older patients as a special population similar to pediatric patients [1]. This concept is especially relevant to drug therapies in this special population.

Pharmacologic use is highly valued in the treatment of acute and chronic conditions in older adults. Yet the balance of the benefit of pharmacologic interventions must be evaluated with knowledge of the risk and harm drugs may cause in this delicate population. The need for practitioners to create harmony between avoiding medications with adverse effects, while at the same time providing access to therapies which may have beneficial effects on morbidity, mortality, function, and quality of life in older patients is challenging.

"Aged heterogeneity" is a principle in gerontology describing inter-individual variability in health, disease, and disability, and how these factors change with age [2]. This heterogeneity results in a wide range of health status of older people, from those who are fit to those who are frail. This makes generalization of prescribing decisions difficult for practitioners. Variables affecting the use of drugs in this heterogeneous older population include comorbidities, limited evidence for efficacy, increased risk of adverse drug reactions, polypharmacy, altered pharmacokinetics, functional status, cognitive impairment, and social support.

Older patients often are involved in a vicious cycle described by Rochan as the "prescribing cascade" [3,4]. This cascade begins when an adverse drug reaction is misinterpreted as a new medical condition. A drug is prescribed to treat this new "medical condition" and another adverse drug effect occurs. This interpretation of a side effect as a new condition results in the patient being subjected to unnecessary treatment and additional adverse effects of another drug. Since older patients have multiple medical problems, they are prescribed multiple medications leading to increased risk of adverse effects. Many of these adverse effects go unrecognized as such and lead to new drugs being added. This perpetuates the continued cycle of adverse effects.

This chapter describes the scope of the problem of drug prescribing in the older adult. It looks at the concept of adverse drug reactions and events, principles underlying clinical geriatric pharmacology, and the impact on admissions, and reviews drugs that commonly cause adverse drug reactions. It includes recommendations about drugs to be avoided, substitutes, and suggests approaches to evaluating the evidence for risk and benefits when selecting medications for older patients.

Epidemiology

Drug prescribing in the older population is important to consider for many reasons. These include the growth of the aging population, the existence of chronic illness, and the use of multiple medications. In addition, since pharmacokinetics and pharmacodynamics may be altered by age and disease, this group is at high risk to be affected. All of these points increase the susceptibility for adverse drug reactions.

In the year 2010, there were 40.4 million people over the age of 65 years in the US, which represented a 5.4 million increase (15.3%) since 2000 [5]. This group received approximately 30% of prescribed drugs, which is twice as much as their younger counterparts [5]. They also use at least 25% of over-the-counter drugs. It is anticipated that significant growth will occur in this age group during the years 2011 to 2030 when baby boomers, the people born between 1946 and 1964, turn 65 years old [5]. By 2030, there will be 72.1 million older persons in the US, twice the number in 2000. Worldwide in developed countries, people are living longer and having fewer children, so the population balance is rapidly changing. Therefore any issues that affect this growing population will continue not only to exist but to become more pronounced.

As stated, the incidence of chronic illness and pathology increases with age leading to polypharmacy in this group. Although the term carries negative connotations, use of numerous medications is sometimes necessary [6]. Despite the view that there is widespread underuse of beneficial therapies in the elderly, drugs with known value in decreasing mortality in clinical trials are being offered more and more frequently to this population. These include mainstays of therapy such as statins in hypercholesterolemia, aspirin in coronary artery disease and stroke prevention (especially in patients unable to take

---

Geriatric Emergency Medicine, ed. Joseph H. Kahn, Brendan G. Magauran Jr., and Jonathan S. Olshaker. Published by Cambridge University Press.
© Cambridge University Press 2014.

Table 5.1. Herbal medications and supplements used by the elderly*

Herb/supplement	Reasons for use	Drugs which commonly interact
Vitamins	General health	Aspirin, Calcium 600, Crestar
Vitamin D	Osteoporosis prevention	Aluminum, Calcipotriene
Vitamin E	Prevention of Alzheimer's, Parkinson's diseases	Aspirin, Calcium
Vitamin C	Anti-cancer, heart disease prevention	Aspirin, Aluminum
Multivitamins		Aspirin, Calcium, Colace
Supplements		
Lutein	Macular degeneration and antioxidant	Beta-carotene
Lycopen	Antioxidant, cancer prevention, prevention of heart disease and diabetes	Cancer chemotherapeutics, Cipro/Oxacen
Glucosamine/Chondroitin	Osteoarthritis, pain relief, and prevention	Anti-inflammatory agents
Fish oil/flaxseed	Beneficial for heart health, flexible joints, the immune system, good mood, and mental health	None
Allium sativum (garlic)	Immune-enhancing, anti-cancer	Warfarin/Antiplatelet drugs, Protease inhibitors
Ginkgo biloba extract	Prevention of vascular dementia	Anticonvulsant medication, Aspirin
Coenzyme Q	Alzheimer's disease, peripheral vascular disease, tinnitus	Warfarin, Acetaminophen
Ginseng	Cure-all herb	Warfarin, Alcohol
Senna, cascara	Laxative	Can decrease all drug availability

* In order of decreasing frequency.

warfarin), thiazide diuretics, beta blockers and angiotensin-converting enzyme (ACE) inhibitors in hypertension, as well as ACE inhibitors in heart failure, antiplatelet agents in atrial fibrillation, and antiplatelet agents and beta blockers in those with myocardial infarction [7–10].

Older people have more adverse drug events than any other age group because their exposure to a greater number of medications provides more opportunities for medication errors and adverse effects. The Slone Survey, which is a phone survey of a random sample of the non-institutionalized US population, reported data on the range of drugs used by the general public. For patients aged at least 65 years in 2006, this survey found that during the preceding week, 57% of women and 59% of men had taken at least 5 medications and 17% of women and 10% of men had taken more than 10 medications [11]. Others have reported similar numbers, with community-dwelling elders taking between 2 and 6 medications and 1 to 3 non-prescription medications on a routine basis [12].

The Slone Survey also reported on common vitamin, herbal, and over-the-counter medication use by this age group. The most common over-the-counter drug used is aspirin. Vitamins used by both sexes in patients 65 years of age and older were multivitamins, vitamin E, and vitamin C. In addition, women used calcium and vitamin D. Common herbal supplements are listed in Table 5.1 [11]. Awareness of the use of the full range of medications, both prescription and non-prescription, is essential for patient safety and to reduce risks associated with their consumption.

The use of medications not documented or revealed to the physician while in the hospital may contribute to adverse outcomes. It has been described that on average about 1.5 additional drugs are not mentioned on an initial assessment of drug history and will be discovered on a second interview. This has been verified by actual urine sampling of patients, with analgesics, benzodiazepines, and ranitidine being reported as most commonly not disclosed [13]. This widespread phenomenon, of physicians being unaware of medication used by the patient, has been described in emergency departments, surgical settings, and in office visits as well [14].

Definitions

Adverse drug reactions (ADRs) are defined by the World Health Organization (WHO) as "any noxious, unintended, and undesired effect of a drug which occurs at doses used in humans for prophylaxis, diagnosis or therapy" [15]. This does not include therapeutic failures, poisonings (whether accidental or intentional), overprescribing, abuse of drugs, errors in administration, or noncompliance. Therefore, the term adverse drug reaction probably underestimates the true incidence of events related to drugs.

Other terms are used rather than adverse drug reaction. "Adverse drug event" refers to any injury resulting from administration of a drug. A "drug-related problem" includes the above definitions but also includes failure to receive drugs for a medical problem (underprescribing) and drug use without indication (misprescribing). Most literature, however, tends not to use these broader definitions.

Recent literature suggests it may be better to define "appropriate prescribing." Three important domains in determining appropriateness include what the patient wants, scientific and

Table 5.2. Mechanisms of drug clearance in the elderly

Route of clearance	Example of common drugs
Renal	Cardiovascular: Atenolol, digoxin, furosemide, hydrochlorothiazide, procainamide, enalapril, lisinopril
	Antibiotics: Ampicillin, ceftriaxone, gentamycin, penicillin, ciprofloxacin, levofloxacin, ofloxacin
	Gastrointestinal: Cimetidine, ranitidine, famotidine
	Neurologic: Amantadine, lithium, pancuronium, phenobarbital
	Hypoglycemic drugs: Chlorpropamide, glyburide
Hepatic	Cardiovascular: Labetolol, lidocaine, prazosin, propranolol, quinidine, salicylates, warfarin
	Analgesics: Acetaminophen, ibuprofen, codeine
	Pulmonary: Theophylline
	Neurologic: Amitriptyline, barbiturates, phenytoin, benzodiazepines

technical rationalism, and the general good (family and societal values) [2]. Appropriate prescribing in older patients is more complex since drug trials on efficacy may be scarce, goals of treatment are not the same as in younger counterparts, and social and economic factors may be different as well. One of the major goals of this topic has to be to alert physicians about the preventability of these reactions. However, one must keep in mind that literature on adverse drug reactions demonstrates that even when drugs are used properly there are still a large number of serious adverse drug reactions that occur.

Pharmacokinetics

Drug absorption, distribution, metabolism, excretion, and the physiologic response to drugs are altered in older people. The impairment of drug absorption due to resection of the gut, bacterial overgrowth, or achlorhydria is felt to have minimal clinical implications [7]. However, drug interactions do occur where one drug changes the absorption characteristics of another. The classic example of one drug binding another is the use of antacids containing calcium and magnesium. Absorption of drugs such as antibiotics, aspirin, and digoxin can be significantly impaired by concurrent administration of antacids. Also, changes in gastrointestinal transit time may consequently change a drug's pharmacological action. Practitioners should be aware of drugs which alter transit time, and monitor patients on these medications.

Body composition in the older adult has decreased lean body mass, decreased total body water, and increased proportion of body fat and may alter drug distribution significantly [9,10]. These changes lead to a decrease in the volume of distribution and an increase in the serum concentrations of drugs. Drugs which are water soluble such as coumadin, digoxin, and propranolol will have higher plasma concentrations at a given dose in older patients. In drugs with a low or narrow therapeutic window such as digoxin, aminoglycosides, lithium, and procainamide, this can lead to toxicity.

Serum protein, especially albumin, also decreases with age [10]. There are decreased binding sites for protein-bound medications and higher serum concentrations. Malnutrition is a cause of decreased serum albumin and is common in older patients, especially those who are institutionalized. Competitive inhibition for protein-binding sites by drugs can lead to displacement of one drug by another with increased levels of the drug being displaced. An example is aspirin and warfarin, where aspirin increases the unbound fraction of warfarin.

Metabolism and clearance of drugs also change with aging [7,9,10,16] (Table 5.2). Unfortunately, since older patients with comorbid conditions are often excluded from drug trials, the knowledge of drug metabolism is limited. There are age-related decreases in renal function that are not related to kidney disease. As the kidney ages there is a decrease in glomerular filtration rate and tubular efficiency. A production of vasodilatory renal prostaglandins occurs to compensate for this decreased renal function, and drugs that impair this compensatory mechanism can cause a decrease in the metabolism of renally eliminated drugs. Nonsteroidal anti-inflammatory drugs (NSAIDs) are an example [17].

Nephron loss is a normal aging process leading to a lower glomerular filtration rate, which requires drug doses to be adjusted. Despite the lower glomerular filtration rate, serum creatinine may be normal in older patients due to decreased creatinine intake and lower muscle mass [18]. It is recommended that creatinine clearance be calculated with correction for age and ideal body weight using the Cockroft–Gault formula (creatinine clearance = ([140 – age] × weight [kg])/[72 × creatinine (mg/dl)]) × 0.85 for females]). Results of decreased renal function include prolonged half-life of renally cleared medications, increased serum levels, and prolonged clinical effects. For some drugs such as antibiotics, renal insufficiency may or may not result in serious effects. However, failing to adjust for others such as metformin puts the patient at risk for life-threatening events.

The other organ that contributes to metabolism of many drugs is the liver. Hepatic metabolism in the elderly is not only related to age, but also to lifestyle, genotype, hepatic blood flow, hepatic disease, and interactions with other medications. It may be reduced up to 30 to 50% in older adults [16]. The evidence as related to age is not completely clear. Hepatic metabolism occurs through two biotransformation systems. Phase I reactions occur through the cytochrome P450 system, which either clears drugs or allows oxidation and activation of drugs. This can occur much more slowly in some older adults. The change in Phase I reactions leads to change in the serum levels and clinical activity of drugs. Inhibitors of the P450 system cause an increase in the serum concentrations of drugs metabolized by the liver by impairing clearance of those drugs. Medications that induce the P450 system lead to decreased levels of medications metabolized by the liver. The metabolizing activity of the P450 system has not always been found to be affected by age and frailty, but is more affected by female sex. Since studies include so few older adults, many of the results are inconclusive although trends showing significant inter-individual variability have been reported [19]. Phase II metabolism, which includes acetylation, sulfonation, conjugation, and glucuronidation, is minimally affected in the older population [16]. Cigarette smoking, alcohol use, and caffeine may also affect hepatic metabolism.

Other physiologic changes occur that affect the pharmacodynamics of many drugs. Age-related changes in cardiovascular function occur and may explain the reduced compensatory capacity effect in the elderly to many drugs. Changes in cardiac morphology with age include a decreased number of myocytes, stiffening of myocardial cells, reduced responsiveness to β-adrenergic stimulation, and decreased contractility of the heart. In parallel to these changes, large arteries dilate with increased wall thickness and increased smooth muscle tone with age [20,21]. This leads to increased systolic blood pressure and elevated left ventricular afterload, resulting in left ventricular wall thickening. This in turn causes loss of left ventricular compliance and impairment of diastolic function. Other changes in the older population include an increase in sympathetic outflow causing decreased sensitivity to β-adrenergic stimulation, as well as autonomic and baroreceptor dysfunction leading to decreased response to posture and hypotension.

The central nervous system (CNS) is the other area where aging changes must be considered. Research now suggests that it is not a simple loss in the number of neurons that occurs with time, but subtler changes occurring at the level of synapses. Alterations in cellular Ca^{2+}, capacity to deal with oxidative stress, reduced regeneration capacity (re-myelination), and decrease in receptor sites as well as changes within these sites have all been identified as explanations for the diminution of CNS functioning and sensitivity to drugs in the elderly [16,20,22].

Outcomes of adverse drug reactions

The outcomes for medication-related problems are profound. In 2004, a collaborative group (the Centers for Disease Control and Prevention, the US Consumer Product Safety Commission, and the US Food and Drug Administration) developed the National Electronic Injury Surveillance System-Cooperative Adverse Drug Event project (NEISS-CADES) to estimate and describe the national burden of adverse drug events (ADEs) that cause emergency department (ED) visits. The most recent data published found an estimate of at least 265,000 ED visits annually in patients 65 years or older for adverse drug events [23]. Hospitalization was needed in 37.5% of these events. International studies reveal similar rates [24–27]. Nearly half of the hospitalizations required involved adults 80 years of age and older. The hospitalization rate per 1000 persons was 3.5-fold higher in patients over 85 years compared with adults aged 65 to 69 years. Emergency department visits resulting in hospitalization in older patients were more likely to involve unintentional overdoses and five or more concomitant medications. For the population older than 65 years of age, the annual population rate of ADEs requiring hospitalization was nearly seven-fold the rate of patients younger than 65 years [28].

The most common drugs implicated in older patients requiring admission in the NEISS-CADES database were warfarin (33.3%), insulins (13.9%), oral antiplatelet agents (13.3%), and oral hypoglycemic agents (10.7%). These four drugs were implicated in two-thirds of all hospital admissions related to ADEs. These remained the most common drugs when stratified by age and sex for patients older than 65 years. In 12 and 15% of cases of warfarin and the insulins, respectively, other drugs in the same category were implicated as contributing to the problem. In regard to warfarin, concomitant use of other antiplatelet drugs contributed to the adverse drug event, and for insulins, concomitant use of oral hypoglycemic agents contributed to adverse drug events.

Therapeutic drug categories most commonly requiring ED visits are listed in Table 5.3 [29,30]. Medications commonly designated as high risk or potentially inappropriate by current national quality measures were rarely implicated. Implementing quality measures to monitor safe use, especially of antithrombotic and antidiabetic agents, must be considered. Caution should be exercised when reviewing these data because in the majority of studies it is difficult to determine what is the overall consumption of drugs. Drugs implicated in causing adverse drug reactions may be more related to how commonly they are used. Between 3 and 28% of hospital admissions can be attributed to drug-related problems or drug toxic effects [29,31]. In patients withADRs requiring hospitalization, the mortality rate is increased by 20% when compared with all admissions.

If fatal ADRs were classified as a distinct entity, they would rank between the fourth and sixth leading cause of death in the US. This would rank ADRs above pneumonia and diabetes as a cause of death. This is not unique to the US, but has also been identified in other nations' health systems [25].

The cost of drug-related morbidity and mortality is estimated to be more than 177 billion dollars in the US [15]. Admissions related to ADRs cost $121 billion, 70% of the total cost. Eighteen percent of the cost was for long-term admissions ($32.8 billion). In the United Kingdom, drug-related problems account for 4% of hospital bed capacity [30]. A review of ADRs related to hospital admission found that "80% are directly responsible for the admission or known as "causal." The other 20% are "coincidental" and, although not directly responsible for the admission, may have contributed to it. Almost three-quarters are considered avoidable [29].

Table 5.3. Drugs implicated in causing hospital admission* [29,30]

Diuretics

Warfarin

Nonsteroidal anti-inflammatory agents (includes aspirin)

Chemotherapeutics

Antidiabetic agents

Cardiotonics

Anti-epileptic drugs

Immunosuppressants

Antibiotics

*In order of frequency.

Table 5.4. Top ten dangerous drug interactions seen in nursing homes [37]

Interaction	Effects
Warfarin–NSAIDs	Increased bleeding
Warfarin–sulfonamides	Prolongation of warfarin's effects due to unknown mechanism. Need to decrease dose of warfarin by 50% during and 1 week after therapy with antibiotic
Warfarin–macrolide antibiotics	Prolongation of warfarin's effects due to inhibition of warfarin metabolism by macrolides
Warfarin–quinolone antibiotics	Prolongation of warfarin's effects due to unknown mechanism. May be due to decrease in vitamin K production and altered warfarin metabolism
Warfarin–phenytoin	Prolongation of phenytoin half-life with increased serum levels
ACE inhibitors–potassium	Hyperkalemia can occur due to decreased aldosterone production caused by ACE inhibitors
ACE inhibitors–spironolactone	Both drugs increase serum potassium and can cause hyperkalemia
Digoxin–amiodarone	Amiodarone decreases the clearance of digoxin leading to toxicity; decrease the dose of digoxin by 50% and monitor levels
Digoxin–verapamil	Both drugs increase serum concentrations leading to bradycardia and heart block
Theophylline–quinolone antibiotics	Some quinolones can affect the metabolism of theophylline and lead to its toxicity

These adverse drug events are not limited to causing admissions. In hospitalized patients, in the United Kingdom it is estimated that 2,216,000 patients experience an adverse drug reaction while being treated and 106,000 of these are fatal [29]. For most hospitals, this translates to about 2 deaths for every 100 admissions. In addition to the increased risk of death associated with an ADR, the increase in cost is significant. These events increase the hospital length of stay and the cost by 20%, and if generalized to the whole US population cost approximately $2 billion [29].

Adverse drug events occur in the nursing home population as well. Rates for ADRs in nursing homes are 1.19 to 7.26 per 100 resident-months [32]. Most are for a direct response to a drug, but therapeutic failures and adverse drug withdrawal events also occur [33]. Data from the largest study on ADRs in nursing homes suggest that more than half of the events are preventable and that 70% are associated with monitoring errors [34]. For every dollar spent on drugs in nursing homes, it is estimated that $1.33 in health care resources are consumed in the treatment of drug-related problems [35].

The most common drugs causing problems in nursing home residents identified by practitioners are listed in Table 5.4 [36]. Warfarin is a drug that is identified as a problem not only in the hospital but in nursing homes as well. Prescribers, however, frequently do not make modifications in the warfarin dose even when drugs with well-established interactions with warfarin are prescribed [36,37]. Other drugs causing problems in the nursing home include psychoactive medications such as antipsychotics, antidepressants, and sedative/hypnotics. Percentages of nursing home patients using these drugs were 17, 36, and 24%, respectively. Neuropsychiatric episodes such as oversedation, confusion, hallucinations, and delirium were the most common types of adverse drug events in this population. Falls and bleeding were half as common and ranked as second and third.

Risk factors for adverse drug reactions

Problems of drug use in the elderly include wrong or unnecessary drugs prescribed, use of medication without appropriate monitoring, dosage too high or too low, adverse drug reactions, non-adherence, and polypharmacy. Most of the time, however, ADRs are an accentuation of the drugs' known pharmacologic effects. Drugs with low therapeutic ratios (ratio between average therapeutic and toxic dose) such as cardiovascular drugs and analgesics are commonly implicated, as stated earlier. Also drugs that are frequently used in the elderly are likely to be associated with ADRs. The actual effect of age alone and its relationship to ADRs has been questioned [38].

The direct relationship between the number of medications taken and ADRs is substantiated [38]. The concept of polypharmacy is challenging. It is known that several conditions can exist in the elder patient, and these conditions may best be treated with multiple drugs resulting in "obligatory or rational pharmacy" [39]. Toxicity of drug combinations may be synergistic and be greater than the sum of the toxicity of either agent alone. This is reflected by the work on ADRs related to hospital admission [28,35,36], which showed the odds ratio for those taking three to nine medications compared with those taking fewer than three medications was 1.8. The odds ratio for those taking ten or more medications compared with those taking three medications or less was 13.4 [40].

Noncompliance is another issue leading to ADRs. Patients may underuse, overuse, or misuse medications. Elderly people who live alone, use two or more medications, have no assistance in taking their medications, and who use more than two pharmacies and physicians are more likely to have noncompliance. Medication regimens with a greater number of pills taken per day, greater number of kinds of medications, as well as a greater number of needed medications are cited as problematic. Noncompliance is felt to be almost equally split, with half being intentional and the other half unintentional. Forgetfulness, unpleasant side effects of medications perceived as unnecessary, confusion, cost, and disliking taking medications are all cited by patients as causes for noncompliance.

Costs of medications are also related to ADRs. This may reflect the use of newer, more costly medications that may have more side effects, more drug interactions, and prescriptions by practitioners with less awareness of potential reactions in this population.

Other risk factors for adverse drug reactions in older outpatients are listed in Table 5.5. Similar characteristics are found in the nursing home population. These include age 85 years and older, more than six active chronic medical diagnoses,

Table 5.5. Risk factors for adverse drug reactions in older outpatients

Polypharmacy (>5 medications)

Multiple (>2) chronic medical problems

Prior adverse drug reaction

Dementia

Renal insufficiency (creatinine clearance <50ml/min)

Advanced age (>85 years)

Multiple prescribers

Table 5.6. Causes of unintentional exposure in the elderly

Taking extra dose of medication

Mistaking external preparations to be given orally

Taking nonmedicines in error

Mistaking eye for ear drops (or vice versa)

Mistaking another person's or the pet's prescription for one's own

Taking non-food substances placed in food containers

low body weight or body mass index, nine or more medications, more than 12 doses of medication per day, and a previous adverse drug reaction [41].

Poisoning in the elderly

Data from poison control centers reveal that therapeutic errors are more common in the elderly (25% compared with 14.5% in younger patients) [42]. Elderly patients also contact poison centers more with acute on chronic conditions, especially women. This suggests this population may not recognize the adverse drug reaction. Further, prescribed drugs may be added or self-medication may occur complicating both the recognition and treatment of the adverse drug event [42]. Misuse of drugs also increases slightly with age but then decreases in the oldest patients. Accidental exposures can be attributed to confusion, dementia, impaired vision, forgetfulness, or lack of knowledge or understanding of products' intended uses. Examples of unintentional exposure are listed in Table 5.6.

Inappropriate medications in the elderly

Consensus criteria have been used to identify safe medication use in older patients [43,44]. Explicit criteria provide useful tools for assessing the quality of prescribing and potential risks from prescribing. The initial criteria developed by Beers were targeted to the frail nursing home patient. The most recent Beers Criteria update was supported by the American Geriatrics Society (AGS) and the work of an interdisciplinary panel of 11 experts in geriatric care and pharmacotherapy, who applied a modified Delphi method to the systematic review and grading to reach consensus [43]. Fifty-three medications or medication classes encompass the final updated Beers Criteria, which are divided into three categories: potentially inappropriate medications and classes to avoid in older adults; potentially inappropriate medications and classes to avoid in older adults with certain diseases and syndromes that the drugs listed can exacerbate; and medications to be used with caution in older

adults. This update has much strength, including the use of an evidence-based approach using the Institute of Medicine Standards. Several stakeholders, including CMS, NCQA, and the Pharmacy Quality Alliance (PQA), have identified the Beers Criteria as an important quality measure. The criteria by Beers were adopted by the Health Care Financing Administration as a guideline for surveyors of long-term care institutions.

Medications with high severity rating for adverse reactions are listed in Table 5.7. Some discussion of the drugs and the reasoning behind the "inappropriate" label are discussed here. Many common themes are revealed in a review of inappropriate drug lists. Anticholinergic drugs and drugs with anticholinergic effects are considered inappropriate. These drugs cause mild side effects (dry mouth, thirst, mydriasis) but can also cause toxicity with urinary retention, agitation, hallucinations, seizures, cardiac arrhythmias, and heart block. Thermoregulation is impaired, causing patients to be more at risk for heatstroke during hot weather. Delirium and cognitive impairment can also occur.

Traditional antihistamines are not used in the older population due to their central nervous system effects and anticholinergic properties. They are present in many over-the-counter medications for insomnia, respiratory symptoms, and allergic conditions. The sedative effects decrease motor reflexes and place older patients at risk for motor vehicle accidents, falls, and hip fractures. Second-generation antihistamines are a better choice if antihistamines are felt to be of benefit to the patient.

Antiparkinsonian drugs, antispasmodics, and phenothiazines are other drugs which have anticholinergic effects. Cyclobenzaprine (Flexeril/Amrix) is a centrally acting muscle relaxant with marginal value and should be avoided in older adults. It is found to be the most common drug with diphenhydramine (Benadryl) used in older veterans discharged from emergency departments [45].

Tricyclic antidepressants (TCAs) are considered inappropriate not only due to their anticholinergic effects, but also to their increased volume of distribution and slowed metabolism in older adults. Cardiac toxicity occurs more frequently in patients with cardiac disease. This may result in heart block and fatal ventricular arrhythmias. Orthostatic hypotension is common. Central nervous system effects such as confusion and seizures are more common in the older patient.

Antipsychotic medications are occasionally prescribed in older patients with behavioral problems associated with dementia. Antipsychotics produce extrapyramidal and anticholinergic effects as well as tardive dyskinesia, which can occur after short-term and low dose use. Newer-generation antipsychotics (resperidone (Resperdal), olanzapine (Zyprexa), and quetiapine (Seroquel)) are available with efficacy similar to that of traditional antipsychotics but with a greater safety record.

Barbiturates, except when used as anticonvulsants, are considered inappropriate in older adults. This is due to their high lipid solubility and prolonged duration of action, which can lead to accumulation and toxicity. Tolerance to their sedating effects and disruption of REM sleep occurs, leading to unnatural sleep. Benzodiazepines are used in anxiety mood

Table 5.7. Inappropriate medications in the elderly [44]

Medication (with example)	Reason for status
Amphetamines/anorexic agents	Potential for dependence, hypertension, angina, myocardial infarction
Analgesics	
Pentazocine	CNS adverse effects, also mixed agonist–antagonist
Indomethacin	Has most adverse effects of all NSAIDs
Keterolac	Potential for GI bleeding
NSAIDs	Potential for GI bleeding, renal failure, high blood pressure, heart failure
Anti-anxiety agents/sedatives/ hypnotics	
Long-acting benzodiazepines	Highly addictive, cause more side effects than sedative/hypnotics; better alternatives available
Short-acting benzodiazepines	Smaller doses are safer
Nonbenzodiazepine hypnotics	Adverse events similar to benzodiazepines
Barbiturates	Highly addictive; better alternatives available
Meprobamate	Highly sedating anxiolytic; need to withdraw slowly
Chloral hydrate	Risks outweigh benefits
Antiarrhythmic agents	**Avoid antiarrhythmic drugs as a first-line treatment for atrial fibrillation**
Disopyramide	Negative inotropes, can cause heart failure; strong anticholinergic
Amiodarone	Lack of efficacy in older patients; prolongs QT interval/torsades
Droneadarone	Worse outcomes reported in patients with atrial fibrillation and heart failure
Digoxin >0.125 mg/day	Higher doses have no additional benefit and increased risk of toxicity
Spironolactone >25 mg/day	Hyperkalemia, especially with other drugs (NSAIDs, ACE, angiotensin receptor blockers, or potassium)
Nifedipine (short-acting)	Potential for orthostatic hypertension and CNS adverse effects
Anticoagulants	
Dipyridamole	May cause orthostatic hypotension
Ticlopidine	No better than aspirin, may be more toxic
Antidepressants/tertiary TCAs	
Amitriptyline, chlordiazepoxide, imipramine, clomipamine, doxepin >6 mg/day	Anticholinergic effects (arrhythmia, dry mouth and eyes, urinary retention)
Antimicrobials	
Nitrofurantoin	Potential for renal impairment
Antiparkinsonian	
Benztropine	More effective agents
Antispasmodics/muscle relaxants	
Dicyclomine, hyoscyamine, belladonna alkaloids, cyclobenzaprine, orphenadrine	Antiocholinergic effects, questionable effectiveness
Blood glucose regulators	
Sulfonylureas (chlorpropamide, glyburide)	Prolonged half-life leads to prolonged hypoglycemia
Insulin, sliding scale	Higher risk of hypoglycemia without better control of blood sugar
Cardiovascular drugs	
Alpha-1 blockers (prazosin, doxazosin)	High risk of orthostatic hypertension; not recommended as routine treatment for hypertension
Alpha-blockers, central (clonidine, methyldopa)	High risk of CNS effects, may cause bradycardia; not recommended as routine first-line antihypertensive treatment
First- and second-generation antipsychotics	
Thioridazine, resperidine, mesoridazine, ziprasidone	CNS adverse effects, extrapyramidal effects. Better alternatives available
First-generation antihistamines	
Diphenhydramine, hydroxine	Confusion and sedation
Gastrointestinal	
Mineral oil	Potential for aspiration

Table 5.7. *(cont.)*

Medication (with example)	Reason for status
Trimethobenzamide	Extrapyramidal side effects
Endocrine	
Estrogens with or without progesterone	Evidence of cardiogenic potential
Growth hormone	Avoidance recommended except as hormone replacement after pituitary gland removal
Methyltestosterone	Potential for prostatic hypertrophy and cardiac problems
Thyroid (dessicated)	Cardiac effects

Not all drugs are listed. See www.americangeriatrics.org/health_care_professionals/clinical_practice/clinical_guidelines_recommendations/2012 for full 2012 guideline.

disorders. They are categorized according to half-life and the presence or absence of active metabolites. The older benzodiazepines (diazepam (Valium), chlordiazepoxide (Librium), and flurazepam (Dalmane)) have an increased volume of distribution in the elderly. This is due to their lipid solubility and increase in adipose stores that increase with age. Also, since benzodiazepines are degraded by the liver and hepatic function changes with age, their half-life can increase up to four- to five-fold in an older patient compared with a younger patient [17]. Low-lipid soluble benzodiazepines (lorazepam (Ativan) and oxazepam (Serax)) have less risk for accumulation and toxicity. Use of benzodiazepines should be avoided in older patients. If needed, they should be prescribed in low doses, be short acting, and only used for short-term therapy.

NSAIDs are commonly used in the elderly for symptom management. NSAIDs are highly lipid-soluble drugs with extensive protein binding. In the elderly, there is widespread distribution of NSAIDs due to increased adipose stores. Unbound drug is also increased due to the reduction in plasma protein found in many older persons. NSAIDs are renally cleared and since there may be decreased renal function in older patients, there is potential for excessive drug levels and toxicity.

Complications from NSAIDs are reported, with gastropathy being the most common [46]. These effects occur not only in the stomach, duodenum, and esophagus but also in the small intestine and colon. Bleeding occurs and is increased in patients taking anticoagulants and prednisone. NSAIDs may also inhibit the action of antihypertensive agents whose activity is via renal prostaglandins such as β-blockers and angiotensin-converting agents. NSAIDs can also produce renal insufficiency, hyperkalemia, and fluid retention.

There is not adequate evidence to label NSAIDs as a class as inappropriate for use in the elderly population. Beers specifically delineated indomethacin, due to its CNS toxicity and phenylbutazone, because of its risk of bone marrow suppression as inappropriate. However, because NSAIDs benefit so many people it is felt that cautious use with low doses and short-term therapy is appropriate.

Avoiding certain analgesics is recommended by the Beers guidelines. Pentazocine is a mixed opiate agonist/antagonist with adequate efficacy but with increased risk of seizures and CNS effects compared with other analgesics.

Dipyridamole had been classified as inappropriate. However, this was before there was evidence that it benefits some patients by preventing strokes. Its designation as being inappropriate for the elderly was due to hypotension seen early in therapy. However, the risk should not preclude its use if it is felt there is potential benefit.

Preventability

Despite the guidelines, inappropriate medications are still being prescribed with little or no evidence of improvement over time [47]. Improving drug benefits and limiting harm should be the goal of prescribers. The use of a large number of pharmaceuticals will always be an important component of the medical care of the older patient. Resolving the tension of avoiding excessive use of medications and providing access to therapies that are beneficial will only continue to be more difficult.

It is important to note that drug interactions accounted for one in six of ADRs [48]. Therefore, regular review of prescriptions, the use of computerized prescribing, and pharmacists' review of prescribing behavior may limit adverse drug reactions [47,49,50]. Factors which may have prevented hospital admission in patients with adverse drug reactions included documentation of serum blood levels or laboratory tests in over two-thirds of cases [48]. Other preventable factors included inappropriate dose for an individual, noncompliance, and drug interactions. The majority of events, however, involved more than one preventability factor.

Efforts must be made to expand the knowledge of benefits and risks in the elderly by including them in clinical trials. This is especially true for elderly patients with comorbid conditions. Without adequate research information on this population, clinicians are unable to decide whether drugs are beneficial for them and may withhold medication for fear of doing harm. The federal government has begun some programs to monitor drugs. The Food and Drug Administration's program MedWatch collects voluntary reports on suspected adverse drugs effects in the general population, but it is not adequate to develop a large database for the elderly.

The use of interdisciplinary teams to care for complex elderly patients may improve the quality of care for these patients and avoid inappropriate prescribing [50]. This has been beneficial for management of diseases such as congestive heart failure [51]. However this approach needs to be comprehensive and not only consider medical and pharmacologic issues, but also social and financial components to be successful.

The other factor that is crucial to avoid inappropriate medications is a linked information system that allows physicians to easily review and prescribe medications. Computerized decision support systems would allow physicians and pharmacists to be alerted to use of inappropriate medications and allow easy access to alternative suggestions. Electronic medical record interventions, including pharmacy and laboratory data, sending alerts to physicians that new medications have been started, and laboratory monitoring should be done, helping to minimize ADR incidence. Links which would accommodate individual status of the patient, accounting for their age-related physiologic changes and concomitant diseases, will improve care.

Useful general concepts for prescribing are based in the ethical principles of beneficence, nonmaleficence, and autonomy. Practitioners need to ask, "How will this medication benefit this particular patient?" If evidence does not exist at all or is not based in the elder population, practitioners may trial the medication and make a clinical decision if there is overall good that has been achieved. Another question that may be asked is, "How will this harm this particular patient?" The high rate of adverse drug reactions should be balanced against the efficacy or uncertain efficacy in older people before a decision to prescribe is finalized. Finally, prescribers need to include the concept of what the patient wants in the decision to prescribe [2]. Older patients may be concerned about their independence and side effects of medication rather than whether their disease or risk factors are managed according to a published guideline. Lastly, close oversight and continuous re-evaluation for benefits and risks need to become the norm of practice.

Conclusion

The challenge for the practitioner is to balance incomplete evidence about the efficacy of medications in frail older people against the problems related to adverse drug reactions without denying people potentially valuable pharmacotherapeutic interventions. Prescribers need to be diligent in reviewing medications periodically as well as when new medications are being considered. Review of updated explicit criteria is essential to understand and prescribe appropriately in this special population.

Pearls and pitfalls

Pearls

- Heightened awareness of the issue of polypharmacy and adverse drug effects is essential in older patients, with special attention to warfarin, hypoglycemic agents, antiplatelet agents, and insulin.
- Use the Beers list to avoid potentially harmful drugs.
- Start with lower doses and go slow.
- Consider non-pharmacologic measures.

Pitfalls

- Not doing a risk–benefit analysis especially when using anticoagulants in patients at risk for falls.

- Using complicated scheduling regimens.
- Not limiting the use of PRN medications.

References

1. Wilber S, Blanda M. Inappropriate medication use in older emergency department patients: results of a national probability sample. *Acad Emerg Med.* 2003;10:493.

2. Spinewine A, Schmader K, Barber N, et al. Appropriate prescribing in elderly people: how well can it be measured and optimised? *Lancet.* 2007;370:173–84.

3. Rochon PA, Gurwitz JH. Drug therapy. *Lancet.* 1995;346(8966):32–6.

4. Rochon PA, Gurwitz JH. Optimising drug treatment for elderly people: the prescribing cascade. *BMJ.* 1997;315(7115):1096–9.

5. *A Profile of Older Americans* (Washington, DC: US Department of Health and Human Services Administration on Aging, 2008, accessed from www.aoa.gov/AoAroot/Aging_Statistics/Profile/2008/docs/2008profile.pdf).

6. Chutka DS, Takahashi PY, Hoel RW. Inappropriate medication use in the elderly. *Essent Psychopharmacol.* 2005;6(6):331–40.

7. Delafuente J. Arthritis. In *Therapeutics in the Elderly*, ed. Delafuente J, Stewart R (Cincinnati, OH: Harvey Whitney Books Co., 2001), pp. 499–513.

8. Lindley RI. Drug trials for older people. *J Gerontol A Biol Sci Med Sci.* 2012;67(2):152–7.

9. Crome P. What's different about older people. *Toxicology.* 2003;192(1):49–54.

10. Grandison MK, Boudinot FD. Age-related changes in protein binding of drugs: implications for therapy. *Clin Pharmacokinet.* 2000;38(3):271–90.

11. *Patterns of Medication Use In The United States: 2006* (A report from the Slone Survey, 2006, accessed from www.bu.edu/slone/SloneSurvey/AnnualRpt/SloneSurveyWebReport2006.pdf).

12. Yang C, Tomlinson G. Medication lists for elderly patients. *J Gen Intern Med.* 2001;16(2):112–15.

13. Rieger K, Scholer A, Arnet I, et al. High prevalence of unknown co-medication in hospitalised patients. *Eur J Clin Pharmacol.* 2004;60(5):363–8.

14. Chung MK, Bartfield JM. Knowledge of prescription medications among elderly emergency department patients. *Ann Emerg Med.* 2002;39(6):605–8.

15. World Health Organization (WHO). *International Monitoring: The Role of the Hospital* (Geneva, Switzerland: World Health Organization, 2008).

16. Zeeh J, Platt D. The aging liver: structural and functional changes and their consequences for drug treatment in old age. *Gerontology.* 2002;48(3):121–7.

17. Swedko PJ, Clark HD, Paramsothy K, Akbari A. Serum creatinine is an inadequate screening test for renal failure in elderly patients. *Arch Intern Med.* 2003;163(3):356–60.

18. Vuyk J. Pharmacodynamics in the elderly. *Best Pract Res Clin Anaesthesiol.* 2003;17(2):207–18.

19. Liukas A, Hagelberg NM, Kuusniemi K, Neuvonen PJ, Olkkola KT. Inhibition of cytochrome P450 3A by clarithromycin uniformly affects the pharmacokinetics and pharmacodynamics of oxycodone in young and elderly volunteers. *J Clin Psychopharmacol.* 2011;31(3):302–8.

20. Gardin JM, Arnold AM, Bild DE, et al. Left ventricular diastolic filling in the elderly: the cardiovascular health study. *Am J Cardiol*. 1998;82(3):345–31.

21. Toescu EC, Verkhratsky A. Parameters of calcium homeostasis in normal neuronal aging. *J Anat*. 2000;197(Pt 4):563–9.

22. Joseph JA, Denisova NA, Bielinski D, Fisher DR, Shukitt-Hale B. Oxidative stress protection and vulnerability in aging: putative nutritional implications for intervention. *Mech Aging Dev*. 2000;116(2–3):141–53.

23. Budnitz DS, Lovegrove MC, Shehab N, Richards CL. Emergency hospitalizations for adverse drug events in older Americans. *N Engl J Med*. 2011;365(21):2002–12.

24. Ventura MT, Laddaga R, Cavallera P, et al. Adverse drug reactions as the cause of emergency department admission: focus on the elderly. *Immunopharmacol Immunotoxicol*. 2010;32(3):426–9.

25. Lai S-W, Lin C-H, Liao K-F, et al. Association between polypharmacy and dementia in older people: A population-based case-control study in Taiwan. *Geriatr & Gerontol Int*. 2012;12(3):491–8.

26. Nguyen JK, Fouts MM, Kotabe SE, Lo E. Polypharmacy as a risk factor for adverse drug reactions in geriatric nursing home residents. *Am J Geriatr Pharmacother*. 2006;4:36–41.

27. Monastero R, Palmer K, Qiu C, Winblad B, Fratiglioni L. Heterogeneity in risk factors for cognitive impairment, no dementia: population-based longitudinal study from the Kungsholmen Project. *Am J Geriatr Psychiat*. 2007;15(1):60–9.

28. Budnitz DS, Pollock DA, Weidenbach KN, et al. National surveillance of emergency department visits for outpatient adverse drug events. *JAMA*. 2006;296(15):1858–66.

29. Mirmohamed M, James S, Meakin S, et al. Adverse drug reactions as cause of admission to hospital: prospective analysis of 18820 patients. *BMJ*. 2004;329(7456):15–19.

30. Wiffen P, Gill M, Edwards J, Moore A. Adverse drug reactions in hospital patients. *Bandolier Extra*. 2002;1–15.

31. Bond CA, Raehl C. Adverse drug reactions in United States hospitals. *Pharmacotherapy*. 2006;26(5):601–8.

32. Handler SM, Wright RM, Ruby CM. Epidemiology of medication-related adverse events in nursing homes. *Am J Geriatr Pharmacother*. 2006;4:264–72.

33. Hanlon JT, Schmader KE, Ruby CM et al. Suboptimal prescribing in older inpatients and outpatients. *J Am Geriatr Soc*. 2001;49:200–9.

34. Gurwitz JH, Field TS, Avorn J et al. Incidence and preventability of adverse drug events in nursing homes. *Am J Med*. 2000;109:87–94.

35. Bootman JL, Harrison DL, Cox E. The health care cost of drug-related morbidity and mortality in nursing facilities. *Arch Intern Med*. 1997;157(18):2089–96.

36. Gurwitz JH, Field TS, Avorn J, et al. Incidence and preventability of adverse drug events in nursing homes. *Am J Med*. 2000;109(2):87–94.

37. Davidsen F, Haghfelt T, Gram LF, et al. Adverse drug reactions and drug noncompliance as primary causes of admission to a cardiology department. *Eur J Clin Pharmacol*. 1988;34:83–6.

38. Gurwitz JH, Avorn J. The ambiguous relation between aging and adverse drug reactions. *Ann Intern Med*. 1991;114(11):956–66.

39. Hajjar ER, Hanlon JT, Artz MB, et al. Adverse drug reaction risk factors in older outpatients. *Am J Geriatr Pharmacother*. 2003;1(2):82–9.

40. Routledge PA, O'Mahony MS, Woodhouse KW. Adverse drug reactions in elderly patients. *Br J Clin Pharmacol*. 2004;57(2):121–6.

41. Williams CM. Using medications appropriately in older adults. *Am Fam Physician*. 2002;66(10):1917–24.

42. Skarupski K, Mrvos R, Krenzelok E. A profile of calls to a poison information center regarding older adults. *J Aging Health*. 2004;16(2):228–47.

43. American Geriatrics Society 2012 Beers Criteria Update Expert Panel. American Geriatrics Society updated Beers Criteria for potentially inappropriate medication use in older adults. *J Am Geriatr Soc*. 2012;60(4):616–31.

44. *When Medicine Hurts Instead of Helps: Preventing Medication Problems in Older Patients* (Washington, DC: Alliance for Aging Research, 1998, accessed from www.agingresearch.org/content/article/detail/706/).

45. Hastings SN, Sloane RJ, Goldberg KC, Oddone EZ, Schmader KE. The quality of pharmacotherapy in older veterans discharged from the emergency department or urgent care clinic. *J Am Geriatr Soc*. 2007;55(9):1339–48.

46. Lanza FL, Umbenhauer ER, Melsom RS, et al. A double blind randomized placebo controlled gastroscopic study to compare the effects of indomethacin capsules and indomethacin suppositories on the gastric mucosa of human volunteers. *J Rheumatol*. 1982;9:415–19.

47. Goulding MR. Inappropriate medication prescribing for elderly ambulatory care patients. *Arch Intern Med*. 2004;164:305–12.

48. Le Couteur DG, Hilmer SN, Glasgow N, et al. Prescribing in older people. *Aust Fam Physician*. 2004;33(10):777–81.

49. Anderson WK, Wahler R. Pharmacy management can reduce Medicare – and human costs. *Aging Today*. 2001;January/February.

50. Schmader KE, Hanlon JT, Pieper CF, et al. Effects of geriatric evaluation and management on adverse drug reactions and suboptimal prescribing in the frail elderly. *Am J Med*. 2004;116:394–401.

51. Hanlon JT, Lindblad CI, Gray SL. Can clinical pharmacy services have a positive impact on drug-related problems and health outcomes in community-based older adults? *Am J Geriatr Pharmacother*. 2004;2(1):3–13.

Chapter

6

Generalized weakness in the elderly

(Mary) Colleen Bhalla

Introduction

Generalized weakness and fatigue are common nonspecific complaints of older emergency department patients. Generalized weakness and fatigue can be presenting complaints of a serious medical issue, contribute to a chief complaint such as a fall, or be the complaint that causes readmission after discharge. A review of the National Hospital Ambulatory Medical Care Survey (NHAMCS) representing 181,786 visit observations found that generalized weakness and fatigue was the 5th most common chief complaint after trauma, dyspnea, chest pain, and abdominal pain [1]. Generalized weakness or fatigue as a chief complaint often prompts an extensive work-up and often leads to admission [1]. Generalized weakness is also associated with several geriatric syndromes including frailty, sarcopenia, functional decline, failure to thrive, frequent falls, incontinence, and inability to ambulate. Many of these syndromes have shared risk factors, associated findings and overlapping diagnostic features (Table 6.1). We will discuss generalized weakness and fatigue both as a presenting complaint and as associated with other geriatric syndromes.

Generalized weakness and fatigue

As a chief complaint, generalized weakness and fatigue have not been extensively researched. The Basel Nonspecific Complaints (BANC) study found that 20% of older emergency department (ED) patients have no specific complaint and that 50% were found to have an acute medical problem [2]. This study looked at adult patients with an emergency severity score of 2 or 3 and excluded those with a specific complaint, a clinical presentation suggestive of a working diagnosis, a known terminal medical condition, or who were hemodynamically unstable or had vitals outside normal range (systolic blood pressure <90 mmHg, heart rate >120 beats/min, temperature >38.4°C (101.1°F) or less than 35.6°C (96.1°F)) [2]. The majority of patients with nonspecific complaints were older adults with a median age of 82 years [2]. The most frequent chief complaints were generalized weakness, feeling exhausted, and recent falls [2]. They found that gait disturbance, lack of appetite, history of falls within three months, and a history of chronic hypertension were significant predictors of a serious medical condition

[2]. The study also found that 77% of the patients had a final diagnosis made in the ED, but did not elaborate on specific diagnoses [2]. The mortality rate for those patients was 9% and the admission rate was 82% [2]. Another study with the same inclusion and exclusion criteria found a mortality rate of 6.4% and an admission rate of 87.7% [3]. Overall, patients with nonspecific chief complaints tended to be older (85.6% were ≥65 years) and 43.4% were dependent on at least one activity of daily living (ADL) [3].

A review of NHAMCS found 6.4% of all ED patients over 65 years and 7.7% of those over 85 years had a chief complaint of weakness and fatigue [1]. Those with weakness and fatigue had longer ED lengths of stay and higher admission rates than those without weakness or fatigue. In this study, fever and hypotension were more common in those with weakness and fatigue [1]. The most common final diagnosis was "other malaise and fatigue" followed by pneumonia, urinary tract infection, congestive heart failure, volume depletion, fever, anemia, dehydration, and hemorrhage of the gastrointestinal tract [1]. A descriptive study of patients over the age of 65 years with a nonspecific chief complaint of "home care impossible" found that this represented 9.3% of visits and an acute medical condition was found in 51% [4]. The most common medical conditions found were infection (24%) and cardiovascular disorders (14%) [4].

Although patients with generalized weakness and fatigue do not always receive a specific diagnosis, they are often still admitted to the hospital [1]. One study found that the chief complaint of generalized weakness had an odds ratio predictive of admission of 2.0 and an "admit and return within 30 days" odds ratio of 1.57 [5]. It is still important to identify those without a specific diagnosis because of their need for additional resources both in the hospital and after discharge. One study comparing rehabilitation efficiency of patients with debility impairment such as hip fracture to patients with nondebility generalized weakness (ICD-9 728.2 muscle wasting and disuse atrophy; 728.87 muscle weakness; 780.79 other malaise and fatigue/asthenia) looked at patients admitted for acute inpatient rehabilitation [6]. They assessed patients using the functional independence measure and found that the rehabilitation efficiency of nondebility generalized weakness was significantly

---

Geriatric Emergency Medicine, ed. Joseph H. Kahn, Brendan G. Magauran Jr., and Jonathan S. Olshaker. Published by Cambridge University Press.
© Cambridge University Press 2014.

Table 6.1. Features of geriatric syndromes associated with generalized weakness

	Failure to thrive	Sarcopenia	Frailty	Functional decline	Delirium
↓Muscle mass/↑Fat mass		D	A		A
Weight loss >5% of baseline	D	A	D		A
Decreased appetite	D				
Poor nutrition	D		A		A
Low cholesterol levels	D				
Low physical activity level		A	D		
Increased infection	A	A			
Decubitus ulcer	A			A	
Incontinence				A	
Recurrent falls		A	A	A	
Difficulty with ADL*	A	A	A	D	A
Slow gait speed		A	D		
Weak grip strength		A	D		
Poor endurance			D		
Acute change in attention/cognition					D

*ADL (activities of daily living)
A = associated feature, D = diagnostic feature.

greater than that of the debility group and that the rates of discharge home, transfer to acute care hospital, and mortality were the same [6].

The clinical presentation of generalized weakness may lead you to a diagnosis or help you to focus your work-up. Often, however, the presentation and the exam are nonspecific. When gathering a history, the focus should be on both the symptoms of specific diseases and the change from baseline that prompted the evaluation. One must also try to get the patient to further characterize their weakness: Is it really general debility, light-headedness, fatigue, muscle aches, focal weakness, sleepiness, confusion, depression, loss of appetite, pain, difficulty with ADL, loneliness, hunger, abuse, neglect, or fear? The exam must include all organ systems, as dysfunction of any could lead to generalized weakness or fatigue. The general appearance may suggest ability to care for oneself and nutritional status. General behavior, alertness, and orientation may show signs of delirium, dementia, intoxication, medication reaction, and mental illness. Neurologic exam may reveal signs of stroke, electrolyte disturbance, medication toxicity, or central nervous system infection. A thorough evaluation of the skin may show infection, trauma, abuse, compression ulcers, jaundice, anemia, or coagulopathy. Cardiovascular, pulmonary, urinary, and gastrointestinal examinations are also needed to rule out serious medical conditions and to help guide evaluation. Most patients, depending on their goals of care, require laboratory work and often radiologic tests. If the history and physical does not point to a specific diagnosis, at minimum a urinalysis, blood count, chemistry panel, and chest X-ray should be done. The need for additional tests such as electrocardiogram (ECG), cardiac enzymes, computed tomography (CT) scan of the head, liver function tests, lumbar puncture, and specific

medication levels such as digoxin depends on the history and presentation. Consider the need for additional specialty input such as psychiatry, social work, pharmacy, physical therapy, or financial aid. The need for admission depends on the seriousness of the medical condition, diagnosis, ability to be cared for at home, financial situation, availability of follow-up, and the overall goals of care.

When evaluating a patient in the ED with a chief complaint of generalized weakness or fatigue it is important to keep a broad differential diagnosis. One must also identify those patients requiring an extensive work-up in the ED and recognize the patients that need to be admitted for further evaluation and resources even when the work-up does not result in a diagnosis.

Failure to thrive

Failure to thrive, generalized weakness, functional decline, and frailty are terms often used interchangeably, but adult failure to thrive has its own ICD-9 code (783.7) separate from associated conditions of generalized weakness (780.79); muscle weakness (728.87); other malaise and fatigue (780.79); cachexia (799.4); debility, nonspecific (799.3); senility without mention of psychosis (797); and urinary incontinence (788.3) [7]. There are no ICD-9 codes for frailty or functional decline. Adult failure to thrive is defined as weight loss greater than 5% of baseline, decreased appetite, poor nutrition, and low cholesterol levels [8]. It is often associated with increased infection rates, diminished cell-mediated immunity, hip fractures, decubitus ulcers, and increased surgical mortality rates [8]. Depending on the study, failure to thrive is found in 35% of community-dwelling older adults, 25 to 40% of nursing home residents, and 50 to 60%

of hospitalized veterans [8]. The in-hospital mortality reaches almost 16% [8]. In patients with failure to thrive, impaired function, malnutrition, depression, and cognitive impairment are all predictive of adverse events [8]. Many of these features are also associated with frailty and functional decline. Patients suspected of failure to thrive should have an assessment of their ADL and instrumental activities of daily living (IADL) needs, along with their work-up for specific medical conditions to assess for functional decline and need for additional resources. Because failure to thrive often occurs at the end of a person's life, the diagnosis should prompt an end-of-life discussion to prevent needless or unwanted interventions [8]. The complaints that are associated with adult failure to thrive often prompt an ED referral for "home care impossible" [4]. This is often the chief complaint when a patient can no longer be cared for at home either by himself or herself or by family. A study of those with a chief complaint of "home care impossible" found that 67% had falls, 48% had incontinence, and 61% had cognitive decline [4].

When evaluating a patient with generalized weakness, it is important to recognize that failure to thrive may be a contributing factor requiring additional resources such as physical or nutritional therapy, help with housework or meals, or visiting nursing for the patient to return home. Alternatively, the failure to thrive may have progressed to the point where the patient may need to receive rehabilitation or long-term placement in a skilled nursing facility. These should be coordinated prior to discharge to prevent further decline. Elder abuse and neglect must also be considered as potential causes of failure to thrive, and their presence must prompt further investigation and consideration for disposition. It is important for the emergency physician to know the local laws regarding reporting suspected elder abuse and neglect.

Sarcopenia

Sarcopenia is an age-associated loss of skeletal muscle mass and function caused by disuse, altered endocrine function, chronic diseases, inflammation, insulin resistance, and/or nutritional deficiencies [9]. There is an expected loss of muscle mass associated with age as seen even in master athletes. Performance in marathon runners and weight lifters declines after the age of 40 and there is a 50% decrease in performance by age 80 [10]. From age 20–80, there is a 30% reduction in muscle mass and a decline in cross-sectional area of 20% [9]. Sarcopenia is associated with a loss of muscle mass alone or in conjunction with an increased fat mass, and is diagnosed in men with an appendicular fat lean mass/height^2 of ≤7.23 kg/m^2 and in women of ≤5.67 kg/m^2 measured by dual X-ray absorptiometry (DXA) [9]. The initial presentation of sarcopenia is often associated with a decline in function, strength, and health status; self-reported mobility-related difficulty; history of recurrent falls; recent unintentional weight loss of greater than 5%; post-hospitalization; and chronic medical conditions [9]. The prevalence is approximately 12% for patients 60–70 years of age and 30% for those over 80 years. Sarcopenia should be suspected in any patient who is bedridden, cannot independently rise from a chair, has difficulties in performing ADL, has a history of

falls, documented recent weight loss, has a history of a chronic condition associated with muscle loss such as chronic kidney disease, or has a gait speed of less than 1 m/s [9]. Sarcopenia is predictive of falls and nosocomial infection and thus should be studied and identified in all older patients.

The causes of sarcopenia are multifactorial and involve multiple signaling pathways [9,11]. Age-related muscle wasting is characterized by loss of skeletal muscle mass, decrease in force-producing capacity, maximum velocity of muscle shortening, and general slowing of muscle contraction and relaxation [11]. There are age-related biological processes of oxidative stress associated with motor unit remodeling involving denervation of muscle fibers, preferential loss of fast motor units, and neuromuscular junction remodeling involving fast motor units greater than slow twitch units. These processes cannot be prevented by exercise alone [11]. There is an age-related inflammatory response in skeletal muscle seen in sarcopenia associated with tumor necrosis factor alpha (TNF-α) and interleukin-6 (IL-6) [11]. TNF-α increases apoptosis and impairs inflammatory response to injury in skeletal muscle, and high levels of IL-6 initiate muscle wasting [11]. There may also be an age-related decline in muscle regeneration capacity as a consequence of a decreased number or function of quiescent skeletal muscle precursor cells [11]. These processes may be a result of a decline in hormonal systems as defined by a decrease in hormones such as testosterone, dehydroepiandrosterone (DHEA), growth hormone (GH), IGF-I (insulin like growth factor-1), catecholamines, TSH, and T3 [11].

Identification and treatment of sarcopenia is currently an area of investigation, though it is not actually recognized by the United States Center for Medicare and Medicaid Services (CMS) or the United States Federal Drug Administration (FDA) as a treatable condition [9]. Current treatment options being studied are physical activity, nutritional therapies, and androgen therapy. Studies involving master athletes and previously sedentary adults show that age-associated atrophy, weakness, and fatigability can be slowed but not halted. The most successful programs last longer than 12 weeks, occur at least three times per week, involve three types of muscle contractions (shortening, isometric, and lengthening), and increase the weight load incrementally [10].

When evaluating a patient in the ED with suspected sarcopenia, it is important to relay this suspicion to the admitting team or the follow-up physician so that the patient can be evaluated for their access to and appropriateness for a physical conditioning program. The combination of sarcopenia and predisposing factors that decrease skeletal muscle reserve, added to acute physiologic insults that cause patients to seek care in the ED may lead to muscle weakness and a cascade of detrimental outcomes (Figure 6.1). Further research aimed at initiating interventions in the ED to prevent and treat sarcopenia may help guide patient care.

Geriatric syndromes

Geriatric syndromes are terms used to capture clinical conditions in older persons that do not fit discrete disease categories. These include delirium, falls, frailty, dizziness, syncope, urinary

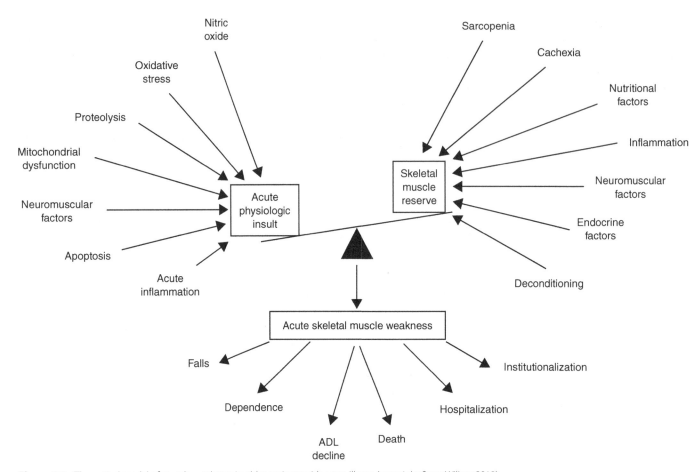

Figure 6.1. Theoretical model of muscle weakness in older patients with acute illness (copyright Scott Wilber, 2012).

incontinence, pressure ulcers, and functional decline [12]. All of these syndromes are preventable, multifactorial, and associated with morbidity and poor outcomes [12]. Studies have shown that these syndromes have several shared risk factors including baseline cognitive impairment, baseline functional impairment, impaired mobility, and older age [12]. Because of these shared risk factors it is suspected that there is a shared pathophysiologic mechanism involving multisystem dysregulation, inflammation, sarcopenia, and atherosclerosis. These are often found linked, although they often involve distant and distinct organ systems such as in the case of a urinary tract infection. Urinary tract infection may cause inflammation and multisystem dysregulation, leading to altered neural function in the form of cognitive and behavioral changes associated with delirium. A patient with underlying frailty and generalized weakness from sarcopenia may develop worsening functional decline with a urinary tract infection causing incontinence, and suddenly may no longer be able to live independently performing his or her ADL. The delirium, generalized weakness, or functional decline that ensues may cause a fall, leading the patient to further weakness and debility. The debility could then cause immobility and a pressure ulcer, worsened by incontinence.

Falls

Patients present to the emergency department with injuries from falls, functional limitations as the result of falls, fear

of falling limiting activity, and return to the ED with decline in function after discharge. As a geriatric syndrome, falls are the leading cause of unintentional injury and the 6th highest cause of death among the elderly [12]. Falls occur in 30% of adults over 65 and 40% over 80, leading to functional decline, hospitalization, institutionalization, and increased health care costs [12]. Falls are commonly associated with severe injury, and even those whose injuries allow them to return home are at high risk for functional decline [13,14]. Different studies have sought to identify fall risk factors with varying success in finding modifiable common conditions. Polypharmacy, home hazards, decreased balance, and arthritis were found to be associated in one study, while another only found nonhealing foot sores, prior fall history, self-reported depression, and the inability to cut one's own toenails to be risk factors for a fall. Obesity in older adults is a risk factor for poor lower extremity mobility, and body mass index (BMI) and waist circumference were predictors of onset or worsening mobility disability [15,16]. Physical fatigue may also represent a risk factor for falls. One study looked at patients purposely fatigued by a repeated sit-to-stand task and compared their gaits at different speeds to a cohort that was not fatigued. The gait changes that they observed following the fatiguing task agree with gait changes found in older persons at risk for falls [17].

Fear of falling is common after a fall, with a prevalence up to 85% depending on how it is measured [18]. Patients with fear of falling causing activity restriction often have a history of an injurious fall, slow-timed physical performance, two or more chronic conditions, and depressive symptoms [19]. Fear of falling leads to decline in physical and mental performance, increased risk of falling, and progressive loss of health-related quality of life [18]. One fall prevention program found an increase in the physical function of health-related quality of life, measured with short form 36 (SF-36), on completion of the program [20]. Women with fear of falling change the way they walk half a mile, have difficulty rising from a chair, have activities limited due to eyesight, often suffer from acute hospitalization, visit their primary care physician frequently, and have low habitual physical activity [21]. Given that low physical activity is associated with sarcopenia and other geriatric syndromes, screening and addressing fear of falling after discharge may be important to prevent further deterioration in function.

Many patients who present to the ED have a history of recurrent falls. Age, mobility disorder, osteoporosis, incontinence, fear of falling, and orthostatic hypotension are all associated with recurrent falls [14]. After a fall or blunt injury, many patients have functional decline or need for repeat visits to the ED [13,22]. Functional decline is associated with fractures, functional independence before the fall, and slower timed up-and-go (TUG) scores [22]. Future research may investigate interventions that address prevention of functional decline after a fall to prevent recurrent falls.

Prior to dispositioning a patient with a history of fall or an injury or condition that may make them prone to falls, it is important to consider his or her living conditions and available resources. Some patients with minor injuries may need to be admitted or referred to home nursing because they cannot care for themselves alone due to their physical limitations. It is also important to counsel the patient on fall prevention or give them a referral to a hospital, home-based balance clinic, or fall prevention program.

Frailty

Frailty is a state of heightened vulnerability to acute and chronic stressors as a consequence of reduced physiologic reserve [23–25]. Frailty is defined in the Cardiovascular Health Study Collaborative Research Group as three or more of 1) shrinking or unintentional weight loss in the previous year; 2) weakness of grip strength; 3) poor endurance and energy as self-reported exhaustion; 4) slowness defined as time to walk 15 feet (5 m); and 5) low physical activity level defined by a weighted score of kilocalories expended per week [23]. There are several other frailty identification tools such as the Clinical Frailty Scale, Frailty Index-Comprehensive Geriatric Assessment, and Canadian Study of Health and Aging Frailty Index, all of which correlate with functional decline, increased risk of institutionalization, and mortality [25]. It is important to identify frailty since it is associated with other geriatric syndromes of falls, osteoporotic fractures, incontinence, cognitive decline, malnutrition, muscle wasting, and anemia [25]. Frail patients are at increased risk of hospitalization, nursing home placement, and death [23]. One study found mortality was six times higher than in non-frail patients over three years and three

times higher over seven years [23]. Hospitalized frail patients develop further functional decline and dependence for ADL [25]. The prevalence of frailty is between 7 and 36.6% depending on population studied and definition criteria [25].

Risk factors for frailty include diagnoses such as congestive heart failure, history of myocardial infarction, diabetes, hypertension, depression, chronic obstructive pulmonary disease (COPD), silent strokes, and subclinical atherosclerotic disease found with carotid stenosis and low ankle–brachial index [25]. Also associated are excessive drinking, smoking cigarettes, low physical activity, self-perceived poor or fair physical health, BMI <18.5 or >25, and ADL limitations [25]. One might have a preconception that a frail patient is cachectic, but obese patients can be frail as well. It is the relative sarcopenia or loss of muscle mass that is more important than overall weight. Although there is an association with comorbidity and disability, these terms are not synonymous with frailty. There are patients with these risk factors who do not become frail and there are those with disabilities who are not frail. There are also frail patients with no risk factors. One study found that 72% of frail patients reported difficulty with mobility, 60% had difficulty with an IADL, but only 27% had difficulty with an ADL [23]. Frailty causes disability independent of clinical and subclinical disease [23].

There are two main theories on how people develop frailty. The first is that frailty arises from an accumulation of severe and separate diseases. The other is that frailty is a result of physiologic changes of aging that are not disease based [23,26]. With aging, the adaptive strategies of normal homeostasis become progressively limited. Inflammation and coagulation pathways seem to play a role in normal aging and development of frailty. Several studies show that C-reactive protein, leukocytosis, IL-6, and TNFα are increased in normal aging. Higher IL-6 is associated with loss of mobility and the development of disability and frailty [25]. C-reactive protein is also associated with frailty [25]. Mediators of inflammation also contribute to sarcopenia [25]. Procoagulation markers such as D-dimer, fibrinogen, and factor VIII increase with age and are found to be higher in frail versus non-frail patients [25]. Increased D-dimer was found to be associated with limitations of IADL, lower extremity function, and lower performance on cognitive testing [25]. Inflammatory and coagulation pathways feed back in a positive manner and thus form a self-perpetuating cycle.

Mobility decline is associated with both falls and frailty. Slow walking speed, easy exhaustion, and poor grip strength are all components of frailty. We know that maximal energy expenditure (VO_{2max}), the upper limit of energy available, or the capacity to perform vigorous activities declines with age [26,27]. A decline in VO_{2max} starts at age 30 and continues thus by about 10% per decade depending on health and activity level [27]. One theory describing the link between aging and mobility loss supposes that as VO_{2max} approaches the energy required for usual walking, walking speed declines as an adaptation to allow the individual to remain within the limits of energetic boundary [27]. When aerobic capacity declines, an individual must access anaerobic pathways to meet energy demands which trigger feelings of fatigue [27]. Thus one enters the frailty cycle of decreased activity due to fatigue leading to loss of muscle

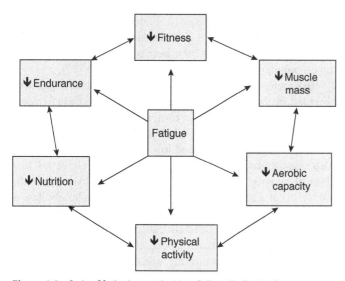

Figure 6.2. Cycle of frailty (copyright Mary Colleen Bhalla, 2012).

mass, sedentary behavior, undernutrition, less endurance, and further decline in fitness (Figure 6.2) [23,26,27].

Frailty may present in association with delirium. Although frailty and delirium seem to be two separate processes, they share common pathophysiologic processes involving inflammation, atherosclerosis, and chronic nutritional deficiencies [28]. Preoperative frailty is a risk factor for postoperative delirium, and the occurrence of delirium can stress fat and protein stores and potentiate sarcopenia [28]. Delirious patients are vulnerable to underfeeding and weight loss. Patients with persistent delirium have been shown to be less likely to regain ADL function, resulting in new or increasing frailty [28].

There is a pre-frail state that implies a progression from robustness to frailty [23–25]. As the frailty cycle progresses and a patient develops sarcopenia, the perception of exercise effort increases causing avoidance of physical activity, downregulation of physiologic systems, and decline in general function leading to further sarcopenia and increased restriction of physical activity [24]. Frailty begins by affecting mobility tasks before causing end-stage function debility in ADL, so frailty and pre-frailty should be screened for early [23]. Undernutrition, sarcopenia, and obesity are important precursors in the progression from pre-frail to frail. Frailty is hallmarked by slow and incomplete recovery after any new stress [24]. In the pre-frail state there are physiologic reserves sufficient to respond to stresses with complete recovery. Once a patient has developed end-stage function debility in ADL, it is unlikely that he/she will regain these abilities and will need additional resources to meet ADL needs. Undernutrition, sarcopenia, and obesity are important precursors in the progression from pre-frail to frail, and thus are potential areas to target for prevention [24,25]. Different frailty prevention strategies involve diet, regular exercise, monitoring of abilities, prevention of infection, anticipation of stressful events, and rapid reconditioning after stressful events [24]. To date, only physical activities studies have been found to benefit patients with moderate frailty but not those with severe frailty [24]. The greatest benefit was seen in resistance training programs which increase strength and improve risk factors for frailty [26]. Prevention of sarcopenia and

preservation of fat-free mass should help prevent the decrease in metabolic rate associated with frailty [26]. Nutritional intervention alone was not beneficial [24].

When evaluating a patient in whom you suspect frailty, it is important to note the heightened vulnerability and need for additional resources both at home and in the hospital. It is also important to recognize those patients in a pre-frail state to take steps to prevent frailty. For instance, a patient with a broken humerus may be sent home in a sling. The sling may prevent him or her from cooking full meals and their nutritional status may suffer. If their family or senior services are made aware of their need for help with meals while wearing the sling, an increase in frailty may be prevented. Conversely a patient with a broken foot may give up on any exercise while recovering because he or she can no longer participate in his or her senior aerobics class, but might start an exercise regimen involving a hand cycle if he or she understands the importance of keeping to a fitness program.

Functional decline

Functional decline or the decreased ability to perform ADL can be either a consequence of illness or injury after hospital admission or a visit to the ED or a precursor that prompts a visit to the ED [13,29,30]. ADL can be divided into IADL and physical activities of daily living (PADL). PADL include walking, dressing, transferring, bathing, grooming, continence, and eating [30]. IADL include shopping, housework, transportation, meals, medicine, money, and telephone use [30]. One study looking at functional decline prompting a visit to the ED found that 74% of patients 75 years and older with an illness or injury more than 48 hours had a decline in their PADL or IADL [30]. Two-thirds of those with IADL decline and three-fourths of those with PADL decline said that it had contributed to their visit to the ED. Another study looked at older adults who lived without help for their PADL disability and their hospital admission rate [29]. When additional resources were provided to the patients at home to meet their PADL needs, their hospitalization rate dropped to that similar to older adults with no unmet PADL needs [29]. Living with unmet PADL needs is associated with falling, pressure ulcers, contractures, and an increasing use of primary, emergency, and acute health care services [29]. Older patients without a specific complaint requiring admission often cannot return home because of an unmet PADL or IADL need [4]. A study of patients labeled as "home care impossible" in the ED found 90% to have a problem with an IADL, 75% to have a communication problem, 67% had suffered falls, 48% had incontinence, and 61% had cognitive decline [4].

Functional decline might also occur after discharge from the hospital or ED [30,31]. A study of ED patients over 64 years of age with blunt injury who were discharged home found that in one week 40% had developed functional decline, 49% had new services initiated, and 33% had an unscheduled medical contact. At four weeks, 15% had a repeat ED visit and 11% were hospitalized [13]. The majority of the patients had new services initiated by family members [13]. Predictors of functional decline were female gender, IADL dependence, extremity fracture or dislocation, trunk injury, or head injury [13].

Table 6.2. Tools to predict functional decline

Identification of seniors at risk (ISAR) Self-reported, Yes/No response	Triage risk screening tool (TRST) Completed by nurses, Yes/No response
In general, do you have serious problems with your memory?	Presence of cognitive impairment?
Since the illness or injury that brought you to the ED, have you needed more help than usual to take care of yourself?	Difficulty walking, transferring, or recent fall?
Before the illness or injury that brought you to the ED, did you need someone to help you on a regular basis?	Lives alone with no available caregiver?
Do you take more than 3 different medications every day?	Five or more prescription medications?
Have you been hospitalized for one or more nights during the past 6 months (excluding a stay in the ED)?	ED use in last 30 days or hospitalization in last 90 days?
In general, do you see well?	Registered Nurse concern?

There are several tools to predict functional decline, two examples being the Identification of Seniors at Risk (ISAR), which is a self-completed, six-item measure and the Triage Risk Screening Tool (TRST), which is completed by triage nurses (Table 6.2) [31,32]. Both identify patients who are likely to return to the ED due to functional decline. Patients that are found to be positive with either tool could be referred to a primary care physician, home care, or social services for a more detailed functional assessment.

When evaluating a patient in the ED it is important to consider the role that functional decline played in his or her reason for coming to the ED so that it can be addressed prior to disposition. It is important also to consider potential decline after discharge so that steps can be taken to prevent it by educating family or ensuring the patient has access to appropriate resources such as senior services or physical therapy.

Summary

Generalized weakness can be a presenting chief complaint that requires an extensive evaluation to elicit the cause, or may be associated with other geriatric syndromes such as failure to thrive, functional decline, sarcopenia, frailty, and falls. When evaluating any older ED patient, one must always consider their functional status and goals of care when considering a work-up and planning a disposition. The main goal is always to consider the patient not as a specific diagnosis but as part of a larger social and health care delivery system.

Pearls and pitfalls

Pearls

- Recognize that generalized weakness and fatigue may be caused by a specific disease or condition or be part of a geriatric syndrome.
- Remember to think of a patient's goals of care before proceeding with an extensive work-up.
- Consider a patient's home situation when planning for discharge.
- Know your hospital, governmental, and local resources to assist you with evaluation, discharge planning, and caregiver support.

Pitfalls

- Do not forget the importance of a mental health evaluation.
- Always be suspicious of elder abuse and neglect and know your local reporting responsibility.
- Do not forget to involve the patient's family and friends in history taking.
- Always consider polypharmacy and drug interactions when considering a differential diagnosis and discharge planning.

References

1. Bhalla M, Stiffler K, Gerson L, Wilber S. Abstracts of the SAEM (Society for Academic Emergency Medicine) Annual Meeting, June 1–5, 2011, Boston, MA. *Acad Emerg Med.* 2011;18(Suppl. 1):S221–2.
2. Nemec M, Koller MT, Nickel CH, et al. Patients presenting to the emergency department with nonspecific complaints: the Basel Nonspecific Complaints (BANC) study. *Acad Emerg Med.* 2010;17(3):284–92.
3. Nickel CH, Ruedinger J, Misch F, et al. Copeptin and peroxiredoxin-4 independently predict mortality in patients with nonspecific complaints presenting to the emergency department. *Acad Emerg Med.* 2011;18(8):851–9.
4. Rutschmann OT, Chevalley T, Zumwald C, et al. Pitfalls in the emergency department triage of frail elderly patients without specific complaints. *Swiss Med Wkly.* 2005;135(9–10):145–50.
5. LaMantia MA, Platts-Mills TF, Biese K, et al. Predicting hospital admission and returns to the emergency department for elderly patients. *Acad Emerg Med.* 2010;17(3):252–9.
6. Haley R, Sullivan DH, Granger CV, et al. Inpatient rehabilitation outcomes for older adults with nondebility generalized weakness. *Am J Phys Med Rehabil.* 2011;90(10):791–7.
7. Anon. *International Classification of Diseases, Ninth Revision, Clinical Modification (ICD-9-CM)* (accessed May 8, 2012 from www.cdc.gov/nchs/icd/icd9cm.htm).
8. Robertson RG, Montagnini M. Geriatric failure to thrive. *Am Fam Physician.* 2004;70(2):343–50.
9. Fielding RA, Vellas B, Evans WJ, et al. Sarcopenia: an undiagnosed condition in older adults. Current consensus definition: prevalence, etiology, and consequences. International working group on sarcopenia. *J Am Med Dir Assoc.* 2011;12(4):249–56.

10. Faulkner JA, Larkin LM, Claflin DR, et al. Age-related changes in the structure and function of skeletal muscles. *Clin Exp Pharmacol Physiol.* 2007;34(11):1091–6.

11. Ryall JG, Schertzer JD, Lynch GS. Cellular and molecular mechanisms underlying age-related skeletal muscle wasting and weakness. *Biogerontology.* 2008;9(4):213–28.

12. Inouye SK, Studenski S, Tinetti ME, et al. Geriatric syndromes: clinical, research, and policy implications of a core geriatric concept. *J Am Geriatr Soc.* 2007;55(5):780–91.

13. Wilber ST, Blanda M, Gerson LW, et al. Short-term functional decline and service use in older emergency department patients with blunt injuries. *Acad Emerg Med.* 2010;17(7):679–86.

14. van Nieuwenhuizen RC, van Dijk N, van Breda FG, et al. Assessing the prevalence of modifiable risk factors in older patients visiting an ED due to a fall using the CAREFALL Triage Instrument. *Am J Emerg Med.* 2010;28(9):994–1001.

15. Vincent HK, Vincent KR, Lamb KM. Obesity and mobility disability in the older adult. *Obes Rev.* 2010;11(8):568–79.

16. Marsh AP, Rejeski WJ, Espeland MA, et al. Muscle strength and BMI as predictors of major mobility disability in the Lifestyle Interventions and Independence for Elders pilot (LIFE-P). *J Gerontol A Biol Sci Med Sci.* 2011;66(12):1376–83.

17. Helbostad JL, Leirfall S, Moe-Nilssen R, et al. Physical fatigue affects gait characteristics in older persons. *J Gerontol A Biol Sci Med Sci.* 2007;62(9):1010–15.

18. Scheffer AC, Schuurmans MJ, van Dijk N, et al. Fear of falling: measurement strategy, prevalence, risk factors and consequences among older persons. *Age Aging.* 2008;37(1):19–24.

19. Murphy SL, Williams CS, Gill TM. Characteristics associated with fear of falling and activity restriction in community-living older persons. *J Am Geriatr Soc.* 2002;50(3):516–20.

20. Vind AB, Andersen HE, Pedersen KD, et al. Effect of a program of multifactorial fall prevention on health-related quality of life, functional ability, fear of falling and psychological well-being. A randomized controlled trial. *Aging Clin Exp Res.* 2010;22(3):249–54.

21. Martin FC, Hart D, Spector T, et al. Fear of falling limiting activity in young-old women is associated with reduced functional mobility rather than psychological factors. *Age Aging.* 2005;34(3):281–7.

22. Russell MA, Hill KD, Blackberry I, et al. Falls risk and functional decline in older fallers discharged directly from emergency departments. *J Gerontol A Biol Sci Med Sci.* 2006;61(10):1090–5.

23. Fried LP, Tangen CM, Walston J, et al. Frailty in older adults: evidence for a phenotype. *J Gerontol A Biol Sci Med Sci.* 2001;56(3):M146–6.

24. Lang PO, Michel JP, Zekry D. Frailty syndrome: a transitional state in a dynamic process. *Gerontology.* 2009;55(5):539–49.

25. Kanapuru B, Ershler WB. Inflammation, coagulation, and the pathway to frailty. *Am J Med.* 2009;122(7):605–13.

26. Fried LP, Walston JD, Ferrucci L. Frailty. In *Hazzard's Geriatric Medicine and Gerontology*, 6th edn (McGraw-Hill Professional).

27. Schrack JA, Simonsick EM, Ferrucci L. The energetic pathway to mobility loss: an emerging new framework for longitudinal studies on aging. *J Am Geriatr Soc.* 2010;58(Suppl. 2):S329–36.

28. Quinlan N, Marcantonio ER, Inouye SK, et al. Vulnerability: the crossroads of frailty and delirium. *J Am Geriatr Soc.* 2011;59(Suppl. 2):S262–8.

29. Sands LP, Wang Y, McCabe GP, et al. Rates of acute care admissions for frail older people living with met versus unmet activity of daily living need. *J Am Geriatr Soc.* 2006;54(2):339–44.

30. Wilber ST, Blanda M, Gerson LW. Does functional decline prompt emergency department visits and admission in older patients? *Acad Emerg Med.* 2006;13(6):680–2.

31. Hustey FM, Mion LC, Connor JT, et al. A brief risk stratification tool to predict functional decline in older adults discharged from emergency departments. *J Am Geriatr Soc.* 2007;55(8):1269–74.

32. McCusker J, Cardin S, Bellavance F, et al. Return to the emergency department among elders: patterns and predictors. *Acad Emerg Med.* 2000;7(3):249–59.

Chapter

7

Management of trauma in the elderly

Deborah R. Wong and Todd C. Rothenhaus

Background

Trauma in the elderly presents significant challenges for the clinician. The incidence of serious injury is high and occult injury is common. Injury patterns differ from those in younger adults and require unique consideration. Physiologic changes associated with aging confound clinical assessment and impact morbidity and mortality. Patients may present with significant co-existing medical conditions or may be taking medications that can complicate assessment and resuscitation.

Knowledge of the physiology of aging, the unique patterns of injury in the elderly, the impact of co-existing acute and chronic medical conditions, and the classic pitfalls of geriatric trauma care are critical to good outcomes. This chapter reviews the epidemiology, mechanisms of injury, pre-hospital considerations, initial assessment, and emergency department (ED) management and disposition of elderly victims of trauma.

Epidemiology

The elderly are one of the fastest growing segments of the US population [1]. By 2035, the number of people over the age of 85 will have doubled to more than 14 million. People are living longer and are more active. Between 1982 and 2005, the number of non-disabled people rose in all age groups above 65, with the greatest increase being 32% in those aged 85 and older [2].

In the US, trauma is the fifth leading cause of death, and the seventh leading cause of death in patients over 65 [3]. Most lethal injuries in this age group arise from motor vehicle collisions [4]. The elderly have disproportionately higher mortality and hospitalization rates when compared with younger cohorts. They are more severely injured, develop more complications (54 versus 34%), and die more frequently (17 versus 4.7%). Length of hospitalization is also longer, translating to higher medical expenses [5].

Currently, the leading cause of injury in older patients is falls from standing. However, over the next few decades, we are likely to see an increase in the number of high-energy injuries due to motor vehicle collisions and falls from heights as the older population continues to drive and lead more dynamic lifestyles.

Mechanisms of injury

Falls

Approximately 30% of persons aged >65 years fall each year, and this increases to at least 40% by age 80 [6,7]. Falls are by far the most common cause of injury in the elderly, and resulting complications are a frequent cause of death. Low-level falls (from a standing position or lower) are the most prevalent. The incidence of falls increases with age and varies according to living status: 30 to 40% of community-dwelling seniors sustain a significant fall in their lifetime, and approximately 50% of individuals living in a long-term care facility will sustain a fall. This percentage climbs to 60 if there has been a fall within the previous year [8–11]. Of those older than 75 who fall, 7% seek care in the ED and at least 40% of those are admitted [12].

Major risk factors for falls include past history of a fall, female gender, gait deficits, use of assistive device, muscle weakness, arthritis, and sedative medications including psychotropics and benzodiazepines. Other etiologies to consider include visual impairment, cognitive impairment, chronic medical conditions such as anemia, environmental hazards, and orthostatic hypotension [13]. Multiple risk factors significantly increase the risk of falling, and falls are often multifactorial in nature. In their classic study on falls in the elderly, Tinetti et al. showed that patients with four or more established risks for falls had a 78% risk of subsequent fall compared with 27% in patients with zero or one risk factor [7].

Not only does the risk of falling increase with age, but the severity of injury also worsens. Injuries to the head, pelvis, and lower extremities are more common in the geriatric patient than in younger patients with a similar mechanism of injury. Elderly patients account for less than 15% of trauma admissions due to falls; however, they account for more than half of deaths due to falls. Overall mortality is approximately 11%. Falls from a height greater than 15 feet (5 m) are less common but about a quarter of these are fatal [14].

In the ED, it is imperative that acute medical conditions precipitating falls such as syncope, transient ischemic attacks, metabolic derangements, and infection be considered in tandem with the acute trauma evaluation.

Geriatric Emergency Medicine, ed. Joseph H. Kahn, Brendan G. Magauran Jr., and Jonathan S. Olshaker. Published by Cambridge University Press.
© Cambridge University Press 2014.

Motor vehicle collisions

The pathophysiology of aging and concomitant medical conditions affecting vision, hearing, reflexes, balance, and cognition place elderly drivers at high risk for motor vehicle collisions. Drivers over the age of 75 are second only to those under 25 in the incidence of crashes, and have the highest mortality of any age group. The majority of collisions occur in scenarios where the driver is making a left turn or merging, as these situations require more attuned cognitive function, reflexes, and vision [15]. Poor weather conditions and night driving are also more challenging for the elderly driver. Many elderly drivers are not aware of their functional impairment but, if educated, do change their behavior and exposure to risk.

Pedestrians struck by automobiles

The elderly represent some of the most seriously injured patients in trauma with mortality greater than 25%. In 2005, 20% of the 4881 pedestrian fatalities in the US involved those aged 65 and over despite that demographic comprising only 12.4% of the population [16]. Fatalities tend to be from severe head injury or major vascular damage, with the majority occurring at the scene or in the ED. Non-fatal injuries in this population tend to be more severe than in other populations. In a recent paper, Richards and Carroll showed a significant increased risk of pedestrian head injury in those older than 70 versus their younger counterparts [17]. Injuries to the spine and thorax, and fractures, also increase dramatically with age although injuries to the abdomen do not [18,19].

Elderly patients are frequently struck within marked crosswalks or walk directly into the path of an oncoming vehicle. Often they misjudge the speed of oncoming traffic and cannot accelerate their own pace to compensate [20]. Urban settings are most dangerous, with the majority of injuries occurring in situations involving merging or turning vehicles. Elderly pedestrian trauma is also greater in the winter when it is darker and more difficult to visually discern objects [21].

Burns

Burns are relatively common in the elderly. Physiologic changes associated with aging, acute and chronic medical conditions, and social isolation (resulting in accidental fires) have been associated with morbidity and mortality from burns in the geriatric population. Elderly individuals represented approximately 13% of patients admitted to burns units. Total body surface area burned, mortality, and hospital length of stay are all higher in the elderly. Mortality has been shown to be 100% in patients over the age of 60 who sustain a body surface area burn of 50% or greater [22–24].

As with other forms of trauma, burn treatment in the elderly is complicated by co-existing disease and impaired functional reserve [25]. Curiously, however, one study demonstrated improved outcomes in patients who were taking beta blockers at the time of their burn despite the comorbidities implicit in taking a cardiovascular medication [26].

Elder abuse and neglect

Elder abuse is far more common than most physicians realize. One in four vulnerable elders are at risk of abuse, and when studied, over 6% of the older general population report abuse in the previous month. A significant proportion of elderly are abused or neglected by family members and reluctant to report them. Perpetrators were most likely related to the victim (44%) and most often the adult child of the victim (33%). Risk factors for abuse include female gender, age >80, and Caucasian race. Females are more likely to be the abusers than males [27].

Evaluation of all geriatric injury victims in the ED should include an assessment for signs and symptoms of abuse. Bruises in multiple stages of healing, unexplained fractures, untreated injuries, signs of neglect such as dehydration, malnutrition, and bedsores are important clues to the possibility of abuse or neglect. Elder abuse is covered in more detail in a separate chapter.

Physiology of aging and trauma

Aging is the normal, predictable, and irreversible decline of organ system function over time. These changes affect patients in a number of ways, but usually manifest as a loss of function, functional reserve, and decreased ability to meet metabolic demands of stress or injury. Although distinguishing the effects of aging from the effects of disease may be difficult, the presence of comorbidity impacts the morbidity and mortality from trauma independent of the normal process of aging [28,29].

Cardiovascular

Cardiac functional reserve is diminished with age. Myocardium degenerates and myocytes are replaced by collagen and fat. The cells that do remain have decreased contractility and compliance, resulting in a 50% reduction in baseline cardiac output by 80 years of age. The cardiac outflow tract also stiffens with age leading to increased afterload. In addition, there is a decrease in the chronotropic response to catecholamines due to aging of the conducting system, as well as the potential effects of prescribed beta blockers or calcium channel blockers.

Elderly patients have a blunted cardiovascular response to stress. Compensatory tachycardia, seen almost universally in young patients in response to hypovolemia or shock, is often absent [30,31]. In a classic study on severely injured elderly, approximately half of patients with normal blood pressure had occult shock and poor outcomes. These outcomes were improved with aggressive management of volume resuscitation (preload), inotropic agents, and afterload reduction [32].

Superimposed on the normal effects of age on the heart can be the presence of heart failure, which may diminish cardiac output further; heart block, which can further blunt the rate response to stress; and coronary artery disease, which may manifest as demand ischemia during the stress of trauma. The risk of an acute cardiac event must be considered in every case of trauma in the elderly. An electrocardiogram (ECG) is recommended early in the work-up.

Pulmonary

Pulmonary function also declines with age. Loss of elasticity in the chest wall and lungs leads to decreased compliance and an increase in work of breathing, which can become more apparent during acute illness or injury. Alveolar loss and decreased diffusion capacity result in an age-dependent decline in arterial oxygen tension such that patients approximately 80 years of age can have an expected baseline PaO_2 between 78 and 92 mmHg. There is no similar change in $PaCO_2$, and therefore hypercarbia should always be considered pathologic. Mucociliary clearance declines as well leading to a decreased ability to clear the bronchial tree and increased incidence of pulmonary infections. Vital capacity, forced expiratory volume, and functional reserve are also compromised with age and need to be considered in evaluation of breathing [33].

Gastrointestinal

Age per se is not associated with physiologic changes that alter management in the ED. However, co-existing hepatic disease significantly impacts mortality in trauma patients [34]. Patients with end-stage liver disease and cirrhosis have a much higher mortality from the risk of bleeding and uncontrolled hemorrhage.

Renal

The number of functioning nephrons decreases with age, as does renal blood flow, leading to an age-related decline in creatinine clearance that is nearly always underappreciated in elderly patients, since muscle mass (the primary source of creatinine) also decreases significantly with age. The clinician should be aware that a "normal creatinine" in an elderly patient may actually reflect a significant reduction in renal function. This should be kept in mind when one is administering intravenous contrast for imaging, and intravenous volume expansion should be considered to reduce contrast-induced nephropathy [35].

Central nervous system

The brain atrophies with aging, leading to an approximately 200 g decrease in brain weight and a concomitant decrease in brain volume. Bridging vessels are stretched over the surface of the brain and are more susceptible to tearing under rapid acceleration or deceleration, resulting in a subdural hematoma. Cerebrovascular autoregulation in the brain also declines with age, potentially resulting in labile intracranial pressure after head injury [17,36].

Musculoskeletal

With age, the ratio of lean body mass to total body weight decreases. Muscle strength decreases by one-third after the age of 60, leading to difficulty with mobility and balance. Women are known to have accelerated loss of bone mass compared with men, but by age 60 the rates of bone loss are comparable. Overall, changes in bone mass and bone construction conspire to make bones more fragile and vulnerable than in younger populations [37].

Skin

Skin functions deteriorate with age. The numbers of Langerhans cells and melanocytes decrease, and the dermal–epidermal junction becomes flattened. Keratinocyte proliferation is reduced, and the time required for these cells to migrate from the basal layer to the skin surface doubles. In addition, the dermis has reduced vascularity.

Aging of the skin leads to increased susceptibility to injury. Reduction in nerve endings reduces pain sensation, increasing the risk of burns and mechanical injury, and increased fragility leads to higher incidence of laceration or avulsion due to mechanical forces. Wound healing is delayed across all phases of wound healing: hemostasis, inflammation, proliferation, and tissue remodeling [38].

Endocrine

Elderly patients have diminished glucose tolerance, leading to the possibility of stress-induced hyperglycemia (SIH) after injury. SIH has been associated with a twofold increase in mortality in multi-trauma patients and has been associated with poor outcomes in patients with head injury [39,40]. Intensive insulin therapy is associated with a decrease in mortality, and the effect increases with injury severity and age [41]. Finger stick glucose should be obtained on initial evaluation, and at regular intervals post-injury if elevated.

Pre-existing medications

A number of medications are strongly associated with trauma in the elderly, including psychotropics, antihypertensives, and, less frequently, anti-epileptic and glaucoma agents. Over 80% of patients evaluated after accidental falls are found to be on medications typically implicated in falls [42]. The presence of four or more chronic medications seems to correlate well with an increasing risk of falls [43].

Identification of medications that can impact management and outcome is critical to management of geriatric trauma. Antihypertensive medications may make resuscitation more difficult. Beta blockers, in one retrospective study, were associated with increased mortality in patients over 65 [44]. While antihypertensive overdose may be considered, hypotension should not be attributed to blood pressure medications until hemorrhage and ischemia have been ruled out.

Anticoagulants and antiplatelet agents

Chronic therapy with oral warfarin (Coumadin), new oral anticoagulants such as dabigatran etexilate (Pradaxa) and rivaroxaban (Xarelto), aspirin, and other platelet inhibitors such as clopidogrel (Plavix) has become commonplace. Use of warfarin is indicated in a number of medical conditions including venous thromboembolism, atrial fibrillation, stroke, and valve replacement [45]. The incidence of warfarin use increases with age. Unfortunately, the risk of major bleeding complications and supratherapeutic International Normalized Ratios (INRs) due to warfarin increases as well.

Warfarin significantly worsens outcome from severe head injury, but has a less dramatic impact on mortality in injured patients without head injury [46–49]. Similarly, aspirin and clopidogrel seem to increase the risk of death in patients who sustain intracranial injury [50,51]. This may be because they present with higher-grade bleeds than controls. It appears that both the size of the initial bleed and the Glasgow Coma Score (GCS) upon admission are the greatest predictors of mortality in patients with intracranial hemorrhage (ICH) taking antiplatelet agents. In contrast, patients taking warfarin more often are found to present with low-grade hemorrhage which then transforms to high-grade bleeding and death. Transfusion of platelets does not seem to have any effect on outcomes in patients with ICH taking antiplatelet agents. However, rapid reversal of INR does improve outcomes of those taking warfarin [52].

Treatment of patients taking warfarin who sustain injury needs to be individualized, based on the need to continue therapy (i.e., mechanical valve and risk of embolic stroke), the need for immediate reversal (i.e., life-threatening hemorrhage or intracranial bleeding), the need for non-urgent reversal (i.e., elective preoperative), or a decision to simply discontinue warfarin (i.e., subsequent risk of falls).

For patients requiring immediate reversal of warfarin in the emergency department, published guidelines suggest the administration of four-factor prothrombin complex concentrate (PCC) rather than fresh frozen plasma (FFP) and vtamin K [53]. Unfortunately, at this time, only three-factor PCCs are available in the US. These PCCs (Bebulin VH and Profilnine SD) contain factors II, IX, and X but minimal concentrations of factor VII. There are some concerns that they are not as effective in reversing anticoagulation as four-factor PCC [54]. However, the benefit of PCC in comparison with FFP and vitamin K is clear in terms of volume infused and time to reversal. It generally takes 6–10 units (1500–2500 ml) of FFP to reverse a 70 kg patient. This is a large volume for a patient who may have underlying heart failure or isolated head injury. FFP also takes, on average, 30 hours for reversal of warfarin, while vitamin K takes up to 12–24 hours to achieve its desired effect. In contrast, it takes about 20 ml of reconstituted PCC to achieve the same effect with an onset of 15 minutes. In the past, there was some reluctance to use PCCs because they might cause thromboembolic events. These data were derived from prior experience in hemophiliacs. A recent small study in Sweden found that the risk of thromboembolic events in cases of warfarin coagulopathy was small (3.8%) and the efficacy of PCC was good in most patients [54].

If prothrombin complex concentrate is unavailable, FFP and vitamin K (10 mg IV) are indicated. Repeat treatment may be necessary, depending on the result of subsequent INR measurements. For non-emergent reversal of warfarin, administration of a single (1–2.5 mg) oral or parenteral dose of vitamin K may be considered, but should generally be made in conjunction with the patient's primary care or admitting physician [55].

The newer oral anticoagulants, Pradaxa and Xarelto, are currently approved for the treatment of atrial fibrillation and deep venous thrombosis (DVT), respectively. They have the advantage of being easier to manage for both the patient and

clinician in that they require no blood testing for levels and have an improved medication and food interaction profile versus warfarin. However, there are no antidotes available in case of severe or life-threatening bleeding. The current recommendation is to discontinue the drug (which has a relatively short half-life and should clear in 1–2 days), provide supportive care, and to consider PCC (though there is currently a lack of human studies to support this) [53].

Pre-hospital considerations

Patients who sustain serious injury are best managed in trauma centers, including the elderly [56]. Historically, development of statewide trauma systems has led to improved survival for geriatric trauma patients [57]. However, studies remain inconclusive over whether age per se should be a criterion for transfer to a trauma center. At all levels of injury severity, patients older than 60 years have an increased risk for morbidity and mortality. In fact, the risk of death and morbidity from minor injuries is far higher in the elderly than the young. In a recent study, elderly patients with minor Injury Severity Score (ISS) had a threefold increase in morbidity and a fivefold increase in mortality, and elderly patients with a major ISS demonstrated a twofold increase in morbidity and a fourfold increase in mortality when compared with younger cohorts [58].

Advocates suggest trauma team activation for all patients over age 75 [59]. Some argue that triage of isolated injuries (i.e., hip fractures) to trauma centers overburdens the trauma system, while others support the concept of a team approach for all geriatric trauma [60,61]. Current guidelines put forth by the Eastern Association for the Surgery of Trauma endorse a lower threshold for transfer to a trauma center in injured patients >70 years and in those >65 with a known pre-existing medical condition or Abbreviated Injury Scale (AIS) ≥3 [62]. The Centers for Disease Control (CDC) and ACS currently recommend that the following conditions prompt field triage of geriatric patients directly to trauma centers: age >55, systolic blood pressure (SBP) <110 (which might indicate shock in elderly), and use of anticoagulants. The CDC also recognize low-level falls as having the propensity to lead to severe injury and recommend a low threshold for direct transport to a trauma center [63].

Evaluation and management

Initial evaluation

Failure to appropriately manage the airway, breathing, and circulation (ABC) in geriatric trauma victims will lead to hypoxia, respiratory failure, shock, and death. Aggressive care is warranted. Evaluation of the ABC in geriatric patients includes a number of important considerations [64].

The elderly have decreased airway reflexes, and expeditious management of the airway should be considered to prevent aspiration. Anatomically, the geriatric airway can be difficult to manage. Mouth opening may be impaired, dentures are often present, and, coupled with the need to maintain in-line stabilization of the spine, the presence of kyphosis, or impaired mobility make laryngoscopy difficult. Use of glidescope, C-MAC, or other airway adjuncts may facilitate intubation in these patients.

Pharmacologic therapy for rapid-sequence intubation in the geriatric patient requires modification. While the dosages of neuromuscular blocking agents should not be reduced, dosages of nearly all sedatives, including barbiturates, benzodiazepines, and etomidate, should be reduced in the elderly to avoid hypotension. Doses of lidocaine and opiates, used as premedication prior to intubation of patients suffering head injury, should also be reduced. Priming or administration of a defasciculating dose of a non-depolarizing neuromuscular blocker may abolish respirations prematurely, resulting in apnea with inadequate relaxation.

It may be difficult to detect impending respiratory failure in geriatric patients with trauma. Ventilatory responses to hypoxia and hypercarbia are blunted in the elderly, leading to occult respiratory insufficiency. Consider early, elective intubation in patients leaving the ED for diagnostic tests. If intubation is not immediately indicated, arterial blood gas analysis is recommended in seriously injured geriatric patients, and should be considered mandatory in patients with any signs of difficulty breathing, thoracic trauma, altered mental status, or the need for supplemental oxygen to maintain oxygenation.

Perhaps the most common mistake in the management of geriatric patients with trauma is under-resuscitation – the clinical presentation is underappreciated, small-bore IVs are placed, and fluids held out of fear that the patient "will end up in CHF." Unrecognized shock and under-resuscitation lead to extremely poor outcomes. Standard hemodynamic parameters are inadequate to determine the stability of geriatric patients. Cardiac monitoring, frequent vital signs determinations, and intensive care throughout the ED work-up and stay should be the rule. Resuscitation should begin with crystalloid, though emergent transfusion should begin in patients who present with hypotension. Metabolic acidosis, base-deficit on arterial blood gas (ABG), or elevated lactate suggest shock and mandate an emergent search for hemorrhage. Conversely, absence of metabolic acidosis or a normal lactate do not rule out serious injury in elderly patients [65].

Intensive care unit admission should be strongly considered in patients with base deficit ≤6 [66]. The elderly are at increased risk for the development of hypothermia during resuscitation, and external warming devices should be considered [66].

Central nervous system

Computed tomography (CT) of the brain should be obtained liberally in elderly patients sustaining head injury. In a subgroup analysis of the NEXUS study, significant intracranial injury was more common in elderly patients (12.5%) than in those under 65 (7.9%) [67]. Studies have revealed significant intracranial injury despite minor head injury mechanism, normal mental status, and normal neurological examination [68,69]. This incidence, while small, is further increased if the patient is taking warfarin, other anticoagulants, or antiplatelet agents [70]. Although not the current standard in the US, the European Federation of Neurological Societies (2002)

recommendation is to obtain an initial CT, admit for observation for 24 hours, and obtain a second CT prior to discharge. One prospective study found this protocol sufficient to detect most occurrences of delayed bleeding and in fact found that 6% of patients did have bleeding on follow-up CT [71]. This same study found that the relative risk of delayed hemorrhage with an INR greater than 3 was 14. Therefore, our recommendation is to obtain a head CT, as well as assess the coagulation profile as soon as possible, and to start reversing any supratherapeutic anticoagulation within two hours of admission for elderly patients sustaining head injury.

Spine

Elderly patients undergoing radiography of the cervical spine after trauma have at least twice the likelihood of cervical spine fracture than younger patients [72]. Elderly patients who fall from low heights are at significantly increased risk of injury between the occiput and C2, while patients in motor vehicle collisions and high falls are more likely to injure lower cervical vertebrae. Injuries to the cervical spine at multiple levels are common [73].

In the Canadian C-spine rule, age greater than 65 is an exclusion criterion, offering no data to guide cervical spine imaging in geriatric trauma patients [74]. In contrast, the NEXUS clinical decision rule was validated in a cohort of geriatric patients. NEXUS investigators estimated that application of the decision rule could reduce the need for cervical spine imaging by 14%. Of note, 15% of injured geriatric patients were considered intoxicated at time of evaluation [72].

Given the high incidence of injuries to the atlantoaxial (C1–C2) complex, and the low sensitivity of plain films, a quite justifiable strategy is to CT the cervical spine of all elderly trauma patients requiring CT of the head. Some centers have advocated CT of C1–C2 in all patients undergoing head CT for trauma, regardless of indications for imaging the cervical spine. This recommendation may be challenged in younger adults as awareness of sensitivity to radiation dose in the neck has grown. However, CT should be considered the primary imaging modality of the cervical spine in most elderly patients [73,75].

Spinal cord injury without radiologic abnormality (SCIWORA) on plain radiographs (or even CT) may present in patients with cervical spondylosis owing to narrowing of the spinal canal and subsequent spinal cord compression with hyper-extension of the neck. Patients present with either a central cord or Brown–Séquard-like syndrome [76]. Emergent magnetic resonance imaging (MRI) should be obtained to rule out disk herniation requiring decompression.

Thorax

Rib fractures are both an important injury per se and a marker of injury severity in multiply injured geriatric patients. They are quite common, occurring in up to two-thirds of cases of chest trauma, and may be underreported due to occult fractures in up to 50% of radiographs [77]. Elderly patients with rib fractures have nearly twice the mortality of younger victims, despite a lower ISS and higher GCS. In addition, mortality rises significantly with the number of rib fractures, from 12% in patients sustaining 1–2 fractures, to nearly 40% in patients with 7 or more fractures. The risk of pneumonia increases with each additional rib fracture. Even the presence of a single rib fracture in the elderly carries significant morbidity and mortality [78–80]. This should be considered when contemplating discharge from the ED, and social supports, primary care follow-up, and adequate oral analgesia should be in place when outpatient management is deemed appropriate. In those hospitalized, early intervention with epidural analgesia improves pain and pulmonary function and has become the standard treatment [77].

Abdomen

While abdominal examination has been historically considered less reliable in the elderly, abdominal injury per se has not been found to be more frequent in the elderly when compared with younger cohorts. Anatomically, the spleen is smaller owing to involution and is injured less frequently. When solid organ injury is present, data suggest that age alone is not a contraindication to non-operative management [81]. For elderly patients in extremis with abdominal injury, survival after damage control laparotomy exceeds 50% [82].

Musculoskeletal

Hip fractures are quite common in elderly patients who sustain injuries after a fall [83]: in the US, 250,000 patients with hip fractures present to the ED each year and this is expected to double over the next 30 years [37]. Patients sustaining isolated hip fracture have similar injury severity scores, and a similar incidence of severe complications, as the trauma population in general [60].

There have been numerous studies examining the impact of multidisciplinary orthogeriatric hospital care on the morbidity and mortality of elderly hip fracture patients. These studies have consistently shown significant improvements in both mortality and functional outcome [37]. Failure to appreciate the morbidity and mortality associated with isolated hip fracture is a key mistake. As most patients with isolated hip fractures in the US are seen primarily by an emergency physician and admitted to either an orthopedist or the patient's primary care physician, creation of care guidelines and protocols for hospitalization that ensure highest-level care in community hospital settings should be considered.

Failing to consider occult fracture in patients with persistent hip pain and negative radiographs is a common pitfall. Standard AP and cross-lateral projections obtained in the ED are only 90% sensitive in detecting fractures [84]. In a study of patients presenting to the ED with hip pain and negative plain films, 4.4% were diagnosed with fracture. Of those, over 90% were over 65 years of age. MRI is the imaging modality of choice to rule out occult fractures with sensitivity and specificity approaching 100%. MRI may also provide evidence of an alternate diagnosis or pathologic finding which is not visible on plain imaging [85]. If MRI is unavailable or if the patient is unable to undergo MRI scanning, CT may also be used to rule out an occult hip fracture.

Acetabular fractures can be easily missed on plain radiographs. CT or MRI of the pelvis should be considered.

Periprosthetic fractures must be considered in patients with a history of hip replacement and hip or pelvic pain after trauma, as these can result in numerous complications [86].

Vertebral fractures in elderly patients are common even after minor or unapparent trauma. The prevalence of vertebral fractures in the general population increases dramatically with age. Patients present with pain at the level of fracture which may radiate outward along the associated dermatome. There is generally tenderness to palpation of the spine and worsening of the pain with certain movements (such as sitting or standing) that increase axial loading. Three types of fractures are common: anterior wedge, biconcave, and crush. Elderly patients who present with back pain should undergo radiographs to evaluate for fracture; however, a negative radiograph does not definitively rule out a fracture. If a fracture is present, it is still difficult to discern acuity without comparison films and a MRI or delayed bone scan [87–89].

Pelvic fractures result in significant morbidity and mortality in the elderly. Fractures of the pubic rami are most common (56%), followed by fractures of the acetabulum (19%) and ischium (11%). Multiple fractures are common and mortality is substantially higher than in younger patients [90]. Elderly patients with pelvic fractures are more likely to hemorrhage and require angiography. In addition, the elderly are more likely to sustain lateral compression fractures as opposed to anterior compression fractures, are more likely to require transfusion, and have a higher mortality [91,92].

Failure to identify and splint all extremity injuries is an error of omission that may lead to worsening injury during patient handling and movement through the work-up.

Prognosis

Elderly patients who arrive in the ED moribund have a dismal prognosis. However, while early mortality is clearly high in elderly patients who sustain serious injury, patients surviving hospitalization have reasonable long-term survival and many return home despite major injuries. At this point, there seem to be few if any decision points that would warrant anything but aggressive resuscitation on the basis of age alone.

Geriatric patients involved in serious trauma have high admission rates to intensive care and correspondingly high morbidity and mortality rates [93]. Most deaths occur in the first 24 hours of admission [94,95]. Geriatric trauma patients have longer hospital stays, incur higher overall hospital charges, and require longer periods of rehabilitation [4,96]. Recovery from injury can be prolonged, but with aggressive management over 90% of patients survive and many can return home [97,98]. Prolonged ICU stay is not associated with an unfavorable long-term outcome [97].

Disposition

Patients who sustain multiple injuries should be admitted, and evidence strongly suggests that multiply injured geriatric trauma patients are best served in a trauma center [4,99,100]. Patients requiring general surgical, neurosurgical intensive care, or burn care should be transferred once best attempts to stabilize the victim have occurred. Patients requiring repeat operation or particular orthopedic or other surgical expertise should also be considered for transfer. Lengthy attempts at defining all injuries in the initial receiving hospital are not warranted if they will not significantly change management or will delay transfer for definitive care of more life-threatening injuries.

Identification of a medical cause for fall or motor vehicle collision, such as syncope, MI, seizure, or infection is crucial. Once admitted, elucidation of potential precipitating medical factors, and management of co-existing medical issues and complications may be suboptimal. Therefore it is incumbent on the emergency physician to complete his or her work-up prior to transfer of care to a surgeon or other specialist. Fallon et al. found that a geriatric consultation service improved outcomes by identifying issues such as alcoholism and delirium as well as decreasing falls, functional decline, and death [61].

Selected patients sustaining isolated injuries after falls may be considered for discharge from the ED. Patients who report recurrent falls, have an abnormal mental status, or exhibit gait instability upon evaluation are poor candidates for discharge, and should undergo falls assessment by a geriatric specialist. Patients with lower extremity injuries are particularly high risk: canes and walkers have been shown to substantially increase the risk of falls [12,101]. Even those who meet discharge criteria should have close outpatient follow-up to try to mitigate risk of a subsequent fall. Comprehensive geriatric assessment can provide concrete recommendations for medication changes, environmental changes, physical therapy, and also provide the emotional support needed after the trauma of a fall. This type of multidisciplinary approach has been shown to reduce the rate of hospital admission, reduce ED visits, and improve outcomes in patients discharged from the ED [102].

Pearls and pitfalls

Pearls

- Search for a medical precipitant of trauma, such as syncope, MI, seizure, or infection.
- There is significant morbidity and mortality associated with isolated hip fracture.
- Remember to identify and splint all injuries.

Pitfalls

- Failure to aggressively manage the airway and breathing may lead to hypoxia and death.
- Under-resuscitation of hypovolemia/shock for fear that fluids will push patient into CHF.
- Failure to appreciate the increased risk of morbidity and mortality in elderly patients with less severe injury.

References

1. Vincent G, Velkoff V. The next four decades: The older population in the United States: 2010 to 2050. US Bureau of the Census. *Current Population Reports*. 2010;P25–1138.

2. Manton KG, Gu X, Lamb VL. Change in chronic disability from 1982 to 2004/2005 as measured by long-term changes in function and health in the US elderly population. *Proc Natl Acad Sci.* 2006;103(48):18374–9.

3. Miniño AM, Murphy SL. *Death in the United States, 2010.* NCHS data brief, no. 99 (Hyattsville, MD: National Center for Health Statistics, 2012).

4. Bergen G, Chen LH, Warner M, Fingerhut LA. *Injury in the United States: 2007 Chartbook* (Hyattsville, MD: National Center for Health Statistics, 2008).

5. Newell MA, Rotondo MF, Toschlog EA, et al. The elderly trauma patient: an investment for the future? *J Trauma.* 2009;67(2):337–40.

6. Stevens JA, Ryan G, Kresnow MS. Fatalities and injuries from falls among older adults – United States, 1993–2003 and 2001–2005. *MMWR.* 2006;55(45):1221–4.

7. Tinetti ME, Speechley M, Ginter SF. Risk factors for falls among elderly persons living in the community. *N Engl J Med.* 1988;319:1701–7.

8. Graafmans WC, Ooms ME, Hofstee HM, et al. Falls in the elderly: A prospective study of risk factors and risk profiles. *Am J Epidemiol.* 1996;143:1129–36.

9. Campbell AJ, Borrie MJ, Spears GF. Risk factors for falls in community-based prospective study of people 70 years and older. *J Gerontol.* 1989;44(4):M112–17.

10. Thapa PB, Brockman KG, Gideon P, Fought RL, Ray WA. Injurious falls in non-ambulatory nursing home residents: a comparative study of circumstances, incidence, and risk factors. *J Am Geriatr Soc.* 1996;44:273–8.

11. Sattin RW. Falls among older persons: A public health perspective. *Annu Rev Public Health.* 1992;13:489–508.

12. Thomas DC, Edelberg HK, Tinetti ME. Falls. In *Geriatric Medicine: An Evidence-based Approach*, ed. Cassel CK, Liepzig R, Cohen H, et al. (New York: Springer, 2003).

13. Nevitt MC, Cummings SR, Hudes ES. Risk factors for injurious falls: A prospective study. *J Gerontol.* 1991;46:M164–70.

14. Demetriades D, Murray J, Brown C, et al. High-level falls: type and severity of injuries and survival outcome according to age. *J Trauma.* 2005;58:342–5.

15. Stapin L, Lococo KH, Martell C, Stutts J. *Taxonomy of Older Driver Behaviors and Crash Risk.* National Traffic Highway Safety Administration, Report No DOT HS 811 468A, February 2012.

16. Zegeer C, Henderson D, Blomberg R, et al. *Evaluation of the Miami-Dade Pedestrian Safety Demonstration Project* (Washington, DC: USA National Highways Transport Safety Administration, 2008).

17. Richards D, Carroll J. Relationship between type of head injury and age of pedestrian. *Accid Anal Prev.* 2012;47:16–23.

18. Demetriades D, Murray J, Martin M, et al. Pedestrians injured by automobiles: relationship of age to injury type and severity. *J Am Coll Surg.* 2004;199:382–7.

19. Sklar DP, Demarest GB, McFeeley P. Increased pedestrian mortality among the elderly. *Am J Emerg Med.* 1989;7(4):387–90.

20. Rolison JJ, Hewson PJ, Hellier E, et al. Risk of fatal injury in older adult drivers, passengers, and pedestrians. *J Am Geriatr Soc.* 2012;60:1504–8.

21. Cleven AM, Blomberg RD. *A Compendium of NHTSA Pedestrian and Bicyclist Research Projects: 1969–2007* (accessed from NHTSA website, July 2007).

22. Manktelow A, Meyer AA, Herzog SR, Peterson HD. Analysis of life expectancy and living status of elderly patients surviving burn injury. *J Trauma*. 1989;29(2):203–7.

23. Anous MM, Heimbach DM. Causes of death and predictors in burned patients more than 60 years of age. *J Trauma*. 1986;26:135–9.

24. Linn BS. Age differences in the severity and outcome of burns. *J Am Geriatr Soc*. 1980;28:118123.

25. Zanni GR. Thermal burns and scalds: clinical complications in the elderly. *Consult Pharm*. 2012;27(1):16–22.

26. Arbabi S, Ahrns KS, Wahl WL, et al. Beta blocker use is associated with improved outcomes in adult burn patients. *J Trauma*. 2004;56(2):265–9.

27. Cooper C, Selwood A, Livingston G. The prevalence of elder abuse and neglect: a systematic review. *Age Aging*. 2008;37:151–60.

28. McMahon DJ, Schwab CW, Kauder D. Comorbidity and the elderly trauma patient. *World J Surg*. 1996;20:1113–20.

29. Milzman DP, Boulanger BR, Rodriguez A, et al. Pre-existing disease in trauma patients: a predictor of fate independent of age and injury severity score. *J Trauma*. 1992;32:236–43.

30. Martin JT, Alkhoury F, O'Connor JA et al. 'Normal' vital signs belie occult hypoperfusion in geriatric trauma patients. *Am Surg*. 2010;76(1):65–9.

31. Heffernan D, Thakkar RK, Monaghan SF, et al. Normal presenting vital signs are unreliable in geriatric blunt trauma victims. *J Trauma*. 2010;69:813–20.

32. Scalea TM, Simon HM, Duncan AO, et al. Geriatric blunt multiple trauma: Improved survival with early invasive monitoring. *J Trauma*. 1990:30:129–34.

33. Menaker J, Scalea TM. Geriatric care in the surgical intensive care unit. *Crit Care Med*. 2010;38(9)(Suppl.):S452–9.

34. Grossman MD, Miller D, Scaff DW, Arcona S. When is an elder old? Effect of pre-existing conditions on mortality in geriatric trauma. *J Trauma*. 2002;52:242–6.

35. Laville M, Juillard LJ. Contrast-induced acute kidney injury: how should at-risk patients be identified and managed? *Nephrology*. 2010;23(4):387–98.

36. Czosnyka M, Balestreri M, Steiner L, et al. Age, intracranial pressure, autoregulation, and outcome after brain trauma. *J Neurosurg*. 2005;102:450–4.

37. Carpenter CR, Stern ME. Emergency orthogeriatrics: Concepts and therapeutic alternatives. *Emerg Med Clin N Am*. 2010;28:927–49.

38. Sgonc R, Gruber J. Age-related aspects of cutaneous wound healing: A mini-review. *Gerontology*. 2012, accessed from http://content.karger.com/produktedb/produkte.asp?DOI=10.1159/000342344.

39. Jeremitsky E, Omert LA, Dunham CM, Wilberger J, Rodriguez A. The impact of hyperglycemia on patients with severe brain injury. *J Trauma*. 2005;58(1):47–50.

40. Kerby JD, Griffin RL, MacLennan P, Rue LW 3rd. Stress-induced hyperglycemia, not diabetic hyperglycemia, is associated with higher mortality in trauma. *Ann Surg*. 2012;256(3):446–52.

41. Eriksson E, Christianson D, Vanderkolk W, et al. Tight blood glucose control in trauma patients: Who really benefits? *J Emerg Trauma Shock*. 2011;4(3):359–64.

42. Sterke CS, Ziere G, van Beeck EF, et al. Dose-response relationship between selective serotonin re-uptake inhibitors and injurious falls: A study in nursing home residents with dementia. *Br J Clin Pharmacol*. 2012;73(5):812–20.

43. Nordell E, Jarnlo GB, Jetsen C, Nordstrom L, Thorngren KG. Accidental falls and related fractures in 65–74 year olds: a retrospective study of 332 patients. *Acta Orthop Scand*. 2000;71:175–9.

44. Neideen T, Lam M, Brasel KJ. Preinjury beta blockers are associated with increased mortality in geriatric trauma patients. *J Trauma*. 2008;65:1016–20.

45. Hirsh J, Fuster V, Ansell J, et al. American Heart Association/ American College of Cardiology Foundation guide to warfarin therapy. *Circulation*. 2003;107:1692–711.

46. Williams TM, Sadjadi J, Harken AH, Victorino GP. The necessity to assess anticoagulation status in elderly injured patients. *J Trauma*. 2008;65:772–7.

47. Kirsch MJ, Vrabec GA, Marley RA, Salvator AE, Muakkassa FF. Preinjury warfarin and geriatric orthopedic trauma patients: a case-matched study. *J Trauma*. 2004;57:1230–3.

48. Lavoie A, Ratte S, Clas D, et al. Preinjury warfarin use among elderly patients with closed head injuries in a trauma center. *J Trauma*. 2004;56:802–7.

49. Mina AA, Bair HA, Howells GA, Bendick PJ. Complications of preinjury warfarin use in the trauma patient. *J Trauma*. 2003;54:842–7.

50. Ohm C, Mina A, Howells G, Bair H, Bendick P. Effects of antiplatelet agents on outcomes for elderly patients with traumatic intracranial hemorrhage. *J Trauma*. 2005;58:518–22.

51. Ivascu FA, Howells GA, Junn FS et al. Predictors of mortality in trauma patients with intracranial hemorrhage on preinjury aspirin or clopidogrel. *J Trauma*. 2008;65:785–8.

52. Holbrook A, Schulman S, Witt DM, et al. Evidence-based management of anticoagulant therapy: Antithrombotic therapy and prevention of thrombosis. 9th ed. American College of Chest Physicians Evidence-based Clinical Practice Guidelines. *Chest*. 2012;141:e152–84s.

53. Kaatz S, Kouides PA, Garcia DA, et al. Guidance on the emergent reversal of oral thrombin and factor Xa inhibitors. *Am J Hematol*. 2012;87:S141–5.

54. Majeed A, Eelde A, Agren A, et al. Thromboembolic safety and efficacy of prothrombin complex concentrates in the emergency reversal of warfarin coagulopathy. *J Thromb*. 2012;129:146–51.

55. Ansell J, Hirsh J, Dalen J, et al. Managing oral anticoagulant therapy. *Chest*. 2001;119:22–38S.

56. Pracht EE, Langland-Orban B, Flint L. Survival advantage for elderly trauma patients treated in a designated trauma center. *J Trauma*. 2011;71(1):69–77.

57. Mann NC, Cahn RM, Mullins RJ, Brand DM, Jurkovich GJ. Survival among injured geriatric patients during construction of a statewide trauma system. *J Trauma*. 2001;50:1111–16.

58. Shifflette VK, Lorenzo M, Mangram AJ, et al. Should age be a factor to change from a level II to a level I trauma activation? *J Trauma*. 2010;69(1):88–92.

59. Demetriades D, Sava J, Alo K, et al. Old age as a criterion for trauma team activation. *J Trauma*. 2001;51(4):754–6.

60. Bergeron E, Lavoie A, Belcaid A, Ratte S, Clas D. Should patients with isolated hip fractures be included in trauma registries? *J Trauma.* 2005;58:793–7.

61. Fallon WF, Rader E, Zyzanski S, et al. Geriatric outcomes are improved by a geriatric trauma consultation service. *J Trauma.* 2006;61:1040–6.

62. Calland JF, Ingraham AM, Martin ND, et al. *Geriatric Trauma Practice Management Guideline (Update* 2010) (Chicago, IL: Eastern Association for the Surgery of Trauma, accessed from www.east.org/resources/treatment-guidelines/geriatric-trauma-(update)).

63. Centers for Disease Control and Prevention. Guidelines for Field Triage of Injured Patients Recommendations of the National Expert Panel on Field Triage, 2011. *MMWR.* 2012;61:1–21.

64. Milzman DP, Rothenhaus TC. Resuscitation of the geriatric patient. *Emerg Clin North Am.* 1996;14:233–45.

65. Demetriades D, Karaiskakis M, Velmahos G, et al. Effect of early intensive management of geriatric trauma patients. *Br J Surg.* 2002;89:1319–22.

66. Wang HE, Callaway CW, Peitzman AB, Tisherman SA. Admission hypothermia and outcome after major trauma. *Crit Care Med.* 2005;33(6):1296–30.

67. Rathlev NK, Medzon R, Lowery D, et al. Intracranial pathology in elders with blunt head trauma. *Acad Emerg Med.* 2006;13(v):302–7.

68. Mack LR, Chan SB, Silva JC, Hogan TM. The use of head computed tomography in elderly patients sustaining minor head trauma. *J Emerg Med.* 2003;24:157–62.

69. Li J, Brown J, Levine M. Mild head injury, anticoagulants, and risk of intracranial injury. *Lancet* 2001;357:771–2.

70. Reynolds FD, Dietz PA, Higgins D, Whitaker TS. Time to deterioration of the elderly, anticoagulated, minor head injury patient who presents without evidence of neurologic abnormality. *J Trauma.* 2003;54:492–6.

71. Meditto VG, Lucci M, Polonara S, et al. Management of minor head injury in patients receiving oral anticoagulant therapy: A prospective study of a 24-hour observation protocol. *Ann Emerg Med.* 2012;59(6): 451–5.

72. Touger M, Gennis P, Nathanson N, et al. Validity of a decision rule to reduce cervical spine radiography in elderly patients with blunt trauma. *Ann Emerg Med.* 2002;40(3):287–93.

73. Lomoschitz FM, Blackmore CC, Mirza SK, Mann FA. Cervical spine injuries in patients 65 years old and older: epidemiologic analysis regarding the effects of age and injury mechanism on distribution, type, and stability of injuries. *AJR Am J Roentgenol.* 2002;178:573–7.

74. Stiell IG, Wells GA, Vandemheen K, et al. Variation in emergency department use of cervical spine radiography for alert, stable trauma patients. *CMAJ.* 1997;156:1537–44.

75. Schrag SP, Toedter LJ, McQuay N. Cervical spine fractures in geriatric blunt trauma patients with low-energy mechanism: Are clinical predictors adequate? *Am J Surg.* 2008;195:170–3.

76. Regenbogen VS, Rogers LF, Atlas SW, Kim KS. Cervical spinal cord injuries in patients with cervical spondylosis. *AJR Am J Roentgenol.* 1986;146:277–84.

77. Simon B, Cushman J, Barraco R. Pain management guidelines for blunt thoracic trauma. *J Trauma.* 2005;59:1256–67.

78. Bulger EM, Areneson MA, Mock CN, Jurkovich GJ. Rib fractures in the elderly. *J Trauma.* 2000;48(6):1040–7.

79. Stawicki SP, Grossman MD, Hoey BA, Miller DL, Reed JF 3rd. Rib fractures in the elderly: a marker of injury severity. *J Am Geriatr Soc.* 2004;52:805–8.

80. Bergeron E, Lavoie A, Clas D, et al. Elderly trauma patients with rib fractures are at greater risk of death and pneumonia. *J Trauma.* 2003;54(3):478–85.

81. Victorino GP, Chong TJ, Pal JD. Trauma in the elderly patient. *Arch Surg.* 2003;138:1093–8.

82. Newell MA, Schlitzkus LL, Waibel BH, et al. "Damage control" in the elderly: futile endeavor or fruitful enterprise? *J Trauma.* 2010;69(5):1049–53.

83. Nordell E, Jarnlo GB, Jetsen C, Nordstrom L, Thorngren KG. Accidental falls and related fractures in 65–74 year olds: a retrospective study of 332 patients. *Acta Orthop Scand.* 2000;71:175–9.

84. Dominguez S, Liu P, Roberts C, Mandell M, Richman PB. Prevalence of traumatic hip and pelvic fractures in patients with suspected hip fracture and negative initial standard radiographs – a study of emergency department patients. *Acad Emerg Med.* 2005;12(4):366–9.

85. Hossain M, Barwick C, Sinha AK, et al. Is magnetic resonance imaging necessary to exclude occult hip fracture? *Injury.* 2007;38:1204–08.

86. Della Rocca GJ, Leung KS, Pape HC. Periprosthetic fractures: epidemiology and future projections. *J Orthop Trauma.* 2011;25(Suppl. 2):S66–70.

87. Papaioannou A, Watts NB, Kendler DL, et al. Diagnosis and management of vertebral fractures in elderly adults. *Am J Med.* 2002;113(3):220–8.

88. Chapman J, Bransford R. Geriatric spine fractures: An emerging health care crisis. *J Trauma.* 2007;62:S61–2.

89. Pottenger L. Orthopedic problems of aging. In *Geriatric Medicine: An Evidence-based Approach*, ed. Cassel et al. (New York: Springer, 2003).

90. Alost T, Waldrop RD. Profile of geriatric pelvic fractures presenting to the emergency department. *Am J Emerg Med.* 1997;15(6):576–8.

91. Henry SM, Pollak AN, Jones AL, Boswell S, Scalea TM. Pelvic fracture in geriatric patients: a distinct clinical entity. *J Trauma.* 2002;53(1):15–20.

92. O'Brien DP, Luchette FA, Pereira SJ, et al. Pelvic fracture in the elderly is associated with increased mortality. *Surgery.* 2002;132(4):710–14.

93. Zietlow SP, Capizzi PJ, Bannon MP, Farnell MB. Multisystem geriatric trauma. *J Trauma.* 1994;37(6):985–8.

94. Finelli FC, Jonsson J, Champion HR, Morelli S, Fouty WJ. A case control study for major trauma in geriatric patients. *J Trauma.* 1989;29(5):541–8.

95. Oreskovich MR, Howard JD, Copass MK, Carrico CJ. Geriatric trauma: Injury patterns and outcome. *J Trauma.* 1984;34(7):565–72.

96. Ferrera PC, Bartfield JM, D'Andrea CC. Outcomes of admitted geriatric trauma victims. *Am J Emerg Med,* 2000;18(5):575–80.

97. Richmond TS, Kauder D, Strumpf N, Meredith T. Characteristics and outcomes of serious traumatic injury in older adults. *J Am Geriatr Soc.* 2002;50:215–22.

98. Carrillo EH, Richardson JD, Malias MA, Cryer HM, Miller FB. Long term outcome of blunt trauma care in the elderly. *Surg Gynecol Obstet.* 1993;176:559–64.

99. McConnell KJ, Newgard CD, Mullins RJ, Arthur M, Hedges JR. Mortality benefit of transfer to level I versus level II trauma centers for head-injured patients. *Health Serv Res.* 2005;40(2):435–57.

100. Sampalis JS, Denis R, Frechette P, et al. Direct transport to tertiary trauma centers versus transfer from lower level facilities: impact on mortality and morbidity among patients with major trauma. *J Trauma.* 1997;43(2):288–95.

101. American Geriatrics Society, British Geriatrics Society, and American Academy of Orthopedic Surgeons Panel on Falls Prevention. Guideline for the Prevention of Falls in Older Persons. *J Am Geriatr Soc.* 2001;49:664–72.

102. Caplan GA, Williams AJ, Daly B, Abraham K. A randomized, controlled trial of comprehensive geriatric assessment and multidisciplinary intervention after discharge of elderly from the emergency department – the DEED II study. *J Am Geriatr Soc.* 2004;52(9):1417–23.

Chapter

Pain management in the elderly

Ula Hwang and Timothy Platts-Mills

Pitfalls

Undertreatment

It has been repeatedly demonstrated that older adults face disparities in pain care when compared with younger adults. Although older adults have acute and chronic pain as often as if not more than the general population, they frequently receive less treatment and experience less pain relief than younger adults [1–4]. This is particularly true in the emergency department (ED) setting, where oligoanalgesia among older adults has been described based both on high rates of pain at the end of the ED visit and lower rates of treatment for older versus younger adults [5–10]. While increased attention to this issue has resulted in some improvement in pain care documentation and use of analgesics in older adults [11], older adults with acute pain are still less likely to receive treatment than younger patients and still often leave the ED with pain.

Unrelieved pain has negative consequences for physiological, functional, and psychological outcomes resulting in an unnecessary burden on patients and the health care system [12]. Pain in older adults interferes with day-to-day functioning as indicated by difficulty or dependence in the ability to perform basic activities of daily living [13,14]. Unrelieved pain can result in impaired gastrointestinal and pulmonary function, nausea and dyspnea, increased metabolic rate (and in the case of cancer, increased tumor growth and metastases), impaired immune response, insomnia, delayed healing, and inability to walk or move about [12,15,16]. Pain has been identified as a risk factor for functional decline and increased dependency in older adults [17]. Psychological changes associated with persistent pain include anxiety and depression [18]. Unrelieved acute pain is associated with poor outcomes during hospitalization and with the development of chronic pain [19,20]. For older adults, it has been shown that unrelieved hip fracture pain is associated with longer hospital length of stay, missed or shortened physical therapy sessions, and delays to ambulation [21)]. Inadequate analgesia for older adults after surgery has been shown to be a risk factor for developing delirium [22,23]. For patients with hip fractures who do not receive adequate analgesia, severe pain increases the risk of delirium greater than ninefold [24].

Drug sensitivity and clearance in older adults

There are a number of factors which make effective pain management in older adults more difficult than in younger individuals. Age-related changes in metabolism and body mass distribution impact how drugs are absorbed and eliminated. These changes begin at 20–30 years of age and impact both pharmacodynamics (how a drug acts at receptor sites) and pharmacokinetics (how drugs are distributed and eliminated) [25]. Decreased lean body mass and total body water, and increased fatty tissue, coupled with decreased liver and renal clearance result in decreased drug elimination. As a result of these changes, analgesics, and in particular opioids, should be administered less frequently and in lower doses in older adults than in younger adults [26].

Adverse drug events

A second factor complicating the treatment of pain in older adults is the high prevalence of polypharmacy. Among ED patients aged 65 or older, over 90% are on at least 1 medication [27] and up to 50% receive a new medication upon discharge from the ED [28]. The increased risk of drug reactions in older adults is not caused by age, but is instead secondary to the physiologic changes that occur with aging, compounded by the higher rates of polypharmacy, comorbidities, severe illness, and prior drug reactions in older adults [29]. Adults aged 65 and older make up more than one-quarter of all ED visits due to adverse drug events and are more than twice as likely to have an adverse drug event when compared with younger patients [30].

Beers Criteria and analgesic risks

Since the early 1990s, to assist in medication prescribing for older adults, an interdisciplinary panel of experts in geriatric care, clinical pharmacology, and psychopharmacology has developed guidelines and criteria for appropriate medication use in older adults. These are known as the Beers Criteria. Using a modified Delphi approach for safe medication use, the medical literature has been reviewed for potentially inappropriate medications that have been incorporated into quality measures in the nursing home, community, outpatient, and acute care settings. The most recent update was completed in 2012 and

Table 8.1. 2012 AGS Beers Criteria for potentially inappropriate medication use in older adults – analgesics and muscle relaxants. Adapted with permission from reference [31]. See reference for further information

Drug category	Rationale	Recommendations
Meperidine	Not effective oral analgesic; may cause neurotoxicity; safer alternatives available	AVOID
Non-COX, NSAIDs (oral) Aspirin (>325 mg/day) Diclofenac Diflunisal Etodolac Fenoprofen Ibuprofen Ketoprofen Meclofenamate Mefenamic acid Meloxicam Nabumetone Naproxen Oxaprozin Piroxicam Sulindac Tolmetin	Increased GI bleeding risk (especially >75 years old or taking corticosteroids, anticoagulants, or antiplatelet agents). Upper GI ulcers, gross bleeding, or perforation caused by NSAID use in 1% of patients treated for 3–6 months, 2–4% for those treated > 1 year. Use of proton pump inhibitor or misoprostol reduces but does not eliminate risk	AVOID CHRONIC USE unless other alternatives not effective and patient can take gastroprotective agents
Indomethacin Ketorolac (both oral and parenteral)	Increased risk of GI bleed and peptic ulcer disease. Indomethacin has most adverse effects	AVOID
Pentazocine	Opioid analgesic that causes adverse CNS effects (confusion, hallucinations); safer alternatives available	AVOID
Skeletal muscle relaxants Carisoprodol Chlorzoxazone Cyclobenzaprine Metaxalone Methocarbamol Orphenadrine	Most muscle relaxants poorly tolerated because of anticholinergic adverse effects, sedation, risk of fracture	AVOID

identifies the following best practice guidelines: 1) medications to avoid in older adults regardless of disease or conditions; 2) medications considered potentially inappropriate in older adults with certain diseases or syndromes; and 3) medications to be used with caution [31].

The American Geriatrics Society (AGS) 2012 Beers Criteria Updated Expert Panel identified 53 medications, of which 26 are considered analgesic or muscle relaxant medications that fall under the categories of opioids, non-cyclooxygenase (COX)-selective, nonsteroidal anti-inflammatory drugs (NSAIDs), and skeletal muscle relaxants. For a list of these drugs, the rationales for why they should be avoided, and the expert panel's recommendation on use, please see Table 8.1. For a list of analgesics and muscle relaxants that are considered potentially inappropriate for patients with specific diseases or syndromes, please see Table 8.2.

Analgesic options

Unfortunately no guidelines currently exist on acute analgesic treatment and dosing for older adults. Evidence-based guidelines in pain treatment for older adults have been primarily focused on

treatment of chronic or persistent pain with medication recommendations divided into short- (<6 weeks) and long-term (> 6 weeks) treatments [32]. There is insufficient evidence at present to support guidelines further characterizing which patients with acute pain are most likely to benefit from alternative therapies including non-opioids and regional anesthesia. It is our general recommendation, however, that the World Health Organization (WHO) analgesic "pain ladder" [33,34] is a good model to follow for the treatment of acute ED pain in older adults:

- Mild pain should be treated with non-opiates (e.g., acetaminophen).
- Moderate pain should be treated with an oral opioid (e.g., oxycodone).
- Severe pain should be treated with an opioid (preferably parenteral) that can be easily titrated.

Non-opioids

Acetaminophen

Acetaminophen is perhaps the safest analgesic in older ED patients because of the ability to control dosing (i.e., nurses

Table 8.2. 2012 AGS Beers Criteria for potentially inappropriate medication use in older adults – analgesics and muscle relaxants that may exacerbate specific diseases or syndromes. Adapted with permission from reference [31]. See reference for further information

Disease or syndrome	Drug category	Rationale	Recommendations
Cardiovascular Heart failure	NSAID and COX-2 inhibitors	Potential to promote fluid retention and exacerbate heart failure	AVOID
Central nervous system Chronic seizures or epilepsy	Tramadol	Lowers seizure threshold; may be acceptable in patients with well-controlled seizures	AVOID
Central nervous system Delirium	Meperidine	Avoid in older adults with high risk of delirium because of inducing or worsening delirium	AVOID
Gastrointestinal History of gastric or duodenal ulcers	Aspirin (>325mg/day) Non-COX-2 selective NSAIDs	Exacerbate existing or cause new ulcers	AVOID unless other alternatives are not effective and patient can take gastroprotective agent (PPI or misoprostol)
Renal Chronic kidney disease stage IV, V	NSAIDs	May increase risk of kidney injury	AVOID

administer medications) and the absence of gastrointestinal, renal, and cardiovascular risks with appropriate dosing. Effective for musculoskeletal pain, it is recommended by the American Geriatrics Society (AGS) as a first-line agent for mild ongoing and persistent pain, with increased dosing if pain relief is not satisfactory (up to 4000 mg/24 h) before moving onto a stronger alternative [32]. Risks of hepatic toxicity with acetaminophen are minimal and have primarily been observed with long-term use [35]. Nonetheless, acetaminophen should be avoided in patients with liver disease or a history of heavy alcohol use. Unfortunately, it is not as effective for inflammatory pain, and patients presenting to the ED with acute pain frequently experience more than mild pain.

NSAIDs

All commonly used NSAIDs are on the Beers list of inappropriate medications for older adults. Even short-term use of NSAIDs should be considered unacceptable in older adults with diabetes, impaired kidney function, or taking medications that may impair kidney function (diuretics, ACE inhibitors) or metformin [36]. Both renal and gastrointestinal toxicity from NSAIDs are dose- and time-dependent. The patient's risk factors for side effects and recent history of NSAID exposure should be reviewed prior to administering or prescribing NSAIDs.

Despite these concerns, ibuprofen and ketorolac are commonly used in the treatment of acute pain in older ED patients. Ketorolac (both its oral and parenteral forms) is listed as a Beers Criteria drug that is inappropriate for use in older adults and is an analgesic to avoid. It is suggested that the remaining non-selective NSAIDs (e.g., ibuprofen, naproxen, aspirin >325mg) be avoided if used on a long-term basis (>4 weeks): "Key issues in the selection of NSAID therapy are pain amelioration, cardiovascular risk, nephrotoxicity, drug interactions, and gastrointestinal toxicity" [32].

For these reasons, NSAIDs may still be used judiciously in the acute setting for older patients who do not have contraindications (decreased renal function, gastropathy, cardiovascular disease, congestive heart failure). Reduced doses

and limitations on frequency (e.g., prescribing ibuprofen 200 mg maximally three times a day [32]) should be considered if NSAIDs are to be used and prescribed from the ED. When NSAIDs are administered, patients should be informed of the risks and warning signs of adverse effects (decreased urination, abdominal pain, nausea) [37]. Gastric acid suppression with a proton pump inhibitor should also be considered [32].

Opioids

Opioids are recommended for the treatment of moderate to severe pain in older adults by the AGS for persistent pain [32] and by the WHO pain ladder [33,34]. It is our recommendation that for those who present in moderate pain (pain score 4–7 on a scale of 0–10), oral opioids (e.g., oxycodone) be given initially. For those in severe pain (pain score 8–10), parenteral opioids such as morphine or hydromorphone should be considered as these are more effective and easily titrated.

Fortunately, unlike many non-opioids (e.g., acetaminophen), opioid analgesics do not have a ceiling effect: There is no maximal dose for opioids and their use is constrained only by the development of common side effects including nausea, vomiting, dizziness, constipation, and somnolence. For these reasons, if an oral opioid such as oxycodone is prescribed from the ED upon discharge for outpatient use, it is our recommendation that it should not be prescribed as a combination medication (e.g., Percocet – acetaminophen and oxycodone) secondary to the ceiling dose limitation of the non-opioid drug (i.e., no more than 4000 mg of acetaminophen is recommended on a daily basis [32]). Instead, older adults who are sent home with analgesics from the ED should receive a recommendation for a maximal dose of acetaminophen and a separate prescription for an opioid to take as needed. Additionally, if opioids are prescribed from the ED in older adults, because of the constipating effects of opioids it is also recommended that a bowel regimen be concurrently given. One that consists of both a stool softener (e.g., docusate) and laxative (e.g., senna) is suggested.

Unfortunately, use of opioids has also been associated with increased rates of falls and fall-related injuries in older adults

[38]. More recently, a publication of opioid safety in an adult veteran population found that higher doses of opioids were associated with increased risk of overdose death. Veterans who received as-needed (PRN) and regularly scheduled doses, however, had no significant risk of overdose [39]. The potential for serious adverse events should be reviewed at the time of discharge, with older adults initiating outpatient treatment with an opioid.

Specific opioids have been associated with specific risks. When compared with hydrocodone, codeine carried an increased cardiovascular event risk after 180 days, and oxycodone and codeine had higher all-cause mortality at 30 days [40]. QT prolongation and torsades de pointes are more commonly seen with methadone than other opioids [41]. Opioids have also been associated with an increased risk for fractures, adverse events resulting in hospitalizations, and mortality. In particular, increased rates of injuries have been associated with methadone, propoxyphene, and fentanyl [42]. Although potentially important for long-term pain management, these results are based on analyses of observational data and, despite appropriate methods for adjustment, may still be confounded by indication (i.e., patients with a greater risk of death being more likely to receive opioids). As a result, it remains unclear how these results should inform pain care treatment in older adults [43].

With the growing recognition for the need for better pharmacologic management of pain in older adults, the National Institutes of Health Pain Consortium has identified several significant research priorities: 1) long-term safety and efficacy of commonly used analgesics; 2) optimal approaches to minimize side effects; and 3) understanding of risk factors and methods of detection of opioid abuse/misuse [44].

Regional anesthesia

Femoral nerve blocks are a feasible and effective primary or adjunctive therapy for acute pain due to hip fractures. Usually this involves administration of a long-acting local anesthetic (e.g., bupivacaine) under ultrasound guidance [45]. Regional anesthesia has the important advantage of limiting the patient's exposure to systemic analgesics. Unfortunately, many forms of acute pain are not easily amenable to regional anesthesia.

Geriatric ED pain care quality indicators

Quality indicators are operational metrics used to determine whether or not care is delivered well or poorly. They set a minimum standard for the care expected from clinicians. Following the Assessing Care of Vulnerable Elders (ACOVE) quality indicator approach [46], a task force convened by the Society for Academic Emergency Medicine (SAEM) and the American College of Emergency Physicians (ACEP) developed the following indicators to measure the quality of geriatric pain care received in the ED setting [47]:

1. Formal assessment for the presence of acute pain should be documented within 1 hour of ED arrival.
2. If a patient remains in the ED for >6 hours, a second pain assessment should be documented.
3. If a patient receives pain treatment, a pain reassessment should be documented prior to discharge from the ED.
4. If a patient has moderate to severe pain, pain treatment should be initiated (or a reason documented why it was not initiated).
5. Meperidine (Demerol) should not be used to treat pain in older adults.
6. If a patient is prescribed opioid analgesics upon discharge from the ED, a bowel regimen should also be provided.

Goals of pain care management

Ultimately, goals of care should include assessment of pain, treatment of the pain, and reduction in pain. Akin to the management of diabetic ketoacidosis in the ED setting, where frequent measurements of glucose and electrolyte levels are necessary to appropriately manage the patient's hyperglycemia, effective management of acute pain in older adults requires frequent reassessments of pain and often requires retreatment. Because of concerns about drug sensitivity, decreased clearance, and a greater risk of adverse drug events, the maxim "start low and go slow" is recommended when dosing analgesics for older adults. Careful titration with frequent reassessment will allow for optimal acute pain care in older adults [48].

Pain assessment

Studies have demonstrated that documentation of pain scores improves analgesic administration patterns in the ED [49] and that documentation is less likely to occur for older adults [50]. The need for titration of analgesic dosing requires frequent assessment and reassessment of pain in older adults. Thus, the assessment of pain is critical for the safe and effective treatment of acute pain.

Pain scores

Numerous pain assessment methods have been described and studied in older adults [26]. For patients who are cognitively intact, the verbal numeric rating scale is the most easily administered method of assessing pain and the one preferred by patients [51,52]. The Verbal Descriptor Scale may serve as a more sensitive and reliable instrument for measuring pain in older adults than the numeric rating scale [52], but the marginal benefit of using a descriptor scale rather than a numeric rating scale in cognitively intact older adults is unclear. Several tools have been proposed for the assessment of pain in cognitively impaired patients. These tools are generally based on observation of behaviors indicative of pain and include the Abbey Pain Scale (Abbey) [53], assessment of discomfort in dementia (ADD) protocol [54], checklist of nonverbal pain indicators (CNPI) [55], Noncommunicative Patient's Pain Assessment Instrument (NOPPAIN) [56], Pain Assessment Checklist for Seniors with Limited Ability to Communicate (PACSLAC) [57], and pain assessment in advanced dementia (PAINAD) [58]. Although many of these tools demonstrate potential, most are still in the early stages of development and testing. More important than which scale is used is the point that an effort should be made to assess pain in all cognitively impaired patients and treat it when present.

Patient goals of pain care

Incorporating patient preferences and goals of care for treatment and pain relief is also a priority of quality geriatric patient care [59,60]. Because pain control in older adults almost always involves some trade-off between pain relief and the risk of unwanted side effects, an open discussion with the patient can help the provider understand the manner and degree to which the pain causes problems for the patient and what they perceive to be their risks of various side effects. Many older adults have prior experience with analgesics, and these experiences can help guide decision making.

Among patients with acute severe pain, most patients desire that pain be treated in the ED, would like to be treated early on, are agreeable to having a nurse administer medication prior to physician evaluation, and would prefer pain control without sedation [61]. These preferences support the use of protocols for nurse-administered analgesia. They also indicate the need for a titrated approach to pain management in older adults in order to balance pain control with side effects such as sedation.

Summary

The effective management of acute pain in older adults is a common challenge faced by emergency providers. Because of the profound impact of pain on the health and function of older adults, pain management is an important priority in this population. However, the high frequency of analgesic side effects in older adults demands a cautious approach. Acetaminophen, NSAIDs, opioids, and regional anesthesia each have a role to play in acute pain management. Knowledge of the limitations, contraindications, and risks of these medications is essential for selecting the appropriate analgesic for both ED and early outpatient treatment in older patients. Communication about risks and close outpatient follow-up with a primary physician are essential to optimize the safe and effective treatment of pain in older adults.

Pearls

Keys to the successful treatment of pain in older adults are as follows.

- Assess for, treat, reassess for pain.
- Start low and go slow with analgesic dosing and titration.
- Use non-opioids for mild pain, oral opioids for moderate pain, and opioids that can be rapidly titrated for severe pain.
- Patients who require analgesic treatment at home should receive a maximal dose of acetaminophen (if no contraindication) and an opioid as needed.

References

1. Honori S, Patterson DR, Gibbons J, et al. Comparison of pain control medication in three age groups of elderly patients. *J Burn Care Rehab*. 1997;18:500–4.

2. Federman AD, Litke A, Morrison RS. Association of age with analgesic use for back and joint disorders in outpatient settings. *Am J Geriatr Pharmacother*. 2006;4:306–15.

3. Elliott AM, Smith BH, Penny KI, Smith WC, Chambers WA. The epidemiology of chronic pain in the community. *Lancet*. 1999;354(9186):1248–52.

4. Blyth FM, March LM, Brnabic AJ, et al. Chronic pain in Australia: a prevalence study. *Pain*. 2001;89(2–3):127–34.

5. Terrell KT, Hui SL, Castelluccio P, et al. Analgesic prescribing for patients who are discharged from an emergency department. *Pain Med*. 2010;11:1072–7.

6. Heins A, Grammas M, Heins JK, et al. Determinants of variation in analgesic and opioid prescribing practice in an emergency department. *J Opioid Manag*. 2006;2:335–40.

7. Hwang U, Richardson LD, Harris B, Morrison RS. The quality of emergency department pain care for older adult patients. *J Am Geriatr Soc*. 2010;58:2122–8.

8. Iyer RG. Pain documentation and predictors of analgesic prescribing for elderly patients during emergency department visits. *J Pain Symptom Manage*. 2010;c:367–73.

9. Arendts G, Fry M. Factors associated with delay to opiate analgesia in emergency departments. *J Pain*. 2006;7:682–6.

10. Platts-Mills TF, Esserman DA, Brown L, et al. Older US emergency department patients are less likely to receive pain medication than younger patients: results from a national survey. *Ann Emerg Med*. 2012;60(2):199–206.

11. Herr K, Titler M. Acute pain assessment and pharmacological management practices for the older adult with a hip fracture: review of ED trends. *J Emerg Nurs*. 2009;35:312–20.

12. Berry P, Dahl J. The new JCAHO pain standards: Implications for pain management nurses. *Pain Manage Nurs*. 2000;1:3–12.

13. Ferrell B, Ferrell B, Osterweil D. Pain in the nursing home. *J Amer Gerontol Soc*. 1990;38:409–14.

14. Jaycox A, Carr D, Payne R, et al. *Management of Cancer Pain. Clinical Practice Guidelines No. 9* (Rockville, MD: Agency for Health Care Policy and Research, 1994).

15. Sasamura T, Nakamura S, Iida Y, et al. Morphine analgesia suppresses tumor growth and metastasis in a mouse model of cancer pain produced by orthotopic tumor inoculation. *Eur J Pharmacol*. 2002;441(3):185–91.

16. Harimaya Y, Koizumi K, Andoh T, et al. Potential ability of morphine to inhibit the adhesion, invasion and metastasis of metastatic colon 26-L5 carcinoma cells. *Cancer Lett*. 2002;187(1–2):121–7.

17. Hughs S, Gibbs J, Dunlop D, et al. Predictors of decline in manual performance in older adults. *J Am Geriatr Soc*. 1997;45:905–10.

18. Siddall P, Cousins M. Persistent pain as a disease entity: implications for clinical management. *Anesth Analg*. 2004;99:510–20.

19. Dworkin R. Which individuals with acute pain are most likely to develop a chronic pain syndrome? *Pain Forum*. 1997;6:127–36.

20. Desbiens N, Mueller-Rizner N, Connors A, Hamel M, Wenger N. Pain in the oldest-old during hospitalization and up to one year later. *J Am Geriatr Soc*. 1997;45:1167–72.

21. Morrison RS, Magaziner J, McLaughlin MA, et al. The impact of post-operative pain on outcomes following hip fracture. *Pain*. 2003;103(3):303–11.

22. Duggleby W, Lander J. Cognitive status and postoperative pain: older adults. *J Pain Sympt Manage.* 1994;9:19–27.

23. Lynch E, Lazor M, Gelis J, et al. The impact of postoperative pain on the development of postoperative delirium. *Anesth Analg.* 1998;86:781–5.

24. Morrison RS, Magaziner J, Gilbert M, et al. Relationship between pain and opioid analgesics on the development of delirium following hip fracture. *J Gerontol.* 2003;58:76–81.

25. Evans R, Ireland G, Morely J, et al., ed. *Pharmacology and Aging* (Pasadena, CA: Beverly Cracom Publications, 1996).

26. Hwang U, Jagoda A. Geriatric emergency analgesia. In *Emergency Department Analgesia*, ed. Thomas S. (Cambridge, UK: Cambridge University Press, 2008).

27. Hohl C, Dankoff J, Colacone A, Afilalo M. Polypharmacy, adverse drug-related events, and potential adverse drug interactions in elderly patients presenting to an emergency department. *Ann Emerg Med.* 2001;38:666–71.

28. Beers MH, Storrie M, Lee G. Potential adverse drug interactions in the emergency room. An issue in the quality of care. *Ann Intern Med.* 1990;112:61–4.

29. Beyth R, Schorr R, ed. *Medication Use* (Philadelphia, PA: W.B. Saunders, 1998).

30. McDonnell PJ, Jacobs MR. Hospital admissions resulting from preventable adverse drug reactions. *Ann Pharmacother.* 2002;36:1331–6.

31. American Geriatrics Society 2012 Beers Criteria Update Expert Panel. American Geriatrics Society updated Beers Criteria for potentially inappropriate medication use in older adults. *J Am Geriatr Soc.* 2012;60(4):616–31.

32. American Geriatrics Society Panel on the Pharmacological Management of Persistent Pain in Older Persons. Pharmacological management of persistent pain in older persons. *J Am Geriatr Soc.* 2009;57:1331–46.

33. WHO. *WHO Pain Ladder* (accessed January 4, 2007 from www.who.int/cancer/palliative/painladder/en/).

34. National Comprehensive Cancer Network. *NCCN Clinical Practice Guidelines in Oncology* (accessed January 4, 2007 from www.nccn.org/professionals/physician_gls/f_guidelines.asp#care).

35. Watkins PB, Kaplowitz N, Slattery JT, et al. Aminotransferase elevations in healthy adults receiving 4 grams of acetaminophen daily: A randomized controlled trial. *JAMA.* 2006;296:87–93.

36. Platts-Mills TF, Richmond NL, Hunold KM, Bowling CB. Life-threatening hyperkalemia following two days of ibuprofen. *Am J Emerg Med.* 2012;13(2):465.

37. Bocing CB, O'Hare AM. Managing older adults with CKD: Individualized versus disease-based approaches. *Am J Kidney Dis.* 2012;59:293–302.

38. Huang AR, Mallet L, Rochefort CM, et al. Medication-related falls in the elderly: causative factors and preventive strategies. *Drugs Aging.* 2012;29:359–76.

39. Bohnert AS, Valenstein M, Bair MJ, et al. Association between opioid prescribing patterns and opioid overdose-related deaths. *JAMA.* 2011;305:1315–21.

40. Solomon DH, Rassen JA, Glynn RJ, et al. The comparative safety of opioids for nonmalignant pain in older adults. *Arch Int Med.* 2010;170:1979–86.

41. Chan BK, Tam LK, Wat CY, et al. Opioids in chronic non-cancer pain. *Expert Opin Pharmacother.* 2011;12:705–20.

42. Blackwell SA, Montgomery MA, Waldo D, et al. National study of medications associated with injury in elderly Medicare/Medicaid dual enrollees. *J Am Pharm Assoc.* 2003;49(6):751–9.

43. Hwang U, Morrison RS, Richardson LD, Todd KH. A painful setback: Misinterpretation of analgesic safety in older adults may inadvertently worsen pain care. *Arch Int Med.* 2011;171(12):1127.

44. Reid MC, Bennett DA, Chen WG, et al. Improving the pharmacologic management of pain in older adults: identifying the research gaps and methods to address them. *Pain Medicine.* 2011;12(9):1336–57.

45. Beaudoin FL, Nagdev A, Merchant RC, Becker BM. Ultrasound-guided femoral nerve blocks in elderly patients with hip fractures. *Am J Emerg Med.* 2010;28(1):76–81.

46. Wenger N, Shekelle P. Assessing care of vulnerable elders: ACOVE project overview. *Ann Intern Med.* 2001;135(8, Part 2):642–6.

47. Terrell KT, Hustey FM, Hwang U, et al. Quality indicators for geriatric emergency care. *Acad Emerg Med.* 2009;16:441–50.

48. Fine PG. Treatment guidelines for the pharmacological management of pain in older persons. *Pain Med.* 2012;13(Suppl. 2):s57–66.

49. Silka PA, Roth MM, Moreno G, Merrill L, Geiderman JM. Pain scores improve analgesic administration patterns for trauma patients in the emergency department. *Acad Emerg Med.* 2004;11:264–70.

50. Iyer RG. Pain documentation and predictors of analgesic prescribing for elderly patients during emergency department visits. *J Pain Sympt Manage.* 2010;41:367–73.

51. Ware LJ, Epps CD, Herr K, Packard A. Evaluation of the Revised Faces Pain Scale, Verbal Descriptor Scale, Numeric Rating Scale, and Iowa Pain Thermometer in older minority adults. *Pain Management Nursing.* 2006;7(3):117–25.

52. Herr K, Spratt K, Mobiliy P, Richardson G. Pain intensity assessment in older adults: use of experimental pain to compare psychometric properties and usability of selected pain scales with younger adults. *Clin J Pain.* 2004;20:207–19.

53. Abbey J, Piller N, DeBellis A, et al. The Abbey Pain Scale. A 1-minute numerical indicator for people with late-stage dementia. *Int J Palliat Nurs.* 2004;10:6–13.

54. Krovach C, Weissman D, Griffie J, Matson S, Machka S. Assessment and treatment of discomfort for people with late-stage dementia. *J Pain Sympt Manage.* 1999;18:412–19.

55. Feldt K. The checklist of nonverbal pain indicators (CNPI). *Pain Management Nursing.* 2000;1:13–21.

56. Snow A, Weber J, O'Malley K, et al. NOPPAIN: a nurse assistant-administered pain assessment instrument for use in dementia. *Dement Geriatr Cogn Disord.* 2004;17:240–6.

57. Fuchs-Lacelle S, Hadjistavropoulos T. Development and preliminary validation of the pain assessment checklist for seniors with limited ability to communicate (PACSLAC). *Pain Management Nursing.* 2004;5:37–49.

58. Warden V, Hurley A, Volicer L. Development and psychometric evaluation of the pain assessment in advanced dementia (PAINAD) scale. *J Am Med Dir Assoc.* 2003;9–15.

59. Isaacs CG, Kistler C, Hunold KM, et al. *Shared Decision Making in the Selection of Outpatient Analgesics for Older Emergency Department Patients* (Chicago, IL: Society of Academic Emergency Medicine, 2012).

60. Bowling CB, O'Hare AM. Managing older adults with CKD: Individualized versus disease-based approaches. *Am J Kidney Dis*. 2012;59:293–302.

61. Beel TL, Mitchiner JC, Frederiksen SM, McCormick J. Patient preferences regarding pain medication in the ED. *Am J Emerg Med*. 2000;18:376–80.

Chapter

9

Chest pain in the elderly

Joseph R. Pare and Jeffrey I. Schneider

Introduction

This chapter will cover the evaluation of the geriatric patient presenting to the emergency department (ED) with chest pain. Although potentially an indication of acute cardiac ischemia, there are a number of alternative etiologies for the elderly individual with chest pain that will be discussed. These include several pulmonary, vascular, musculoskeletal, and gastrointestinal sources of chest pain syndromes. As with many other disease entities, geriatric patients may present with "atypical" symptoms, later in the course of their disease process, or with vague and/or constitutional complaints. Clinicians would be wise to keep their differential diagnoses broad when evaluating elderly patients with complaints of chest pain.

Cardiac causes of chest pain

Acute coronary syndrome

Approximately 8 to 10% of ED visits are for the evaluation of chest pain [1], and between 2 and 8% of these patients will be discharged from the ED despite having underlying cardiac etiology of their symptoms [2]. Approximately 20% of those older than 65 and nearly 30% of those over 75 will have at least one ED visit annually [3]. It is easy to appreciate from this that the financial and resource burden of geriatric patients with chest pain in the ED is substantial.

While clinicians generally consider acute coronary syndrome (ACS) as a potential cause of chest discomfort in patients with a chief complaint of chest pain, physicians must also recognize that elderly patients may present with vague symptoms such as dyspnea, fatigue, malaise, nausea, and vomiting in the absence of chest pain in the setting of acute cardiac ischemia [4]. Although some have suggested that research aimed at investigating myocardial ischemia in the elderly has been limited, there are some data which demonstrate differences in the presentation of elderly patients with ACS. Specifically, examination of a national registry of myocardial infarctions indicates that the complaint of chest pain was present in nearly 90% of patients age <65 years with ACS. However, only 57% of patients

>85 years old reported chest pain [4]. In addition the Worcester Heart Attack Study reported that amongst all patients with ACS, approximately 63% reported chest pain, whereas less than half of women >75 years old with ACS complained of chest pain [5].

Some have hypothesized that "atypical" presentations (e.g., malaise, nausea, or dyspnea in the absence of chest pain) occur more frequently in the elderly due to the physiologic effects of ACS on an aging body. For example, elderly patients may be more likely to present with dyspnea from ACS due to associated lung disease or acute left ventricular dysfunction. Other alternative theories include an elderly patient's potential inability to accurately recall and report symptoms [5].

Ischemic cardiac disease can be classified in several ways, but this chapter will break the topic into five etiologies of cardiac ischemia. All of these types of cardiac ischemia are due to primary cardiac lesions except for demand ischemia. Demand ischemia in other literature has been termed Type II MI by the 2007 Clinical Classification and there are limited data on its evaluation and treatment.

ST elevation myocardial infarction

As with all patients, irrespective of age, the goal of ST elevation myocardial infarction (STEMI) care is rapid reperfusion therapy. This can be accomplished by either pharmacologic or mechanical means. In general, percutaneous coronary intervention (PCI) is the preferred method for re-establishing coronary blood flow in geriatric patients with a STEMI [6]. While the administration of thrombolytics continues to play an important role in some instances of STEMI care, providers must be cognizant of absolute and relative contraindications to its use. For example, the elderly may be more likely to have a recent ischemic stroke, previous intracerebral hemorrhage, current anticoagulant use, or recent internal bleeding [5]. Similarly, in patients older than 75 years, the risk of complications associated with the administration of intravenous thrombolytics (e.g., intracerebral hemorrhage) is greater [5]. While the mortality benefit of PCI over fibrinolysis is known to decrease with an increase in door-to-balloon time, this effect is delayed in those

Geriatric Emergency Medicine, ed. Joseph H. Kahn, Brendan G. Magauran Jr., and Jonathan S. Olshaker. Published by Cambridge University Press.
© Cambridge University Press 2014.

patients older than 65 years. Specifically, the survival advantage associated with PCI was lost after 71 minutes for those less than 65 years, compared with 155 minutes for those older than 65 years of age [6]. In those patients for whom STEMI is complicated by cardiogenic shock, the SHOCK trial showed that there was a 15% reduction in 30-day mortality for patients age <75 years who undergo PCI. For those over the age of 75 years, however, the data are less clear [7].

Research has also looked at the utility of PCI for the very elderly patient (VEP), defined as age greater than 80 years. One report indicated that for the VEP, mortality could be cut from 62 to 34% if PCI was performed for acute myocardial infarction (AMI). Interestingly, nearly 40% of those aged >80 years that did not undergo PCI reported family/patient preference as the reason for refusing intervention. In comparison, renal dysfunction and cognitive impairment precluded PCI in 18 and 14% of cases, respectively [8].

Similarly, other analyses have demonstrated that PCI is valuable in patients older than 85 years of age [9]. A different but similar study looked at outcomes of PCI in the very elderly, but the cutoff was age greater than 85 years rather than 80. In regard to unadjusted in-hospital mortality for age >85 (102 cases) and those <85 (1597 cases), this was 3.9 and 0.68%, respectively. Additional important findings to note are that of those patients >85 who presented with STEMI, 26.6% died whereas those <85 presenting with STEMI had an in-hospital mortality rate of only 3.7%. However, in elderly patients presenting with non-ST elevation myocardial infarction (NSTEMI), post-STEMI, or other coronary syndrome there was no associated mortality with PCI in this trial [9].

NSTEMI

In addition to the variability in interventional therapy between geriatric and non-geriatric patients described above, there are also data to suggest that various medical therapies are utilized differently in elderly patients with NSTEMI or unstable angina, when compared with younger patients. Older individuals are less likely to receive antiplatelet therapy such as aspirin and clopidogrel, and they are less likely to receive early (within two days) revascularization procedures. Relatedly, they are more likely to suffer recurrent MI, congestive heart failure, stroke, and need for transfusion. Not surprisingly, patients older than 85 years of age had an adjusted odds ratio of 3 for the endpoint of in-hospital death [10]. While delays in definitive therapy or lack of administration of some therapies in the elderly might be partially explained by their atypical presentations, there is likely room for improvement in the care of geriatric patients with ACS.

Although their presentation may be atypical, most elderly patients with ACS have positive biomarkers upon initial presentation to the ED. In the CRUSADE Trial, 92% of those over 85 years old with ACS had laboratory evidence of such upon hospital arrival [10]. Additionally these very elderly patients had fewer cardiac risk factors, were more likely to have coronary artery disease (CAD), and nearly 42% of these patients had congestive heart failure on presentation when compared with those younger than 85 with NSTEMI who were enrolled in the study.

Demand ischemia

There are several instances in which elderly patients may have positive cardiac biomarkers in the absence of ACS. For example, "demand ischemia" may be seen in geriatric patients with sepsis, aortic dissection, stroke, large burns, toxic ingestions, cardiac trauma, cardiomyopathies, and renal failure. While the exact pathophysiology of this is poorly understood, it is thought to occur in the absence of true ACS [11,12]. Despite this, many of these patients do have underlying CAD and the clinical outcomes of those with positive biomarkers is poorer when compared with those who do not have a measureable troponin leak [13]. There are scant data on demand ischemia, and even fewer in elderly patients. The best recommendations at this time are to treat the suspected cause of demand ischemia rather than treating the patient for ACS.

Post-MI complications

While the risk of MI increases with age, so too does the risk of death. Older patients are more likely to exhibit the mechanical complications of MI (e.g., papillary muscle rupture, free wall rupture, and septal necrosis leading to ventricular septal defect), and the frequency of post-MI cardiac arrest also increases. Similarly, congestive heart failure (CHF) is a common consequence of MI in the elderly, with significant associated morbidity and mortality [14].

In the US, CHF affects approximately 5.7 million people and its care presents a significant cost burden with estimates of nearly $39 billion annually [15]. MI, which can cause ventricular remodeling and poor contractility, is a leading cause of CHF. It is known to be more prevalent in men than women, and the incidence increases from 1.9% in men aged 40–49 to 14.7% in men aged >80 years [15]. For women the rate increases from 1.4 to 12.8%, respectively for the same age groups. In addition to MI as a risk factor for the development of CHF, other factors such as hypertension and diabetes, which are thought to contribute to the development of CHF, are also more prevalent in the elderly [15].

Pericarditis

It has been suggested that pericarditis makes up as much as 5% of non-ACS chest pain visits [16]. Pericarditis is generally divided into infectious and non-infectious causes, and many of the risk factors for the development of pericarditis are common among elderly patients. For example, pericarditis is seen in as many as 5–10% of patients after transmural infarction (Dressler's syndrome) [16]. Similarly, 20% of patients who undergo cardiac surgery will develop pericarditis postoperatively [16].

Other, non-infectious causes of pericarditis are also frequently encountered in the geriatric population. These include pericarditis related to malignancy, dialysis, uremia, gout, and various vasculitides [16]. The elderly may also have infectious etiologies of pericarditis such as HIV disease, tuberculosis, and related to viruses such as enterovirus, adenovirus, or influenza. As with other syndromes, the elderly patient with pericarditis may present with a paucity of symptoms or atypical symptoms when compared with their younger counterparts [17].

As with all age groups, the treatment of pericarditis is tailored according to the etiology of the disease. Careful consideration of the use of nonsteroidal anti-inflammatory medications (NSAIDs) is warranted in the elderly given the potential for side effects such as worsening heart failure and/or renal failure, or gastrointestinal bleeding. In individuals with constrictive pericarditis, pericardiectomy may be warranted. As with many other disease processes, elderly patients tend to have poorer outcomes [16].

Pulmonary causes of chest pain

Pneumonia

Chest pain may be the sole presenting complaint in an elderly patient with pneumonia, and as many as 10% of elderly patients with pneumonia may present without any of the classic triad of symptoms of dyspnea, cough, and fever [18]. Among infectious etiologies, community-acquired pneumonia (CAP) is the most common cause of death in the US over the last 20 years, and the incidence of CAP in those over 80 years of age has been rising [19]. In 2005, of patients over age 65 years treated for CAP, nearly half were over the age of 80 years (47.5%) [19]. For a variety of reasons, increasing numbers of these patients are being treated as outpatients – admission rates have fallen from 63% in 1987 to 56% in 2005. Interestingly, despite an aging population and an increase in the total number of elderly patients being treated outside of a hospital setting, there has been a total decrease in the mortality associated with CAP in the geriatric patient population in recent years [19].

It has been postulated that two specific interventions have led to the improved outcomes of patients treated for CAP over the last 20 years. The first is that antibiotic-driven guidelines and clinical decision tools have helped physicians to make informed choices about management and care, and the second is the development and administration of vaccines against the influenza virus and pneumococcus bacterium [19].

Geriatric patients at long-term care facilities (e.g., nursing homes, assisted living, or skilled nursing facilities) are also prone to develop health care-related pulmonary infections. These infections may be a result of more virulent or drug-resistant organisms, and the reported mortality among patients in long-term assisted care facilities has been reported to be about 1 in 1000 patient-days (all causes) [20]. Underlying lung disease (e.g., chronic obstructive pulmonary disease, COPD), limited functional status, and a higher risk of aspiration make the geriatric population more susceptible to respiratory tract infections [20]. In addition to the common bacterial pathogens, viral infections are also associated with significant morbidity and mortality in this age group. For example, influenza and respiratory syncytial virus (RSV) are associated with mortalities that range from 5 to 40% in elderly patients [20]. As with CAP, clinical status, functional status, and the ability and capability of a particular chronic care facility may determine whether a geriatric patient with a viral lung infection is cared for in an inpatient hospital setting.

Pulmonary embolism

Pulmonary embolism (PE) is a disease that affects patients of all ages and its clinical presentation can be varied. As with many other causes of chest pain, rapid evaluation and treatment can be life saving. Within the medical literature, there is documentation of risk factors for PE [21] as well as guidelines that aid clinicians in determining which patients with chest pain may require further evaluation for PE [22–24].

In general, risk factors for the development of a PE are related to underlying health diseases or environmental causes. Venous stasis and endothelial damage both increase the risk for PE, therefore it is not surprising that age itself is also a risk factor [23]. Additional risk factors for PE that are common among elderly patients include obesity, hypertension, immobility, cancer, COPD, diabetes, stroke with paralysis, implanted cardiac device, CHF, and recent orthopedic surgery such as hip repair.

There are specific treatment considerations for elderly patients with PE. In a manner similar to ACS, the risk of bleeding with anticoagulation therapy is higher in geriatric patients than in younger patients [25], and the decision to administer one anticoagulant over another may be informed by a patient's comorbidities. For example, low-molecular weight heparin (LMWH) has been demonstrated to be superior to warfarin in reducing the rate of recurrent PE in those with cancer [25]. Relatedly, clinicians must be wary of LMWH dosing in the elderly, as dosing should take into account creatinine clearance [26]. Additionally, physicians would be wise to consider occult malignancy in geriatric patients who are found to have a PE without clear cause, as the discovery of an undetected malignancy in this group is not uncommon [24].

As previously noted, PE can be difficult to diagnose due to vague and variable complaints. Studies have demonstrated that this may be especially true in the geriatric population who are less likely to present with pleuritic chest pain than their younger counterparts (60 versus 87%) [27]. In addition, older patients may be more likely to present with syncope, cyanosis, and/or hypoxia [27]. PE is also known to be a fairly common complication after hip fractures; a review of a Medicare database demonstrated that nearly 2% of patients with hip fractures were subsequently diagnosed with a PE [28].

Although there is variation amongst centers, the diagnosis of PE is more and more frequently made via computed tomography pulmonary angiogram (CTPA). In many institutions this has replaced conventional angiography and ventilation–perfusion imaging as the diagnostic tool of choice. While some clinicians may use a D-dimer as a screening test in determining which patients require additional testing for the evaluation of potential PE, this may be less useful in an elderly patient. In one study which enrolled an unselected cohort of patients who underwent D-dimer testing (indication for testing not reported), patients up to the age of 40 had an average value of 294 ng/ml, those aged 60–80 averaged 854 ng/ml, and those over the age of 80 had an average value of nearly 1400 ng/ml. Importantly, less than 5% of patients greater than age 80 suspected of having deep venous thrombosis (DVT) or PE had a value of less than 500 ng/ml, the cutoff for not pursuing further testing [29]. This suggests that D-dimer may have a much more limited role in the diagnostic evaluation of venous thromboembolism in the geriatric population. Further prospective studies, including those which might suggest a higher threshold value for D-dimer in the elderly, are needed.

While the radiation exposure of a CTPA may be of less concern to clinicians caring for elderly patients, the prevalence of renal insufficiency (precluding the administration of intravenous contrast) and post-CT contrast nephropathy is an important consideration in the geriatric patient population. As many as 30% of patients with a glomerular filtration rate (GFR) of less than 60 ml/min/1.73 m^2 will develop contrast-induced nephropathy (CIN) [30]. These patients often require prolonged hospitalization, and have a reported mortality as high as 35% if hemodialysis is necessary [30]. Some have advocated for the administration of potential renal protective therapies such as intravenous hydration, theophylline, bicarbonate, N-acetylcysteine, and ascorbic acid in elderly patients who undergo intravenous contrast-enhanced CT – the data supporting this are beyond the scope of this chapter [30].

Geriatric patients may have one or more factors associated with poor outcomes in patients with PE based on the Geneva prognostic index. These include cancer, heart failure, hypoxia, hypotension, and previous or current DVT on ultrasound [21]. In patients with evidence of shock related to PE, urgent embolectomy or thrombolysis may be considered. As is true for the administration of thrombolytics for other indications (e.g., myocardial infarction), the elderly have an increased risk of bleeding complications [25].

Pneumothorax

Pneumothorax should also be considered in the evaluation of the elderly patient with chest pain. Although the diagnosis of secondary spontaneous pneumothorax, such as in the setting of COPD or underlying lung disease (e.g., malignancy), has been described frequently in the literature, there are scant published data comparing pneumothorax in elderly and younger patients. One small series reported that in patients less than 65 years old, two-thirds presented with sudden-onset pleuritic chest pain while only 18% (2/11) of those older than 65 years had a similar presentation. Six of the eleven elderly patients complained of atypical pain or no pain at all, and 9/11 had dyspnea as their primary presenting symptom. In comparison, only 1 of the 15 younger patients had a primary complaint of dyspnea. Similarly, time from onset of symptoms to seeking medical treatment was longer in the older patient group (1 versus 5 days). Physical exam was less reliable in the geriatric cohort – all but one of the younger patients had the diagnosis of pneumothorax made clinically compared with 5/11 elderly patients [31].

Vascular causes

Geriatric patients with aortic catastrophes, such as aortic dissection or aortic aneurysm, may present to the emergency department with a chest pain syndrome that can be difficult to distinguish from other etiologies of acute chest pain. These diagnoses portend high morbidity and mortality for patients – particularly when they are not recognized and treated promptly. In addition, misdiagnosis of acute aortic dissection as acute coronary syndrome can have fatal repercussions if therapies such as anticoagulation or thrombolytics are administered. Elderly patients may have difficulty describing the precise nature of the pain, further complicating the diagnostic picture.

Aortic dissection

Aortic dissection is a disease process that largely affects older individuals, with the majority of cases occurring in those between the ages of 60 and 80 years old [32–35]. As life expectancy of the general population increases, it is anticipated that a rise in the incidence of cardiovascular disease, including aortic dissection, will be seen [34,36]. Men are generally affected more frequently than women, but this male preponderance tends to dissipate in the elderly, likely a result of the relatively longer life expectancy of women. While aortic dissection remains a life-threatening illness, advances in surgical therapies have led to a significant reduction in fatality rates. Patients with proximal dissections who undergo expeditious surgery in experienced centers have a 30-day survival rate as high as 80–85% and a 10-year survival rate of 55% [33]. Similarly, patients with a dissection of the descending aorta who are treated medically with aggressive antihypertensive medications have a 30-day survival rate over 90% and a 10-year survival rate of 56% [33,37]. Some risk factors for the development of aortic dissection may be more common in the elderly, including hypertension [32,34], giant cell arteritis [38], intra-aortic catheterization [39], and a history of cardiac surgery – especially aortic valve replacement [34,40]. However, history and physical exam findings (irrespective of patient age) are believed to be insufficiently sensitive to rule out a diagnosis of aortic dissection [41,42]. In one large study group, patients older than 70 were less likely to report an abrupt onset of tearing or ripping pain, have a pulse deficit, or a murmur of aortic regurgitation [43] – findings which are described as classically being found in patients with aortic dissection. Conversely, hypotension was more often seen at presentation among the older patient cohort [34].

Aortic dissection remains a difficult diagnosis to make – particularly in the elderly who, as discussed above, may not present in a "classic" fashion. It should be considered in patients with chest pain, particularly of acute onset, and in hypertensive males with any of the risk factors listed above. Importantly, it should also be part of the differential diagnosis as an underlying etiology of patients with any chest pain syndrome that is seen in combination with acute stroke, syncope, spinal cord syndromes, or mesenteric ischemia. While history and physical exam may be important in making the diagnosis of aortic dissection, there are few prospective data from blinded studies which examine the true sensitivities of these modalities. Most patients with thoracic dissection have severe pain of abrupt onset, and pulse deficits or focal neurologic deficits, in the appropriate clinical scenario, are associated with the diagnosis. While electrocardiography (ECG) and chest radiography are critical testing modalities for patients with chest pain, neither has findings which are sensitive or specific for aortic dissection. Although clinical history, physical examination, and chest radiography may assist the physician in making the diagnosis of aortic dissection, none are sufficiently accurate to enable the disease to be ruled out. CT angiography, magnetic resonance imaging (MRI), and transesophageal echocardiography are instrumental in making the diagnosis [41].

Although a thorough discussion of the clinical presentation, classification, diagnostic algorithm, and treatment of aortic dissection is beyond the scope of this chapter, the mortality of a type A (ascending) dissection is known to increase with time from presentation, and immediate surgical intervention is generally recommended. Operative repairs have significant associated morbidity and mortality, and increased age has been shown to be a strong independent predictor of in-hospital cardiovascular interventions, including the surgical repair of a type A dissection [34,43,44].

There are conflicting data in the literature as to whether surgical repair of type A dissections should be attempted in those over 70 years of age. The literature is limited in that much of it is observational and retrospective, and reports rely on relatively small numbers of subjects at single centers. Some authors describe operative mortality for dissections of the ascending aorta in patients over 70 years as similar to those younger than 70 [43,45–47], while others suggest a significant increased risk of intraoperative or perioperative death [43,48–50].

An analysis of the International Registry of Acute Aortic Dissection, a multicenter, large-database registry, reveals that surgery was more frequently performed in those younger than 70 years of age with ascending dissections than those older than 70 years, and that the reasons listed for medical treatment included only advanced age, intramural hematoma, severe comorbidities, and refusal of surgery by patients, families, or the care team. Surgical and medical treatment was utilized equally for octogenarians, and medical therapy was offered to all five patients in the cohort who were older than 90 years of age. The in-hospital mortality rate for surgically managed patients increased with age, while the in-hospital mortality rate of those treated medically remained relatively constant (nearly 60%). For patients less than age 80, the in-hospital mortality rate was significantly lower after surgical management when compared with medical management. For those between 80 and 90 years of age the mortality rates were not statistically different. Irrespective of the specific therapy provided, age greater than 70 years was found to be an independent predictor for in-hospital mortality for patients with type A dissections. Importantly, all data from this registry were collected retrospectively, making it impossible to know whether particular therapies or interventions were administered or withheld based on factors other than the patients' age [34].

In summary, there are conflicting data regarding the appropriateness of surgical therapy for geriatric patients with type A dissections. There are no prospective, randomized comparisons of medical and surgical interventions, and mortality rates for both approaches remain high for elderly patients. Increasing age is believed to be a risk factor for poor outcome in those who have surgery, but seems to have little effect on those treated medically (perhaps because outcomes are poor irrespective of age). Most experts suggest that an aggressive surgical approach is a reasonable treatment plan in selected geriatric patients with a type A dissection, and that age alone should not be a reason to exclude elderly patients from undergoing surgical repair [43]. There is a paucity of data examining whether endovascular stents provide benefit while mitigating the risk of surgical interventions in the elderly [51]. With no intervention, and resultant aortic rupture, mortality approaches 100% [36].

Medical management of type A dissections (in either those who decline surgery or who are being prepared for surgical intervention), as well as type B dissections involves aggressive control of blood pressure and heart rate. Parenteral therapy with nitrates, beta blockers, and pain medication should be utilized in an effort to decrease shear forces on the aortic wall.

Aortic aneurysm

Although aneurysmal disease of the aorta is often asymptomatic, patients may present with complaints of upper abdominal or chest pain. In those with large untreated aneurysms, complications arising from their aneurysm (e.g., rupture) are more likely to result in death of those individuals than any other cause [47]. Ultrasound screening studies have demonstrated that abdominal aortic aneurysm (AAA) can be found in 4–8% of older men, and that the incidence of the disease rises substantially in those over 60 years of age [52–54]. Although one might expect that the prevalence of AAA would rise as the population ages and life expectancy increases, some screening programs have seen a decrease in the presence of the disease – perhaps related to decreased rates of tobacco use [55–57].

The majority of aortic aneurysms are asymptomatic and are identified during focused screening or as part of an evaluation for an unrelated complaint [58]. However, those who do present with symptoms (e.g., pain or hemodynamic instability due to rupture) related to their aneurysm require rapid evaluation and management. Irrespective of patient age, the risk of rupture is believed to increase as the diameter of the aneurysm increases, as the rate of expansion increases, and with female gender [59–61]. The mortality associated with rupture is significant – in some series the 30-day mortality of emergent thoracoabdominal aortic aneurysm repair was greater than 40% [62,63]. Large case studies of elective repairs have shown that mortality is associated with age over 75 years, a previous history of coronary artery disease (especially with congestive heart failure, chronic pulmonary disease, and creatinine >2.0) [59].

Although specific guidelines for management and details of surgical approaches for the treatment of ascending and descending aortic aneurysms are beyond the scope of this chapter, published guidelines indicate that surgical repair should be considered in males with aneurysms larger than 5.5 cm (smaller in females). However, for some, such as the elderly who may be poor surgical candidates, have limited life expectancy, or have significant comorbid illnesses which make surgical intervention particularly challenging or risky, delay in repair may be indicated – particularly if endovascular repair is not feasible [59]. As with aortic dissection, aggressive blood pressure control is important in patients who are symptomatic or awaiting emergent surgical repair. Conversely, blood pressure support with crystalloids or colloids (blood products) may be necessary in those with small, contained leaks.

Chest wall pathology

Costochondritis

Musculoskeletal chest pain is another cause of chest pain that can be very difficult to differentiate from chest pain due to more critical etiologies, such as that arising from coronary artery disease. While there are few published data on costochrondritis specifically in the geriatric patient, it is worth noting that the presence of costochondral or costosternal tenderness should not prevent the clinician from considering more life-threatening causes of chest pain. While the diagnosis of costochondritis is generally a diagnosis of exclusion, it generally is based on the finding of reproducible point tenderness over the costocondral junction. In one study of 122 ED patients with atraumatic chest pain who had anterior chest tenderness and were admitted to the hospital, a discharge diagnosis of MI was reported in 6% [64].

Malignancy

The diagnosis of cancer should also be considered in elderly patients presenting with chest pain. While metastatic disease is more common than primary neoplasm of the ribs or sternum, both primary malignancy and metastatic disease can affect the bones of the thorax. Long bones are known to be important in hematopoiesis, but so too is the sternum. As such, the chest pain may be related to metastatic disease presenting in the sternum. Primary cancers of the sternum, ribs, and clavicles are rare but may include plasma cell myeloma, lymphoma, and chondrosarcoma[65]. While a variety of cancers can metastasize to bone in adults, metastases from prostate, breast, renal, and lung primaries make up about 75% of skeletal metastasis [66]. The cancers known to commonly spread to the bones of the chest wall are cancers also common among elderly patients.

While skeletal metastases will usually present as multifocal disease, renal and thyroid tumors specifically are known to produce solitary lesions. The axial skeleton is most frequently the site of bony metastasis, which includes vertebrae, pelvis, skull, and the ribs and sternum [66].

Chest trauma

While trauma is covered in detail elsewhere in this text, falls are a source of significant morbidity in the elderly. As many as 32% of those aged 65–74, 35% of those aged 75–84, and 51% of those older than 85 suffer falls annually [67]. These falls result in fracture in approximately 5% of instances, and cause 12% of all deaths in patients older than 65 years [67]. Polypharmacy, as well as certain commonly prescribed medications, has been associated with increased risk of falls due to drowsiness, alterations in balance, or the induction of postural hypotension. Other factors, including the physical functional loss as part of the aging process, progressive weakness, and vision loss,

environmental factors such as poor lighting, slick surfaces, and loose rugs have also been associated with an increased incidence of falls in the elderly [67].

Although extremity fractures after a fall may be clinically apparent or clearly present on radiographs, rib fractures and associated chest wall injuries may be more subtle. Importantly, there is significant morbidity and mortality associated with rib fractures in the elderly. In a single study when compared to their younger counterparts, geriatric patients were more likely to require prolonged ventilator support, have longer intensive care unit (ICU) stays, and were more likely to die as a result of their injuries [68]. Additionally both morbidity and mortality increased significantly with each rib fractured. Mortality increases by 19%, and the risk of developing pneumonia by 27% for each additional rib fracture. The same study also showed infectious complications, such as pneumonia, are more common for elderly patients when compared with younger patients (31 versus 17%). The use of aggressive pain management with epidural analgesia for patients who were hospitalized more than two days was associated with a decreased mortality from 16 to 10%. In a younger group with similar hospital length of stay, mortality with and without epidural was 0 and 5%, respectively. Data such as these suggest that careful evaluation, inpatient admission, and aggressive pain management are important in the care of the elderly with rib fractures.

Herpes zoster

Elderly patients may have chest pain associated with herpes zoster infection – more than 50% of infections are in those older than 50 years of age [69]. This increase in disease burden with age has been attributed to the progressive weakening of cell-mediated immunity as one gets older [70]. The prodrome of pain may precede the rash by as much as 4–14 days, and approximately 50% of all zoster infections involve a dermatome of the thorax [70]. Other risks factors for the development of zoster include cancer, trauma, immunocompromised status (e.g., chronic steroids or other immunosuppressive agents), HIV, and psychological stress [70]. Elderly patients, much like with other causes of chest pain, may describe the pain in a variety of different ways ranging from burning pain to sharp or stabbing. The pain may be constant or intermittent in nature.

The most frequent complication of herpes zoster is postherpetic neuralgia (PHN), and it is known to develop more commonly in the elderly [70]. The herpes zoster vaccine has been recommended for patients over the age of 60 and has been shown to reduce primary zoster infections as well as postherpetic neuralgia [70]. It is important for physicians to perform a careful skin exam on patients with chest pain with the understanding that the pain may precede the rash by several days.

Gastrointestinal causes of chest pain

Esophageal rupture

Patients with esophageal perforation may present with chest pain. Generally as a result of forceful vomiting, esophagitis from pills, caustic ingestions, Barrett's ulcers, or infectious ulcers associated with AIDS, or iatrogenic (as a result of instrumentation, for example with esophageal dilation), esophageal perforation is associated with significant morbidity and mortality, and is fatal if left untreated [71–73]. Chest radiographs should be performed if esophageal rupture is suspected. A single study has shown that 97% of radiographs with rupture are abnormal, however, mediastinal air is only seen in about 27%. The most common finding was pleural effusion (seen in 61% of patients) [71]. There is very little in the literature regarding the specifics of the geriatric patient with esophageal perforation – most series involve small numbers of patients, precluding focused analysis of those who are older.

Abdominal etiologies

Elderly patients with disease processes that are generally considered to be of "abdominal" etiology may present with poorly localized chest pain or upper abdominal pain. While these are discussed further in Chapter 11 of this text, it should be noted that diagnoses such as pancreatitis, peptic ulcer disease, gastrointestinal malignancies, and disorders of the biliary system should be included in the differential diagnosis of the geriatric patient with any chest pain syndrome.

Pearls and pitfalls

- Physicians should maintain a broad differential diagnosis for the geriatric patient with chest pain. Potential causes range from the immediately life-threatening to the benign.
- Vague, nonspecific, and constitutional complaints may be more common in the elderly than in younger patients and do not necessarily suggest a benign etiology.
- Although literature is often lacking, patient age may impact the effectiveness of various interventions and therapies. Conversely, advanced age, per se, is not necessarily a contraindication to invasive or aggressive treatment.
- In general, outcomes for elderly patients with serious causes of chest pain are worse than in their younger counterparts.

References

1. Pitts SR, Niska RW, Xu J, Burt CW. National Hospital Ambulatory Medical Care Survey: 2006 Emergency Department summary. National health statistics reports, No. 7 (Hyattsville, MD: National Center for Health Statistics, 2008).

2. Pope JH, Aufderheide TP, Ruthazer R, et al. Missed diagnoses of acute cardiac ischemia in the emergency department. *N Engl J Med.* 2000;342(16):1163–70.

3. Garcia TC, Bernstein AB, Bush MA. *Emergency Department Visitors and Visits: Who used the emergency room in 2007? NCHS data brief, No. 38* (Hyattsville, MD: National Center for Health Statistics, 2010).

4. Rogers WJ, Bowlby LJ, Chandra NC, et al. Treatment of myocardial infarction in the United States (1990 to 1993). Observations from the National Registry of Myocardial Infarction. *Circulation.* 1994;90(4):2103–14.

5. Carro A, Kaski JC. Myocardial infarction in the elderly. *Aging Dis.* 2011;2:116–37.

6. Pinto DS, Kirtane AJ, Nallamothu BK, et al. Hospital delays in reperfusion for ST-elevation myocardial infarction: Implications when selecting a reperfusion strategy. *Circulation.* 2006;114(19):2019–25.

7. Hochman JS, Sleeper LA, Webb JG, et al. Early revascularization in acute myocardial infarction complicated by cardiogenic shock. SHOCK investigators. Should we emergently revascularize occluded coronaries for cardiogenic shock. *N Engl J Med.* 1999;341(9):625–34.

8. Kashima K, Ikeda D, Tanaka H, et al. Mid-term mortality of very elderly patients with acute myocardial infarction with or without coronary intervention. *J Cardiol.* 2010;55(3):397–403.

9. Oqueli E, Dick R. Percutaneous coronary intervention in very elderly patients. In-hospital mortality and clinical outcome. *Heart Lung Circ.* 2011;20(10):622–8.

10. Alexander KP, Roe MT, Chen AY, et al. Evolution in cardiovascular care for elderly patients with non-ST-segment elevation acute coronary syndromes. *J Am Coll Cardiol.* 2005;46(8):1479–87.

11. O'Connor RE, Brady W, Brooks SC, et al. Part 10: Acute coronary syndromes: 2010 American Heart Association Guidelines for Cardiopulmonary Resuscitation and Emergency Cardiovascular Care. *Circulation.* 2010;122(18, Suppl. 3):S787–817.

12. Senter S, Francis GS. A new, precise definition of acute myocardial infarction. *Cleveland Clinic J Med.* 2009;76(3):159–66.

13. Wu A. Increased troponin in patients with sepsis and septic shock: myocardial necrosis or reversible myocardial depression? *Intensive Care Med.* 2001;27(6):959–61.

14. Ezekowitz JA, Kaul P, Bakal JA, et al. Declining in-hospital mortality and increasing heart failure incidence in elderly patients with first myocardial infarction. *J Am Coll Cardiol.* 2009;53(1):13–20.

15. Shih H, Lee B, Lee RJ, Boyle AJ. The aging heart and post-infarction left ventricular remodeling. *J Am Coll Cardiol.* 2011;57(1):9–17.

16. Troughton RW, Asher CR, Klein AL. Pericarditis. *Lancet.* 2004;363(9410):717–27.

17. Spodick DH. Evaluation and management of acute pericarditis. *ACC Current Journal Review.* 2004;13(11):15–19.

18. Janssens JP, Krause KH. Pneumonia in the very old. *Lancet Infect Dis.* 2004;4(2):112–24.

19. Ruhnke GW, Coca-Perraillon M, Kitch BT, Cutler DM. Marked reduction in 30-day mortality among elderly patients with community-acquired pneumonia. *Am J Med.* 2011;124(2):171–8

20. Muder RR. Pneumonia in residents of long-term care facilities: epidemiology, etiology, management, and prevention. *Am J Med.* 1998;105(4):319–30.

21. Goldhaber SZ. Pulmonary embolism. *Lancet.* 2004;363(9417):1295–305.

22. Wells PS, Anderson DR, Rodger M, et al. Derivation of a simple clinical model to categorize patients probability of pulmonary embolism: increasing the models utility with the SimpliRED D-dimer. *Thromb Haemost.* 2000;83(3):416–20.

23. Singh B, Parsaik AK, Agarwal D, et al. Diagnostic accuracy of pulmonary embolism rule-out criteria: A systematic review and meta-analysis. *Annals Emerg Med.* 2012;59(6):517–20.

24. Kline JA, Mitchell AM, Kabrhel C, Richman PB, Courtney DM. Clinical criteria to prevent unnecessary diagnostic testing in emergency department patients with suspected pulmonary embolism. *J Thromb Haemost.* 2004;2(8):1247–55.

25. Capodanno D, Angiolillo DJ. Antithrombotic therapy in the elderly. *J Am Coll Cardiol.* 2010;56(21):1683–92.

26. Verbeeck RK, Musuamba FT. Pharmacokinetics and dosage adjustment in patients with renal dysfunction. *Eur J Clin Pharmacol.* 2009;65(8):757–73.

27. Timmons S, Kingston M, Hussain M, Kelly H, Liston R. Pulmonary embolism: differences in presentation between older and younger patients. *Age Aging.* 2003;32(6):601–5.

28. Barrett JA, Baron JA, Beach ML. Mortality and pulmonary embolism after fracture in the elderly. *Osteoporosis Intl.* 2003;14(11):889–94.

29. Harper PL, Theakston E, Ahmed J, Ockelford P. D-dimer concentration increases with age reducing the clinical value of the D-dimer assay in the elderly. *Int Med J.* 2007;37(9):607–13.

30. Sinert R, Doty CI. Prevention of contrast-induced nephropathy in the emergency department. *Annals Emerg Med.* 2007;50(3):335–45.

31. Liston R, McLoughlin R, Clinch D. Acute pneumothorax: A comparison of elderly with younger patients. *Age Aging.* 1994;23(5):393–5.

32. Larson EW, Edwards WD. Risk factors for aortic dissection: a necropsy study of 161 cases. *Am J Cardiol.* 1984;53(6):849–55.

33. Hagan PG, Nienaber CA, Isselbacher EM, et al. The International Registry of Acute Aortic Dissection (IRAD): New insights into an old disease. *JAMA.* 2000;283(7):897–903.

34. Trimarchi S, Eagle KA, Nienaber CA, et al. Role of age in acute type A aortic dissection outcome: Report from the International Registry of Acute Aortic Dissection (IRAD). *J Thoracic Cardiovasc Surg.* 2010;140(4):784–9.

35. Yanagisawa S, Yuasa T, Suzuki N, et al. Comparison of medically versus surgically treated acute type A aortic dissection in patients <80 years old versus patients ≥80 years old. *Am J Cardiol.* 2011;108(3):453–9.

36. Olsson C, Thelin S, Stahle E, Ekbom A, Granath F. Thoracic aortic aneurysm and dissection: Increasing prevalence and improved outcomes reported in a nationwide population-based study of more than 14 000 cases from 1987 to 2002. *Circulation.* 2006;114(24):2611–18.

37. Masuda Y, Yamada Z, Morooka N, Watanabe S, Inagaki Y. Prognosis of patients with medically treated aortic dissections. *Circulation.* 1991;84(5, Suppl.):III7–13.

38. Säve-Söderbergh J, Malmvall BE, Andersson R, Bengtsson BA. Giant cell arteritis as a cause of death. Report of nine cases. *JAMA.* 1986;255(4):493–6.

39. Ohmoto Y, Ikari Y, Hara K. Aortic dissection during directional coronary atherectomy. *Int J Cardiol.* 1996;55(3):289–91.

40. von Kodolitsch Y, Loose R, Ostermeyer J, et al. Proximal aortic dissection late after aortic valve surgery: 119 cases of a distinct clinical entity. *Thorac Cardiovasc Surg.* 2000;48(6):342–6.

41. Klompas M. Does this patient have an acute thoracic aortic dissection? *JAMA.* 2002;287(17):2262–72.

42. Sullivan PR, Wolfson AB, Leckey RD, Burke JL. Diagnosis of acute thoracic aortic dissection in the emergency department. *Am J Emerg Med.* 2000;18(1):46–50.

43. Mehta RH, O'Gara PT, Bossone E, et al. Acute type A aortic dissection in the elderly: clinical characteristics, management, and outcomes in the current era. *J Am Coll Cardiol.* 2002;40(4):685–92.

44. Tan MESH, Morshuis WJ, Dossche KME, et al. Long-term results after 27 years of surgical treatment of acute type A aortic dissection. *Annals Thoracic Surg.* 2005;80(2):523–9.

45. Stamou SC, Hagberg RC, Khabbaz KR, et al. Is advanced age a contraindication for emergent repair of acute type A aortic dissection? *Interact Cardiovasc Thorac Surg.* 2010;10(4):539–44.

46. Shrestha M, Khaladj N, Haverich A, Hagl C. Is treatment of acute type A aortic dissection in septuagenarians justifiable? *Asian Cardiovasc Thorac Ann.* 2008;16(1):33–6.

47. Rylski B, Suedkamp M, Beyersdorf F, et al. Outcome after surgery for acute aortic dissection type A in patients over 70 years: data analysis from the German Registry for Acute Aortic Dissection Type A (GERAADA). *Eur J Cardio-Thoracic Surg.* 2011 (accessed June 20, 2012 from www.sciencedirect.com/science/article/pii/S1010794010010535).

48. Chavanon O, Costache V, Bach V, et al. Preoperative predictive factors for mortality in acute type A aortic dissection: an institutional report on 217 consecutives cases. *Interact Cardiovasc Thorac Surg.* 2007;6(1):43–6.

49. Ehrlich M, Fang WC, Grabenwöger M, et al. Perioperative risk factors for mortality in patients with acute type A aortic dissection. *Circulation.* 1998;98(19, Suppl.):II294–8.

50. Neri E, Massetti M. Acute type A dissection and advanced age. *Ann Thorac Surg.* 2005;80(1):384–5; author reply, 385.

51. Slonim SM, Nyman U, Semba CP, et al. Aortic dissection: percutaneous management of ischemic complications with endovascular stents and balloon fenestration. *J Vasc Surg.* 1996;23(2):241–21; discussion, 251–3.

52. Scott RA, Ashton HA, Kay DN. Abdominal aortic aneurysm in 4237 screened patients: prevalence, development and management over 6 years. *Br J Surg.* 1991;78(9):1122–5.

53. Lederle FA, Johnson GR, Wilson SE, et al. Prevalence and associations of abdominal aortic aneurysm detected through screening. Aneurysm Detection and Management (ADAM) Veterans Affairs Cooperative Study Group. *Ann Intern Med.* 1997;126(6):441–9.

54. Sicgh K, Bønaa KH, Jacobsen BK, Bjørk L, Solberg S. Prevalence of and risk factors for abdominal aortic aneurysms in a population-based study: The Tromsø Study. *Am J Epidemiol.* 2001;154(3):236–44.

55. Svensjö S, Björck M, Gürtelschmid M, et al. Low prevalence of abdominal aortic aneurysm among 65-year-old Swedish men indicates a change in the epidemiology of the disease. *Circulation.* 2011;124(10):1118–23.

56. Sandiford P, Mosquera D, Bramley D. Trends in incidence and mortality from abdominal aortic aneurysm in New Zealand. *Br J Surg.* 2011;98(5):645–51.

57. Lederle FA. The rise and fall of abdominal aortic aneurysm. *Circulation.* 2011;124(10):1097–9.

58. van Walraven C, Wong J, Morant K, et al. Incidence, follow-up, and outcomes of incidental abdominal aortic aneurysms. *J Vasc Surg.* 2010;52(2):282–9.e1–2.

59. Brewster DC, Cronenwett JL, Hallett JW, et al. Guidelines for the treatment of abdominal aortic aneurysms: Report of a subcommittee of the Joint Council of the American Association for Vascular Surgery and Society for Vascular Surgery. *J Vasc Surg*. 2003;37(5):1106–17.

60. Nevitt MP, Ballard DJ, Hallett JW Jr. Prognosis of abdominal aortic aneurysms. A population-based study. *N Engl J Med*. 1989;321(15):1009–14.

61. Katz DA, Littenberg B, Cronenwett JL. Management of small abdominal aortic aneurysms. Early surgery vs watchful waiting. *JAMA*. 1992;268(19):2678–86.

62. Mastroroberto P, Chello M. Emergency thoracoabdominal aortic aneurysm repair: clinical outcome. *J Thorac Cardiovasc Surg*. 1999;118(3):477–81; discussion 481–2.

63. Cowan JA, Dimick JB, Henke PK, et al. Epidemiology of aortic aneurysm repair in the United States from 1993 to 2003. *Annals N Y Acad Sci*. 2006;1085(1):1–10.

64. Disla E, Rhim HR, Reddy A, Karten I, Taranta A. Costochondritis: A prospective analysis in an emergency department setting. *Arch Int Med*. 1994;154(21):2466–9.

65. Habib P, Huang G-S, Mendiola J, Yu J. Anterior chest pain: musculoskeletal considerations. *Emergency Radiology*. 2004;11(1) (accessed July 19, 2012 from http://springerlink. metapress.com/openurl.asp?genre=article&id=doi:10.1007/ s10140-004-0342-7).

66. Kumar V, Fausto N, Abbas AK, Cotran RS, Robbins SL. *Robbins and Cotran's Pathologic Basis of Disease* (Philadelphia, PA; London: Elsevier Saunders, 2004).

67. Baraff LJ, Della Penna R, Williams N, Sanders A. Practice guideline for the ED management of falls in community-dwelling elderly persons. *Ann Emerg Med*. 1997;30(4):480–92.

68. Bulger EM, Arneson MA, Mock CN, Jurkovich GJ. Rib fractures in the elderly. *J Trauma*. 2000;48(6):1040–6; discussion, 1046–7.

69. Oxman MN, Levin MJ, Johnson GR, et al. A vaccine to prevent herpes zoster and postherpetic neuralgia in older adults. *N Engl J Med*. 2005;352(22):2271–84.

70. Weinberg JM. Herpes zoster: Epidemiology, natural history, and common complications. *J Am Acad Dermatol*. 2007;57(6):S130–5.

71. Pate JW, Walker WA, Cole FH, Owen EW, Johnson WH. Spontaneous rupture of the esophagus: A 30-year experience. *Ann Thorac Surg*. 1989;47(5):689–92.

72. Michel L, Grillo HC, Malt RA. Esophageal perforation. *Annals Thoracic Surg*. 1982;33(2):203–10.

73. Flynn AE, Verrier ED, Way LW, Thomas AN, Pellegrini CA. Esophageal perforation. *Arch Surg*. 1989;124(10):1211–14; discussion, 1214–15.

Chapter 10

Dyspnea in the elderly

Denise Law and Ron Medzon

Introduction

According to the 2010 Census, there were over 30 million people over the age of 65 in the US, which was a 15.1% increase over the 2000 census. This growth rate was the highest ever in US history and significantly higher than the overall population growth rate of 9.7%. It is expected that this rate will continue to increase over the next 20 years due to the "baby boom" era of the mid 1940s–60s. The geriatric population is estimated to comprise 12–21% of emergency department (ED) visits [1] with 30–50% of those visits requiring admission. The elderly also have a higher likelihood of requiring admission to an intensive care unit (ICU) [2].

It follows that the increasing geriatric population presents many challenges to the emergency physician, largely due to physiologic changes associated with aging. Specifically, there is an increased incidence of acute pulmonary and cardiac disease along with an increased prevalence of multiple comorbidities in the elderly as compared with the general population.

Dyspnea is one of the most frequent complaints among older adults. Diagnosing the cause and managing acute dyspnea is complicated because the symptoms and physical findings vary considerably. A recent epidemiologic study named congestive heart failure (CHF) (43%), community-acquired pneumonia (CAP) (35%), chronic obstructive pulmonary disease (COPD) exacerbation (32%), and pulmonary embolism (PE) (18%) as the four most common causes of acute respiratory distress [3]. Other etiologies include causes of metabolic acidosis including diabetic ketoacidosis, acute renal failure, and sepsis.

When approaching the elderly patient with acute respiratory distress, the physician should keep a wide differential. By history, acuteness in onset with recent immobilization favors PE as the diagnosis, while a past history of CHF or coronary artery disease (CAD) along with orthopnea, peripheral edema, and paroxysmal nocturnal dyspnea will likely be flash pulmonary edema. Older patients do have asthma and COPD exacerbations, and these are frequently accompanied by a history of chest pain in addition to wheezing and shortness of breath. Wheezing may also be the manifestation of cardiac asthma.

Initial evaluation should always begin with assessment of the patient's airway, breathing, and circulation (ABCs). It is especially important to place the elderly patient on a monitor, establish an IV, and place them on supplemental oxygen if they appear short of breath or have a low oxygen saturation. Physical examination should include a complete set of vital signs, comprehensive pulmonary and cardiac examination including lung auscultation, and assessment for jugular venous distension and extremity edema. Absence of fever does not rule out infection, so pneumonia is on the differential diagnosis even if the patient is afebrile. Diagnostic evaluation includes obtaining blood samples, and specific laboratory tests should be determined on a case-by-case basis. Appropriate tests may include, but are not limited to, a complete blood count, comprehensive metabolic panel, B-natriuretic peptide (BNP), and cardiac markers. If the patient appears dyspneic or ill, an arterial blood gas (ABG) should be obtained since it can provide valuable information on a patient's respiratory status. A D-dimer may also be obtained if there is a suspicion of a pulmonary embolism, but the clinician should keep in mind that the value is often falsely elevated in the elderly population due to underlying multiple comorbidities. An electrocardiogram and chest X-ray should also be performed in all elderly patients presenting with acute dyspnea. Patients presenting with low oxygen saturation, retractions on physical exam, tachycardia, or appearing diaphoretic and tachypneic should be initially stabilized and then moved to an acute care area of the department for further evaluation and treatment.

In this chapter, we will first discuss the physiologic changes in the respiratory and circulatory systems that occur during aging, and then address some of the major disease processes that lead to respiratory distress.

Respiratory system structural mechanics

Because the entire respiratory system undergoes anatomic changes throughout life, even those people without underlying pulmonary disease see deterioration in pulmonary function with age. The respiratory system is comprised of the thoracic cage, lungs, and diaphragm, all of which contribute to total system compliance. Compliance is defined as the change in volume relative to the change in pressure. Structural changes as one ages cause a decrease in compliance.

Geriatric Emergency Medicine, ed. Joseph H. Kahn, Brendan G. Magauran Jr., and Jonathan S. Olshaker. Published by Cambridge University Press.
© Cambridge University Press 2014.

Table 10.1. Age-related structural changes in the lung that contribute to loss of compliance and ability to exchange gases

Structural change	Mechanism	Outcome
Osteoporosis	Kyphosis will ↓ height	↓ Volume
Calcification of rib cage	↓ Expansion of chest wall	↓ Volume
Weakening of diaphragm	↓ Atrophy of fast-twitch fibers	↑ Resp. failure when ill
Stiffening of pulmonary artery	Change in supporting connective tissue in bronchioles	↑ Peripheral vasc. resistance
Reduction in number of alveoli	↑ Ratio of collagen to elastic tissue	↓ Surface area, ↓ gas exchange
↑ Inflammation of lower resp. tract	↑ Ratio CD_4:CD_8 lymphocytes, ↑ release of superoxides	↓ Gas exchange

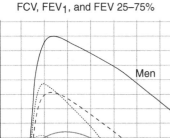

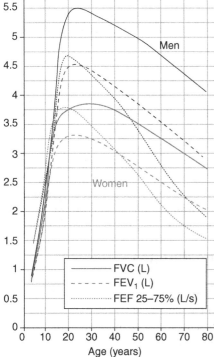

Figure 10.1. Normal values for forced vital capacity (FVC), forced expiratory volume in 1 second (FEV$_1$), and forced expiratory flow 25–75% (FEF 25–75%). Y-axis denotes FVC and FEV$_1$ in L, and FEF 25–75% in L/s. Reprinted with permission of the American Thoracic Society. Copyright © 2012 American Thoracic Society. Stanojevic S, Wade A, Stocks J, et al. Reference ranges for spirometry across all ages: a new approach. *Am J Respir Crit Care Med.* 2008;177(3):253–60.

Age-related osteoporosis of the thoracic cage causes reduced height and kyphosis which reduces lung volume. Calcification of the rib cage causes stiffening, reducing the ability of the lung to expand, diminishing volume, and decreasing compliance. This decrease in chest wall compliance is associated with a higher residual volume [4]. The diaphragm, which is an essential component of respiratory mechanics, weakens with age. This reduction in strength has been attributed to muscle atrophy as well as to failure in fast-twitch fibers. The diaphragm fatigues earlier, which subsequently leads to ventilatory failure during times of increased stress to the cardiopulmonary system [4].

Structural changes to the lung also occur with age, due to a combination of destruction of the lung parenchyma and loss of supporting structures within the lung parenchyma [4]. These include a shrinking of bronchiolar airway size as well as dilation of the alveolar ducts and sacs. All of these changes lead to hyperinflation of the lungs.

There is a decrease in the extensibility of the pulmonary artery which increases stiffness of the pulmonary vasculature, leading to increased peripheral vascular resistance (PVR). This is believed to be due to alterations to the supporting connective tissue in the bronchioles [4]. The PVR appears to be more affected than the systemic vascular resistance [5]. An increase in the proportion of collagen and decrease in that of elastic tissue results in a smaller number of alveoli and thus a decrease in surface area available for gas exchange (Table 10.1).

Effects on lung function

The changes discussed above combine to produce the decline in pulmonary function in the elderly including the rate of airflow while breathing, resting lung volumes, and gas exchange. Lung function begins to decline around 35 years of age (Figure 10.1). The decline in dynamic flow is quantified by a decrease in the forced vital capacity (FVC), the forced expiratory volume in one second (FEV$_1$), and the ratio of FEV$_1$ to FVC [6]. The estimated rate of decline is 25–30 ml/year, but can double after age 70 [4]. These changes are mainly due to the increased rigidity in the chest wall and loss of elastic recoil in the lungs leading to decreased force generated by the muscles of respiration [6]. There is also a change in static lung capacity in that functional residual capacity and residual volume increase, so the vital capacity decreases. Lastly, impairment in gas exchange develops with age. This has been attributed to many factors including a loss of the number of capillaries perfusing the lungs, a decrease in alveolar surface area, and a collapse of peripheral bronchioles, all of which increase ventilation–perfusion mismatching and thus total pulmonary diffusing capacity [4,5].

To summarize, all of the structural changes mentioned cause the aging pulmonary system to undergo progressive deterioration. This can be seen in an almost linear decline of PaO$_2$ of 2–3 mm per decade of life starting in one's 30s. A healthy 80-year-old can have a baseline PaO$_2$ between 78 and 92 mmHg. The lower baseline oxygen saturation and decline in pulmonary function in the elderly make it more difficult for that patient to successfully combat an acute injury to the lungs.

Cardiovascular changes in the elderly

There are significant cardiovascular changes that occur as one ages, independent of genetic and lifestyle factors. These changes

Table 10.2. Age-related changes in the structure of the heart that contribute to decreasing contractility and arrhythmias

Structural change	Mechanism	Outcome
↓ Number of myocytes	Cell death	↓ Contractility
↑ Size of myocytes	Filling space from cell death	Left ventricular hypertrophy
↓ Number of myocytes in SA node	Cell death	↑ Arrhythmias
Fibrotic foci appear	↑ Collagen, elastic tissue, fat deposition	↓ Contractility
Thickening of blood vessel walls	Sclerosis of intima and subendothelium	↓ Blood-carrying ability

contribute to an increased prevalence of cardiopulmonary disease, often presenting with dyspnea in the elderly.

Structural changes

A number of changes occur to the musculature of the heart as one ages. There is a decrease in the number of cardiac myocytes, as well as an increase in size. Collagen, elastic tissue, and fat are deposited, and fibrotic foci begin to show up in the aging myocardium. This eventually leads to hypertrophy of the left ventricle and diminished myocyte contractility. The number of myocytes in the sinoatrial node decreases dramatically, heightening susceptibility and frequency of dysrhythmias [7]. All of these changes can occur independently of, but are accentuated by, the presence of coronary artery disease [7].

In terms of vasculature, the proximal portion of an artery tends to exhibit age-related changes first, with these changes eventually spreading to involve the entire vessel. Age-related changes that are independent of the development of atherosclerosis occur in the intima and subendothelial layer. The intimal wall thickens, and there is greater stiffness throughout the vessel walls [7,8].

All of these structural changes combine to worsen cardiovascular function in the elderly (Table 10.2).

Physiological changes

Cardiac output (CO) is a measure of heart rate and stroke volume. The overall CO, both at rest and with exercise, decreases due to a myriad of causes. Some of the determinants of cardiac output that may be influenced by age are heart rate, preload and afterload, intrinsic muscle performance, and neurohumoral regulation. Interestingly, while the heart rate decreases with aging, the maximum stroke volume is preserved via the Frank–Starling mechanism [8]. There is stiffening of the arteries, especially the ascending aorta, and decreased surface area of small vascular beds, leading to increased peripheral vascular resistance, which translates into increased afterload. The result of this increase in afterload is increased cardiac workload, which is likely a large contributing factor to left ventricular hypertrophy [7].

Myocyte hypertrophy and the excitation-contraction coupling mechanism contribute to diastolic dysfunction by causing a prolonged relaxation phase. Both the prolonged relaxation and the increased stiffness of the myocardium retard ventricular filling, and contribute to higher left ventricular diastolic pressures at rest and during exercise. This can lead to pulmonary and venous congestion and cause symptoms of heart failure. Diastolic dysfunction is also accentuated by changes on a cellular level. Calcium homeostasis is disrupted with age. The sarcoplasmic reticulum loses its capacity to sequester calcium efficiently. This creates an age-associated increase in net transsarcolemmal calcium influx leading to a prolonged and less forceful myocyte contraction as well as an increased relaxation phase. This causes impaired contraction, arrhythmias, and cell death [8]. Decreased oxidative phosphorylation and cumulative mitochondrial peroxidation may further impair myocardial function [7]. In the absence of cardiovascular disease, diastolic dysfunction is often seen prior to systolic dysfunction in the elderly.

Vascular system changes

In addition to the changes in cardiac function, changes in the cardiovascular system lead to an increase in the resting systolic blood pressure in the elderly. While there is no change in the resting heart rate, the maximal heart rate during exercise lessens with age. There is also a delay or insufficiency in the cardiovascular compensatory mechanisms leading to an increase in postural, postprandial, and vasovagal syncopal episodes, in part due to a significant drop in systolic blood pressure not seen in the younger population.

Conditions causing dyspnea
Congestive heart failure

An estimated 5.7 million adults in the US are living with heart failure, with 75% of those over the age of 65. It is the leading cause of hospitalization amongst older adults and the most costly to the Medicare system [9,10]. Multiple studies have demonstrated a positive correlation between age and heart failure prevalence. In fact, age itself has been shown to be the strongest predictor of one's risk of heart failure due to the changes in the cardiovascular system. With age, a higher prevalence of hypertension and coronary artery disease is seen, which are the two largest modifiable risk factors of heart failure [11]. The elderly heart has trouble remodeling after a myocardial infarction (MI), making it more likely to develop ischemic heart failure. The risk of inpatient mortality from CHF in the geriatric population is almost double that of younger patients (10.7 versus 5.6%) [11].

Two types of CHF exist, systolic and diastolic (defined by a preserved ejection fraction), the latter of which is more prevalent in those older than 70 years of age. Systolic HF occurs when there is a decrease in the force of myocyte contraction. In contrast, diastolic heart failure leads to venous congestion due to impaired left ventricular relaxation.

Both types of heart failure can present similarly with exertional dyspnea, paroxysmal nocturnal dyspnea, and orthopnea. Signs include jugular venous distension, presence of an S3 on cardiac exam, pulmonary crackles, and lower extremity edema [12]. Laboratory results that can be especially helpful are BNP <100, which can exclude CHF as a cause of dyspnea [13], while a value >500 can be suggestive of CHF exacerbation. However, many other comorbidities seen in the elderly, including renal failure, can falsely elevate BNP. Obtaining a BNP in the ED has been shown to decrease time to disposition, inpatient cost, and 30-day mortality rate [2,3].

Mainstays of ED treatment include diuretics, morphine, and high-dose nitrates for veno- and arteriodilation [14]. High-dose nitrates have been shown to decrease mortality whereas furosemide alone has not [14]. Beta blockers should be avoided in acute heart failure due to their negative inotropic effects. Noninvasive positive pressure ventilation (NIPPV) (both continuous and biphasic positive airway pressure) is now being used more frequently for heart failure. NIPPV reduces the work of breathing and improves both oxygenation and alveolar ventilation [15,16]. It improves oxygenation, reduces work of breathing, sometimes prevents intubation, and decreases mortality [14]. However, NIPPV can also be dangerous in those exhibiting delirium and dementia and should be used with caution since these states can cause a decreased level of alertness and cooperation, which increases the risk of aspiration and poor tolerance of NIPPV [2].

Pulmonary embolism

The geriatric population is at increased risk of thromboembolic events as defined by Virchow's triad of hypercoagulative state, endothelial injury, and increased stasis. This is due to a combination of decreased mobility, hypercoagulability via increased levels of coagulation factors and impaired fibrinolysis, increased central venous pressure states, and increased endothelial injury from atherosclerotic changes [17,18]. It has been estimated that 12% of mortality in the elderly is attributed to a pulmonary embolism with up to 40% undiagnosed until autopsy [19].

The most common presenting symptoms are dyspnea, followed by tachypnea, pleuritic chest pain, cough, hemoptysis, and syncope [18,19]. However, diagnosis can be made difficult in older patients as compared with the younger population. Clinicians should consider a PE in any elderly patient who presents with a history of acute presentation of dyspnea or suddenly deteriorates while in the ED. Young patients tend to present more frequently with pleuritic chest pain, while older patients are more likely to present with isolated dyspnea or syncope, probably as a result of poor cardiorespiratory reserve [20]. The Wells and/or Geneva Score is used to assess the pretest probability of a PE [19].

Diagnostic tests are less sensitive in the elderly. While D-dimer results maintain a high sensitivity for thromboembolic disease, their specificity falls dramatically with age. This results in a higher proportion of elderly patients needing to undergo second-line testing to exclude PE. What is clinically more useful is a negative D-dimer result in someone with a low pretest probability. This has a very high negative predictive value [19]. ECG findings are often nonspecific and can include sinus tachycardia (most common), right bundle branch block,

and nonspecific ST-T wave abnormalities [19]. CT pulmonary angiogram is the modality of choice in diagnosing PE [18,21]. If unable to give IV contrast due to poor renal function, other modalities including ventilation–perfusion scans and lower extremity Doppler ultrasounds can be utilized. However, it is important to note that ventilation–perfusion scans are often nondiagnostic due to interference from underlying cardiopulmonary disease [18,21]. Sensitivity of extremity venous ultrasonography in detecting deep venous thrombosis (DVT) increases with age [22,23]. There is evidence that in the setting of acute dyspnea and suspicion of a PE, the presence of a recent DVT seen on ultrasound supports the diagnosis of a PE and should prompt initiation of anticoagulation [24].

Acute coronary syndrome

Ischemic heart disease (IHD) is the leading cause of death in First World countries. In 2004, IHD accounted for 35% of all deaths in those over 65 years of age in the US. The elderly population also accounted for 83% of all deaths from IHD.

The elderly tend to present more with atypical symptoms (defined as absence of chest pain) in non-ST-elevation acute coronary syndromes (NSTE ACS) as compared with the general population. More common primary presenting symptoms include dyspnea (reported as 49% from the Global Registry of Acute Coronary Events) [25], diaphoresis, nausea, vomiting, and syncope, sometimes leading to delayed or missed recognition of an MI. Atypical presentations have been associated with worse outcomes, in part from delayed diagnosis and treatment as well as from reduced use of evidence-based medicine. Silent MIs have been shown to account for anywhere from 21 to 68% of MIs in those over 85 years old. The geriatric population is also more likely to develop ACS in the setting of another acute illness. Because of all these factors, clinicians should have a high index of suspicion for ACS in the elderly.

The ACC/AHA guidelines recommend that a 12-lead ECG be obtained in all patients complaining of chest pain or other symptoms consistent with ACS within 10 minutes of arrival in the ED [26]. This is very important considering that in the presence of other disease states, the elderly population has a relatively higher risk of short-term death or non-fatal MI [6].

COPD

Chronic obstructive pulmonary disease encompasses a range of disease states including chronic bronchitis and emphysema, which are characterized by a reduction in expiratory flow measured as an increase in residual volume and FEV_1. Acute respiratory failure is defined as hypercapnia ($PaCO_2$ >50 mmHg), which is due to poor alveolar ventilation, or hypoxemia (PaO_2 <60 mmHg). The latter is the more common and can be attributed to many lung pathologies. Age itself is an independent risk factor for acute exacerbations and the need for hospitalization in the setting of an acute exacerbation. There has been shown to be an increase in the number of exacerbations of 20% for each 10 years of life. For every 5 years over the age of 65, there also exists an additional 36% increase in hospitalization [27].

The elderly tend to have delayed presentations, which have been attributed to multiple causes including a blunted perception of dyspnea and an assumption that symptoms are from mere deconditioning [18]. Common presenting symptoms include dyspnea, cough, chest tightness, sputum production, and wheezing [18,28]. However, the elderly are less likely to endorse a change in sputum production [29]. Signs include tachypnea, tachycardia, and a prolonged expiratory phase. In acute exacerbations, decreased or absent breath sounds are seen more frequently than wheezing. In severe, long-standing COPD, pulmonary artery hypertension may develop with subsequent right ventricular enlargement (cor pulmonale) leading to jugular venous distension (JVD), tender hepatomegaly, and peripheral edema [28]. Other signs may include evidence of cyanosis including nailbed clubbing and decreased mental status. Worsening peripheral edema and co-existent underlying pneumonia are more prevalent in the geriatric population [29]. It is important to consider a spontaneous pneumothorax in patients with a history of COPD who suddenly deteriorate.

There are no definitive laboratory tests or imaging that can be done to diagnose a COPD exacerbation, rather tests such as a BNP and chest X-ray can exclude other diagnoses such as heart failure and pneumonia. However, age, performance status, blood urea nitrogen (BUN), serum albumin, and arterial oxygen saturation have been shown as independent predictors of mortality [29].

Emergency treatment of exacerbations should be directed at reversing hypoxemia and airflow obstruction. Mainstays of therapy include supplemental oxygen, inhaled beta-2 adrenergic agonists, ipratropium bromide, and corticosteroids. The goal is to maintain an arterial oxygen saturation of >90%. Treatment of COPD exacerbations in the geriatric population can be difficult in that therapeutic response to inhaled bronchodilators decreases with advancing age due to the decline in number of beta-2 receptors [28]. Bronchodilators also cause a dose-dependent drop in serum potassium that could cause prolongation of the QT segment, which can be worrisome in those who are already on multiple medications which prolong the QT segment. In COPD patients, corticosteroids have been shown to decrease relapse rate and to decrease inflammation in asthma exacerbations. For patients with increase in sputum or change in color, antibiotics are recommended [27]. NIPPV has become an increasingly utilized form of oxygenation in acute COPD exacerbations and works by decreasing $PaCO_2$ by supporting the respiratory muscles and supplementing alveolar ventilation. In acute hypoxemia, it also helps maintain an adequate PaO_2 [2,30]. NIPPV has been shown to reduce the need for intubation, ventilator-associated pneumonia, duration of ICU stays, and in-hospital mortality [2,30]. Initial studies on NIPPV were done in middle-aged patients. However, more recent studies have shown that the same conclusions can be applied to the elderly population as well [2,3].

Asthma exacerbation

Asthma is an inflammatory disease of the upper airway that leads to diffuse airway narrowing from mucous secretions, bronchospasm, and airway edema. Diagnosis is made in an outpatient setting with pulmonary function tests demonstrating obstruction via an increase in FEV_1 and its reversibility with bronchodilators.

Its prevalence in the elderly population may currently be underestimated due to the multiple underlying comorbidities seen in this population that can cause similar symptoms as asthma [31,32]. While a smaller percentage of asthmatics are elderly, they account for a disproportionate percentage of hospitalizations and mortality [32,33]. There is an increased variability in presentation and duration of acute exacerbations and an irreversibility of obstruction that is unique to the elderly population [34]. This is thought to be due to airway remodeling, relative increase in number of neutrophils leading to increased protease secretion and thus mucus production, as well as other underlying pulmonary comorbidities including COPD, bronchiectasis, and pulmonary fibrosis [34].

Presentation of acute asthma exacerbations and diagnostic work-up are similar to that of COPD exacerbations and are addressed in the COPD section above. Again, as in those with COPD, the clinician should consider a pneumothorax in those with underlying asthma.

Treatment of acute asthma exacerbations is similar to that in the younger population. Mainstays of treatment are inhaled short-acting beta-2 adrenergic agonists (albuterol), inhaled anticholinergics (ipratropium), and corticosteroids. However, symptom relief can be more difficult to achieve in the elderly population. Decreased lung function, especially stiffening of the chest wall, reduced respiratory muscle function, and an increase in residual volume from loss of elastic recoil leads to a reduced response to bronchodilators and corticosteroids [34]. The elderly are also more prone to side effects of beta-2 adrenergic agonists including tachycardia, tremors, QTc prolongation, and decreased serum potassium [33]. NIPPV has not been shown to be as effective in asthma exacerbations as it is in CHF and COPD exacerbations [35].

Pneumonia

The elderly are at an increased risk for developing pneumonia for a myriad of reasons including multiple comorbidities, poor nutrition, recent hospitalization, home care, institutionalization, and general worsening of health [28,36]. Almost one million episodes of community-acquired pneumonia are diagnosed in the elderly each year, with over two-thirds of these requiring hospitalization. In 2008, pneumonia was the fifth leading cause of death in the geriatric population in the US [37].

Over half of patients who develop pneumonia are more than 65 years old [36,38]. Nursing home patients especially have an increased mortality from pneumonia, which has been reported as high as 44% [36,38]. Bacterial pneumonia often originates from the nasopharynx, but the elderly are also predisposed to aspiration due to an ineffective cough reflex, esophageal peristaltic dysfunction, and decreased mental status [28]. These structural changes, which also include decreased muscle strength and subsequent inability to clear secretions, along with a decline in the immune response, make older patients more susceptible to infection and more likely to become critically ill when infection occurs. These factors lead to a higher morbidity and mortality in the geriatric population in the setting of pneumonia.

The elderly often present with atypical symptoms, most commonly dyspnea (reported as 58–74%) [37], followed by cough, fever, and sputum production [18]. It is important to note that half of patients older than 70 years diagnosed with pneumonia presented with nonrespiratory symptoms including failure to thrive, confusion, weakness, and decreased mental status [39].

Work-up of pneumonia in the elderly is similar to that in the general population, which includes complete blood count (CBC), blood cultures when warranted, chest X-ray, and, if possible, sputum cultures. Diagnosis is made more difficult due to the frequent absence of classic signs and symptoms such as fever, leukocytosis, and sputum production [37]. Chest X-ray has been demonstrated to have a low sensitivity and negative predictive value in identifying pulmonary opacities [40], thus a negative chest X-ray cannot rule out the diagnosis of pneumonia.

For multiple reasons, the causative organism is identified less than 50% of the time in the elderly population [28]. However, the most common organisms isolated in the community are *Streptococcus pneumoniae* followed by *Haemophilus influenzae*, and *Moraxella catarrhalis* [37,41]. In the nursing home population there is a higher incidence of multidrug resistance as well as a larger proportion of atypical bacteria such as *Legionella pneumophila*, *Chlamydia pneumoniae*, and *Mycoplasma* [37,42].

The higher morbidity and mortality rate seen in CAP in the elderly is thought to be primarily due to functional status rather than the infecting organism [36]. While Gram-negative rods and multidrug-resistant *Staphylococcus aureus* (MRSA) are less common causes of pneumonia, they are more frequently seen in those who are seriously ill. MRSA has an increased incidence in the setting of a preceding viral illness [37]. Emergency treatment of pneumonia consists of initially stabilizing the patient's respiratory status including maintaining adequate oxygenation, reversing dehydration, and administering antimicrobial therapy. Most recent antibiotic guidelines for nursing home-acquired pneumonia include a fluoroquinolone or amoxicillin/clavulanic acid plus a macrolide for initial treatment in the nursing home. If inpatient treatment is required, an antipseudomonal cephalosporin plus a macrolide is recommended. In those with severe pneumonia, the recommendation is a cephalosporin and ciprofloxacin plus vancomycin [42]. In those with low-risk, community-acquired pneumonia, monotherapy with a macrolide is currently recommended as standard outpatient therapy, both due to its atypical coverage and anti-inflammatory properties [43]. However, certain populations, seen more in Western Europe, are demonstrating increased resistance to macrolides and thus amoxicillin or amoxicillin/clavulanic acid are recommended in such cases [41]. In severe CAP that requires hospitalization, a combination of broad-spectrum antibiotics should be used due to significantly improved outcomes including decreased mortality [43]. However, there are minimal data to support one specific combination of antibiotics to be significantly more

effective than another. Multiple observational studies have shown that combination therapy should include a macrolide. There has been no proven difference in using a macrolide/fluoroquinolone versus a macrolide/beta-lactam combination [43] or between a macrolide/beta-lactam versus fluoroquinolone/beta-lactam combination [44]. It is also unclear whether there is a difference in efficacy among the different macrolides [43]. Other studies also recommend adding piperacillin/tazobactam if concerned about *Pseudomonas aeruginosa* [41]. Treatment duration should be five to seven days, except in the case of proven infections of *P. aeruginosa*, in which a 15-day course of antibiotics has been shown to be more appropriate [41]. Institutional-based prevalence and sensitivities should also be taken into account when determining appropriate antibiotic choices.

Summary

Acute dyspnea is a common presenting symptom of the elderly and can lead to significant morbidity and mortality. Structural, mechanical, and physiologic changes to both pulmonary and cardiovascular systems make the elderly more vulnerable to significant acute injury. Not only are they more susceptible to developing illness, but are less likely to present with classic symptoms and signs and have difficulty with mounting an adequate response to injury.

Given this, the clinician should maintain a wide differential when evaluating the geriatric patient with shortness of breath. The most common causes of acute dyspnea are briefly discussed above. However, there are other disease processes that should be included in the differential for dyspnea in the geriatric population. These include, but are not limited to, pneumothorax, metabolic acidosis in the setting of diabetic ketoacidosis, acute intra-abdominal or renal pathology, and sepsis. The presence of primary metabolic acidosis causes a compensatory increase in respiratory rate. Given the decreased pulmonary function and lower baseline PaO_2 seen in the elderly, they are unable to compensate as efficiently. Also, this increased work of breathing can exacerbate other underlying comorbid conditions that were discussed above. For further details on specific disease processes please refer to Section 3 of this book.

In summary, the clinician should be aware that there are significant changes in the pulmonary and cardiovascular systems as one ages, which alters the approach and treatment of the elderly who present with acute dyspnea.

Pearls and pitfalls

Pearls

- Age-related structural and physiologic changes in both pulmonary and cardiovascular systems make the elderly population more susceptible to and have a more difficult time overcoming acute physiologic stressors.
- Older lungs have decreased functional capacity, lower reserve volume, and decreased baseline PaO_2.
- Older hearts have decreased cardiac output both at baseline and with exercise, as well as a higher resting

systolic blood pressure and increased prevalence of peripheral vascular disease.

- In those with underlying asthma and COPD who report a history of or show sudden deterioration while in the ED, the clinician should always keep pneumothorax in the differential.
- Elderly patients with acute dyspnea tend to not exhibit classic signs or symptoms seen in the younger population. Keep your differential broad.

Pitfalls

- Acute dyspnea in the elderly is more likely to be due to multiple causative factors, including non-cardiopulmonary causes, and necessitates a more extensive work-up.
- Even the relatively healthy elderly patient is unable to compensate as effectively in the setting of acute lung or cardiac injury. Have a lower threshold to admit or to obtain close follow-up of acutely dyspneic elderly patients.
- When initiating treatment for the suspected cause of acute dyspnea, the clinician must take into account the patient's other comorbid conditions and mental status in order to provide the most appropriate care.
- Always consider an acute coronary event as the cause of dyspnea in the elderly population even if the patient does not present with chest pain.

References

1. Aminzadeh F, Dalziel WB. Older adults in the emergency department: a systematic review of patterns of use, adverse outcomes, and effectiveness of interventions. *Ann Emerg Med.* 2002;39:238–47.

2. Ray P, Birolleau S, Lefort Y, et al. Acute respiratory failure in the elderly: etiology, emergency diagnosis and prognosis. *Critical Care (London).* 2006;10:R82.

3. Ray P, Birolleau S, Riou B. Acute dyspnoea in elderly patients. *Revue Des Maladies Respiratoires.* 2004;21:8S42–54.

4. Sharma G, Goodwin J. Effect of aging on respiratory system physiology and immunology. *Clinical Interventions Aging.* 2006;1:253.

5. Taylor NAS. Pulmonary function in aging humans. In *Handbook of the Biology of Aging*, ed. Masoro EJ, Austed SN (Amsterdam: Elsevier, 2010), p. 421.

6. Williams JM, Evans TC. Acute pulmonary disease in the aged. *Clin Geriatr Med.* 1993;9:527–45.

7. Wei JY. Age and the cardiovascular system. *N Engl J Med.* 1992;327:1735–9.

8. Lakatta, E. Changes in cardiovascular function with aging. *Eur Heart J.* 1990;11:22.

9. Thomas S, Rich MW. Epidemiology, pathophysiology, and prognosis of heart failure in the elderly. *Heart Failure Clinics.* 2007;3:381–7.

10. Carek S. Heart failure in older people. *Generations.* 2006;30:25–32.

11. Baker S, Ramani GV. *Heart Failure in the Elderly* (Bethesda, MD: National Institutes of Health, 2006).

12. Michelson E, Hollrah S. Evaluation of the patient with shortness of breath: an evidence based approach. *Emerg Med Clin N Am.* 1999;17:221–37.

13. Wang CS, FitzGerald JM, Schulzer M, Mak E, Ayas NT. Does this dyspneic patient in the emergency department have congestive heart failure? *JAMA.* 2005;c4:1944–56.

14. Delerme S, Ray P. Acute respiratory failure in the elderly: diagnosis and prognosis. *Age Aging.* 2008;37:251–7.

15. Archambault P, St-Onge M. Invasive and noninvasive ventilation in the emergency department. *Emerg Med Clin N Am.* 2012;30:421–49.

16. Bersten AD. Best practices for noninvasive ventilation. *CMAJ.* 2011;183:293–4.

17. Kim DY, Kobayashi L, Barmparas G, et al. Venous thromboembolism in the elderly: the result of comorbid conditions or a consequence of injury? *J Trauma Acute Care Surg.* 2012;72:1286–91.

18. Moayedi S. Approach to dyspnea among older adults. *Geriatrics Aging.* 2008;11:347–50.

19. Masotti L, Ray P, Righini M, et al. Pulmonary embolism in the elderly: a review on clinical, instrumental and laboratory presentation. *Vasc Health Risk Management.* 2008;4:629–36.

20. Castelli R, Bergamaschini L, Sailis P, Pantaleo G, Porro F. The impact of an aging population on the diagnosis of pulmonary embolism: comparison of young and elderly patients. *Clin Appl Thromb/Hemostasis.* 2009;15:65–72.

21. Calvo-Romero JM, Lima-Rodrguez EM, Bureo-Dacal P, Perez-Miranda M. Predictors of an intermediate ventilation/perfusion lung scan in patients with suspected acute pulmonary embolism. *Eur J Emerg Med.* 2005;12:129.

22. Righini M, Goehring C, Bounameaux H, Perrier A. Effects of age on the performance of common diagnostic tests for pulmonary embolism. *Am J Med.* 2000;109:357–61.

23. Righini M, Le Gal G, Perrier A, Bounameaux H. Clinical probability assessment of pulmonary embolism by the Wells' score: is the easiest the best? *J Thromb Haemost.* 2006;4:702–4.

24. Le Gal G, Righini M, Roy PM, et al. Prediction of pulmonary embolism in the emergency department: the revised Geneva score. *Ann Intern Med.* 2006;144:165–71.

25. Goodman SG, Huang W, Yan AT, et al. The expanded Global Registry of Acute Coronary Events: baseline characteristics, management practices, and hospital outcomes of patients with acute coronary syndromes. *Am Heart J.* 2009;158:193–201.

26. Wright RS, Anderson JL, Adams CD, et al. 2011 ACCF/AHA Focused update incorporated into the ACC/AHA 2007 Guidelines for the management of patients with unstable angina/non-ST-elevation myocardial infarction: a report of the American College of Cardiology Foundation/ American Heart Association Task Force on Practice Guidelines. *J Am Coll Cardiol.* 2011;57:e215.

27. Abbatecola AM, Fumagalli A, Bonardi D, Guffanti EE. Practical management problems of chronic obstructive pulmonary disease in the elderly: acute exacerbations. *Curr Opin Pulmon Med.* 2011;17:S49.

28. Imperato J, Sanchez LD. Pulmonary emergencies in the elderly. *Emerg Med Clin N Am.* 2006;24:317–38.

29. Stone RA, Lowe D, Potter JM, et al. Managing patients with COPD exacerbation: does age matter? *Age Aging.* 2012;41:461–8.

30. Ray P, Al-Harty A. *Management of Acute Respiratory Failure in Elderly Patients: Prognosis and Risk Factors* (accessed from www.touchemergencymedicine.com/.../private/articles/10513/pdf/ray.pdf).

31. Bellia V, Battaglia S, Catalano F, et al. Aging and disability affect misdiagnosis of COPD in elderly asthmatics: the SARA study. *Chest.* 2003;123:1066–72.

32. Enright PL, McClelland RL, Newman AB, Gottlieb DJ, Lebowitz MD. Underdiagnosis and undertreatment of asthma in the elderly. *Chest.* 1999;116:603–13.

33. Hanania NA, King MJ, Braman SS, et al. Asthma in the elderly: Current understanding and future research needs: a report of a National Institute on Aging (NIA) workshop. *J Allergy Clin Immunol.* 2011;128:S4–24.

34. Reed CE. Asthma in the elderly: diagnosis and management. *J Allergy Clin Immunol.* 2010;126:681–7.

35. Bhattacharyya D, Prasad B, Rajput A. Recent advances in the role of non-invasive ventilation in acute respiratory failure. *Med J Armed Forces India.* 2011;67:187–91.

36. Ewig S, Welte T, Chastre J, Torres A. Rethinking the concepts of community-acquired and health-care-associated pneumonia. *Lancet Infect Dis.* 2010;10:279–87.

37. Caterino JM. Evaluation and management of geriatric infections in the emergency department. *Emerg Med Clin N Am.* 2008;26:319–43.

38. Adedeipe A, Lowenstein LR. Infectious emergencies in the elderly. *Emerg Med Clin N Am.* 2006;24:433–48.

39. Feldman C. Pneumonia in the elderly. *Emerg Med Clin N Am.* 2001;85:1441.

40. Self WH, Courtney DM, McNaughton CD, Wunderink RG, Kline JA. High discordance of chest X-ray and computed tomography for detection of pulmonary opacities in ED patients: implications for diagnosing pneumonia. *Am J Emerg Med.* 2012;31:401–5.

41. Thiem U, Heppner HJ, Pientka L. Elderly patients with community-acquired pneumonia: optimal treatment strategies. *Drugs Aging.* 2011;28:519–37.

42. Mylotte JM. Nursing home-acquired pneumonia: update on treatment options. *Drugs Aging.* 2006;23:377–90.

43. Waterer GW, Rello J, Wunderink RG. Management of community-acquired pneumonia in adults. *Am J Resp Crit Care Med.* 2011;183:157–64.

44. Wilson BZ, Anzueto A, Restrepo MI, Pugh MJV, Mortensen EM. Comparison of two guideline-concordant antimicrobial combinations in elderly patients hospitalized with severe community-acquired pneumonia. *Crit Care Med.* 2012;40:2310–14.

Abdominal pain in the elderly

Joseph P. Martinez and Amal Mattu

Background

The elderly patient presenting to the emergency department (ED) with acute abdominal pain remains one of the most complex, time-consuming, and perilous patients that the practitioner will encounter. These patients consume more time and resources than any other ED patient presentation [1]. Compared with younger patients with the same complaints, the elderly patient with abdominal pain will stay in the ED 20% longer, require admission nearly half the time, and require urgent surgical intervention in nearly one-third of cases [2]. The mortality rate approaches 10% and is nearly ninefold higher than in younger patients. Elderly patients that are discharged home have a recidivism rate of one-third. Many practitioners in emergency medicine become skilled at recognizing patients as "sick or not sick." While a valuable skill, this recognition is not sufficient in the case of the geriatric patient with abdominal pain. Failure to diagnose a surgical condition in the ED greatly increases the patient's mortality, even if that patient is admitted to the hospital for continued observation [2]. As the world's population continues to age, practicing clinicians will encounter more of these cases with each shift. A healthy appreciation of the perilous nature of this complaint in this age group is important. Combining this with a structured approach and an understanding of the atypical presentation of serious disease is the key to providing high-quality, life-saving care.

History

Taking an accurate history is crucial in patients with abdominal pain. This seemingly straightforward skill can be problematic in the geriatric patient. Decreased hearing, decreased memory, and stoicism are some of the challenges faced. Geriatric patients often have multiple comorbidities and are on multiple medications. Some patients will actually withhold aspects of the history out of fear that they will be hospitalized, leading to a loss of independence.

The history itself should focus on the same red flags that would be sought in a younger patient with abdominal pain. These include abrupt onset, significant associated symptoms such as syncope, gross blood in vomit or stool, and fever, among

others. Certain differences are important to remember. The incidence of vascular disease is higher in the elderly. Vascular emergencies should always be considered early in the course, as the window to intervene is small. Elderly patients often present later than young patients, even with surgical pathology. Over a quarter of all elderly patients with appendicitis present after more than three days of symptoms, and a significant proportion will have symptoms for more than one week before seeking medical care [3].

Medication lists are often lengthy in this age group. Medications may cause abdominal pathology, mask its symptoms, and alter the vital sign abnormalities one would expect. Adverse drug reactions lead to nearly 15% of all admissions in the elderly [4]. Nonsteroidal anti-inflammatory drugs (NSAIDs) should be specifically asked about, as these greatly increase the risk for peptic ulcer disease (PUD). Steroids are often used for conditions such as rheumatoid arthritis, temporal arthritis, and lung disease. The use of these medications may blunt the inflammatory response to peritonitis, and they also contribute to the development of PUD. Beta blockers may mask the tachycardia that one expects to see with intra-abdominal sepsis. Digitalis, metformin, and colchicine (among many others) may actually cause abdominal pain. An accurate medication list including over-the-counter medication, herbs, and supplements is crucial. If the patient cannot provide one, it should be sought from the family, primary care provider, or pharmacy.

Physical examination

The physical examination is equally challenging. Vital signs become less reliable. Elderly patients may not mount a fever as expected. They are equally likely to be normothermic or hypothermic, even with serious intra-abdominal pathology [5]. Hypertension affects 1 billion people worldwide. A seemingly normal blood pressure may actually reflect significant hypotension in someone with preceding hypertension. Acquired conduction system abnormalities may prevent tachycardia, in addition to the medications mentioned earlier.

The abdomen should be carefully assessed and noted specifically for the presence or absence of masses or bruits. Surgical scars should be explained. The skilled practitioner

Geriatric Emergency Medicine, ed. Joseph H. Kahn, Brendan G. Magauran Jr., and Jonathan S. Olshaker. Published by Cambridge University Press. © Cambridge University Press 2014.

will not be falsely reassured by the absence of a rigid, board-like "surgical abdomen." With aging, the abdominal musculature loses mass. Rigidity and guarding is often much less than expected in this age group. Rigidity may be absent in up to 80% of perforated ulcers [6]. Hernias should be searched for, remembering that femoral hernias are a more common cause of small bowel obstruction in women of this age group.

The physical examination should not be limited to the abdomen. General appearance of the patient is important, as are clues such as pallor or icterus. The cardiopulmonary examination may suggest an alternate diagnosis causing pain, such as a lower lobe pneumonia or congestive heart failure with hepatic congestion. The presence of atrial fibrillation is of particular importance, as its presence increases the likelihood of acute mesenteric ischemia.

Diagnostic tests

An extended array of laboratory tests is often sent in geriatric patients with abdominal pain. One of the common pitfalls is being reassured by "normal" laboratory values. For example, leukocytosis may be absent in up to one-quarter of cases of appendicitis in this age group [7]. Another pitfall is being misled by abnormal values that do not correlate with the patient's clinical picture. Elevated amylase may be seen in pancreatitis, but this nonspecific finding can also be seen in more life-threatening entities such as mesenteric ischemia. Microscopic hematuria may indicate a kidney stone, or it may accompany a ruptured aortic aneurysm. In geriatric patients with appendicitis, 17% will have an elevated bilirubin and up to 40% will have an abnormal urinalysis [8].

An electrocardiogram should be obtained early in the course of any elderly patient with abdominal pain. The physiologic stress of severe intra-abdominal pathology may trigger myocardial ischemia. Elderly patients may also present with abdominal symptoms caused by myocardial infarction. Nearly one-third of elderly women will present with abdominal pain instead of chest pain as the symptoms of their myocardial infarction [9].

Imaging studies

Plain radiographs

Plain radiographs are commonly ordered as one of the first steps in evaluating the geriatric abdomen. If the clinician is considering free intraperitoneal air, bowel obstruction, or foreign body, these may be useful. As a general screen for all patients, they are of limited utility. Normal plain films should not falsely reassure the clinician that there is no serious underlying pathology. Similar to laboratory tests, there may be incidental findings that lead the clinician away from the correct diagnosis. For instance, phleboliths are often misinterpreted as ureteral stones and the patient's pain attributed to this diagnosis, whether or not it fits the clinical picture.

Ultrasound

Ultrasound is becoming more widely available, and more practitioners are being trained in its use. Indications for ultrasound are expanding almost daily. A skill that is quick to obtain, even for inexperienced ultrasound operators, is evaluating the size of the abdominal aorta [10]. This is an invaluable tool in the work-up of acute abdominal pain. Ultrasound may not be able to determine aneurysm rupture, but in the appropriate clinical scenario, presence of aneurysm alone mandates urgent transport to the operating room.

Ultrasound remains the test of choice to evaluate biliary pathology. This is of particular utility as acute cholecystitis is the most common reason for acute abdominal surgery in this age group. As a word of caution, the incidence of choledocholithiasis is higher in this age group as well. This is not well detected by ultrasound. Ultrasound is also useful in the detection of ovarian or testicular pathology.

Computed tomography

Computed tomography (CT) is another modality whose use is expanding. With the advent of multidetector row CT (MDR-CT), resolution is improving and the ability to generate angiographic quality images has arrived.

Computed tomography has been shown to alter decision making in the elderly. In a 2004 study, CT usage altered the diagnosis in 45% of cases and changed the admission decision in one-quarter. It frequently altered the need for antibiotics, the need for surgery, and doubled the diagnostic certainty of the attending physician [11]. Long-term risks from ionizing radiation exposure are negligible in this population, and CT has also been shown to be cost-effective when compared with admission for serial abdominal examinations [12].

Angiography

Angiography is being used less commonly as more practitioners are opting for MDR-CT angiography. Despite its invasive nature and potential for nephrotoxicity, angiography remains an invaluable tool in the evaluation of mesenteric ischemia. It can confirm the diagnosis and is useful for adjunctive or sole treatment.

Differential diagnoses

The differential list for the elderly patient with abdominal pain is extensive. Given the high prevalence of atherosclerosis in this population, vascular catastrophes should always be considered early in the work-up.

Vascular catastrophes

Ruptured abdominal aortic aneurysm

Ruptured abdominal aortic aneurysm (AAA) remains one of the leading causes of death in this age group. The mortality is extremely high. One study found a mortality rate of 70% despite a door to operating room time of only 12 minutes [13]. The classic portrait of ruptured AAA is an elderly patient who presents with abdominal pain, hypotension, and a pulsatile abdominal mass. This straightforward presentation is rarely seen in clinical medicine. Atypical presentations abound. Hypotension is absent in nearly 65% of cases that survive to presentation and palpable mass is absent in one-quarter of cases.

The most common misdiagnosis of ruptured AAA is renal colic. Many of the signs and symptoms of these two disorders overlap: flank pain that may radiate to the groin accompanied by microscopic hematuria from the AAA irritating the ureter. As a general rule, new-onset kidney stones after the age of 50 warrant imaging of the aorta before discharge, either by ultrasound or CT. Other common disorders that are mistakenly diagnosed include musculoskeletal back pain, syncope, and peripheral neuropathy (when the femoral or obturator nerve is compressed).

A careful physical examination is important. As noted above, a pulsatile mass may be absent but its presence helps make the diagnosis. Documentation of peripheral pulses is important. Ecchymosis of the toes may be the result of emboli from a thrombus in the aorta. Unexplained ecchymosis of the abdomen, flank, or groin may also signify AAA rupture. The great majority of aortic aneurysms rupture either intraperitoneally or into the left retroperitoneal space. They may also rupture into the vena cava and present with a continuous abdominal bruit and high-output heart failure. Aortic aneurysms may form an abnormal communication with the GI tract. Patients with a known AAA or a previous AAA repair who present with gastrointestinal bleed should be assumed to have an aortic-enteric fistula (AEF). This entity is much more common after repair (secondary AEF) than with a native AAA (primary AEF). The hemorrhage may initially be mild, similar to the "sentinel bleed" of subarachnoid hemorrhage.

Work-up of suspected AAA rupture depends on the stability of the patient. Unstable patients with known AAA or suspected AAA based on exam or bedside ultrasound should be transported rapidly to the OR. Stable patients can undergo further imaging with contrast-enhanced CT scan.

If evaluation reveals a leaking AAA, operative repair should be pursued. Advanced age does not preclude repair [14]. Open versus endovascular repair should be discussed with the treating surgeon. Aggressive volume repletion in stable patients should be avoided, but large amounts of blood (at least 10 units) should be made available as these patients often have substantial transfusion requirements.

Acute mesenteric ischemia

A devastating disorder, the mortality of acute mesenteric ischemia (AMI) remains high despite better understanding of the pathophysiology and better treatment options. Mesenteric ischemia is a difficult disorder to diagnose in a timely fashion, and is equally difficult to treat. Treatment needs to be multifactorial, addressing issues of reperfusion, vasospasm, and ischemia-reperfusion injury.

Mesenteric ischemia is a generic term. There are at least four different types including superior mesenteric artery (SMA) embolus, SMA thrombosis, mesenteric venous thrombosis (MVT), and nonocclusive mesenteric ischemia (NOMI). Challenges exist with all types, but there are clues that may help point towards the diagnosis (see Table 11.1).

Embolus of the SMA is the most common type of AMI. Patients present with acute abdominal pain. The most common

Table 11.1. Historical clues to assist in the diagnosis of acute mesenteric ischemia

Etiology	Clue
SMA embolus	1/3 of patients have prior embolus
SMA thrombosis	Previous history of intestinal angina (80%)
Mesenteric venous thrombosis	1/2 of patients have personal or family history of VTE
NOMI	Dialysis/digitalis

SMA, superior mesenteric artery; NOMI, nonocclusive mesenteric ischemia; VTE, venous thromboembolic disease.

etiology is atrial fibrillation, but it can be caused by any disorder that leads to stasis in the left ventricle such as ventricular aneurysm from previous myocardial infarction. As the bowel becomes ischemic, it attempts to empty its contents. As such, the pain is often associated with "gut emptying" – vomiting, diarrhea, or both. This explains why the most common misdiagnosis for AMI is gastroenteritis. One-third of patients with SMA embolus will have had a previous embolic event [15]. Patients should be specifically questioned and old records examined for embolic strokes, renal or splenic infarcts, and lower extremity arterial emboli.

Thrombosis of the SMA shares a similar pathophysiology to acute coronary syndrome (ACS). Turbulent flow at the origin of the SMA leads to plaque deposition. Patients tend to have risk factors for atherosclerosis, including smoking. If flow-limiting stenosis develops, patients may develop "intestinal angina," postprandial abdominal pain leading to "food fear," and weight loss. This may persist for months to years and may be accompanied by significant weight loss. Similar to ACS, if plaque rupture occurs, blood flow to the SMA is abruptly reduced and symptoms comparable to SMA embolus occur. A history of intestinal angina makes the diagnosis of AMI much more likely. Patients should be routinely questioned about symptoms consistent with this entity.

Mesenteric venous thrombosis has a number of important differences from the other etiologies of AMI. It tends to occur in a younger cohort of patients, many of whom have an underlying hypercoagulable state. The time course is much more indolent, with time from onset of symptoms to diagnosis being days to weeks [16]. An important historical clue is that one-half of patients with MVT will have a personal or family history of venous thromboembolism [17].

Nonocclusive mesenteric ischemia develops in patients due to low-flow states such as sepsis, severe volume depletion, or cardiogenic shock. It may also be seen in dialysis patients due to transient hypoperfusion. Patients taking digoxin are at increased risk as well. It is often seen in ICU patients where it manifests as abdominal distension and GI bleeding.

Patients with AMI present with pain out of proportion to exam. The work-up includes labs, imaging, and consultation with vascular and general surgery. Laboratory data suggestive of AMI include metabolic acidosis, leukocytosis, and elevated amylase and lactate levels. Plain films are not helpful in the evaluation. Early angiography (before the onset of

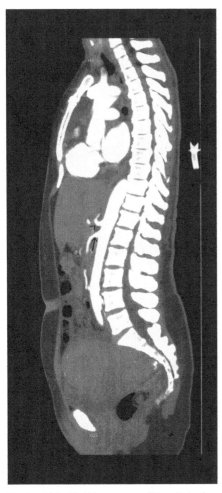

Figure 11.1. Multidetector row CT; sagittal reformatting of normal celiac axis (arrowhead) and normal superior mesenteric artery (arrow).

peritoneal signs) is the only intervention to date that has been proven to reduce mortality [18]. The work-up of suspected AMI has been evolving with the advent of MDR-CT angiography (Figure 11.1). Given the quality of the images and ease of acquisition, many centers are employing a strategy of using MDR-CT angiography to screen suspected cases and following up positive films with traditional angiography to help plan surgical approach and treat associated vasospasm [19]. Patients that are too ill for open surgery may sometimes be treated angiographically with catheter-based therapy.

Bowel obstructions

Small bowel obstruction

Elderly patients with small bowel obstruction (SBO) present in a similar manner to young patients. They typically have nausea, vomiting, distension, and constipation. The prognosis for elderly patients is worse. Mortality rates range from 14 to 35%. The excess mortality may at least partially be due to missed or delayed diagnosis – SBO remains the second most common condition to be inappropriately discharged home, behind appendicitis [2]. This occurs primarily in those cases where SBO presents without significant abdominal pain. This is also a condition where appropriate diagnosis in the ED is essential.

If a patient with SBO is admitted to the medical service for conservative treatment, surgical therapy (when necessary) is delayed with increased morbidity and mortality [20].

Adhesions or hernias cause most cases of SBO in the elderly. While gallstone disease causes only 2% of SBOs in young patients, gallstone ileus accounts for nearly one-quarter of obstructions in women older than 65 [21].

Large bowel obstruction

Cancer, diverticulitis, and volvulus cause most cases of large bowel obstruction (LBO). While LBO is less common than SBO, proportionally more cases of LBO are seen in the elderly as cancers and diverticulitis are more commonly seen in this age group. Patients with LBO typically present with vomiting, constipation or obstipation, and abdominal pain. However, many elderly patients will actually have diarrhea with an LBO and only one-half will complain of constipation or vomiting [22].

Volvulus is a less frequent cause of LBO, often requiring surgical intervention. Volvulus may occur in either the sigmoid colon or cecum, with sigmoid volvulus being slightly more common. Sigmoid volvulus tends to occur in debilitated, chronically ill patients and is of more gradual onset (Figure 11.2). It can initially be treated non-operatively with sigmoidoscopic decompression. Due to the high rate of recurrence, it often subsequently requires a more definitive operation. Cecal volvulus occurs more acutely, usually in a younger age group. Given its anatomic location, it is not amenable to endoscopic decompression and almost always requires acute surgical intervention.

Peptic ulcer disease

It is rare for young patients to have PUD without pain. However, a 1960s' study found that 35% of patients over the age of 60 with endoscopically proven PUD had no associated pain [23]. One-half of all elderly patients with PUD will have their initial presentation as a complication [24]. This is often perforation, but may include hemorrhage, gastric outlet obstruction, or penetration into adjacent structures. Even with these complications, the elderly patient may present atypically. Rigidity is noted in less than 20% of perforations, and less than half of patients will describe the acute onset of pain [6]. Upright chest radiographs are reasonable as a screen for free intraperitoneal air, but this is absent in 40% of elderly patients with perforated viscus [25] (Figure 11.3). The mortality rate approaches 30% when there is a perforation, nearly threefold that of younger patients. The mortality increases eightfold if the diagnosis is delayed by 24 hours [26]. Patients older than 70 are less likely to respond to conservative treatment compared with surgery [27].

Elderly patients with PUD are more likely to bleed than younger patients. They are also more likely to rebleed, to require blood transfusions, and to require surgery to control bleeding [28].

Biliary tract disease

Acute cholecystitis is the most common surgical emergency in this age group [29]. Emergent cholecystectomy carries a fourfold higher mortality rate than elective cholecystectomy. The rate of complications from biliary disease is higher in the

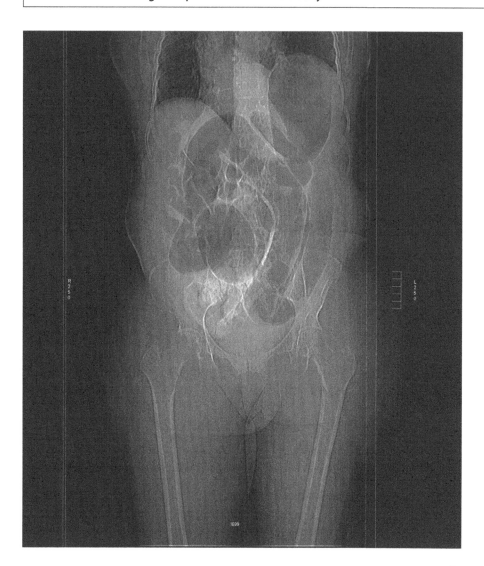

Figure 11.2. Scout image from CT scan showing "bent inner-tube" bowel gas predictive of sigmoid volvulus.

elderly as well. The gallbladder is a poorly vascularized structure and more susceptible to perforation in this population that often has underlying atherosclerosis. The elderly are also more at risk for emphysematous cholecystitis, gallstone-induced pancreatitis, and gallbladder gangrene. Choledocholithiasis is also more common, leading to a higher incidence of ascending cholangitis.

Tenderness with palpation in the right upper quadrant (RUQ) and over the gallbladder is commonly seen with acute cholecystitis, though the patient's complaint of pain may not specifically localize to the RUQ. Many of the other signs and symptoms of acute cholecystitis may be absent, leading to delays in diagnosis and increased complications. Elderly patients are afebrile in half the cases of cholecystitis and often lack nausea and vomiting. Leukocytosis is absent in 30 to 40% and liver function tests are often normal. Given the higher incidence of acalculous cholecystitis in this age group, a normal ultrasound, coupled with a high pretest probability, should prompt further evaluation with a hepatobiliary iminodiacetic acid (HIDA) scan.

Broad-spectrum antibiotics should be initiated when the diagnosis is suspected. Early surgical consultation is imperative, as delays in surgery lead to increased morbidity

and mortality [30]. Ascending cholangitis is also more commonly seen in this population. Acute suppurative cholangitis requires immediate decompression either through open surgery, endoscopic decompression, or percutaneous decompression.

Pancreatitis

The incidence of pancreatitis increases 200-fold after the age of 65 [31]. It is the most common nonsurgical abdominal condition in this population. The mortality rate approaches 40% above the age of 70 [32]. The presentation of pancreatitis in the elderly mirrors that in younger patients, but there is a small group of elderly patients in whom pancreatitis presents merely as altered mental status and hypotension [24]. Pancreatitis in the elderly can sometimes manifest as nausea and vomiting without significant pain. The "older old" (above the age of 80) are at higher risk for necrotizing pancreatitis. This condition often leads to rapid deterioration. The threshold for utilizing CT imaging of suspected pancreatitis in the elderly should be low, especially if they are exhibiting signs of systemic inflammatory response syndrome (SIRS) or impending sepsis. As noted above, hyperamylasemia may also be seen with acute mesenteric ischemia. Prudent clinicians will not attribute

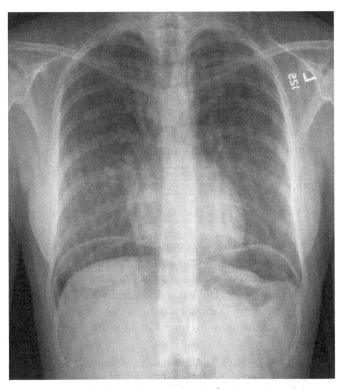

Figure 11.3. Upright chest radiograph showing free intraperitoneal air.

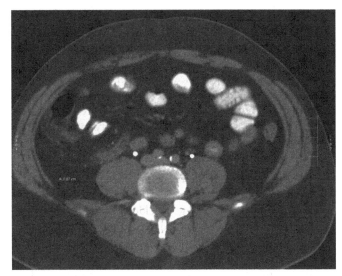

Figure 11.4. CT scan showing dilated appendix that does not fill with oral contrast, consistent with appendicitis.

amylase elevations to pancreatitis without the appropriate clinical picture.

Appendicitis

Appendicitis was once thought to be a disease only of the young. It is now recognized that it can and does occur in the elderly. It is actually the third most common abdominal surgical condition and remains the most common condition that is misdiagnosed and inappropriately discharged [33]. The elderly account for only 14% of all cases of appendicitis but 50% of all the deaths from appendicitis [34]. Appendicitis carries a mortality rate of 4 to 8% in the geriatric population, compared with 1% in the overall population [35]. Morbidity is increased in the elderly as well. Nearly 70% of all cases of appendicitis in the elderly have perforated by the time they go to surgery [36].

The diagnosis of appendicitis in the elderly is challenging. One-quarter of all cases are missed on initial presentation. Many clinicians are familiar with Dr. Alfredo Alvarado's scoring system for suspected appendicitis, commonly referred to as MANTRELS. This encompasses the typical signs and symptoms of appendicitis. Patients receive one point each for the following criteria, with right lower quadrant (RLQ) tenderness and leukocytosis receiving two points each: Migration to the RLQ; anorexia; nausea and vomiting; tenderness in the RLQ; rebound tenderness; elevated temperature; leukocytosis; and shift to the left (bandemia) [37]. This scoring system, while useful, underperforms in the elderly. In a study of 143 patients with surgically proven appendicitis, 12 cases would have been missed using the MANTRELS score. Ten of those 12 cases were above the age of 60 [38].

Atypical presentations of appendicitis appear to be the norm in the elderly population. Only 20% of the elderly will present classically with fever, anorexia, RLQ pain, and leukocytosis [39]. Fever is present in only one-third, one-quarter will have a normal white blood cell count, and 30% will not even have RLQ tenderness on examination [7]. Elderly patients tend to present later in their course as well. One-fifth will present after more than 3 days of symptoms and another 10% after a week of symptoms [3]. This likely contributes to the high rate of perforation. It may also account for part of the high rate of misdiagnosis. Many clinicians are less suspicious of appendicitis when symptoms have been present for a week.

Clinicians should be suspicious of appendicitis in any geriatric patient presenting with abdominal pain and who has not had a prior appendectomy. Liberal use of CT imaging to evaluate for this condition is encouraged (Figure 11.4). In suspicious cases or those that are equivocal, surgical consultation is recommended. Early diagnostic laparotomy improves the outcome in this age group compared with a practice of watchful waiting [40].

Diverticular disease

Similar to many of the previous conditions, the prevalence of diverticular disease increases with age. After the age of 70, the incidence is 50% and rises to 80% after the age of 85 [41]. It may manifest as either lower GI bleeding or diverticulitis.

The most common cause of lower GI bleeding is diverticulosis. Fifteen percent of patients with diverticular disease will have at least one significant episode of bleeding. In the elderly patient, the hemorrhage may be quite significant. The risk of rebleeding in this age group is also high, nearly 25% [42].

Diverticulitis typically presents as fever, nausea, leukocytosis, and a tender mass in the left lower quadrant. In the elderly, one-half will be afebrile and many will not exhibit leukocytosis. There may be other misleading signs and symptoms. Pyuria or hematuria from irritation of the ureter may lead to the diagnosis of kidney stone or urinary tract infection. Right-sided diverticulitis may be thought to be appendicitis. The palpable mass may be misinterpreted as a malignancy. Fully one-half of all cases of diverticulitis are initially misdiagnosed [43].

The elderly are at significantly higher risk for complications from diverticulitis. These include abscess formation, fistula formation, bowel obstruction, and sepsis. Free perforation is also more common and carries a mortality rate as high as 25% [44].

Extra-abdominal causes

The geriatric abdomen does not exist in a vacuum. As previously noted, a significant percentage of elderly patients with myocardial infarction present with GI symptoms. Similarly, other extra-abdominal causes can present with symptoms referable to the abdomen. Pulmonary causes such as pneumonia, pneumothorax, pleural effusions, and pulmonary emboli, especially if they involve the lower lobes, can present with abdominal pain. Other cardiac causes should be considered as well, including pericarditis and decompensated heart failure. Endocrine causes such as diabetic ketoacidosis or hypercalcemia often have associated nonspecific abdominal pain. Herpes zoster, especially in the pre-vesicular phase, may cause abdominal pain depending on the dermatome involved. The astute clinician will remember to consider non-abdominal causes in the differential diagnosis of abdominal symptoms.

Disposition

Geriatric patients presenting with abdominal pain often require long, extensive work-ups. Even after labs and imaging, many patients will require hospital admission or prolonged observation for serial examinations to ensure that a life-threatening condition does not manifest. Those that are discharged to home should have careful discharge instructions with a definite follow-up plan over a definite time period, as opposed to being told to follow up if their symptoms worsen. They should have a number of serial examinations documented on their chart demonstrating improvement, have no concerning findings on laboratory or imaging, be able to tolerate liquids (and their routine medications), and have a reliable adult to assist them at home. Clinicians are urged to avoid using wastebasket terms such as "gastroenteritis" or "stomach flu" for undifferentiated pain. The use of these terms may discourage patients from returning for further evaluation if their symptoms worsen.

Pearls and pitfalls

Pearls

- Many elderly patients with surgical abdominal conditions will have a normal temperature and a normal white blood cell count.
- Patients with acute abdominal pain and reasons for stasis in the left ventricle (such as atrial fibrillation) should be evaluated for mesenteric ischemia, despite a reassuring abdominal examination.

- Peptic ulcer disease in the elderly frequently initially presents with a complication.
- Appendicitis can present in the elderly even after a week of symptoms.
- Given the atypical presentation of serious pathology in the elderly, clinicians should have a low threshold for obtaining advanced imaging, such as a CT scan.
- Up to one-third of women over 65 will have abdominal pain as their presenting symptom of myocardial infarction.

Pitfalls

- Relying on rigidity to diagnose a perforation – rigidity will be absent in 80%.
- Delaying the time to decompression in acute suppurative cholangitis.
- Over-reliance on typical signs and symptoms (e.g., MANTRELS score) to diagnose appendicitis.
- Not considering vascular catastrophes early in their course – the window for intervention is very short in these cases.
- Assigning patients with nonspecific abdominal pain more benign diagnoses such as gastroenteritis.

References

1. Baum SA, Rubenstein Z. Old people in the emergency room: age-related differences in emergency department use and care. *J Am Geriatr Soc.* 1987;35:398–404.

2. Brewer RJ, Golden GT, Hitsch DC, et al. Abdominal pain: an analysis of 1,000 consecutive cases in a university hospital emergency room. *Am J Surg.* 1976;131:219–24.

3. Freund HR, Rubinstein E. Appendicitis in the aged: is it really different? *Am Surg.* 1984;50:573–6.

4. Beijer HJ, deBlaey CJ. Hospitalizations caused by adverse drug reactions (ADR): a meta-analysis of observational studies. *Pharmacy World & Science.* 2002;24(2):46–50.

5. Fenyo G. Diagnostic problems of acute abdominal diseases in the aged. *Acta Chir Scand.* 1974;140:396–405.

6. Fenyo G. Acute abdominal disease in the elderly: experience from two series in Stockholm. *Am J Surg.* 1982;143:751–4.

7. Storm-Dickerson TL, Horattas MC. What have we learned over the past 20 years about appendicitis in the elderly? *Am J Surg.* 2003;185:198–201.

8. Martinez JP, Mattu A. Abdominal pain in the elderly. *Emerg Med Clin North Am.* 2006;24:371–88.

9. Lusiani I, Perrone A, Pesavento R, et al. Prevalence, clinical features, and acute course of atypical myocardial infarction. *Angiology.* 1994;45:49–55.

10. Jehle D, Davis E, Evans T, et al. Emergency department sonography by emergency physicians. *Am J Emerg Med.* 1989;7(6):605–11.

11. Esses D, Birnbaum A, Bijur P, et al. Ability of CT to alter decision making in elderly patients with acute abdominal pain. *Am J Emerg Med.* 2004;22(4):270–2.

12. Romero J, Sanabria A, Angarita M, Varon JC. Cost-effectiveness of computed tomography and ultrasound in the diagnosis of appendicitis. *Biomedica.* 2008;28(1):139–47.

13. Johansen K, Kohler TR, Nicholls SC, et al. Ruptured abdominal aortic aneurysm: the Harborview experience. *J Vasc Surg.* 1991;13:240–5.

14. Barry MC. An "all comers" policy for ruptured abdominal aortic aneurysms: how can results be improved? *Eur J Surg.* 1998;164(4):263–70.

15. Martinez JP, Hogan GJ. Mesenteric ischemia. *Emerg Med Clin N Am.* 2004;22:909–28.

16. Sack J, Aldrete JS. Primary mesenteric venous thrombosis. *Surg Gynecol Obstet.* 1982;154:205.

17. Rhee RY, Gloviczki P, Mendonca CT, et al. Mesenteric venous thrombosis: still a lethal disease in the 1990s. *J Vasc Surg.* 1994;20:688–97.

18. Boley SJ, Sprayregen S, Siegelman SJ, Veith FJ. Initial results from an aggressive roentgenologic and surgical approach to acute mesenteric ischemia. *Surgery.* 1977;82:848.

19. Wasnik A, Kaza RK, Al-Hawary MM, Liu PS, Platt JF. Multidetector CT imaging in mesenteric ischemia – pearls and pitfalls. *Emerg Radiol.* 2011;18:145–56.

20. Schwab DP, Blackhurst DW, Sticca RP. Operative acute small bowel obstruction: admitting service impacts outcome. *Am Surg.* 2001;67(11):1034–8.

21. Sanson TG, O'Keefe KP. Evaluation of abdominal pain in the elderly. *Emerg Med Clin N Am.* 1996;14(3):615–27.

22. Greenlee HB, Pienkos EJ, Vanderbilt PC, et al. Acute large bowel obstruction. *Arch Surg.* 1974;108:470–6.

23. Leverat M. Peptic ulcer disease in patients over 60: experience in 287 cases. *Am J Dig Dis.* 1966;11:279–85.

24. Caesar R. Dangerous complaints: the acute geriatric abdomen. *Emerg Med Rep.* 1994;15:191–202.

25. McNamara RM. Acute abdominal pain. In *Emergency Care of the Elder Person*, ed. Sanders AB (St Louis, MO: Beverly Cracom Publications, 1996), pp. 219–43.

26. Wakayama T. Risk factors influencing the short-term results of gastroduodenal perforation. *Surg Today.* 1994;24(8):681–7.

27. Crofts TJ, Park KG, Steele RJ. A randomized trial of nonoperative treatment for perforated peptic ulcer. *N Engl J Med.* 1989;320(15):970–3.

28. Borum ML. Peptic-ulcer disease in the elderly. *Clin Geriatr Med.* 1999;15:457–71.

29. Rosenthal RA, Anderson DK. Surgery in the elderly: observations on the pathophysiology and treatment of cholelithiasis. *Exp Gerontol.* 1993;28:458–72.

30. Madden JW, Croker JR, Beynon GPJ. Septicemia in the elderly. *Postgrad Med.* 1981;57:502–6.

31. Martin SP, Ulrich CD II. Pancreatic disease in the elderly. *Clin Geriatr Med.* 1999;15:579–605.

32. Paajanen H. AP in patients over 80 years. *Eur J Surg.* 1996;162(6):471–5.

33. Kauvar DR. The geriatric acute abdomen. *Clin Geriatr Med.* 1993;9:547–58.

34. Shoji BT, Becker JM. Colorectal disease in the elderly patient. *Surg Clin N Am.* 1994;74:293–316.

35. Gupta H, Dupuy D. Abdominal emergencies: has anything changed? *Surg Clin N Am.* 1997; 77:1245–64.

36. Yamini D, Vargas H, Bongard F, et al. Perforated appendicitis: is it truly a surgical urgency? *Am Surg.* 1998;64:970–5.

37. Alvarado A. A practical score for the early diagnosis of acute appendicitis. *Ann Emerg Med.* 1986;15:557–64.

38. Gwynn LK. The diagnosis of acute appendicitis: Clinical assessment versus computed tomography evaluation. *J Emerg Med.* 2001;21(2):119–23.

39. Horattas MC, Guyton DP, Wu D. A reappraisal of appendicitis in the elderly. *Am J Surg.* 1990;160:291–3.

40. Koruda MJ. Appendicitis: laparoscopic strategy in diagnosis and treatment. *N Carol Med J.* 1992;53:196–8.

41. Ferzoco LB. Acute diverticulitis [review]. *N Engl J Med.* 1998;338(21):1521–6.

42. Henneman PL. Gastrointestinal bleeding. In *Rosen's Emergency Medicine: Concepts and Clinical Practice, 5th ed*, ed. Marx JA, Hockberger RS, Walls RM, et al. (St Louis, MO: Mosby Inc., 2002), pp. 194–200.

43. Ponka JL, Welborn JK, Brush BE. Acute abdominal pain in aged patients: an analysis of 200 cases. *J Am Geriatr Soc.* 1963;11:993–1007.

44. Krukowski ZH, Matheson NA. Emergency surgery for diverticular disease complicated by generalized and faecal peritonitis: a review. *Br J Surg.* 1984;71:921–7.

12

Altered mental status in the elderly

Scott T. Wilber and Jin H. Han

Introduction

Altered mental status is a common complaint in older emergency department (ED) patients, affecting up to six in ten patients [1–6]. A variety of synonyms are used to describe altered mental status in this population, including confusion, lethargy, MSΔ, ↓LOC, disorientation, delirium, agitation, inappropriate behavior, inattention, hallucination, and lethargy [7]. The lack of standardized terminology may contribute to the difficulty in assessing and appropriately managing this clinical syndrome. Regardless of the terminology used, altered mental status refers to a disturbance in brain function manifested by an alteration in consciousness (the level of awareness of one's environment, or how awake one is) and/or an alteration in cognition (confusion and/or perceptual disturbances).

Alterations in consciousness or cognition can be acute, subacute, or chronic, and each may impact an older patient's ED evaluation. Acute alterations in mental status can be caused by a variety of serious medical conditions and require prompt recognition and treatment for optimal outcomes. In addition, altered mental status can affect other important patient care issues, such as the accuracy of the patient's history and comprehension of their diagnosis and discharge instructions [8].

In this chapter, we review acute disturbances in consciousness (coma, stupor, and delirium) as well as acute (delirium) and chronic (dementia) disturbances in cognition. We discuss the assessment and treatment of these conditions, as well as the assessment of medical decision-making capacity in older ED patients.

Acute disturbances in consciousness

Coma and stupor

Comatose patients have no response to external stimuli or awareness of the external environment, and these patients will have a modified Richmond Agitation and Sedation Scale (mRASS) of –5 (Table 12.1 and Assessing Level of Consciousness, below) [9,10]. Stupor consists of a sleepful level of consciousness from which the patient can only be aroused with maximal stimuli (mRASS –4) [9–11]. The majority of cases of coma (85%) are caused by systemic disease, rather than primary CNS

abnormalities, and the etiologies of coma and delirium are similar [12]. Consequently, there is substantial overlap between the discussion of stupor or coma and that of delirium, which involves an altered level of consciousness that does not reach the level of stupor or coma [13]. As the patient's level of consciousness becomes more depressed in stupor or coma, concern for a life-threatening acute medical illness that precipitated the change in mental status should similarly increase. Although comatose and stuporous patients demand a more rapid evaluation, and at times more aggressive management of life threats, the evaluation is similar to that of delirious patients.

Delirium

Delirium is an acute, fluctuating alteration in consciousness and attention, which is accompanied by impaired cognition or perceptual disturbances, not better explained by a pre-existing dementia [14]. The change in level of consciousness and cognition occurs over a period of hours to days, and the symptoms tend to wax and wane over the course of the day. Delirium is typically caused by an acute medical illness, and may be the first manifestation of such illness.

Subtypes

Delirium can be classified by psychomotor subtype into hypoactive, hyperactive, and mixed delirium. Hypoactive delirium is associated with depressed levels of consciousness (mRASS <0, Table 12.1) [10]. Hypoactive patients are "quiet" and the symptoms may be subtle, so this form of delirium may be attributed to other conditions such as depression or fatigue, and is frequently missed by clinicians [15]. Hyperactive delirium is associated with increased psychomotor activity (mRASS >0, Table 12.1) such as anxiety, agitation, or combativeness, and is therefore easier for clinicians to detect [10]. Mixed delirium has fluctuating levels of consciousness, from hypoactive to hyperactive. Hypoactive and mixed delirium are the most common in older patients, while hyperactive delirium is the least common [16–18]. Recognizing the psychomotor subtype may be helpful in determining the etiology of delirium, as hypoactive delirium is more likely to be caused by infection or metabolic derangement and hyperactive is more likely to be caused by alcohol or benzodiazepine withdrawal [19].

Geriatric Emergency Medicine, ed. Joseph H. Kahn, Brendan G. Magauran Jr., and Jonathan S. Olshaker. Published by Cambridge University Press.
© Cambridge University Press 2014.

Table 12.1. The modified Richmond Agitation and Sedation Scale (mRASS). From reference [10], used with permission

Step 1: State the patient's name and ask patient to open eyes and look at speaker.

Ask, 'Describe how you are feeling today'.

• If answers with short answer (<10 s), cue with second open-ended question

• If no response to verbal cue, physically stimulate patient by shaking their shoulder

Step 2: Score modified RASS below

Score	Term	Description
+4	Combative	No attention; overtly combative, violent, immediate danger to staff
+3	Very agitated	Very distractible; repeated calling or touch required to get or keep eye contact or attention; cannot focus; pulls or removes tube(s) or catheter(s); aggressive; fights environment not people
+2	Slightly agitated	Easily distractible; rapidly loses attention; resists care or uncooperative; frequent non-purposeful movement
+1	Restless	Slightly distractible; pays attention most of the time; anxious, but cooperative; movements not aggressive or vigorous
0	Alert and calm	Pays attention; makes eye contact; aware of surroundings; responds immediately and appropriately to calling name and touch
−1	Wakes easily	Slightly drowsy; eye contact >10 s; not fully alert, but has sustained awakening; eye-opening/eye contact to *voice* >10 s
−2	Wakes slowly	Very drowsy; pays attention some of the time; briefly awakens with eye contact to *voice* <10 s
−3	Difficult to wake	Repeated calling or touch required to get or keep eye contact or attention; needs repeated stimuli (touch or voice) for attention, movement, or eye opening to *voice* (but no eye contact)
−4	Can't stay awake	Arousable but no attention; no response to voice, but movement or eye opening to *physical* stimulation
−5	Unarousable	No response to *voice* or *physical* stimulation

Table 12.2. Prevalence of altered mental status in older ED patients (%)

Undifferentiated cognitive impairment [1–6]	26–60
Cognitive impairment without delirium [2,3,5,6]	16–38
Stupor or coma [2,3]	5–9
Delirium [20]	7–20
Delirium in nursing home residents [37]	38
Delirium in non-nursing home residents [37]	6

Epidemiology and outcomes

Delirium is common, occurring in 7–20% of older ED patients (Table 12.2) [20]. Much of the information on the outcomes of patients with delirium is based on studies of hospitalized older patients. These patients are more likely to die, be institutionalized, develop dementia, have functional decline, have prolonged hospitalization, and generate higher health care expenditures [21–24]. The longer a patient has delirium, the worse the outcome, with every 48 hours of delirium increasing the 3-month risk of death by 11% [25]. This emphasizes the importance of early detection and treatment. In ED patients, delirium is an independent predictor of death at 6 months (37% unadjusted mortality) and hospital length of stay in admitted patients (median increase of 1.5 days), and may be associated with accelerated functional decline [26–28].

Risk factors

The development of delirium is a complex interaction between predisposing and precipitating factors (Table 12.3) [29,30]. Patients with significant predisposing factors are more vulnerable as they have less physiological reserve. These patients

may develop delirium with minor physiological insult, such as a urinary tract infection or a single anticholinergic medication. Patients without significant predisposing factors have a greater physiological reserve, and therefore require a more significant physiological insult (such as severe sepsis or multiple anticholinergic medications) to develop delirium [31].

Dementia is the most consistently observed predisposing factor for delirium, in both ED and hospitalized patients [16,32]. As the severity of the dementia worsens, the risk of delirium increases [33]. Older ED patients with a history of dementia are three times more likely to have delirium, and delirium is more difficult to diagnose in patients with dementia [16]. Other risk factors identified in ED patients include premorbid functional impairment and hearing impairment, advanced age, cerebrovascular disease, and seizure disorder [16,34].

There are many potential precipitating factors for delirium. Regardless of the precipitating factor, those with higher severity of illness, or physiological insult, have a higher risk of developing delirium [23,35,36]. In addition, multiple etiologies may occur concurrently, and sometimes no etiology can be identified [37,38]. Infections are the most common cause of delirium, occurring in up to half of cases [16,36,39]. One study of precipitants of delirium in community-dwelling older patients identified infection in 43%, intracranial disease in 25%, cardiovascular disorders in 18%, and medications in 12% [39].

Medications are both a predisposing and precipitating factor for delirium. Pre-existing medication use including narcotics, benzodiazepines, and anticholinergics may predispose patients to delirium [23,40,41]. A recent systematic review suggested that opioids, benzodiazepines, and antihistamines were associated with delirium [42]. Although opioids can exacerbate or cause delirium, undertreatment of pain can also cause

Table 12.3. Predisposing factors for delirium (modified from references) [29,30]

Predisposing factors	Precipitating factors
Demographics	Systemic Disease
• Advanced age	• Infection /sepsis
• Male gender	• Dehydration
	• Hypoxia
	• Hypercarbia
	• Shock
	• Electrolyte abnormalities
	• Hypo- or hyperglycemia
	• Hypo- or hyperthermia
	• Trauma
	• Acute myocardial infarction
Comorbid disease	Primary central nervous system disease
• Number of comorbidities	• Stroke
• Severity of comorbidities	• Intracerebral hemorrhage
• Visual impairment	• Meningitis
• Hearing impairment	• Encephalitis
• Dementia	• Seizures or post-ictal state
• Depression	• Subdural hemorrhage
• History of delirium	• Epidural hemorrhage
• Cerebrovascular disease	
• Falls	
• Functional impairment	
• Terminal illness	
• Malnutrition	
Drugs	Drugs
• Polypharmacy	• Polypharmacy
• Baseline psychoactive medication use	• Withdrawal from alcohol or sedatives
• Alcohol abuse	• Recreational drug or alcohol use
• Drug abuse	• Anticholinergics
	• Sedative-hypnotics
	• Opioids
	Environmental/Iatrogenic
	• Prolonged ED length of stay
	• Sleep deprivation
	• Physical restraints
	• Indwelling urinary catheter
	• Pain
	• Surgery or procedures

agitation in the delirious patient, so the risks must be assessed and balanced.

One class of medications commonly implicated as a precipitating factor for delirium in older patients is the anticholinergics, which include commonly prescribed ED medications such as antihistamines, muscle relaxants, antiemetics, and GI antispasmodics [43,44]. Of note, some studies have not found an association between these medications and delirium [45] while others have shown an association [46,47]. In addition, these medications may increase the severity of delirium [48].

The recently updated Beers Criteria for Potentially Inappropriate Medication Use in Older Adults recommends avoiding anticholinergics in patients with or at high risk of delirium because these may induce or worsen delirium; this recommendation was based upon moderate quality of evidence and strong strength of recommendation from the consensus panel [43]. This document also provides a list of anticholinergics, and the tables are available in a pocket card format for download at the American Geriatrics Society website. Other medications that the Beers Criteria recommends avoiding in delirium include benzodiazepines and other sedative-hypnotics, corticosteroids, H2-receptor antagonists, and meperidine [43].

Chronic disturbances in cognition

Dementia

In contrast to delirium, dementia involves gradual and progressive cognitive defects in multiple areas, primarily memory [14]. Although delirium and dementia are distinct entities, dementia is an important predisposing factor for the development of delirium, and both can occur concurrently. ED patients with a history of dementia are three times more likely to have delirium, and diagnosing delirium superimposed upon dementia may be more difficult [16]. This is especially true in patients with severe dementia, who may exhibit symptoms of delirium such as inattention, altered level of consciousness, disorganized thinking, sleep–wake cycle disturbances, and perceptual disturbances in the absence of delirium. However, it is important to note that even in those with severe dementia, delirium is still characterized by an acute change in level of consciousness and cognition. Therefore, obtaining information about the patient's baseline mental status from a family member, caregiver, primary care provider, or nursing home is needed to diagnose delirium.

Dementia is typically irreversible and not secondary to an underlying medical illness. However, it is important for emergency physicians to realize that some cases of dementia are secondary to medical illness and may be reversible. Hypothyroidism, vitamin B12 deficiency, and depression may cause a reversible dementia-like illness [49]. Normal pressure hydrocephalus (NPH) is potentially reversible and comprises 6% of dementia cases. NPH is characterized by gait disturbances, urinary incontinence, and cognitive impairment [49]. Findings of dilated ventricles on computed tomography (CT) of the head may suggest this syndrome in older ED patients. Diagnosis is dependent on these clinical findings, neuroimaging, cerebrospinal pressure (CSF) monitoring, and improvement with a trial of CSF drainage [50]. Ventriculoperitoneal shunt placement may reverse the symptoms of NPH [50].

Dementia with Lewy bodies (DLB) is the second most common type of dementia (after Alzheimer's) [49]. In contrast to Alzheimer's dementia, the decline in cognition in DLB can be rapid and may fluctuate over several hours or days. Patients with DLB also commonly have perceptual disturbances. For these reasons, differentiating between DLB and delirium can be difficult for the emergency physician. One distinguishing characteristic is that patients with DLB have Parkinsonian motor symptoms such as cog wheeling, shuffling gait, stiff movements, and reduced arm-swing during walking; these are typically absent in patients with delirium [49]. However, determining the diagnosis in these patients generally requires detailed evaluation by a neurologist or psychiatrist. This evaluation may be accomplished in the ED, inpatient, or outpatient setting depending upon the severity of the presentation, availability of consultants, and other considerations.

Assessment

History

There may be significant limitations in obtaining history from patients with altered mental status in the ED. Those with stupor and coma will be unable to provide any history, and some with delirium and dementia will be unable to provide reliable information. In some cases, though, patients will be able to provide at least some history. Some patients may have recollections of recent perceptual disturbances; one question that may be helpful when assessing patients is, "Over the past few days, have you been seeing or hearing things that weren't really there?"

In many cases of altered mental status, history will need to be obtained from surrogates such as family, caregivers, primary care physician, or nursing home staff. Important aspects of the history include the quality of symptoms (altered level of consciousness, confusion, perceptual disturbances), onset of symptoms, presence of fluctuation ("Did the symptoms you noticed tend to come and go, or get worse and better, over time?"). A thorough medication history, including the possibility of complementary or over-the-counter medications like diphenhydramine, must be obtained because so many medications have been implicated as potentially precipitating delirium. It is important to determine whether any new medications are temporally related to the development of the patient's symptoms, and to assume that the medications may be causative if they are temporally related.

Physical examination

The physical examination is of critical importance in evaluating the patient with altered mental status. In critically ill patients with altered mental status, the physical examination may need to be performed in conjunction with treatment.

Assessing level of consciousness

Using validated scales to evaluate the level of consciousness in patients with altered mental status is helpful for good communication with other caregivers and to allow for the assessment of change over time and between caregivers. A number of different scales are used to evaluate level of consciousness. One of the simplest is the "AVPU" scale, which stands for alert, responsive to verbal stimuli, responsive to painful stimuli, or unresponsive [51]. However, this scale does not evaluate the level of response to the stimuli, limiting its usefulness. For example, patients who respond to painful stimuli by waking and interacting with the examiner differ substantially from those whose response to painful stimuli is withdrawing or posturing. To improve the description of the level of consciousness,

the Glasgow Coma Scale (GCS) may be used. The GCS rates eye opening and motor response to verbal and painful stimuli, and verbal response. Patients with coma do not open their eyes, obey commands, or have understandable conversation [2].

The Confusion Assessment Method (CAM) uses a verbal scale for assessing level of consciousness ranging from alert (normal), vigilant (hyperalert), through lethargic (drowsy, easily aroused), stupor (difficult to arouse), or coma (unarousable) [11]. However, this scale is somewhat subjective.

The mRASS is an objective rating of level of consciousness that is rapid to perform (~10 seconds), reliable, valid, and sensitive to change (Table 12.1) [10,52,53]. Given its brevity, objectivity, and reproducibility, the mRASS is recommended to assess and document level of consciousness in older patients with altered mental status. This tool can be easily integrated into the normal evaluation of the patient without adding extra time, and can be repeated serially to assess change.

Inattention is also a disturbance of consciousness. Inattention can be assessed by informally observing the patient, asking them to count backwards from 20 to 1, recite the months of the year backwards, or days of the week backwards. There are also formal tests of attention such as the Digit-Span Forward or Digit-Span Backwards tests, the Vigilance "A" test, and the Digit Cancellation Test. Each test objectively assesses attention and these tests may be useful in assessing delirium in older hospitalized patients; their use in older ED patients requires further evaluation [54].

Assessing cognition

Cognitive impairment is common and emergency physicians must maintain a high index of suspicion for it in older ED patients. It is common to assume that the patient who is alert and able to carry on a conversation is cognitively intact without formal testing. In practice we find that the common phrase "A&O×3" reflects such an awake and conversational patient, rather than formal testing of cognition. Given the complexity of an older patient's presentation, it is important to perform objective testing of their cognition. However, many of the available tools may be difficult to use in the busy ED setting.

The classic cognitive screening tool since 1975 has been the Mini-Mental State Exam (MMSE) [55]. This comprehensive, 20-question test of orientation, registration, recall, calculation, and ability to follow commands should be familiar to most emergency physicians. However, a number of issues make it unsuitable for routine ED use. In older ED patients, it can take between 5 and 15 minutes to complete. It requires a patient with intact vision, hearing, and ability to write; this may be limited in older ED patients due to forgotten glasses, hearing aids, and injuries to or IVs in the arms. Finally, it is not easily memorized or scored, making the use of instructions and scoring sheets a must.

Many other mental status screens have been developed and validated. Screens studied for ED use include the Clock-drawing Test, the Mini-Cog, the Brief Alzheimer's Screen (BAS), the Caregiver-completed AD8, the Short Blessed Test (SBT, also known as the Orientation Memory Concentration Test), the Six-item Screener, and the Ottawa 3DY (Table 12.4)

Table 12.4. Screening tests for cognitive impairment in older ED patients

Test	Sensitivity (%)	Specificity (%)
Mini-cog [58]	77	85
Brief Alzheimer's Screen [56]	95	52
Short Blessed Test [56]	95	65
Ottawa 3DY [56]	95	52
Caregiver-completed AD8 [56,57]	63–83	63–79
Six-item Screener [57–59]	63–94	77–85

[56–59]. The Clock-drawing Test and the Mini-Cog, which incorporates a clock-drawing test with 3-item recall, also require intact vision and the ability to write, limiting their use in the older ED patient.

A recently published study evaluated the BAS, the SBT, the Ottawa 3DY, and the Caregiver-completed AD8 to assess cognition in older ED patients, in comparison with the MMSE [56]. Of these tools, the BAS, SBT, and Ottawa 3DY had the highest sensitivity, and the SBT also had the highest specificity (Table 12.4). The tools are available as supplements to the article online.

The SBT has been used in other ED-based research studies to evaluate mental status in older ED patients [1,5]. Consisting of six questions, including temporal orientation, counting backwards from 20, saying the months in reverse order, and short-term memory, the test takes 2–5 minutes to perform. Due to the number of questions and the weighted scoring, a scoring sheet, pocket card, or computerized system is necessary for administration [56]. The BAS consists of three-item recall, the date, naming as many animals as possible in 30 seconds, and spelling "world" backwards. Given these components, it would likely require a few minutes to complete and has an even more complicated scoring system, requiring a calculator or computer program for administration and scoring [56]. These issues make the SBT and BAS less useful for incorporation into general ED practice, though the SBT's combination of sensitivity, specificity, and brevity compared with the MMSE could make it a useful tool for more complex patients or in geriatric EDs where ancillary staff may be able to perform the testing [60].

Consisting of asking the patient the **D**ay of the week, spell "world" backward (**D**lrow), the **D**ate, and the **Y**ear, the Ottawa 3DY is rapid, easily remembered, and easily scored (any error is a positive test for cognitive impairment) [56]. The Six-item Screener (SIS) is also a rapid, easily remembered, and easily scored mental status test [57–59]. The SIS consists of three-item recall and orientation to year, month, and day of the week, and scoring is the sum of correct answers. Several studies of the SIS in older ED patients have been performed, using a cutoff of four abnormal /five normal; the SIS has a sensitivity of 63–94% and a specificity of 77–86% when compared with the MMSE (Table 12.4) [57–59]. The SIS takes a median of 1 minute to administer in older ED patients, and the Ottawa 3DY should be similar, so these tests can be incorporated into the physical examination and will not substantially increase the time to evaluate an older patient. Furthermore, their simplicity makes them easy to remember and score, without scoring sheets or pocket cards.

Neurologic examination

In addition to assessing levels of consciousness and cognition, a thorough neurologic examination is necessary in patients with altered level of consciousness. The National Institute of Health Stroke Scale (NIHSS) is an excellent approach to the neurologic examination in patients with altered level of consciousness [61]. In addition to objectively measuring motor strength and sensation, it also assesses cerebellar function, aphasia, and neglect, which may help in reaching a diagnosis of stroke in patients with altered level of consciousness. The NIHSS becomes more complicated to score as the level of consciousness decreases, so it is important to understand the scoring in patients who are unable to follow commands and to have scoring sheets or pocket cards with instructions available. Training is also available online, without cost, through the American Heart Association website.

When evaluating the patient with altered level of consciousness, there are several important features of the neurologic examination that should be emphasized. First, it is important to evaluate for focal, lateralizing findings. The combination of focal, lateralizing findings with stupor or coma suggests intracranial pathology such as stroke, hemorrhage, or mass effect requiring emergent CT scanning and rapid treatment based on the results. Second, it is important to evaluate for subtle signs of seizure, such as repetitive movement of the eyelids, eyes, or extremities. These findings may indicate the need for emergent EEG to evaluate for non-convulsive status epilepticus. In addition, altered mental status associated with seizure is one of the few indications for the administration of benzodiazepines (see Treatment).

General physical examination

A detailed physical examination should be performed in order to help determine the etiology of the altered mental status. After airway, breathing, and circulation are assessed and immediate life threats addressed (see Treatment), a head to toe examination should be performed. Vital signs may provide clues to the etiology: fever or hypothermia suggest an infectious etiology; hypotension may indicate cerebral hypoperfusion; tachycardia may indicate sympathomimetic or anticholinergic toxicity or an infectious etiology; tachypnea may indicate pneumonia. Head examination should evaluate for signs of trauma, which suggest that evaluation for intracranial injury should be suspected. Pupillary abnormalities can be seen with drug intoxication (miosis with opiates, mydriasis with sympathomimetics and anticholinergics); nystagmus may indicate intoxication with alcohol or other drugs. The neck should be examined for meningismus or thyromegaly.

Cardiac, pulmonary, and abdominal examination, should evaluate for evidence of infection or other potential etiologies of the symptoms. A thorough skin examination, including feet, perineum, and sacrum, should be performed to evaluate for signs of infection, jaundice, or medication patches such as fentanyl or scopolamine. Due to the frequency of anticholinergic medications causing delirium, one should be alert for symptoms consistent with an anticholinergic toxidrome (dry mouth, urinary retention, tachycardia, fever). Alcohol or sedative-hypnotic withdrawal is associated with coarse tremors, tachycardia, and low-grade fever.

Assessment of delirium

Despite the fact that it is both common and serious, delirium is frequently not diagnosed by emergency physicians. Studies in EDs have found sensitivities of 11–46%, for physician detection (sensitivity is the percent of patients with delirium diagnosed by emergency physicians) [20]. This leaves a majority of delirious patients in whom the diagnosis will not be made in the ED. This has a significant impact on patients, as the majority (94%) of older ED patients admitted with undiagnosed delirium will not be diagnosed by the hospital physician [16]. In one study, patients with delirium undiagnosed in the ED had a higher 6-month mortality (31%), compared with non-delirious patients (14%) and those in whom delirium was detected (12%) [62]. For these reasons, assessment for delirium has been proposed as a quality indicator for geriatric emergency care [63].

The criteria for delirium are defined by the *Diagnostic and Statistical Manual of Mental Disorders, Fourth Edition* (DSM-IV) [14]. To meet the diagnostic criteria for delirium, a patient must have: 1) a disturbance of consciousness (i.e., reduced clarity of awareness of the environment) with reduced ability to focus, sustain, or shift attention; 2) a change in cognition or the development of a perceptual disturbance that is not better accounted for by a pre-existing, established, or evolving dementia; and 3) development of the disturbance over a short period of time (usually hours to days) and a tendency for it to fluctuate during the course of the day. A fourth criterion in the DSM-IV involves the etiology of delirium [14].

The first DSM-IV criterion indicates that disturbance in consciousness and attention must be present; inattention is considered a disturbance of consciousness and is a cardinal feature of delirium. Patients who are inattentive are easily distractible during the examination and questions directed towards the inattentive patient may have to be repeated. Patients with mRASS scores of +1 to +5 and −1 to −3 are very likely to be delirious.

The second DSM-IV criterion involves cognition, and may also be assessed in the ED using rapid, validated tools (see Assessing cognition). The earliest cognitive deficit to appear is generally impairment of short-term memory, which is nearly universal in patients with delirium [14]. One study found impaired memory to be 100% sensitive and 33% specific for delirium, and disorientation to time or place to be 89% sensitive and 63% specific for delirium [11]. Perceptual disturbances are part of the second criterion and may include delusions, illusions, misperceptions, or hallucinations. Visual hallucinations are most common, though auditory, tactile, gustatory, or olfactory illusions or hallucinations may occur [13]. Perceptual disturbances are less common than memory disturbances, occurring in only 23% of patients with delirium, but are more

specific (90% specific) [11]. The third criterion, acuity and fluctuation, is most easily obtainable from caregivers, family, or others who know the patient well. Fluctuation in course may be apparent during the ED stay or may also require external history, though it may also be observed in the ED.

The CAM was developed by operationalizing the DSM-III criteria for delirium to enable non-psychiatrists to "identify delirium quickly and accurately" [11]. The CAM requires the presence of acute onset *and* fluctuating course *and* inattention, *and* either disorganized thinking *or* altered level of consciousness. The original CAM validation study was conducted in hospitalized patients, and was found to have a sensitivity of 96% and a specificity of 93% [11]. The CAM requires significant training, and may be less sensitive when used by those with less clinical experience [64]. The training manual recommends the use of the Modified Mini-Cog and the Digit Span test, which may require 5 minutes or longer to complete [65]. For these reasons, the CAM may be difficult to apply universally in ED settings to detect delirium.

Shorter delirium screening tools may be more feasible for use in the ED. The Brief Confusion Assessment Method (bCAM) is based upon the CAM and was developed for use in the ICU [66]. The bCAM uses brief objective assessments to test for inattention and disorganized thinking, uses the RASS to evaluate for altered level of consciousness, and allows for early stoppage if the patient does not have altered mental status and a fluctuating course. Because it takes less than 2 minutes to complete, it may be feasible to perform in the ED [66]. Another simple assessment tool for delirium is the Single Question in Delirium (SQiD). This consists simply of asking the patient's family or caregiver the following question: "Do you think [name of patient] has been more confused lately?" Preliminary study of this assessment tool found it to be 80% sensitive and 71% specific in oncology patients compared with a psychiatrist's assessment [67]. Simply evaluating the mRASS for a score of other than zero was 64% sensitive and 93% specific for delirium in a recent study; serial measurements increased this to 74 and 92%, respectively [10]. Both the SQiD and mRASS require evaluation in ED patients, and other brief tools are presently being developed for ED use.

Diagnostic testing

Diagnostic testing in patients with altered mental status is directed at discovering the etiology of the patient's symptoms, so that effective treatment can be provided. Given the wide differential diagnosis, and the possibility of multiple etiologies of altered mental status, this evaluation can be extensive [13]. The diagnostic evaluation of the patient with altered mental status should be based on a careful history and physical examination and should be tailored to the individual patient, rather than a "shotgun" approach [68].

The majority of older patients with altered mental status require, at minimum, a complete blood count, electrolytes, BUN, creatinine, glucose, and ECG to evaluate for common and serious causes including anemia, leukocytosis, electrolyte abnormalities, dehydration, uremia, hypoglycemia, or cardiac ischemia. Infections are the most common cause of delirium in older patients, and these infections may present without fever or elevated white blood cell count. Common sources of infection in older patients include pneumonia, urinary tract infections, skin and soft tissue, and intra-abdominal infections. Chest radiography and urinalysis may be helpful, and abdominal CT scanning is useful in the patient with altered mental status and abdominal pain. Lumbar puncture should be considered in patients with altered mental status combined with headache, fever without an obvious source, or clinical suspicion of meningitis or encephalitis.

Cardiac enzymes should be measured in the patient with symptoms of cardiac ischemia or new ECG changes, as acute myocardial infarction is an etiology of delirium [69]. Patients with chronic lung disease or sleep apnea should have arterial or venous blood gas analysis to evaluate for hypercarbia causing altered mental status. Hepatic function tests and serum ammonia levels are appropriate for those with a history of or examination consistent with liver disease, such as scleral icterus, jaundice, or asterixis. As both hyperthyroidism and hypothyroidism can cause altered mental status, a thyroid-stimulating hormone level can be helpful in patients with signs of these conditions.

Patients with stupor or coma, focal neurological findings, or recent history of head trauma should undergo emergent non-contrast CT of the head [3,70]. However, there is limited evidence on the use of CT in delirious older patients. Two retrospective studies found that approximately 15% of patients with confusion or altered level of consciousness had an abnormal head CT [3,70]. However, in the absence of a coma, trauma, or focal neurological findings, there were no positive CT scans in these patients [3,70]. Routine use of head CT in delirious patients without trauma or new neurological findings is therefore not recommended. However, if no plausible etiology of the delirium has been determined after a thorough history, examination, and the above laboratory studies, head CT should be considered.

The roles of magnetic resonance imaging of the brain (brain MRI) and electroencephalography (EEG) are less clear in ED patients, and emergent access to these tests may not be available to emergency physicians. Brain MRI may be helpful in assessing patients for acute ischemic stroke during the window of time when head CT is non-diagnostic. For example, patients with ischemic strokes in the right parietal lobe can present with delirium as the only symptom of stroke, without any focal neurological findings [71]. Non-convulsive status epilepticus may also present with altered level of consciousness; a systematic review reported that it occurred in 8–30% of patients with altered mental status [72]. EEG is necessary to make this diagnosis, and should be considered in those with stupor and coma without identifiable cause after evaluation. In both ischemic stroke and non-convulsive status epilepticus, early diagnosis and treatment may improve outcomes; neurologic consultation in the ED may help guide diagnostic testing in these challenging patients.

Treatment

In patients with severely impaired levels of consciousness, assessment and treatment may need to be performed simultaneously. Evaluation of the patient's airway, breathing, and circulation should be performed, and problems identified in each area addressed. In particular, patients who are not able to protect their airway may need airway management as appropriate. Assessment of oxygenation and perfusion is also critical so that severe impairments can be addressed.

The most effective method of treating the patient with altered mental status is to identify and treat the underlying cause. In some cases, such as hypoxia or hypoperfusion, this will result in a rapid recovery of normal mentation. However, in other cases recovery may be prolonged. Delirium is traditionally thought of as a transient condition, but recent studies have demonstrated that, in some cases, recovery may be slow and prolonged and symptoms may persist for months to years [29].

Patients suspected of altered mental status due to opioid excess may benefit from the administration of naloxone for diagnostic and therapeutic reasons. We recommend diluting 0.4 mg in 10 ml of normal saline, and administering slowly over several minutes till the desired effect is reached in order to prevent severe withdrawal symptoms. Administration of flumazenil in cases of altered level of consciousness due to benzodiazepine excess is not recommended due to the risk of seizures.

In addition to treating the underlying cause of delirium, there are a variety of non-pharmacological and pharmacological treatments available. Non-pharmacological treatments should be attempted prior to using pharmacological treatment. Many of these recommendations may seem to contradict traditional emergency medical teaching and practice. However, attention to these treatments may improve the care of the older patient with delirium and agitation, while maintaining safety for the patient and providers.

Non-pharmacological treatment of delirium and agitation

There are a variety of techniques to reduce agitation in the delirious patient; these techniques may also be effective in patients with dementia and agitation. "Tethering devices" should be avoided unless absolutely necessary for patient care, and they should not be used for the convenience of staff members. Blood pressure cuffs, pulse oximeters, and cardiac monitoring devices should be discontinued in favor of intermittent measurement when feasible [73]. Intravenous lines can be changed to saline locks if the patient does not require infusions, and intravenous fluids can be given by intermittent bolus rather than continuous infusion. If the patient seems agitated by the saline lock, or tries to remove it, the lock can be hidden by a cast sleeve when not in use. Using a decoy, such as taping a false saline lock on the non-dominant arm, may also help [73].

Indwelling urinary catheters should not be placed without a specific medical indication, as they are associated with increased in-hospital and 90-day mortality, a 2.4-fold higher risk of developing delirium during hospitalization, and a longer hospital length of stay [74,75]. One appropriate indication is acute urinary retention, which itself can cause agitation in the patient with altered mental status. If urine must be obtained as part of the evaluation and the patient is incontinent, straight catheterization should be used rather than an indwelling catheter. Avoiding or removing urinary catheters can reduce agitation, trauma from traumatic self-removal, and also reduces the risk of catheter-associated infections.

Physical restraints are associated with a 4.4-fold higher risk of developing delirium during hospitalization, and are also associated with a greater severity of symptoms in patients with delirium [74]. Physical restraints should be avoided in patients with delirium and agitation unless absolutely necessary for patient or provider safety, and then only used until non-pharmacological or pharmacological alternatives are effective. The use of family or sitters can eliminate the need for physical restraints in many patients by providing feedback to patients when they initiate dangerous behaviors such as attempting to climb out of bed or interfering with therapies.

In addition to avoiding tethers, other non-pharmacological strategies for treating delirium include encouraging the use of sensory aids such as glasses and hearing aids, and providing orientation cues. Large-face clocks and calendars can help with orientation. Reducing artificial light during night hours may also be beneficial in orienting the delirious patient. Families should be encouraged to stay at the bedside with patients and to provide reorientation as necessary, reminding the patient where they are and why. Sitters and other staff can also provide this reorientation while at the bedside [29]. However, some authors note that reorientation and short-term memory questions may agitate the patient, and recommend the "T-A-DA" approach (i.e., "Tolerate, Anticipate, Don't Agitate" [73]. These authors recommend that reorientation be attempted, but if that doesn't work, to use distraction techniques or go along with the disorientation and other behaviors as long as they don't cause harm [73].

Adequate treatment of pain may reduce agitation in the patient with altered mental status. Older patients may have long ED stays, and providing oral hydration and a meal may reduce agitation. Reducing the duration of the ED stay may also reduce the risk of developing delirium in patients who are admitted; those with an ED stay of 12 hours or longer have a 2.1-fold increased risk of developing delirium [74].

Pharmacological treatment of delirium

The first step in the pharmacological management of delirium is to avoid drugs which can exacerbate the condition (see Delirium: Risk factors). For those patients in whom pharmacological treatment of agitation associated with delirium is required, typical or atypical antipsychotics are recommended. Haloperidol, risperidone, olanzapine, and quetiapine have been studied for the treatment of delirium [76,77]. These drugs may reduce both the severity and duration of delirium [77]. Doses of these agents are listed in Table 12.5.

A recent review found that there was no evidence of superiority of the atypical antipsychotics risperidone and olanzapine compared with low-dose haloperidol (<3.5 mg/day) [77]. However, high-dose haloperidol (>4.5 mg/day) was associated with a higher incidence of extrapyramidal side effects [77].

Table 12.5. Antipsychotics for the pharmacological treatment of agitation in altered mental status

Drug	Dose	Notes
Haloperidol (oral)	0.5–1.0 mg twice daily and every 4 h as needed	
Haloperidol (parenteral)	0.5–1.0 mg IM every 30–60 min as needed	IM dosing preferred over IV due to short duration of action IV. Usually patients respond to ≤3 mg
Risperidone	0.5 mg orally twice daily	
Olanzapine	2.5–5.0 mg orally once daily	
Quetiapine	12.5–25.0 mg orally twice daily	Recommended in Parkinson's disease

Advantages of haloperidol also include the ability to administer parenterally. When administered parenterally to older patients with delirium, the initial dose of 0.5–1.0 mg IM or IV is very low (~10% of that often used to treat agitation in younger patients with psychosis). This dose can be repeated every 30 minutes as needed to provide a calm but not overly sedated patient (<3 mg total initial dose is generally required) [78]. Although commonly used in emergency medicine practice, there is no FDA approval for intravenous haloperidol. There may be a higher risk of QTc prolongation with IV use, so cardiac monitoring is recommended [78]. Furthermore, IM dosing is associated with more favorable pharmacokinetics [29,78].

A recent small randomized, controlled trial of quetiapine versus haloperidol in ICU patients with delirium found that the quetiapine group had a shorter duration of delirium and less agitation compared with the haloperidol group [79]. Quetiapine also has a lower incidence of QTc prolongation and fewer extrapyramidal side effects compared with haloperidol [78]. Because haloperidol can worsen extrapyramidal symptoms in patients with Parkinson's disease, quetiapine is especially recommended in this population [78].

Since antipsychotics may cause QTc prolongation, they should be used with caution in those on other medications which may prolong the QTc interval (www.qtdrugs.org).

Benzodiazepines have long been used to treat the agitated patient. However, benzodiazepines may worsen and prolong delirium symptoms [29,80]. A recent Cochrane Collaboration review found no evidence to support the use of benzodiazepines to treat agitation associated with delirium, and stated that they "could not be recommended" for this indication [80]. In critically ill, intubated patients, sedation with dexmedetomidine has been associated with a lower incidence and duration of delirium compared with benzodiazepines [81,82]. The only indications for benzodiazepines for the treatment of agitation in delirium are in patients who are withdrawing from alcohol or benzodiazepines, and those with delirium associated with seizures [80].

Assessment of decision-making capacity

Emergency physicians may need to assess older patients, especially those with altered mental status, for medical decision-making capacity, or the ability to consent or refuse medical care. Two ethical principles guide this decision – autonomy and paternalism. Autonomy, or self-determination, is the ability to make decisions for oneself, regardless of the consequences. Paternalism is limiting autonomy in order to do "what is best" for the patient. Autonomy overrules paternalism unless the patient lacks decision-making capacity [83].

In general, clinicians do not adequately assess patients for medical decision-making capacity, and often do not identify patients with incapacity [84]. However, this skill is important for emergency physicians, as a significant portion of our patients may lack capacity. Healthy older patients generally retain medical decision-making capacity, with only 2.8% lacking capacity [84]. However, in patients with mild cognitive impairment this rises to 20%, to 44% in nursing home residents, and to 54% in Alzheimer's dementia [84]. The severity of cognitive impairment, as measured by formal instruments such as the MMSE, correlates directly with the prevalence of incapacity [84].

There are three elements to consent for medical treatment: 1) the patient must be given adequate information, including risks, benefits, and alternatives, to the proposed medical care; 2) the patient must be free from coercion; and 3) the patient must have medical decision-making capacity [84]. Patients must have four abilities to have medical decision-making capacity: 1) the ability to understand the information presented, including risks, benefits, and alternatives; 2) the ability to appreciate the consequences of their decision; 3) the ability to use reason in their decision-making; and 4) the ability to express their choice [83,84]. These abilities must be assessed in the context of the current medical situation. Patients may have the capacity to make some medical decisions, for instance, those with limited information and risk, but lack capacity to make decisions on more complicated, higher-risk medical decisions.

There are a number of validated tools that can be used to assess medical decision-making capacity. A recent review found the Aid to Capacity Evaluation (ACE) to be the best tool for determining whether a patient has medical decision-making capacity [84]. The ACE is available without cost, and the packet includes a training scenario, instructions for scoring, and a form for clinical use. The ACE assesses seven domains, including the patient's understanding of: 1) their medical condition; 2) the proposed treatment; 3) alternatives; 4) the option of refusing treatment; 5) the consequences of accepting the treatment; 6) the consequences of refusing the proposed treatment; and 7) whether the decision is affected by depression or psychosis. The ACE is a useful and thorough tool; however, administration takes between 10 and 20 minutes, so its use in the ED will be most applicable to those who face complex decisions with significant risk [84].

When a patient lacks medical decision-making capacity, a surrogate must make medical decisions for them. However, the patient may still participate in the discussion, and provide their assent (as opposed to consent) for the medical care provided, in order for outcomes to be optimized [83]. Surrogate decision makers should be advised that they should use "substituted judgment" rather than "best interest" whenever possible in making medical decisions for the patient [83,85]. Substituted judgment maintains autonomy by using one's knowledge of the patient's preferences and beliefs in the decision-making process. The simplest way to impart this information to the surrogate decision maker is to phrase questions as "What would the patient want us to do in this situation?" rather than "What do you want us to do for the patient?" Only when patient preferences are unknown should a surrogate act in the "best interest" of the patient [83,85].

Disposition

The causes of altered mental status are generally serious and the symptoms are not usually immediately reversible. Because of the potential adverse consequences of these conditions and the altered mental status itself, admission to a general medical floor or intensive care unit is usually necessary. In cases where the cause of the altered mental status has been identified and eliminated and the patient has recovered to baseline mental status, patients may be considered for discharge after a suitable observation period.

Summary

Altered mental status is a common and serious condition in older ED patients. The use of objective, validated tools will help clinicians detect and correctly classify patients with altered mental status and allow for optimal treatment. We recommend the use of the modified Richmond Agitation and Sedation Scale (mRASS) to assess level of consciousness, the Ottowa 3DY or the Six-Item Screener to assess for altered cognition, and the SQiD as a part of the "geriatric review of symptoms" when family or caregivers are available. These can be incorporated into the general evaluation of the older patient used by emergency physicians without substantially increasing the time required for evaluation. Use of these tools should provide enough information to allow for the diagnosis of delirium using either the DSM-IV criteria or the CAM. Alternatively, emergency physicians may use the bCAM in complex patients.

Treatment of altered mental status is focused on treatment of the underlying condition, avoiding risky medications, and the non-pharmacological and pharmacological treatment of agitation associated with delirium. Non-pharmacological treatment is focused on eliminating sources of agitation such as tethers or restraints, and providing reorientation. Pharmacological management is indicated only if non-pharmacological treatment is unsuccessful and is primarily through the use of antipsychotics; benzodiazepines have limited indications.

Pearls and pitfalls

Pearls

- Acute disturbances in consciousness are fluid; patients who are stuporous or comatose will often transition to delirium, or vice versa.

- Dementia and delirium are distinct conditions, but may occur concomitantly as dementia is an important predisposing factor for delirium.
- Delirium can be more subtle in clinical presentation than stupor or coma, and is often missed by emergency physicians. Use of objective, validated tools to evaluate older ED patients will minimize the risk of missed delirium.
- The evaluation and treatment of patients with altered mental status should be focused on identifying and treating the underlying etiology.
- The more depressed the level of consciousness (stupor or coma), the more concern the emergency physician should have for an acute life-threatening illness. In these patients, rapid assessment and treatment are critically important.
- For patients who are agitated (hyperactive delirium), non-pharmacologic interventions should initially be attempted to calm the patient. Tethers such as physical restraints and urinary bladder catheters should be minimized as these may exacerbate agitation.
- Anticholinergic medications should be avoided when possible as this class of medications may cause delirium or increase its severity.

Pitfalls

- Assuming that the altered mental status is secondary to dementia or psychiatric illness rather than delirium may lead to a delay in diagnosis, missed medical illness, and increased mortality.
- Treating agitation with benzodiazepines in those who are not withdrawing from ethanol or benzodiazepines.
- Avoiding narcotic pain medication in a delirious patient with poor pain control, as this can precipitate or worsen delirium.
- Treating with antipsychotics at doses used in younger psychiatric patients with agitation. The dose in older patients with agitation due to delirium is approximately 1/10 that in younger patients.

References

1. Gerson LW, Counsell SR, Fontanarosa PB, Smucker WD. Case finding for cognitive impairment in elderly emergency department patients. *Ann Emerg Med*. 1994;23(4):813–17.

2. Naughton BJ, Moran MB, Kadah H, Heman-Ackah Y, Longano J. Delirium and other cognitive impairment in older adults in an emergency department. *Ann Emerg Med*. 1995;25(6):751–5.

3. Naughton BJ, Moran M, Ghaly Y, Michalakes C. Computed tomography scanning and delirium in elder patients. *Acad Emerg Med*. 1997;4(12):1107–10.

4. Hustey FM, Meldon SW, Palmer RM. Prevalence and documentation of impaired mental status in elderly emergency department patients. *Acad Emerg Med*. 2000;7(10):1166.

5. Hustey FM, Meldon SW. The prevalence and documentation of impaired mental status in elderly emergency department patients. *Ann Emerg Med*. 2002;39(3):248–53.

6. Hustey FM, Meldon SW, Smith MD, Lex CK. The effect of mental status screening on the care of elderly emergency department patients. *Ann Emerg Med*. 2003;41(5):678–84.

7. Morandi A, Solberg LM, Habermann R, et al. Documentation and management of words associated with delirium among elderly patients in postacute care: a pilot investigation. *J Am Med Dir Assoc*. 2009;10(5):330–4.

8. Han JH, Bryce SN, Ely EW, et al. The effect of cognitive impairment on the accuracy of the presenting complaint and discharge instruction comprehension in older emergency department patients. *Ann Emerg Med*. 2011;57(6):662–71.e2.

9. Posner JB, Plum F. *Plum and Posner's Diagnosis of Stupor and Coma* (Oxford; New York: Oxford University Press, 2007).

10. Chester JG, Beth Harrington M, Rudolph JL. Serial administration of a modified Richmond Agitation and Sedation Scale for delirium screening. *J Hosp Med*. 2011;7(5):450–3.

11. Inouye SK, van Dyck CH, Alessi CA, et al. Clarifying confusion: the confusion assessment method. A new method for detection of delirium. *Ann Intern Med*. 1990;113(c2):941–8.

12. Wolfe RE, Brown DFM. Coma and depressed level of consciousness. In *Rosen's Emergency Medicine: Concepts and Clinical Practice*, ed. Marx J (St. Louis, MO: Mosby, 2002), pp. 137–44.

13. Anon. Practice guideline for the treatment of patients with delirium. American Psychiatric Association. *Am J Psychiatry*. 1999;156(5 Suppl.):1–20.

14. American Psychiatric Association. Task Force on DSM-IV. *Diagnostic and Statistical Manual of Mental Disorders: DSM-IV-TR* (Washington, DC: American Psychiatric Association, 2000).

15. Farrell KR, Ganzini L. Misdiagnosing delirium as depression in medically ill elderly patients. *Arch Intern Med*. 1995;155(22):2459–64.

16. Han JH, Zimmerman EE, Cutler N, et al. Delirium in older emergency department patients: recognition, risk factors, and psychomotor subtypes. *Acad Emerg Med*. 2009;16(3):193–200.

17. Liptzin B, Levkoff SE. An empirical study of delirium subtypes. *Br J Psychiatry*. 1992;161:843–5.

18. O'Keeffe ST. Clinical subtypes of delirium in the elderly. *Dement Geriat Cognit Disord*. 1999;10(5):380–5.

19. Ross CA, Peyser CE, Shapiro I, Folstein MF. Delirium: phenomenologic and etiologic subtypes. *Int Psychogeriatr*. 1991;3(2):135–47.

20. Barron EA, Holmes J. Delirium within the emergency care setting, occurrence and detection: a systematic review. *EMJ*. 2012 (accessed July 31, 2012 from www.ncbi.nlm.nih.gov/pubmed/22833596).

21. Witlox J, Eurelings LSM, de Jonghe JFM, et al. Delirium in elderly patients and the risk of postdischarge mortality, institutionalization, and dementia: a meta-analysis. *JAMA*. 2010;304(4):443–51.

22. Inouye SK, Rushing JT, Foreman MD, Palmer RM, Pompei P. Does delirium contribute to poor hospital outcomes? A three-site epidemiologic study. *J Gen Intern Med*. 1998;13(4):234–42.

23. Francis J, Martin D, Kapoor WN. A prospective study of delirium in hospitalized elderly. *JAMA*. 1990;263(8):1097–101.

24. Leslie DL, Marcantonio ER, Zhang Y, Leo-Summers L, Inouye SK. One-year health care costs associated with delirium in the elderly population. *Arch Intern Med*. 2008;168(1):27–32.

111

25. Gonzalez M, Martinez G, Calderon J, et al. Impact of delirium on short-term mortality in elderly inpatients: a prospective cohort study. *Psychosomatics*. 2009;50(3):234–8.

26. Han JH, Shintani A, Eden S, et al. Delirium in the emergency department: an independent predictor of death within 6 months. *Ann Emerg Med*. 2010;56(3):244–52.e1.

27. Han JH, Eden S, Shintani A, et al. Delirium in older emergency department patients is an independent predictor of hospital length of stay. *Acad Emerg Med*. 2011;18(5):451–7.

28. Vida S, Galbaud du Fort G, Kakuma R, et al. An 18-month prospective cohort study of functional outcome of delirium in elderly patients: activities of daily living. *Int Psychogeriatr*. 2006;18(4):681–700.

29. Inouye SK. Delirium in older persons. *N Engl J Med*. 2006;354(11):1157–65.

30. Han JH, Wilson A, Ely EW. Delirium in the older emergency department patient: a quiet epidemic. *Emerg Med Clin N Am*. 2010;28(3):611–31.

31. Inouye SK. Predisposing and precipitating factors for delirium in hospitalized older patients. *Demen Geriatr Cogn*. 1999;10(5):393–400.

32. Pompei P, Foreman M, Rudberg MA, et al. Delirium in hospitalized older persons: outcomes and predictors. *J Am Geriatr Soc*. 1994;42(8):809–15.

33. Voyer P, Cole MG, McCusker J, Belzile E. Prevalence and symptoms of delirium superimposed on dementia. *Clin Nurs Res*. 2006;15(1):46–66.

34. Kennedy M, Enander RA, Wolfe RE, Marcantonio ER, Shapiro NI. Identification of delirium in elderly emergency department patients. *Acad Emerg Med*. 2012;19(Suppl. 1)(s1):S147.

35. Inouye SK, Viscoli CM, Horwitz RI, Hurst LD, Tinetti ME. A predictive model for delirium in hospitalized elderly medical patients based on admission characteristics. *Ann Intern Med*. 1993;119(6):474–81.

36. Rockwood K. Acute confusion in elderly medical patients. *J Am Geriatr Soc*. 1989;37(2):150–4.

37. Han JH, Morandi A, Ely W, et al. Delirium in the nursing home patients seen in the emergency department. *J Am Geriatr Soc*. 2009;57(5):889–94.

38. Lipowski ZJ. Delirium in the elderly patient. *N Engl J Med*. 1989;320(9):578–82.

39. Rahkonen T, Makela H, Paanila S, et al. Delirium in elderly people without severe predisposing disorders: etiology and 1-year prognosis after discharge. *Int Psychogeriatr*. 2000;12(4):473–81.

40. Schor JD, Levkoff SE, Lipsitz LA, et al. Risk factors for delirium in hospitalized elderly. *JAMA*. 1992;267(6):827–31.

41. Gustafson Y, Berggren D, Brannstrom B, et al. Acute confusional states in elderly patients treated for femoral neck fracture. *J Am Geriatr Soc*. 1988;36(6):525–30.

42. Clegg A, Young JB. Which medications to avoid in people at risk of delirium: a systematic review. *Age Aging*. 2011;40(1):23–9.

43. Anon. American Geriatrics Society updated Beers Criteria for potentially inappropriate medication use in older adults. *J Am Geriatr Soc*. 2012;60(4):616–31.

44. Anon. Drugs that may cause cognitive disorders in the elderly. *Med Lett Drugs Ther*. 2000;42(1093):111–12.

45. Campbell N, Perkins A, Hui S, Khan B, Boustani M. Association between prescribing of anticholinergic medications and incident delirium: a cohort study. *J Am Geriatr Soc*. 2011;59(Suppl. 2):S277–81.

46. Agostini JV, Leo-Summers LS, Inouye SK. Cognitive and other adverse effects of diphenhydramine use in hospitalized older patients. *Arch Intern Med*. 2001;161(17):2091–7.

47. Luukkanen MJ, Uusvaara J, Laurila JV, et al. Anticholinergic drugs and their effects on delirium and mortality in the elderly. *Demen Geriatr Cogn Extra*. 2011;1(1):43–50.

48. Han L, McCusker J, Cole M, et al. Use of medications with anticholinergic effect predicts clinical severity of delirium symptoms in older medical inpatients. *Arch Intern Med*. 2001;161(8):1099–105.

49. Craft S, Cholerton B, Reger M. Cognitive changes associated with normal and pathological aging. In *Hazzard's Geriatric Medicine & Gerontology*, 6th edn, ed. Halter J, Ouslander J, Tinetti M, et al. (McGraw-Hill Professional, 2009), pp. 751–65.

50. McGirt MJ, Woodworth G, Coon AL, et al. Diagnosis, treatment, and analysis of long-term outcomes in idiopathic normal-pressure hydrocephalus. *Neurosurgery*. 2005;57(4):699–705; discussion, 699–705.

51. Sanders AB. *Emergency Care of the Elder Person* (St Louis, MO:Beverly Cracom Publications, 1996).

52. Sessler CN, Gosnell MS, Grap MJ, et al. The Richmond Agitation-Sedation Scale: Validity and reliability in adult intensive care unit patients. *Am J Respir Crit Care Med*. 2002;166(10):1338–44.

53. Ely EW, Truman B, Shintani A, et al. Monitoring sedation status over time in ICU patients: reliability and validity of the Richmond Agitation-Sedation Scale (RASS). *JAMA*. 2003;289(22):2983–91.

54. O'Keeffe ST, Gosney MA. Assessing attentiveness in older hospital patients: global assessment versus tests of attention. *J Am Geriatr Soc*. 1997;45(4):470–3.

55. Folstein MF, Folstein SE, McHugh PR. "Mini-mental state." A practical method for grading the cognitive state of patients for the clinician. *J Psychiatr Res*. 1975;12(3):189–98.

56. Carpenter CR, Bassett ER, Fischer GM, et al. Four sensitive screening tools to detect cognitive dysfunction in geriatric emergency department patients: brief Alzheimer's Screen, Short Blessed Test, Ottawa 3DY, and the caregiver-completed AD8. *Acad Emerg Med*. 2011;18(4):374–84.

57. Carpenter CR, Despain B, Keeling TN, Shah M, Rothenberger M. The Six-Item Screener and AD8 for the detection of cognitive impairment in geriatric emergency department patients. *Ann Emerg Med*. 2011;57:653–61.

58. Wilber ST, Lofgren SD, Mager TG, Blanda M, Gerson LW. An evaluation of two screening tools for cognitive impairment in older emergency department patients. *Acad Emerg Med*. 2005;12(7):612–16.

59. Wilber ST, Carpenter CR, Hustey FM. The Six-Item Screener to detect cognitive impairment in older emergency department patients. *Acad Emerg Med*. 2008;15(7):613–16.

60. Carpenter CR, Griffey RT, Stark S, Coopersmith CM, Gage BF. Physician and nurse acceptance of technicians to screen for geriatric syndromes in the emergency department. *West J Emerg Med*. 2011;12(4):489–95.

61. Adams HP, Zoppo G del, Alberts MJ, et al. Guidelines for the Early Management of Adults With Ischemic Stroke. A Guideline From the American Heart Association/ American Stroke Association Stroke Council, Clinical Cardiology Council, Cardiovascular Radiology and Intervention Council, and the Atherosclerotic Peripheral Vascular Disease and Quality of Care Outcomes in Research Interdisciplinary Working Groups: The American Academy of Neurology affirms the value of this guideline as an educational tool for neurologists. *Stroke.* 2007;38(5):1655–711.

62. Kakuma R, du Fort GG, Arsenault L, et al. Delirium in older emergency department patients discharged home: effect on survival. *J Am Geriatr Soc.* 2003;51(4):443–50.

63. Terrell KM, Hustey FM, Hwang U, et al. Quality indicators for geriatric emergency care. *Acad Emerg Med.* 2009;16(5):441–9.

64. Wei LA, Fearing MA, Sternberg EJ, Inouye SK. The Confusion Assessment Method: a systematic review of current usage. *J Am Geriatr Soc.* 2008;56(5):823–30.

65. Inouye SK. *The Confusion Assessment Method (CAM): Training Manual and Coding Guide*, 2003 (accessed October 24, 2011 from www.hospitalelderlifeprogram.org/pdf/TheConfusionAssessmentMethod.pdf).

66. Han JH, Wilson A, Vasilevskis EE. Diagnosing Delirium in older emergency department patients: Validity and reliability of the Delivium Triage Screen and the Brief Confusion Assessment Method. *Ann Emerg Med* 2013 (forthcoming).

67. Sands MB, Dantoc BP, Hartshorn A, Ryan CJ, Lujic S. Single Question in Delirium (SQiD): testing its efficacy against psychiatrist interview, the Confusion Assessment Method and the Memorial Delirium Assessment Scale. *Palliat Med.* 2010;24(6):561–5.

68. Inouye SK. The dilemma of delirium: clinical and research controversies regarding diagnosis and evaluation of delirium in hospitalized elderly medical patients. *Am J Med.* 1994;97(3):278–88.

69. Bayer AJ, Chadha JS, Farag RR, Pathy MS. Changing presentation of myocardial infarction with increasing old age. *J Am Geriatr Soc.* 1986;34(4):263–6.

70. Hardy JE, Brennan N. Computerized tomography of the brain for elderly patients presenting to the emergency department with acute confusion. *Emerg Med Australas.* 2008;20(5):420–4.

71. Mesulam MM, Waxman SG, Geschwind N, Sabin TD. Acute confusional states with right middle cerebral artery infarctions. *J Neurol Neurosurg Psychiatr.* 1976;39(1):84–9.

72. Zehtabchi S, Abdel Baki SG, Malhotra S, Grant AC. Nonconvulsive seizures in patients presenting with altered mental status: an evidence-based review. *Epilepsy Behav.* 2011;22(2):139–43.

73. Flaherty JH, Little MO. Matching the environment to patients with delirium: lessons learned from the delirium room, a restraint-free environment for older hospitalized adults with delirium. *J Am Geriatr Soc.* 2011;59(Suppl. 2):S295–300.

74. Inouye SK, Charpentier PA. Precipitating factors for delirium in hospitalized elderly persons: Predictive model and interrelationship with baseline vulnerability. *JAMA.* 1996;275(11):852–7.

75. Holroyd-Leduc JM, Sen S, Bertenthal D, et al. The relationship of indwelling urinary catheters to death, length of hospital stay, functional decline, and nursing home admission in hospitalized older medical patients. *J Am Geriatr Soc.* 2007;55(2):227–33.

76. Tahir TA, Eeles E, Karapareddy V, et al. A randomized controlled trial of quetiapine versus placebo in the treatment of delirium. *J Psychosomat Res.* 2010;69(5):485–90.

77. Lonergan E, Britton AM, Luxenberg J, Wyller T. Antipsychotics for delirium. *Cochrane Database Syst Rev.* 2007;(2):CD005594.

78. Fosnight S. Delirium in the elderly. In *Geriatrics (Pharmacotherapy Self-Assessment Program Book 7)*, in ed. Chant C, Chessman K, Richardson M (Rockville, MD: American College of Clinical Pharmacology, 2011), pp. 73–96.

79. Devlin JW, Roberts RJ, Fong JJ, et al. Efficacy and safety of quetiapine in critically ill patients with delirium: a prospective, multicenter, randomized, double-blind, placebo-controlled pilot study. *Crit Care Med.* 2010;38(2):419–27.

80. Lonergan E, Luxenberg J, Areosa Sastre A, Wyller TB. Benzodiazepines for delirium. *Cochrane Database Syst Rev.* 2009;(1):CD006379.

81. Pandharipande PP, Pun BT, Herr DL, et al. Effect of sedation with dexmedetomidine vs lorazepam on acute brain dysfunction in mechanically ventilated patients: the MENDS randomized controlled trial. *JAMA.* 2007;298(22):2644–53.

82. Riker RR, Shehabi Y, Bokesch PM, et al. Dexmedetomidine vs midazolam for sedation of critically ill patients: a randomized trial. *JAMA.* 2009;301(5):489–99.

83. Drickamer M, Lai J. Assessment of decisional capacity and competencies. In *Hazzard's Geriatric Medicine & Gerontology, 6th edn*, ed. Halter J, Ouslander J, Tinetti M, et al. (McGraw-Hill Professional, 2009), pp. 171–6.

84. Sessums LL, Zembrzuska H, Jackson JL. Does this patient have medical decision-making capacity? *JAMA.* 2011;306(v):420–7.

85. Karlawish J, James B. Ethical issues. In *Hazzard's Geriatric Medicine & Gerontology*, 6th edn, ed. Halter J, Ouslander J, Tinetti M, et al. (McGraw-Hill Professional, 2009), pp. 399–406.

Chapter 13

Syncope in the elderly

Teresita M. Hogan and Lindsay Jin

Introduction

Syncope is a sudden transient loss of consciousness (LOC) and postural tone. True syncope is caused by rapid global cerebral hypoperfusion, is of short duration, self-limited, and has recovery to normal function. Cerebral hypoperfusion represents failed cerebral blood flow autoregulation. Other causes of sudden transient LOC that should be differentiated from syncope are hypoxemia, hypoglycemia, seizure, and vertebrobasilar ischemia. Although the definition above is quite specific, it defines a symptom with numerous etiologies. Syncope is a symptom, not a diagnosis per se. Prognosis varies depending on the etiology of syncope, from a mortality of 0% with vasovagal syncope to 30% in the presence of cardiac etiology [1]. The most dangerous cardiac causes are myocardial ischemia, Wolff–Parkinson–White syndrome, long QT syndrome, Brugada syndrome, and polymorphic ventricular tachycardia. Meta-analysis has shown approximately 42% of all syncope patients are hospitalized, a third are discharged without diagnosis, another third are diagnosed with situational, orthostatic, or vasovagal syncope, and 10.4% are diagnosed with a cardiovascular etiology, including bradydysrhythmia and tachydysrhythmia. Risk of death in all-cause hospitalized patients is 4.4% [2]. However, one-year incidence of sudden death increases to 24% in patients with cardiac cause of syncope [3,4].

The emergency evaluation of syncope has several goals:

- to distinguish syncope from other causes of transient LOC;
- to determine the need for further diagnostic evaluation;
- to institute emergent treatment;
- to diagnose the etiology;
- to establish prognosis – risk stratify those in danger of short-term adverse events;
- to appropriately admit those in need of hospitalization.

Aging

The frequency and etiology of syncope are highly age dependent [5]. Age-related changes that predispose elders to syncope are shown in Table 13.1.

Persons <40 years of age experience syncope at a rate of <2/1000, with <10% hospitalized; however the rate rises to

Table 13.1. Age-related changes causing syncope

Reduced cerebral blood flow
a. Hypertension-induced autoregulatory shift
b. Diabetic-related chemoreceptor response
Reduced cardiac output
Reduced thirst mechanism
Altered homeostasis of water
Altered homeostasis of salt
Autonomic dysfunction
Altered baroreceptor function
Carotid sinus hypersensitivity
Structural heart disease

nearly 19.5/1000 in elders, with nearly 60% hospitalized [6,7]. Mortality in syncope rises with increasing age, but no single age cutoff can identify a point of increasing risk. Age distribution shows a sharp rise in syncope after 70 years [8], with incidence of cardiac syncope peaking from 61 to 70 years [9]. An overall incidence of 23% is seen in institutionalized elders [7]. Higher incidence of ED visits for syncope occurs in elders with both age and cardiac disease, which are independently linked to adverse outcomes [10,11,12,13].

The diagnosis of syncope in elders is difficult. First, in older adults the cause of syncope is often multifactorial. Additionally, its evaluation overlaps with that of TIA, dizziness, both orthostatic and postprandial hypotension, drug interactions, and falls. Falls in elders is an epic problem. There is an annual incidence of a fall in up to 30% of elders, with up to 30% of fall events caused by syncope [14].

The epidemiology of syncope varies intensely with age. The primary causes of syncope in older adults are orthostatic hypotension (OH), carotid sinus hypersensitivity (CSH), neurally mediated, and dysrhythmia [13,15]. OH causes syncope in 20–30% of older adults [15,16]. Hospitalization for OH syncope increases with age from 4.2% at 65–74 years to 30.5% in those >75 years [17]. Because treatment for OH (midodrine and fludrocortisones) typically exacerbates supine hypertension, the management of these concurrent conditions is often difficult. Twenty-five percent of elders with OH have OH on the basis of aging physiology alone, while in the remaining

Geriatric Emergency Medicine, ed. Joseph H. Kahn, Brendan G. Magauran Jr., and Jonathan S. Olshaker. Published by Cambridge University Press.
© Cambridge University Press 2014.

75%, drug effect is causative. Syncope in older adults must prompt a complete search for single drug effect and drug–drug or drug–disease interactions, as well as abnormal responses of aging physiology. Cardiac dysrhythmia incidence dramatically increases with age. Prevalence in patients over age 80 years is nearly 9% for atrial fibrillation/flutter alone [18]. Anyone with history of rheumatic fever, congestive heart failure (CHF), or hypertension is at greater risk.

A full syncope assessment and intervention is recommended in all patients regardless of advancing age. In mobile, cognitively intact older adults syncope evaluation is identical to that of younger adult patients [19]. In all elders, the emergency assessment of syncope must broaden not only to determining existence of a life-threat, but also to prevent physical harm from recurrent events or falls. This is especially true in the frail elder. In frail elders orthostatic measurements and carotid sinus massage (CSM) testing are well tolerated. The incidence of CSM-induced neurologic sequelae is extremely low, ranging from only 0.17 to 1.0% even in advanced age [20,21,22,23,24]. Exclusions should include those with known carotid stenosis, or with transient ischemic attack (TIA), cerebrovascular accident (CVA), or MI in the last 3 months. At the end of life, the level of evaluation and treatment should be guided not by age, but by goals of care and prognosis.

The diagnostic value of symptoms in the differentiation of cardiac versus neurally mediated syncope is controversial in older adults. Therefore the value of history in establishing an etiology may be both more difficult as well as more limited in this population. One study noted that the diagnosis of syncope etiology by history alone is possible in only 5% of elders [25]. However, others have noted a careful history, physical, and screening ECG leads to the diagnosis in 34–50% of those >65 years [13,16]. The symptom of dyspnea was predictive of cardiac syncope in elders, while non-cardiac predictive symptoms were noted to be nausea, blurred vision, and diaphoresis [25]. Additionally, in older patients syncope while supine and during exertion is more often associated with cardiac than with neurally mediated syncope [26]. This same study cited blurred vision as being associated with cardiac cause.

Despite the high numbers admitted for evaluation, 54% of elders are discharged without a conclusive diagnosis [27,28]. In patients with known coronary artery disease (CAD) and syncope, risk of death is directly proportional to the severity of left ventricular dysfunction [1]. Evaluation for ischemia, structural heart disease, and dysrhythmia is indicated in these patients. Those who have an ejection fraction of <0.35 realize substantial survival gains with implantable defibrillators [29]. Of note is that the underlying damage causing dysrhythmia is not necessarily resolved with revascularization and may require evaluation after correction of the ischemia [1].

Recurrent syncopal episodes within 3 years of the index event occur in 31–35% of those patients over 85 years [4]. However, it has been demonstrated that these recurrent syncopal events are not linked with increased mortality and that readmission of these patients leads to new diagnosis in only 9% [30]. Patients over 85 years with recurrent syncope experience the highest rates of cardiac cause and the poorest survival. However, these

findings correlate with the high comorbidity burden noted in this population and not with syncope itself [9].

Although the majority of elders with syncope survive without intervention to hospital discharge, they may experience significant morbidity. Even a benign diagnosis, such as vasovagal syncope, may have a serious impact on a patient's well-being. Quality of life studies show elders with syncope develop significant functional impairments [31]. Fear of recurrence resulted in patients' decreased driving and walking, as well as lower overall vitality and social functioning. These effects were most pronounced within the first six months after a syncopal episode, and led to further functional decline. Those with recurrent episodes experienced greater decline. The need for admission, consultation, and further testing were related to poorer functional outcomes. Emergency physicians should consider the negative impact on quality of life experienced by elder syncope patients. Therefore if we determine a benign cause we should attempt to mitigate functional decline through comprehensive patient education and discussions.

Epidemiology

In the ED, syncope is responsible for 1–3% of all patient visits and 6% of total hospital admissions [32,33]. However the elder population experiences disproportionally high hospitalization rates, with 58% of those over age 80 years admitted to the hospital when they present with complaint of syncope [6]. Over 70% of hospital-wide syncope admissions originate in the ED. Consensus panels recommend admission for patients with cardiac history or advanced age [34,35]. Despite the high numbers hospitalized, 60% of admitted patients receive no therapeutic intervention or treatment for syncope and 39–50% of these individuals are sent home without identification of any formal etiology [27,28]. The annual cost of syncope in the US ranges from 2.4 to 2.6 billion dollars, with a mean cost of $5400 per hospitalization [36,37]. For this investment, the one-year morbidity and mortality in all syncope cases, including those of cardiac etiology, is minimally impacted [38].

In the Framingham study, cardiac syncope doubled the risk of death from any cause and increased the risk of non-fatal and fatal cardiovascular events, compared with those without syncope [8]. However, syncope itself has not been found to increase risk of overall cardiac events or death except in the presence of existing heart disease, especially CHF [39].

Causes

The causes of syncope can be classified into three main categories: neurally mediated, cardiac, and orthostatic hypotension. See Table 13.2 for listing of causes of syncope.

Neurally mediated

The most common cause of syncope is neurally mediated. This describes a group of functional disorders resulting from the disruption of cardiac rhythm, usually in the form of bradycardia or through vasodilation. Therefore it is also termed reflex syncope. These neural mechanisms can be subdivided into vasovagal, the single largest overall cause of syncope, situational,

Table 13.2. Causes of syncope

Neurally mediated

• Vasovagal

  • Vagus nerve reacts to a trigger causing bradycardia and hypotension

  • Requires intact autonomic nervous system

• Situational

  • Cough, laughter, defecation, micturition

• Carotid sinus hypersensitivity

  • Results from either an inhibitory signal causing asystole, vasodepression causing hypotension, or a mixture due to hypersensitivity of carotid pressure (shaving, tight collar, turning head, etc.)

Cardiac

• Electrophysiological

  • Dysrhythmia – usually from ischemic or hypertensive disease

  • Stokes–Adams attack – asystole from intermittent AV block

• Structural

  • Valvular disease (aortic stenosis is the classic example), myocardial ischemia, hypertrophic and other cardiomyopathies, cardiac masses such as atrial myxoma, and pericardial effusions

Cerebrovascular

  • Vascular steal syndromes

  • Very rare without focal neurological deficits or seizure-like activity

  • May have transient ischemic attack secondary to vertebrobasilar insufficiency

Orthostatic hypertension

• Simple volume depletion

  • Poor intake, GI loss, hemorrhage, Addison's disease

• Drugs

  • Drugs from several classes may lower peripheral resistance

  • Key among these are antihypertensive agents of several classes (e.g., alpha-adrenoreceptor antagonists, nitrates and other vasodilators, and calcium channel-blocking agents), antidepressants, phenothiazines, ethanol, narcotics, insulin, dopamine agonists, barbiturates, and alpha blockers for prostatic hypertrophy

• Autonomic dysfunction

  • Primary autonomic failure from neurodegenerative disease

  • Secondary autonomic failure is seen in the setting of systemic diseases (e.g., diabetes, hepatic disease, renal failure, and chronic alcohol abuse)

Psychogenic

  • As many as 20–35% of syncope patients may require psychiatric evaluation to explain causes not evident on medical assessment alone

  • The vast majority of these patients are younger in age

Mixed cause

  • Older adults are at high likelihood to have multiple etiologies of syncope

  • Mixed-cause syncope is an independent risk factor for adverse outcome

and carotid sinus syndrome (CSS). CSH associated with syncope defines CSS.

Vasovagal

A precipitating event, such as fear, severe pain, emotional distress, instrumentation, or prolonged standing is associated with typical prodromal symptoms of diaphoresis, nausea, tunnel vision, and LOC.

Situational

Syncope that occurs during, or immediately after, micturition, defecation, coughing, or swallowing.

CSH

This is the exaggerated response to carotid baroreceptor triggers that cause dizziness or syncope through decreased cerebral perfusion from multiple separate mechanisms. CSH is found primarily in older males and often exists in elder patients with syncope and falls. Some have found that CSH is part of a generalized autonomic disorder [40]. CSH is found in up to 9% of patients with recurrent syncope, 14% of nursing home (NH) patients, and 30% of elders with drop attacks. Although patients with CSH are at increased risk for injury and fractures, they are not at increased risk of mortality [41,42]. CSH may be present in as many as 33% of asymptomatic patients, who remain symptom and syncope free thanks to corrective mechanisms.

Cardiac

The second most common cause of syncope is cardiac, with dysrhythmia as the primary etiology followed by structural heart disease [43]. These mechanisms cause hypoperfusion through decreased cardiac output.

Dysrhythmia

Disorders such as atrial fibrillation/flutter, high grade AV block, ventricular tachycardia, sinus node dysfunction, sick sinus syndrome, and pacemaker malfunction are all cause for concern in the elder population.

Structural heart disease

The presence of severe valvular stenosis or other outflow obstruction can cause syncope. The association of syncope with aortic stenosis is classically known to have an approximate two-year survival without valve replacement [44,45,46].

Vascular steal syndromes

Subclavian steal occurs when there is retrograde blood flow in the vertebral artery resulting from stenosis or occlusion of the ipsilateral subclavian artery. After exercising the ipsilateral arm, patients may experience neurological symptoms due to brain ischemia.

Orthostatic hypotension

Orthostatic hypotension (OH) is an example of a multifactorial geriatric syndrome, and may be an indication of the systemic dysregulation seen in frailty [47]. The prevalence of OH is proportional to age, ranging from 5% in community dwellers older than 65 years to 50% in institutionalized elders. The clinical manifestations of OH depend on its cause and severity. Most patients with OH have either no symptoms or atypical symptoms. However, OH is a leading cause of syncope in the elder population and is also associated with cardiovascular mortality. One recent study found OH to be a predictor of myocardial infarction [48]. Overall, OH is a predictor of poor prognosis [49]. Although the risks and benefits of screening for OH have not been well studied [50], this should be examined as a possible cause in elder patients with syncope.

Unlikely causes of syncope

It is highly doubtful that a TIA can be a true cause of LOC. The only logical situation is when a TIA occurs in the vertebrobasilar circulation. In this case other signs such as paralysis, eye movement disorders, and vertigo should be readily apparent. LOC without any such associated symptoms is highly unlikely to be a manifestation of TIA, and the typical syncope patient does not warrant evaluation for cerebrovascular ischemia.

History

The diagnostic value of a syncope history has been evaluated in prospective and case-controlled studies [3,51,52,53,54]. Three elements are basic to the elder syncope history. The first two help establish the diagnosis while the third is key for risk stratification. Additionally, history will inform the strategy for subsequent evaluation.

1. Is the LOC attributable to true syncope or more likely another etiology?
2. Obtain key data to suggest cause of syncope as described below.
3. Is heart disease present?

Sequence of events

In the complete evaluation of syncope, establishing a sequential series of events immediately preceding LOC is critical. Ask about provocation or trigger events. Question the patient through a clear progression of the prodrome phase, the actual LOC, and length of episode. Length of episode may need to be surmised by time lapse or eyewitness report. Be sure to ask about the recovery phase and what symptoms were experienced on awakening. Establish any trauma related to the LOC [55]. This history requires the patient to be cognitively intact; other features require eyewitness observation. The absence of these historical features will inevitably diminish the ability to establish a diagnosis. Age does not independently affect the historical characteristics of a syncopal event, however up to 40% of elders have complete amnesia of the syncopal event [56]. This also affects reporting of pre- and post-episode symptoms. The frequent absence of these features is frustrating but not an excuse to eliminate such important elements from your history.

Specific data points

Include age, gender, history of diseases, establishment of prior syncopal events, and specific questions regarding current medications. It is especially important to note any drugs acting on the cardiovascular system. A careful history of medications is always important in the geriatric population, and drug-related syncope is more common in elderly patients taking several medications [57]. A careful review for proarrhythmia agents such as class IA and IC antiarrhythmic drugs is essential.

Focused history should uncover factors associated with adverse outcomes, and therefore every syncope history should specifically search for gastrointestinal bleeding, cardiac disease, or intracerebral bleeding.

Preceding symptom frequency, position or activity at the time of the event, and occurrence of post-syncopal injury do not vary significantly with age [9]. Syncopal events that are associated with a prodrome, especially those with vagal symptoms like nausea and vomiting, are more likely to be neurally mediated. A clear precipitating event, such as heat, a crowded area, or prolonged orthostasis indicates neurally mediated events. A cardiac etiology is more likely if syncope occurs while seated or supine or without any prodrome [58] or with exertion [59].

Symptoms distinguishing seizure from syncope

Understanding of the physiology of syncope will help decrease confusion with seizure or transient ischemic events. In syncope, a stereotyped progression of neurologic symptoms occur, including a brief period of confusion or disorientation that is followed by midline eye fixation with a glassy stare appearance. Patients report retinal hypoperfusion as a narrowing of the visual field that becomes gray then black, followed by complete visual loss. Hearing loss may follow. When consciousness is lost eyes may gaze upward. Myoclonic jerking movements are common [60]. Witnesses may commonly report tonic–clonic-like movements, which are typically brief and mild. This convulsive syncope can be seen with any etiology [31]. Once consciousness is regained patients quickly return to normal mental status as compared to the post-ictal period seen with seizures.

The recognition of convulsive syncope adds to the difficulty in differentiating these entities. Sheldon et al. described a point score of historical features that distinguishes syncope from seizure with 94% sensitivity and specificity [61]. The total of 118 questions makes the tool prohibitively long for ED use, but it supports the use of targeted questions. Seizure patients are more likely to experience tongue biting, urinary incontinence, déjà vu, mood changes, hallucinations, and trembling preceding the LOC. Syncope patients were more likely to experience diaphoresis, dyspnea, chest pain, palpitations, warmth, nausea, vertigo, and presyncopal prodromes.

Symptoms suggestive of cardiac etiology

A rapid syncope with no prodrome is a clinical clue suggestive of a primary cardiac etiology. It can also be seen in cardiac inhibition from CSS or ocular pressure. The presentation of CSS depends on the duration of cardiac cycle inhibition stopping forward flow of blood. LOC after the inhibition of the cardiac cycle obviously occurs earlier if the patient is upright. Primary ventricular tachydysrhythmias may result in more gradual LOC as some forward blood flow may be present. Palpitations are strongly indicative of dysrhythmia. Complete history should be used to identify patients with heart failure, coronary artery disease, older age, or structural heart disease [35].

Factors associated with autonomic failure

Consider automonic failure in patients with Parkinson's disease and diabetes. If patients experience symptoms of ischemia to other areas these may be noted in primary autonomic failure. Visual scotomas and hallucinations suggest occipital ischemia [62].

Factors that identify a lower risk of adverse events do not often apply to the elderly population, including younger age, no history or signs of cardiovascular disease, and no comorbidities.

Physical exam

As in all ED evaluations, first and foremost is the establishment of airway, breathing, and circulation. Once these are assured vital signs must be reviewed. Persistent hypotension or tachycardia represent hemodynamic instability, and a cause for the syncope such as hemorrhage, heart failure, sepsis, or volume depletion should be sought. Patients suffering from syncope as a result of serious clinical etiologies such as myocardial infarction or dysrhythmia present with unstable vital signs in approximately 70% of cases.

The portions of the physical examination most useful in the diagnosis of syncope are cardiovascular, neurologic, orthostatic measurements, and evaluation of gait and standing balance.

Orthostatic hypotension is the physical finding of a >20 mmHg decrease in systolic or >10 mmHg decrease in diastolic blood pressure within three minutes of standing. Standing results in decreased venous return as 25–30% of the systemic circulation begins pooling in the lower extremities and splanchnic–mesenteric circulation. This is a common finding in patients with syncope. However, OH is not reliably reproducible in older adults, particularly in cases with medication and age-related causes. Therefore, repeated morning measurements may be the only way to diagnose OH [63]. A careful risk assessment should be done when OH is suspected to determine suitability of discharge in these patients. A recent study warns about the lack of dizziness experienced by elders with documented OH pressure drops and falls [64].

Orthostatic hypotension increases with aging due to baroreceptor sensitivity, decreased cardiac contractility, and autonomic dysfunction. In elders the differential for autonomic dysfunction includes the four primary autonomic degenerative disorders. These are multiple system atrophy (Shy–Drager syndrome), Parkinson's disease, Lewy body dementia, and pure autonomic failure. OH should be considered in any syncopal patient with Parkinson's disease. Secondary autonomic failure occurs due to diabetic neuropathy, hepatic or renal failure, or alcohol abuse. In patients with these histories syncope occurs commonly and is often the result of the underlying disease process.

Autonomic dysfunction occurs in 54–56% of institutionalized elders, in contrast to the 6% found in community-dwelling individuals [47]. Although antihypertensive therapy seems intuitively associated with OH, a recent study showed no significant association between the two [65]. Cognitive impairment is frequently associated with OH. Each one point decrease in the Mini-Mental State Exam (MMSE) increases the risk of OH by nearly 10% [64]. So the greater the level of cognitive impairment the more likely the patient has OH.

Subjective lightheadedness within two minutes of standing is considered as OH and may indicate volume depletion or medication effect. This history is difficult to establish in severe cognitive impairment. OH increases with age, and 40% of healthy controls over age 70 had symptoms of OH as well as 23% of patients less than 60 years of age [66,67]. OH as the cause of syncope should be a diagnosis of exclusion, as both high- and low-risk patients will be orthostatic [68]. Supine hypertension is common in patients with OH due to autonomic failure. When supine hypertension is found in the setting of OH, one must consider autonomic failure in the differential.

A careful cardiopulmonary exam should be done to evaluate for signs of heart failure or structural heart disease. These may include peripheral edema, jugular venous distension, rales, murmur, or S3/S4 heart sounds.

An oropharyngeal exam should be done to look for evidence of tongue biting. Although this has low sensitivity, it is highly specific for seizure activity.

Carotid sinus hypersensitivity is the most commonly reported cause of falls and syncope in older persons, present in 39% of individuals over 65 years of age [69]. Yet CSS is frequently underdiagnosed as the cause of falls (with unreported syncope) and syncope in this population [70]. The finding of CSS and thus the positive yield of carotid sinus massage in elder syncope patients was 17.6% [71]. Therefore, CSM is suggested as the diagnostic maneuver of choice to diagnose this entity [71]. CSM should particularly be targeted at older patients with unexplained syncope and falls. CSM should be considered in elderly patients with unexplained bradycardic or hypotensive symptoms [70].

Performance of CSM has been suggested as a first-line investigation in guidelines and textbooks [73,74,75]. CSM is suggested as part of the initial evaluation for the diagnosis and risk stratification of older adults with syncope. CSM is a class 1B recommendation in patients >40 years with syncope of unknown etiology after initial evaluation [72].

Be aware that the performance of CSM could itself provoke vasovagal syncope in predisposed patients [75]. Therefore, positive CSM alone does not mandate a diagnosis of CSH-induced syncope. However, if CSM testing is positive, this suggests need for further evaluation [76]. CSM has greatest clinical utility in males aged 60–80 years. Although CSM is well described in the literature, it is rarely used in clinical practice in the US.

For completeness one method of CSM is described, which includes the following steps:

1. Ensure the patient has been supine for at least 5 minutes, then slightly extend the neck.
2. Listen for a carotid bruit, abort the test if one is present.
3. Place two fingers just medial to the sternocleidomastoid muscle at the upper level of the thyroid cartilage, just over the point of maximal carotid impulse.
4. Continuously monitor ECG and blood pressure.
5. Massage gently for 5 seconds, wait at least one minute, and repeat massage on the opposite side.

The test is positive if:

>3 seconds of asystole is found.
>50 mmHg systolic blood pressure decrease is found.
A combination of the two above is found.

European studies suggest less sensitive cutoffs for positivity of:

BP drop of >60 mmHg systolic lasting for >6 seconds and
Asystole of >6 seconds [77].

The test is absolutely contraindicated patients with stroke, TIA, or MI in the previous 3 months, or known >70% carotid stenosis. Relative contraindications are history of ventricular tachycardia (VT), ventricular fibrillation (VF), or known carotid bruit. Incidence of neurologic complications with carotid massage is <0.2% [79]. Therefore with the above exclusions, CSM is quite safe. It is important to do a thorough exam for trauma related to the syncope because syncope and resultant head injury are associated with increased one-year mortality [10].

A rectal exam should be performed if gastrointestinal hemorrhage is a reasonable consideration as indicated by careful syncope history, vital signs, and preceding physical examination.

Ancillary studies

The ED diagnostic evaluation for syncope exhibits high practice variation; it is not usually performed according to any standardized algorithm and testing is highly inconsistent across ED practice sites [28]. The 2007 American College of Emergency Physicians Clinical Policy: Critical Issues in the Evaluation and Management of Patients Presenting with Syncope [35] notes low yield of non-directed testing [3]. On admitted syncope patients, the most commonly performed ED studies are ECG (99%), cardiac markers (95%), and head CT (63%). Markers and head CT affected diagnosis or management in less than 5% of cases and were diagnostic in <2% [80]. Orthostatic blood pressure readings were performed in only 38% of these cases yet showed effect on diagnosis in 18–26% and in management in 25–30% of cases, and determined etiology in 15–21% of syncope patients.

Emergency department evaluation should be based on syncope history and physical exam, which is used to inform a careful differential diagnosis. Testing based on this differential would yield more cost-effective and clinically significant results.

Cardiovascular testing

ECG

ECG testing to evaluate malignant cardiac etiology in syncope is a 2007 American College of Emergency Physicians (ACEP) clinical policy Level A recommendation [35]. The gold standard for identification of a dysrhythmia causing syncope is an ECG taken at the time of symptoms. ED elders with syncope and a QTc interval ≥ 500 ms are at risk for increased mortality [81]. However, an ECG establishes a diagnosis in <5% of patients.

Recursive partitioning has been used to identify ECG criteria predictive of adverse cardiac outcomes within 30 days. The criteria were: second degree Mobitz type two or third degree AV block, bundle branch block with first degree AV block, right bundle branch block with left anterior or posterior fascicular block, new ischemic changes, non-sinus rhythm, left axis deviation, or abnormal cardiac monitoring during ED observation [82]. These findings, termed the Ottawa Electrocardiographic Criteria, have yet to be externally validated.

Telemetry monitoring

Monitoring identified various dysrhythmias (bradycardia, PVC, non-sustained SVT, non-sustained VT or short sinus pauses) in 85% of patients, but a definite cause of syncope was found in only 10% [3]. Prior studies have shown that 1–4% of normal control populations had periods of sinus pause and up to 2% of controls had short episodes of ventricular tachycardia while asymptomatic [3]. It is important to note that although abnormalities were frequently found, unless accompanied by syncope or presyncope, the findings are most likely incidental and causation should not be assumed [83].

Holter monitoring is appropriate for frequent (at least daily) symptoms while event monitoring is ideal for less common episodes. Implantable loop recorders can record signals for up to 14 months and have yielded diagnosis in more than 90% of appropriate patients [84].

According to the ACEP clinical policy on syncope, continuous telemetry beyond 24 hours is unlikely to provide a diagnosis [35].

Echocardiography

In patients with a normal ECG and normal physical exam, little evidence exists to support routine use of echocardiography in the evaluation of syncope. Echocardiograms should be reserved for patients with abnormal ECG, abnormal physical exam, as well as those in whom an arrhythmic cause of syncope is suggested.

Autonomic nervous system testing

Some guidelines state that patients with recurrent or severe syncope can benefit from tilt table testing even if they have no history of structural heart disease and a normal ECG. However others report there is no evidence to support tilt testing in initial evaluation of simple syncope [19]. The incidence of positive tilt table testing is about 25% in elder patients, while increased medication use and higher value on the geriatric index of comorbidities scale tend to increase positive results [85].

Electrophysiologic testing

Electrophysiologic (EPS) studies are of very limited value with normal ECG and a structurally normal heart. If noninvasive studies fail to identify the cause, patients with ECG evidence of structural disease such as old MI or left bifascicular block (LBBB), prolonged QT, or those taking antiarrhythmic medications may be considered for EPS studies.

Cardiac catheterization

Cardiac catheterization should not be done on a routine basis but only when indicated by laboratory or ECG abnormalities [52].

Ambulatory blood pressure recording

This is beyond the scope of emergency practice, but 24-hour BP measurement may be helpful if unstable BP from medication or postprandial causes is considered.

Carotid sinus massage

If carotid sinus stimulation causes syncope, this is an American College of Cardiology/American Heart Association/Heart Rhythm Society practice guidelines Class I indication for permanent pacing therapy [86]. Carotid Doppler does not stimulate the carotid receptor adequately and thus is not an appropriate test to rule out dynamic hypersensitivity.

Laboratory testing

Routine blood tests are rarely helpful in identifying the cause of syncope. Specific exceptions are the search for myocardial infarction or anemia. The ACEP clinical policy on syncope in adults does not recommend routine lab work. The one exception to this is the hematocrit, which was demonstrated by Quinn et al. to predict adverse events when <30%. Other lab tests should be used according to physical exam, initial ECG, or clinical impression [35,80].

Neurologic testing

Head CT

Although this test is obtained in approximately 60% of cases of ED syncope, it rarely establishes an etiology. A head CT does, however, have utility in evaluating for trauma secondary to a syncopal event. The 2008 ACEP clinical policy on blunt traumatic brain injury provides level A recommendation to perform a non-contrast head CT in any patient with blunt head trauma with LOC and age greater than 60, or level B recommendation to perform the study on any patient without LOC and age greater than 65 [87].

Electroencephalogram

When an electroencephalogram (EEG) is performed broadly in syncope evaluation it is unlikely to yield a diagnosis. The EEG is a poor screening test for seizure as a cause of syncope because although a fair percentage of syncope patients will have abnormal results, so will a similar percentage of normal controls.

Systems of evaluation

When a clear diagnosis cannot be immediately established, the emergency physician (EP) must determine which patients warrant further monitoring and evaluation and whether this should occur in an inpatient or outpatient setting. A risk stratification approach has been suggested for these patients. Risk-factor stratification becomes more complex with advancing age and frailty. The goal of risk stratification is to differentiate three groups of patients: high-, intermediate-, and low-risk. High-risk patients should typically be admitted to the hospital for further evaluation and therapy, low-risk patients can safely be discharged to the outpatient setting, and intermediate-risk patients pose the greatest difficulty for the EP because there is little evidence to help direct clinical care in these cases.

Clinical practice guidelines are statements from experts to assist clinicians with complex management issues in specific clinical scenarios. Although they attempt to distil all the relevant medical knowledge into a usable format, the expert writers must make judgments on the strengths of study data, weight of risk–benefit evaluations, and the recommendations made. These judgments can be subjective and variable. Guidelines are so numerous and the quality of guideline statements is so inconstant that the Institute of Medicine has attempted to standardize them with rigorous criteria [88]. Additionally, organizations worldwide are slowly adopting the Grading of Recommendations Assessment, Development and Evaluation (GRADE) system to unify standards used to categorize quality of evidence and strength of recommendations [89].

Clinical decision rules (CDR) are derived from original research using three or more variables from the history, physical or typical ED testing that are combined to determine the likelihood of a diagnosis or prognostic outcome. Standards exist to help reduce variability and improve methodology in CDR creation. They focus on six stages in the development and validation of a quality CDR, which are: need, appropriate methodology (definition of outcomes, predictor variables, subjects, power, and statistics), validation, implementation to a clinical setting, cost effectiveness, and dissemination.

A CDR is best suited for a prevalent condition where there is variation in practice and limited clinical accuracy. Such is the case for syncope. Multiple CDRs have been developed utilizing empiric evidence to assist with clinical decision making in the area of syncope [11,90,91]. It is important to note that a CDR is sensible, accurate, and implementable in clinical practice only if its intent is to identify short- or long-term adverse events and define predictor variables and subjects. Unfortunately, the methodology and prognostic accuracy of existing syncope CDRs to date have been limited [92]. Major areas of concern are the large number of patients required to adequately power these studies and the inability to achieve external verification of findings.

Although practice guidelines and CDR for the emergency evaluation and risk stratification of syncope exist from various groups and specialty societies, such resources are incompletely disseminated to clinicians, experience erratic application in clinical practice, are not readily accepted as the standard of care, and are not followed by many physicians [93,94,95]. Additionally, when studied they yielded uncertain benefit and were found to lack methodological quality and prognostic accuracy. There is also concern about a lack of adherence to practice guidelines. In a study by Benditt, European Society of Cardiology Syncope Guidelines were taught and reinforced to a group of EPs over two years; despite knowledge of the admission criteria guidelines and support of evidence-based medicine, ED physicians preferred to conservatively admit syncope patients [96]. Therefore, even the most strenuously evidence-based clinical guidelines and risk stratification models are unlikely to significantly alter clinical practice.

Determining risk

Patients with vasovagal syncope do not have increased risk of cardiovascular events or death as opposed to those with cardiac syncope who are at increased risk of cardiovascular events as well as death from any cause. Those with orthostatic events due to age-related functional autonomic dysfunction also suffer high morbidity and mortality. Long-term morbidity and mortality are affected by underlying cardiovascular disease and not by the mechanism of sentinel syncopal event [97]. The following studies attempt to determine which factors from the history, physical examination, and initial ED work-up predict adverse outcomes while limiting the number of unnecessary hospitalizations and merge them to generate CDRs.

The San Francisco Syncope Rule (SFSR) reported on initial publication that there was a higher likelihood of 7-day mortality with abnormal initial ECG, systolic BP <90 mmHg after ED arrival, hematocrit <30%, shortness of breath, or evidence of CHF on history or examination [90]. The SFSR showed sensitivity of 98% and specificity of 56%. Evaluation of the SFSR by external sources showed poor performance with sensitivity of 90%, specificity of 33%, and five occurrences of death, three of which were after ED discharge. The SFSR did not identify

five serious outcomes with four occurring in the ED. All of this transpired despite an increased percentage of patients admitted when the SFSR was followed [98]. The SFSR has therefore not proven to reliably predict adverse events nor reduce admissions [99]. Additionally, the SFSR did not prove valid in the elder population where it had lower sensitivity and specificity [100].

The Risk Stratification of Syncope in the Emergency Department (ROSE) study found B-natriuretic peptide (BNP) ≥300 pg/ml a major predictor of poor outcome, including death. Other indicators of poor outcome requiring admission were: bradycardia <50 beats/min, digital rectal exam (DRE) positive for fecal occult blood, hemoglobin <9 g/dl, chest pain with syncope, Q waves on ECG, and O_2 saturation <94%. Application of the ROSE CDR with BNP reduced admissions by 30%. However, ROSE did not adequately predict one-year adverse outcomes [101]. Elevated BNP was only present in 7% of the validation cohort and this test adds significant cost. The ROSE validation study reported sensitivity of 87% and specificity of 65.5% with a negative predictive value of 98.5%, thereby missing 1.5% of patients with serious adverse outcomes [92].

Emergency physicians were trained to use the Boston Syncope Criteria as a guide for admission decisions. The rules were complex, consisting of 25 items in 8 categories and requiring a training and phase-in period before implementation. The rule was followed in 95.7% of cases. Sensitivity was 100% with 57% specificity and 100% negative predictive value. They achieved an 11% admission reduction while admitting all patients who sustained an adverse outcome. Forty percent of those admitted sustained adverse events during hospitalization and 4% occurred by 30 days [102]. Validation studies are pending.

The Osservatorio Epidemiologico sulla Sincope nel Lazio (OESIL) score, developed in six Italian community hospitals, looked at predictors from a detailed ED history, physical, and ECG. They found significant predictors of mortality to be age >65, known cardiovascular disease, lack of presyncopal prodrome, and abnormal ECG. The higher the score, the higher the mortality rate at one year. This rule had a sensitivity of 95% and specificity of 31%. Although OESIL was able to successfully risk stratify patients, it was not sufficiently sensitive to reduce admissions without missing patients at risk of a serious outcome [10].

Martin et al. showed that mortality and arrhythmia could be predicted by abnormal ECG, history of ventricular arrhythmia, history of CHF, or age greater than 45 years [11]. One-year incidence of dysrhythmia or death was 58–80% in patients with three or more of these factors. Prognostic factors for rehospitalization were diabetes, atrial fibrillation, and smoking [103]. Prognostic factors for time to mortality were diabetes, coronary artery bypass graft surgery, malignancy, narcotics use, smoking, atrial fibrillation, and volume depletion [103].

Meta-analysis review has shown that the most powerful predictors of adverse events are palpitations, syncope during effort, prior CHF or CAD, and an abnormal ECG [2]. Additionally, adverse outcomes are shown to increase with every decade of life.

Table 13.3. Other risk factors

	High risk	Intermediate risk	Low risk
History	• Structural heart disease • Left ventricular dysfunction • CHF • Dysrhythmias	• Recurrent syncope without associated trauma • Correctable drug-related syncope	• No cardiovascular disease • Clear vasovagal event
Presentation	• ACS • Dyspnea • GI Bleed • Syncope on exertion or while supine • Prodrome of palpitations • Total lack of prodrome		
Physical exam	• Unstable vital signs • Systolic BP <90 mmHg • Bradycardia <50 beats/min • Unresolved or symptomatic OH • Concurrent trauma • Positive CSM • Structural heart disease • CHF • DRE + occult blood	• Correctable OH • Dehydration from preventable cause	• Normal stable vitals • Stable gait • Normal get-up-and-go testing
Lab findings	• ECG with active ischemia or dysrhythmia, QTc >500 ms, or any bundle branch block • Hematocrit <30% • Hemoglobin <9 g/dl • BNP >300 pg/ml	• Easily correctable and explainable abnormalities	• Normal ECG • Normal laboratory evaluation

Reed and Gray evaluated current national and international CDRs and guidelines and determined that the most reliable resource specific for ED management of syncope was the ACEP Clinical Policy. There was also evidence that the OESIL score may be helpful for risk stratification in the ED [104].

Implementation of the 2007 ACEP syncope guidelines [35] was studied in 200 patients. Admission was more likely in older age, males, prodromes of dyspnea or vomiting, CAD, CHF, vascular disease, diabetes, or abnormal ECG. A high sensitivity and specificity for cardiac causes was found and a reduction in admissions occurred by applying all level B recommendations over usual institutional practice patterns [105].

In general, patients should be hospitalized if they have known structural heart disease or heart failure, evidence of structural heart disease or failure on exam or work-up, abnormal ECG (signs of ischemia, arrhythmias, or significant conduction abnormalities), hematocrit <30%, or symptoms which suggest ischemia or arrhythmias.

Future risk stratification work may be improved by following suggestions standardizing data elements [106].

Prognosis/risk stratification

In syncope, elder patients are at risk for all-cause morbidity and mortality. Short-term mortality has a different risk profile than long-term mortality. Risk factors for short-term adverse outcomes are: abnormal ECG, concurrent trauma, absence of prodrome, and male gender, while risk factors for long-term issues are age >65 years and history of stroke, malignancy, structural heart disease, and ventricular arrhythmias. Other risk factors listed in Table 13.3 have not been specifically stratified as being associated with either short- or long-term adverse events.

Driving and syncope

Excluding intoxication, the sudden incapacity of a driver is reported as a cause of motor vehicle collisions (MVC) in one per thousand of all collisions [107]. Although syncope is the cause of 21% of accidents with reported driver LOC [108], there is no level A or B evidence to determine fitness for driving after a medical event. Level C guidelines advise: "minimal restrictions and thus only temporarily should patients with heart disease and syncope in this group be advised not to drive" [19].

Patients who were resuscitated from near-fatal ventricular dysrhythmias were asked about resumption of driving. Although they commonly experienced symptoms while driving, accidents occurred less than the rate of 7.1% experienced by the general population [109]. Seventy-eight percent of these patients resumed driving within 6 months. Only 8% of patients with implantable cardioverter-defibrillators reported being shocked while driving. MVCs in this group were preceded by symptoms in 11% and syncope in 5%. The only positive

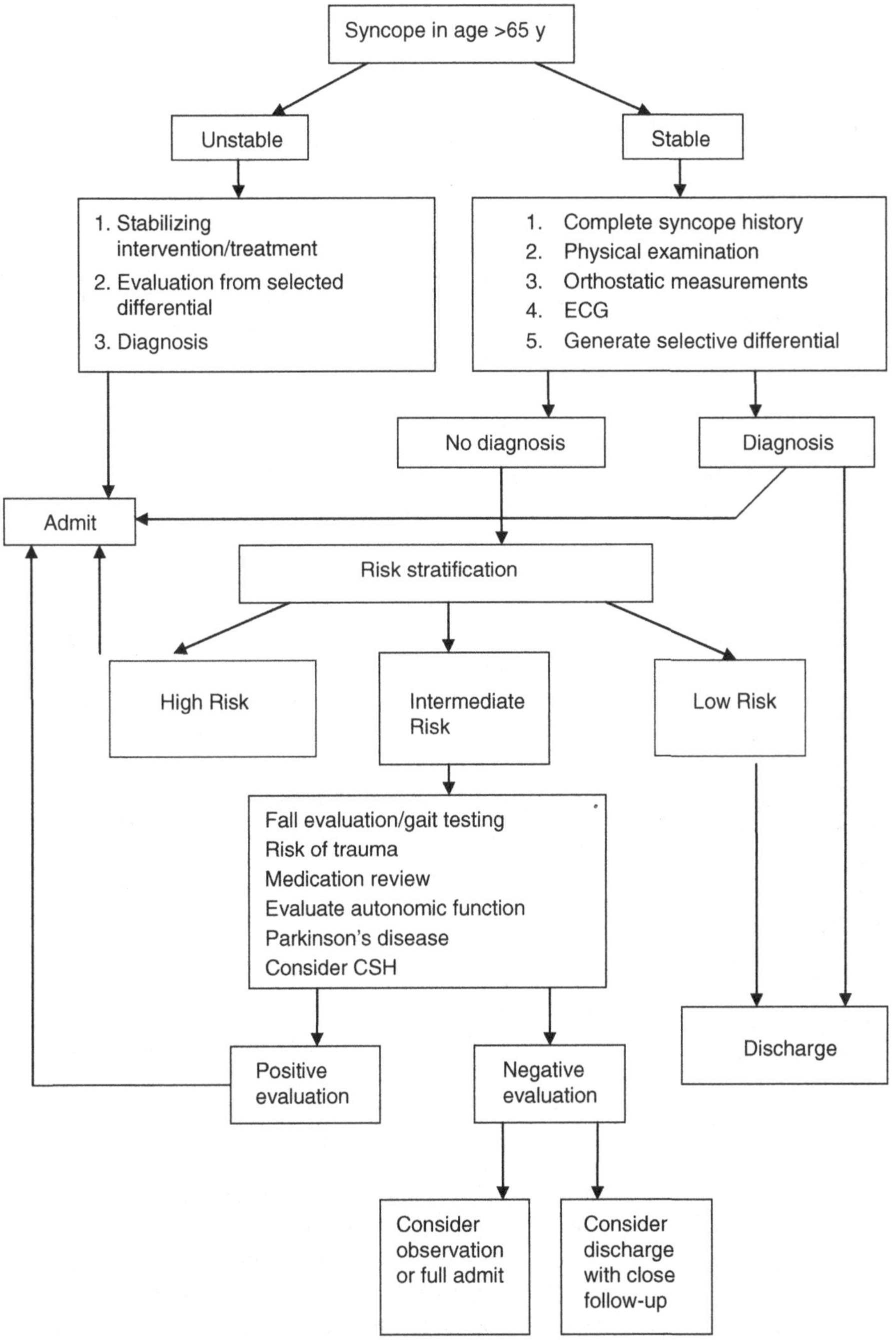

Figure 13.1. The emergency department evaluation of syncope in the older adult.

predictor for MVC was an MVC in the year prior to the implantation. Although symptoms that could result in MVC occurred frequently, most patients were able to maintain control of the vehicle to avoid collision [110].

A study of long-term follow-up for recurrence of syncope found 9.8% had syncope while driving. The probability of recurrence during operation of a car was 7% over 8 years [111]. Therefore risk of syncope while driving in patients with prior episodes of syncope is similar to that in the general population of drivers.

More accurate risk stratification is suggested in elderly drivers with more than four episodes of syncope [112]; however,

no data are provided on how to achieve that stratification. It is left to the individual physician to determine risk. In an opinion statement, authors present a formula to estimate "risk of harm while driving":

Risk = driving time (%) × vehicle type (commercial to private) × annual risk of syncope × probability of injury or accident [113].

California has mandatory Department of Motor Vehicle (DMV) reporting for physicians regarding lapses of consciousness. Only 12% of California EPs are aware of this mandate. Only new-onset seizures are frequently reported and syncope is only occasionally or never reported [114].

Summary and recommendations

Older adult patients should benefit from the same syncope evaluation as younger adults. At the end of life this approach should be guided not by age, but by goals of care and prognosis. As in most other areas, evaluation of the older adult with syncope requires a unique knowledge, assessment, and disposition. Older adults are at high risk for adverse outcomes by virtue of age, but no age cutoff defines a specific inflection point. Risk-factor stratification becomes more complex with advancing age and frailty. Multifactorial causes of syncope should be considered. The EP should be aware of the overlap between falls and syncope.

All patients who present with transient LOC should be differentiated as syncope versus TIA, hypoglycemia, hypoxemia, seizure, or epidural hematoma. A complete directed history and physical exam should be performed on every older adult with syncope to elicit sequence of events, prodrome, duration, and recovery phase. History of structural heart disease, left ventricular dysfunction, CHF, and dysrhythmia should be elicited. A careful evaluation for drug effect, drug–drug, and drug–disease interactions should be done. A physical exam should be performed looking for structural heart disease, OH, CHF, GI bleed, dehydration, signs of trauma, and gait and balance disturbances.

An ECG should be obtained on every elder presenting with syncope. Any further laboratory testing should be selected to support a well-formulated differential diagnosis.

Admission decisions should be informed by knowledge of guidelines and CDRs. Risk stratification should be combined with clinical judgment to maximize both patient safety and resource utilization.

The flow diagram shown in Figure 13.1 attempts to summarize the decision points in the evaluation and disposition of older adults who present to the ED with syncope.

Pearls and pitfalls

Pearls

- Older adult patients should benefit from the same syncope evaluation as younger adults.
- Obtain an ECG in every elder patient presenting with syncope.
- Consider syncope in all elders with falls.
- Cardiac issues are not the most common cause of syncope in elders; always check for orthostatic hypotension and drug effects.

Pitfalls

- Failing to gather a full syncope history.
- Failing to direct evaluation according to full syncope history and physical exam findings.
- Failing to assess goals of care and prognosis to determine need and benefit of hospital admission.
- Missing high-risk features in asymptomatic patients: CAD, CHF, structural heart disease, anemia, abnormal ECG.
- Failing to address elder safety and functional status prior to discharge.

References

1. Strickberger SA, Benson DW, Biaggioni I, et al. AHA/ACCF scientific statement on the evaluation of syncope: from the American Heart Association Councils on Clinical Cardiology, Cardiovascular Nursing, Cardiovascular Disease in the Young, and Stroke, and the Quality of Care and Outcomes Research Interdisciplinary Working Group; and the American College of Cardiology Foundation: in collaboration with the Heart Rhythm Society: endorsed by the American Autonomic Society. *J Am Col Cardiol*. 2006;47:473–84.

2. D'Ascenzo F, Biondi-Zoccai G, Reed MJ, et al. Incidence, etiology and predictors of adverse outcomes in 43,315 patients presenting to the emergency department with syncope: An international meta-analysis. *Int J Cardiol*. 2011;167:57–62.

3. Kapoor W, Karpf M, Wieand S, Peterson J, Levey G. A prospective evaluation and follow-up of patients with syncope. *N Engl J Med*. 1983;309:197–204.

4. Kapoor W. Evaluation and outcome of patients with syncope. *Medicine*. 1990;69:169–75.

5. Manolis AS. Evaluation of patients with syncope: focus on age-related differences. *ACC Curr J Rev*. 1994:13–18.

6. Sun BC, Emond JA, Camargo CA Jr. Characteristics and admission patterns of patients presenting with syncope to US emergency departments, 1992–2000. *Acad Emerg Med*. 2004;11:1029–34.

7. Marrison VK, Fletcher A, Parry SW. The older patient with syncope: Practicalities and controversies. *Int J Cardiol*. 2012;155:9–13.

8. Soteriades ES, Evans JC, Larson MG, et al. Incidence and prognosis of syncope. *N Engl J Med*. 2002;347:878–85.

9. Roussanov O, Estacio G, Capuno M, et al. New-onset syncope in older adults: focus on age and etiology. *Am J Geriat Cardiol*. 2007;16(5):287–94

10. Colivicchi F, Ammirati F, Melina D, et al. Development and prospective validation of a risk stratification system for patients with syncope in the emergency department: the OESIL risk score. *Eur Heart J*. 2003;24:811–19.

11. Martin TP, Hanusa BH, Kapoor WN. Risk stratification of patients with syncope. *Ann Emerg Med*. 1997;29:459–66.

12. Sarasin FP, Hanusa BH, Perneger T, et al. A risk score to predict arrhythmias in patients with unexplained syncope. *Acad Emerg Med*. 2003;10:1312–17.

13. Kapoor W, Snustad D, Peterson J, et al. Syncope in the elderly. *Am J Med*. 1986;80:419–28.

14. Tinetti ME, Williams CS, Gill TM. Dizziness among older adults: a possible geriatric syndrome. *Ann Intern Med*. 2000;132:337–44.

15. McIntosh SJ, da Costa D, Kenny RA. Outcome of an integrated approach to the investigation of dizziness, falls and syncope in elderly patients referred to a syncope clinic. *Age Aging*. 1993;22:53–8.

16. Allcock LM, O'Shea D. Diagnostic yield and development of a neurocardiovascular investigation unit for older adults in a district hospital. *J Gerontol*. 2000;55(8):458–62.

Chapter 13: Syncope in the elderly

17. Linzer M, Pontinen M, Gold DT, et al. Impairment of physical and psychosocial function in recurrent syncope. *J Clin Epidemiol*. 1991;44:1037–43.

18. Wolf PA, Abbott RD, Kannel WB. Atrial fibrillation as an independent risk factor for stroke: The Framingham Study. *Stroke*. 1991;22:983–8.

19. Brignole M, Alboni P, Benditt D, et al. Task Force on Syncope, European Society of Cardiology. Guidelines on management (diagnosis and treatment) of syncope. *Eur Heart J*. 2001;22:1256–306.

20. Davies AJ, Kenny RA. Frequency of neurologic complications following carotid sinus massage. *Am J Cardiol*. 1998;81:1256–7.

21. Munro NC, McIntosh S, Lawson J, et al. Incidence of complications after carotid sinus massage in older patients with syncope. *J Am Geriatr Soc*. 1994;42:1248–51.

22. Richardson DA, Bexton RS, Shaw FE, Kenny RA. Complications of carotid sinus massage – a prospective series of older people. *Age Aging*. 2000;29:413–17.

23. Puggioni E, Guiducci V, Brignole M et al. Results and complications of carotid sinus massage performed according to the 'method of symptoms'. *Am J Cardiol*. 2002;89:599–601.

24. Walsh T, Clinch D, Costelloe A, et al. Carotid sinus massage – How safe is it? *Age Aging*. 2006;35:518–52.

25. Del Rosso A, Alboni P, Brignole M, Menozzi C, Raviele A. Relation of clinical presentation of syncope to the age of patients. *Am J Cardiol*. 2005;96:1431–5.

26. Galizia G, Abete P, Mussi C, et al. Role of early symptoms in assessment of syncope in elderly people: results from the Italian group for the study of syncope in the elderly. *J Am Geriatr Soc*. 2009;57:18–23.

27. Blanc JJ, L'Her C, Touiza A, et al. Prospective evaluation and outcome of patients admitted for syncope over a 1 year period. *EurHeart J*. 2002;23:815–20.

28. Getchell WS, Larsen GC, Morris CD, McAnulty JH. Epidemiology of syncope in hospitalized patients. *J Gen Intern Med*. 1999;14:677–87.

29. Bardy GH, Lee KL, Mark DB, et al. For the Sudden Cardiac Death in Heart Failure Trial (SCD-HeFT) Investigators. Amiodarone or an implantable cardioverter-defibrillator for congestive heart failure. *N Engl J Med*. 2005;352:225–37.

30. Dougnac A, Loyola S, Kychenthal A, et al. Syncope: recurrence and prognosis during 2 years. *Rev Med Chil*. 1990;118:414–22.

31. Van Dijk N, Sprangers MA, Colman N, et al. Clinical factors associated with quality of life in patients with transient loss of consciousness. *J Cardiovas Electrophysiol*. 2006;17:998–1003.

32. Kapoor WN. Evaluation and management of patients with syncope. *JAMA*. 1992;268:2553–60.

33. Quinn JV, McDermott DA, Kramer N, et al. Death after emergency department visits for syncope: how common and can it be predicted? *Ann Emerg Med*. 2008;51:585–90.

34. Linzer M, Yang EH, Estes NA III, et al. Diagnosing syncope part 2: unexplained syncope. Clinical Efficacy Assessment Project of the American College of Physicians. *Ann Intern Med*. 1997;127:76–86.

35. American College of Emergency Physicians. Clinical policy: critical issues in the evaluation and management of patients presenting with syncope. *Ann Emerg Med*. 2007;49:431–44.

36. Getchell WS, Larsen GC, Morris CD, McAnulty JH. A comparison of Medicare fee-for-service and a group-model HMO in the inpatient management and long-term survival of elderly individuals with syncope. *Am J Manag Care*. 2000;6:1089–98.

37. Sun BC, Emond JA, Camargo CA Jr. Direct medical costs of syncope-related hospitalizations in the United States. *Am J Cardiol*. 2005;95:668–71.

38. Crane SD. Risk stratification of patients with syncope in an accident and emergency department. *Emerg Med J*. 2002;19:23–7.

39. Kapoor W, Hanusa B. Is syncope a risk factor for poor outcomes? Comparison of patients with and without syncope. *Am J Med*. 1996;100:646–55.

40. Tan MP, Kenny RA, Chadwick TJ, Kerr SR, Parry SW. Carotid sinus hypersensitivity: disease state or clinical sign of aging? Insights from a controlled study of autonomic function in symptomatic and asymptomatic subjects. *Europace*. 2010;12(11):1630–6.

41. Brignole M, Oddone D, Cogomo S, et al. Long-term outcome in symptomatic carotid sinus hypersensitivity. *Am Heart J*. 1992;123(3):687–92.

42. Hampton JL, Brayne C, Bradley M, Kenny RA. Mortality in carotid sinus hypersensitivity: a cohort study. Geriatric medicine. *BMJ Open*. 2011;1:e000020 doi:10.1136/bmjopen-2010-000020.

43. Freeman R. Syncope. In *Harrison's Principles of Internal Medicine*, 18th edn, ed. Longo DL, Fauci AS, Kasper DL, Hauser SL, Jameson JL, Loscalzo J (New York: McGraw-Hill, 2012, accessed July 10, 2012 from www.accessmedicine.com/content.aspx?aID=9095995).

44. Bhattacharyya S, Hayward C, Pepper J, Senior R. Risk stratification in asymptomatic severe aortic stenosis: a critical appraisal. *Eur Heart J*. 2012;33(19):2377–87.

45. Bonow RO, Carabello B, De Leon AC Jr, et al. ACC/AHA guidelines for the management of patients with valvular heart disease. A report of the American College of Cardiology/American Heart Association Task Force on Practice Guidelines (Committee on Management of Patients with Valvular Heart Disease). *J Am Coll Cardiol*. 1998;32:1486–582.

46. Bonow RO, Carabello B, Chatterjee K, et al. ACC/AHA 2006 guidelines for the management of valvular heart disease. *J Am Coll Cardiol*. 2006;48:e1–148

47. Rockwood MR, Howlett SE, Rockwood K. Orthostatic hypotension (OH) and mortality in relation to age, blood pressure and frailty. *Arch Gerontol Geriatr*. 2010;54(3):255–60.

48. Lin ZQ, Pan CM, Li WH, Huang KQ, Xie ZQ. The correlation between postural hypotension and myocardial infarction in the elderly population. *Zhonghua Nei Ke Za Zhi*. 2012;51(7):520–3.

49. Fenech G, Safar M, Blacher J. Orthostatic hypotension: Marker of severity and management of antihypertensive treatment. *Presse Med*. 2012;Apr 3.

50. Mader SL. Identification and management of orthostatic hypotension in older and medically complex patients. *Expert Rev Cardiovasc Ther*. 2012;10(3):387–95.

51. Hoefnagels WAJ, Padberg GW, Overweg J, Velde E, Roos R. Transient loss of consciousness: the value of the history for distinguishing seizure from syncope. *J Neurol*. 1991;238:39–43.

125

52. Alboni P, Brignole M, Menozzi C, et al. The diagnostic value of history in patients with syncope with or without heart disease. *J Am Coll Cardiol*. 2001;37(7):1921–8.

53. Calkins H, Shyr Y, Frumin H, Schork A, Morady F. The value of clinical history in the differentiation of syncope due to ventricular tachycardia, atrioventricular block and neurocardiogenic syncope. *Am J Med*. 1995;98:365–73.

54. Oh JH, Hanusa BH, Kapoor WN. Do symptoms predict cardiac arrhythmias and mortality in patients with syncope? *Arch Intern Med*. 1999;159:375–80.

55. Numeroso F, Mossini G, Spaggiari E, Cervellin G. Syncope in the emergency department of a large northern Italian hospital: incidence, efficacy of a short-stay observation ward and validation of the OESIL risk score. *Emerg Med J*. 2010;27:653–8.

56. Kaufmann H. Syncope: a neurologist's viewpoint. *Cardiol Clin*. 1997;15:177–94.

57. Hanlon JT, Linzer M, MacMillan JP, Lewis IK, Felder A. Syncope and presyncope associated with probable adverse drug reactions. *Arch Intern Med*. 1990;150:2309–12.

58. Calkins H, Shyr Y, Frumin H, Schork A, Morady F. The value of the clinical history in the differentiation of syncope due to ventricular tachycardia, atrioventricular block, and neurocardiogenic syncope. *Am J Med*. 1995;98:365–73.

59. *The Merick Manual for Health care Professionals. Syncope 2010* (Whitehouse Station, NJ: Merick Sharp and Dohme Corp., accessed November 6, 2012 from www.merckmanuals.com/professional/cardiovascular_disorders/symptoms_of_cardiovascular_disorders/syncope.html#v1145060).

60. Wieling W, Thijs RD, van Dijk N, et al. Symptoms and signs of syncope: a review of the link between physiology and clinical clues. *Brain*. 2009;132(10):2630–42.

61. Sheldon R, Rose S, Ritchie D, et al. Historical criteria that distinguish syncope from seizures. *J Am Col Cardiol*. 2002;40(1):142–8.

62. Ross Russell RW, Page GR. Critical perfusion of brain and retina. *Brain*. 1983;106:419–34.

63. Ward C, Kenny RA. Reproducibility of orthostatic hypotension in symptomatic elderly. *Am J Med*. 1996;100:418–21.

64. Gray-Miceli D, Ratcliffe SJ, Liu S, Wantland D, Johnson J. Orthostatic hypotension in older nursing home residents who fall: are they dizzy? *Clin Nurs Res*. 2012;21(1):64–78.

65. Coutaz M, Iglesias K, Morisod J. Is there a risk of orthostatic hypotension associated with antihypertensive therapy in geriatric inpatients? *Euro Geriat Med*. 2012;3(1):1–4.

66. Atkins D, Hanusa B, Sefcik T, Kapoor W. Syncope and orthostatic hypotension. *Am J Med*. 1990;91:179–85.

67. Rutan GH, Hermanson B, Bild DE, et al. Orthostatic hypotension in older adults. The Cardiovascular Health Study. CHS Collaborative Research Group. *Hypertension*. 1992;19(1):508–19.

68. Sarasin FP, Louis-Simonet M, Carballo D, Slama S, Junod A, Unger P. Prevalence of orthostatic hypotension among patients presenting with syncope in the ED. *Am J Emerg Med*. 2002;20(6):497–501.

69. Kerr SR, Pearce MS, Brayne C, Davis RJ, Kenny RA. Carotid sinus hypersensitivity in asymptomatic older persons: implications for diagnosis of syncope and falls. *Arch Intern Med*. 2006;166(5):515–20.

70. McIntosh SJ, Lawson J, Kenny RA. Clinical characteristics of vasodepressor, cardioinhibitory, and mixed carotid sinus syndrome in the elderly. *Am J Med*. 1993;95(2):203–8.

71. Kenny RA, Traynor G. Carotid sinus syndrome – Clinical characteristics in elderly patients. *Age Aging*. 1991;20:449–54.

72. Kymar NP, Thomas A, Mudd P, Morris RO, Masud T. The usefulness of carotid sinus massage in different patient groups. *Age Aging* 2003;32(6):666–9.

73. Moya A, Sutton R, Ammirati F, et al. Guidelines for the diagnosis and management of syncope (version 2009): the task force for the diagnosis and management of syncope of the European Society of Cardiology (ESC). *Eur Heart J*. 2009;30:2631–71.

74. National Institute for Health and Clinical Excellence. *Transient Loss of Consciousness (Blackouts) Management in Adults and Young People* (accessed September 6, 2012 from www.nice.org.uk/guidance/CG109/FullGuidance).

75. Xiao-Ke Liu, Arshad Jahangir, Win-Kuang Shen. *Hazzard's Geriatric Medicine and Gerontology Part IV. Organ Systems and Diseases Section B. Cardiology. Syncope in the Elderly*, 6th edn (McGraw-Hill Professional, 2009).

76. Humm AM, Mathias CJ. Abnormal cardiovascular responses to carotid sinus massage also occur in vasovagal syncope – implications for diagnosis and treatment. *Eur J Neurol*. 2010;17(8):1061–7.

77. Cunningham R, Mikhail MG. Management of patients with syncope and cardiac arrhythmias in an emergency department observation unit. *Emerg Med Clin North Am*. 2001;19:105–21.

78. Krediet CT, Parry SW, Jardine DL, et al. The history of diagnosing carotid sinus hypersensitivity: why are the current criteria too sensitive? *Europace*. 2011;13(1):14–22.

79. Parry S, Reeve P, Lawson J, et al. The Newcastle Protocols 2008: an update on head up-tilt table testing and the management of vasovagal syncope and related disorders. *Heart*. 1990;95:416–20.

80. Mendu ML, McAvay G, Lampert R, Stoehr J, Tinetti ME. Yield of diagnostic tests in evaluating syncopal episodes in older patients. *Arch Int Med*. 2009;169(14)1299–305.

81. Aggarwal A, Sherazi S, Levitan B, et al. Corrected QT interval as a predictor of mortality in elderly patients with syncope. *Cardiol J*. 2011;18(4):395–400.

82. Thiruganasambandamoorthy V, Hess EP, Turko E, et al. Defining abnormal electrocardiography in adult emergency department syncope patients: the Ottawa Electrocardiographic Criteria. *CJEM*. 2012;14(4):248–58.

83. Meininger G, Calkins H. The evaluation of syncope: pearls from the front lines. *Acc Cur Rev*. 2005;14:8–11.

84. Assar M, Krahn A, Klein G, Yee R, Skanes A. Optimal duration of monitoring in patients with unexplained syncope. *Am J Cardiol*. 2003;92:1231–3.

85. Vetta F, Ronzoni S, Costarella M, et al. Recurrent syncope in elderly patients and tilt test table outcome: the role of comorbidities. *Arch Gerontol Geriatr*. 2009;49(1):231–6.

86. Epstein AE, DiMarco JP, Ellenbogen KA, et al. ACC/AHA/HRS 2008 Guidelines for Device-Based Therapy of Cardiac Rhythm Abnormalities: a report of the American College of Cardiology/American Heart Association Task Force on Practice Guidelines (Writing Committee to Revise the ACC/AHA/NASPE 2002 Guideline Update for Implantation of Cardiac Pacemakers and Antiarrhythmia Devices) developed in collaboration with the American Association for Thoracic Surgery and Society of Thoracic Surgeons. *J Am Coll Cardiol*. 2008;51(21):e1–62.

87. American College of Emergency Physicians. Clinical policy: neuroimaging and decision making in adult mild traumatic brain injury in the acute setting. *Ann Emerg Med.* 2008;52:714–52.

88. *IOM Clinical Practice Guidelines We Can Trust* (Washington, DC: National Academies PR, 2011).

89. Guyatt G, Oxman A, Vist G, et al. GRADE: an emerging consensus on rating quality of evidence and strength of recommendations. *BMJ.* 2008;336:924–30.

90. Quinn JV, Stiell IG, McDermott DA, et al. Derivation of the San Francisco Syncope Rule to predict patients with short-term serious outcomes. *Ann Emerg Med.* 2004;43:224–32.

91. Reed M.J, Newby DE, Coull AJ, et al. The ROSE (risk stratification of syncope in the emergency department) study. *J Am Col Cardiol.* 2010;55:713–21.

92. Serrano LA, Hess EP, Bellolio MF, et al. Accuracy and quality of clinical decision rules for syncope in the emergency department: a systematic review and meta-analysis. *Ann Emerg Med.* 2010;56(4):362–73.

93. Del Greco M, Cozzio S, Scillieri M, et al. The ECSIT study (Epidemiology and Costs of Syncope in Trento). Diagnostic pathway of syncope and analysis of the impact of guidelines in a district general hospital. *Ital Heart J.* 2003;4:99–106.

94. Farwell DJ, Sulke AN. Does the use of a syncope diagnostic protocol improve the investigation and management of syncope? *Heart.* 2004;90:52–8.

95. Cabana M, Rand C, Powe N, et al. Why don't physicians follow clinical practice guidelines? A framework for improvement. *JAMA.* 1999;282:1458–65.

96. Benditt, D. Syncope Management Guidelines at work: first steps towards assessing clinical utility. *Eur Heart J.* 2006;27:7–9.

97. Ungar A, Del Rosso A, Giada F, et al. Early and late outcome of treated patients referred for syncope to emergency department; the EGSYS 2 follow-up study. *Eur Heart J.* 2010;31: 2021–6.

98. Thiruganasambandamoorthy V, Hess EP, Alreesi A, et al. External validation of the San Francisco syncope rule in the Canadian setting. *Ann Emerg Med.* 2010;55(5):464–72.

99. Birnbaum A, Esses D, Bijur P, Wollowitz A, Gallagher EJ. Failure to validate the San Francisco Syncope Rule in an independent emergency department population. *Ann Emerg Med.* 2008;52(2):151–9.

100. Schladenhaufen R, Feilinger S, Pollack M, Benenson R, Kusmiesz AL. Application of San Francisco syncope rule in elderly ED patients. *Am J Emerg Med.* 2008;26(7):773–8.

101. Reed MJ, Henderson SS, Newby DE, Gray AJ. One-year prognosis after syncope and the failure of the ROSE decision instrument to predict one-year adverse events. *Ann Emerg Med.* 2011;58(3):250–6.

102. Grossman S, Bar J, Fisher C, et al. Reducing admissions utilizing the Boston Syncope Criteria. *J Emerg Med.* 2012;42(3):345–52.

103. Sule S, Palaniswamy C, Aronow WS, et al. Etiology of syncope in patients hospitalized with syncope and predictors of mortality and rehospitalization for syncope at 27 month follow-up. *Clin Cardiol.* 2011;34:35–8.

104. Reed MJ, Gray A. Collapse query cause: the management of adult syncope in the emergency department. *Emerg Med J.* 2006;(8):589–94.

105. Elesber AA, Decker WW, Smars PA, Hodge DO, Shen WK. Impact of the application of the American College of Emergency Physicians recommendations for the admission of patients with syncope on a retrospectively studied population presenting to the emergency department. *Am Heart J.* 2005;149(5):826–31.

106. Sun BC, Thiruganasambandamoorthy V, Dela Cruz J. Standardized reporting guidelines for emergency department syncope risk-stratification research. *Acad Emerg Med.* 2012;19(6):694–702.

107. Herner B, Smedby B, Ysander L. Sudden illness as a cause of motor vehicle accidents. *Br J Int Med.* 1966;23:37–41.

108. Driving and heart disease. Task Force Report. Prepared on behalf of the Task Force by MC Petch. *Eur Heart J.* 1998;19:1165–77.

109. Akiyama T, Powell JL, Mitchell LB, Ehlert FA, Baessler C. Antiarrhythmics versus Implantable Defibrillators Investigators. Resumption of driving after life-threatening ventricular tachyarrhythmia. *N Engl J Med.* 2001;345:391–7.

110. Strickberger SA, Cantillon CO, Friedman PL. When should patients with lethal ventricular arrhythmia resume driving? An analysis of state regulations and physician practices. *Ann Intern Med.* 1991;115:560–3.

111. Sorajja D, Nesbitt G, Hodge D, et al. Syncope while driving: clinical characteristics, causes, and prognosis. *Circulation.* 2009;120:928–34

112. Folino AF, Migliore F, Porta A, et al. Syncope while driving: pathophysiological features and long-term follow-up. *Auton Neurosci.* 2012;166(1–2):60–5.

113. Sorajja D, Shen WK. Driving guidelines and restrictions in patients with a history of cardiac arrhythmias, syncope, or implantable devices. *Curr Treat Options Cardiovasc Med.* 2010;12(5):443–56.

114. Turnipseed SD, Vierra D, DeCarlo D, Panacek EA. Reporting patterns for "lapses of consciousness" by California emergency physicians. *J Emerg Med.* 2008;35(1):15–21.

Dizziness in the elderly

Jonathan A. Edlow and David E. Newman-Toker

Introduction and epidemiology

Dizziness is a common problem in the community [1], especially in elderly patients [2]. In emergency department (ED) studies, dizziness is one of the most common presenting symptoms [3,4], and misdiagnosis is common, even when patients are evaluated by neurologists [5]. Dizziness has numerous causes and the very word "dizziness" means different things to different people. Older dizzy patients have a higher incidence of serious central nervous system (CNS) and cardiovascular causes [6–8]. Furthermore, dizziness is often caused by a variety of non-CNS or cardiovascular symptoms such as toxic-metabolic and infectious disorders. For all these reasons, correct diagnosis is critically important, but can be challenging. The evidence base for our understanding of the diagnosis and treatment of dizziness is weak [9], but has increased substantially in the past several years [10,11].

Some challenges are unique to the elderly. Age-related changes in cardiovascular and vestibular physiology can alter the presentations compared with younger patients. Secondly, the elderly are more likely to be cognitively impaired, which, even when minimal, can adversely affect their ability to provide a cogent history, which is so important in the evaluation of the dizzy patient. As well, older patients are far more likely to take multiple medications, which can cause dizziness or exacerbate dizziness due to another cause. Fourthly, they are more likely to have comorbidities such as cardiac disease and vascular risk factors, expanding the differential diagnosis and increasing the likelihood of cardiovascular and cerebrovascular causes. Finally, even if the etiology of dizziness is benign, resultant falls, hip fractures, and loss of independence have a greater impact in the elderly.

Many of these issues are covered in detail in other chapters. This chapter will focus on diagnosis of acute episodes of dizziness in elderly patients. To a much lesser extent, it will also cover issues related to chronic dizziness and treatment of specific syndromes when germane to the context.

Vestibular physiology

Multiple physiological processes support normal balance. Both cardiovascular and neurological systems play key roles. Various sensory inputs from the peripheral nervous system (PNS) and the cerebellum are processed centrally to maintain normal balance. Not surprisingly, all of the functions that are responsible for balance (vision, hearing, various components of the sensory system, the peripheral vestibular apparatus along with its central connections, and cardiovascular tone and reflexes) all degrade with age [12–15]. To the extent that a patient is aware of these deficits and feels "dizzy," a degree of anxiety about falling may compound the initial dizziness. Each of these factors undoubtedly plays a role in the increased incidence of dizzy symptoms in elderly patients. Even when a specific etiology cannot be found, some have hypothesized that dizziness in the elderly is a distinct "geriatric syndrome" based upon mild dysfunction of all of these different systems [16].

Medication issues

Many older patients take a long list of medications, which exert pharmacological effects, side effects, and may have drug–drug interactions, all of which may be exaggerated in older patients. Of patients older than 65 years, approximately 50% take five or more medications and 12% take ten or more [17]. Reduced hepatic and renal function in older patients may alter pharmacokinetics in these patients [18]. Many of these patients will experience chronic dizziness; however, adding a new medication, increase in dosage of an existing one, or decrease in hepatic or renal function may present as an acute episode of dizziness. Importantly, a medication that is frequently used to treat dizziness – meclizine – can worsen dizziness in many instances and should be used very selectively [19]. Chapter 5 discusses pharmacology in the elderly in much greater detail.

Falls

Falls in the elderly (covered in more detail in Chapter 32) are important for three reasons. First, emergency physicians must consider that dizziness from one cause or another may be the direct cause of the patient's fall, so ascertaining the reason for a fall is always important. Falls in the elderly are common. In 2000, there were over 10,000 fatal falls and 2.6 million non-fatal fall-related injuries in the US in patients over 65 years of age [20]. The estimated direct cost of ED visits alone was $4

Geriatric Emergency Medicine, ed. Joseph H. Kahn, Brendan G. Magauran Jr., and Jonathan S. Olshaker. Published by Cambridge University Press.
© Cambridge University Press 2014.

billion [20]. In another study, falls seem to be increasing in frequency, above and beyond what one would expect purely on demographic factors [21]. Dizzy symptoms account for approximately one-third of elderly falls [22].

Secondly, correctly diagnosing the cause of dizziness and treating it is an important strategy in fall prevention. A large part of the morbidity due to dizziness in the geriatric patient has to do with subsequent falls and the resultant injuries. Wrist and hip fractures and intracranial hemorrhage are among the most common injuries. Finally, falls often impact disposition, and loss of independence for an elderly patient may have huge psychosocial consequences. Even a relatively "minor" injury such as a distal radius fracture and its treatment can have a major impact on an elderly patient's independence, especially if it involves the dominant arm and the patient lives alone.

Overarching diagnostic strategy

The traditional diagnostic approach to dizziness is based upon the clinician starting by asking the question, "What do you mean dizzy?" Based on "symptom quality," this paradigm was first published in 1972, based on limited data from a small number of selected patients evaluated in a specialty clinic [23]. The "symptom quality" paradigm is to ask the patient, "What do you mean dizzy?" and their response will place them into one of four categories – vertigo, presyncope, disequilibrium, or "other" nonspecific dizziness. The implication is that each category has etiologic significance. This approach concludes that vertiginous patients have vestibular causes (usually peripheral), presyncopal patients have cardiovascular causes, those with dysequilibrium have neurological issues, while nonspecific dizziness is caused by psychiatric disease. This approach has been and remains the dominant diagnostic strategy used by both emergency physicians and those of other specialties.

Despite this fact, the "symptom quality" (dizziness "type") approach has serious problems. The first has to do with the methods of the original 1972 paper [23]. Recruited patients had to be fluent in English and available to (and well enough for) return on four separate half-days for further testing in a clinic. Of the 125 enrolled patients, 21 were rejected for inadequate data and another 9 for lack of a diagnosis. Only 95 completed the study. A single author, a neurologist, assigned the diagnoses without independent verification, brain imaging, or any long-term follow-up. Skull plain radiographs were the only "brain" imaging tests available in that era. Furthermore, some diagnoses known now to be common causes of dizziness (e.g., vestibular migraine) had not yet been recognized as diagnostic entities. Nevertheless, when no tests identified a specific diagnosis, the type of dizziness was used to assign the final diagnosis (e.g., vertigo was assigned a peripheral vestibular cause if no other cause was found). Although this paper was an important one in its time, it has serious methodological limitations and the paradigm of "symptom quality" has never been prospectively and properly validated.

In addition, it is obvious that many patients who are seen in an ED for dizziness would never end up in an outpatient specialist-run dizziness clinic, including those with acute

cardiovascular, cerebrovascular, metabolic, infectious, and other causes. The original study was done in an era of fewer medications (propranolol was the only beta blocker, there were many fewer antihypertensive agents) and far less polypharmacy. Thus, the patients in that 1972 study were not at all representative of patients seen in an ED in 2014.

Another generic issue with dizziness is that it is a difficult symptom to describe. A recent research study asked patients a series of questions designed at describing their dizziness type [24,25]. Within ten minutes, they were asked the same questions but given the answer choices in a different sequence. Half the patients changed the category of dizziness that they had initially endorsed just a few minutes before, and most of the patients endorsed multiple dizziness symptom qualities. In addition to this, other data show that patients with cardiac causes of dizziness often use the word "vertigo" to describe what they are feeling [26]. In yet another study of older patients presenting to an ED with dizziness, the use of the word "vertigo" (as opposed to lightheadedness or dizziness) did not predict those who had a cerebrovascular cause [27]. The use of the word "imbalance" did predict a cerebrovascular cause.

The converse is also true. Patients with clear-cut vestibular disease often complain of vague lightheadedness or nonspecific "dizziness." In a study of patients with definite benign paroxysmal positional vertigo (BPPV) with a positive Dix–Hallpike test, primary care physicians referred some of their patients to an ear–nose–throat (ENT) clinic and others to a falls and syncope clinic. Those who were referred to the falls and syncope unit were older, more likely had "dizzy" symptoms other than "vertigo" (including postural lightheadedness on arising quickly from bed), were on more medications, and had more vascular comorbid conditions [28]. Therefore, front-line physicians thought "BPPV" when patients used the word "vertigo," and "near syncope" when patients used less specific terms to describe their dizziness, even though all the patients had the exact same problem.

Taken together, this literature suggests that using the "symptom quality" paradigm for the diagnosis of unselected dizzy patients has serious shortcomings. On the other hand, they begin to suggest an alternative paradigm based on "timing and triggers." In the study showing that patients rapidly and frequently change their type of dizziness, their responses to issues about dizziness timing and triggers were far more reliable [25]. Because the type of dizziness may not be etiologically useful and because many of the major dizziness syndromes have reliable timing and triggers patterns, an alternative paradigm based on "timing and triggers" may be more useful to the clinician.

The "timing and triggers" paradigm can be summarized using the mnemonic of **ATTEST** (see Table 14.1).

A: Associated symptoms, signs, and basic testing (such as finger stick glucose)
TT: Timing and triggers
ES: Exam signs
T: Testing (if needed to confirm the clinical diagnosis)

First, ask about associated symptoms that suggest a particular diagnosis or group of diagnoses (Table 14.2). For example,

Table 14.1. ATTEST: a method for diagnosing dizzy patients

A: Associated symptoms, signs, or abnormal basic tests

Using the history (especially the ROS, PMH, and medications), vital signs, physical examination, and basic labs (e.g., finger stick glucose or ECG), search for abnormalities that suggest a specific diagnosis or group of diagnoses.

T: Timing

Is the dizziness intermittent or persistent? Did it start gradually or suddenly? If persistent, how long has the dizziness lasted and if episodic, how long do episodes last?

T: Triggers

Is there anything that triggers the dizziness (e.g., turning one's head, starting a new medication, or is it spontaneous? That is, does it "just happen" out of the blue?); distinguish "triggers" from "exacerbating factors."

ES: Exam signs

Apply several bedside tests that can be very helpful in clinically distinguishing some dangerous from some benign causes of dizziness (in AVS, "H.I.N.T.S. to I.N.F.A.R.C.T" [1,2]; in PVS, positional tests for BPPV) [3].

T: Testing

After history and physical examination with the appropriate bedside testing, there will be instances in which there is still significant diagnostic ambiguity about serious diseases that persists. Perform whatever confirmatory testing or consultation as needed to try to resolve the ambiguity, erring on the side of patient safety.

Table 14.2. Associated findings (that may suggest a specific diagnosis or group of diagnoses)

History

Has the patient started a new medication or changed the dose of an existing one?

Has there been recent exposure to ototoxic medications (e.g., aminoglycosides)?

Has there been ear surgery or recent middle ear/mastoid infection?

Has there been any recent head injury?

Are co-incident symptoms present?

• Headache

• Neck pain

• Ear pain or discharge

• Chest pain or palpitations

• Dyspnea or other acute respiratory symptoms

• Abdominal pain

• Gastrointestinal blood or fluid loss

• Acute neurological symptoms: diplopia, dysphagia, dysarthria, other

Physical examination

Abnormal vital signs

• Fever

• Bradycardia or tachycardia

• Hypotension or severe hypertension

• Tachypnea or hypoxia

New murmur or gallop

New rales or wheeze

Gastrointestinal blood loss

Any new abnormality in the basic neurological examination

Basic laboratory testing (as indicated)

Pregnancy testing

Urinalysis

Electrocardiogram

dizziness associated with chest pain, or vomiting and diarrhea, or acute neck pain or fever and cough, suggest obvious possible diagnoses. Has the patient started a new medication? It is important to establish what symptoms accompany the dizziness, since a large proportion of ED patients have various medical (and not vestibular or neurological) problems that cause their dizziness [4]. This step will often lead to a clear-cut limited differential diagnosis and work-up for many patients, such as a chest X-ray for a dizzy patient with fever, cough, and green sputum.

Next, ask questions (see History section) designed to place the patient into one of four "timing and triggers" categories (see Table 14.3). These include acute vestibular syndrome (AVS), episodic vestibular syndrome (EVS), positional vestibular syndrome (PVS), and chronic vestibular syndrome (CVS). Use the history to define the onset, duration, constancy, and triggering or exacerbating features. Patients can generally describe these features of their histories more reliably than the "type" of dizziness [25]. Each of these four categories suggests a particular differential diagnosis (see Differential diagnosis section and Table 14.3).

Once the category is defined, then one uses bedside and other routine tests to further narrow the differential diagnosis (see Physical examination section). Some of this testing is part of a normal physical examination. Is the patient mentating normally? Is there obvious nystagmus on primary gaze (staring straight ahead)? Is there a murmur or signs of heart failure? Is there melena or evidence of gastrointestinal bleeding? One of the confirmatory tests is a more detailed, but easy to do (and easy to learn) bedside oculomotor exam that helps to distinguish central from peripheral vestibular disorders.

Confirmation with more sophisticated (non-bedside) tests is the final step. This might mean a computed tomographic angiogram (CTA) of the chest if pulmonary embolism is the target diagnosis or telemetry, serial cardiac enzymes, and electrocardiograms if an acute coronary syndrome is the concern. Many patients will not need these tests because the bedside

Table 14.3. Timing and triggers categories for dizzy patients (and differential diagnosis of more common causes)*

Acute vestibular syndrome: Rapid onset of dizziness that persists for days and is associated with nausea/vomiting, head motion intolerance, nystagmus, and gait disturbance

Benign causes: vestibular neuritis (no auditory symptoms) and labyrinthitis (with auditory symptoms)

Serious causes: cerebellar and brainstem infarction (much less commonly, hemorrhage), Wernicke syndrome, acute infectious conditions (e.g., listeria rhombencephalitis)

Episodic vestibular syndrome: Episodes of dizziness lasting minutes to hours without obvious trigger (occasionally shorter spells)

Benign causes: vestibular migraine, Ménière's syndrome (with auditory symptoms), vasovagal near syncope

Serious causes: cardiac arrhythmias, low-flow states (including PE or ACS), posterior circulation TIA, acute infectious or "toxic-metabolic" conditions

Positional vestibular syndrome: Brief episodes of dizziness that are triggered, often lasting only seconds

Benign causes: BPPV

Serious causes: Orthostatic hypotension from hypovolemia (any cause), central positional vertigo (e.g., cerebellar tumor)

Chronic vestibular syndrome: Prolonged dizziness lasting weeks to years

Benign causes: presbylibrium, chronic bilateral vestibular failure, poorly compensated unilateral vestibular failure

Serious causes: paraneoplastic syndrome (e.g., cerebellar degeneration), posterior fossa tumor

* This is not meant to be an encyclopedic list, but rather a list of the more common and more serious conditions that are seen in the emergency department. BPPV, benign paroxysmal positional vertigo; PE, pulmonary embolism; ACS, acute coronary syndrome; TIA, transient ischemic attack.

exam findings and basic tests can establish some diagnoses (e.g., vestibular neuritis or BPPV or a urinary tract infection).

In the authors' experience, the "timing and triggers" paradigm more often leads to making a specific diagnosis compared with the traditional "symptom quality" approach. The approach to patients with AVS and PVS has been studied fairly extensively [10,11,29], but it is important to acknowledge that the "timing and triggers" or ATTEST approach has not been prospectively validated or systematically studied as a complete diagnostic paradigm.

Differential diagnosis

Without some type of diagnostic strategy or algorithmic approach, diagnosis of the dizzy patient is an exercise in futility since dozens, if not hundreds of individual conditions as well as side effects from nearly every medication available can produce dizziness. As we have seen in the previous section, although the traditional "symptom quality" diagnostic paradigm suggests a limited differential diagnosis based upon the type of dizziness the patient endorses, the evidence base for this is somewhat limited. Using the "timing and triggers" approach, the differential diagnosis is based on various temporal categories. Table 14.3 lists the more common and the more serious potential diagnoses and includes vestibular, CNS, and other conditions.

For patients with AVS, the major differential diagnosis is a peripheral vestibular process (of the eighth cranial nerve or its end organ) versus stroke. The eighth cranial nerve has two components – the vestibular and the cochlear, which can be affected together or individually. Patients with vestibular neuritis have dizziness (but no hearing loss) [30]. Patients with acute sensorineural hearing loss have diminished hearing (and no dizziness) [31,32]. The term labyrinthitis is often used when both systems are affected. Because the organs of balance and hearing are co-located peripherally, co-involvement of dizziness and hearing generally implicates a peripheral process.

However this is not always the case. The labyrinth is supplied by the labyrinthine artery, which is a branch of a branch of the anterior inferior cerebellar artery (AICA – itself originating from the basilar). It is therefore possible that an acute vestibular syndrome or an acute sensorineural hearing loss is due to a stroke, although this mechanism is probably less common than benign peripheral causes. With AICA strokes, both balance and hearing are usually affected [33]. Although "vertigo" has been reported in patients with supratentorial stroke [34,35], patients with dizziness or vertigo as a prominent presenting symptom of cerebrovascular disease usually have posterior fossa strokes. While vestibular neuritis accounts for the majority of patients who present with AVS, cerebellar (or brainstem) stroke is the other important possibility [36]. Bedside testing can help distinguish between these groups of patients and, within the first 48 hours, may be better than MRI in making this important distinction [29]. Some older patients with a toxic-metabolic or infectious problem could present with AVS but the frequency with which this happens is probably low (<1%) [11], and many of these patients will likely be identified by attention to associated symptoms. The other relatively common disease that can present as AVS, multiple sclerosis, is less common to present de novo in the elderly.

For patients who present with EVS, vestibular migraine is overall the most common diagnosis. In older patients *without a history of prior migraine*, one should be hesitant to make this diagnosis since it becomes progressively less typical for geriatric patients to present with new-onset migraines. However, migraine is extremely common in the general population and in one series of dizzy patients older than 65 years, 13% were found to have vestibular migraine [37]. Dizziness from migraine can occur with or without headache [38]. Duration of attacks is often minutes to hours to days but can last seconds in 10% of patients [38]. Head motion intolerance is common [38]. Ménière's disease is another cause of EVS and is associated with episodic dizziness and hearing loss, tinnitus, and ear fullness that lasts between minutes and hours [39].

131

The major serious diagnoses that present with EVS are transient ischemic attack (TIA) of the posterior circulation, cardiac arrhythmias, and transient low-flow states such as from pulmonary embolism (PE), acute coronary syndrome (ACS), or aortic stenosis. A full discussion of the cardiovascular causes is beyond the scope of this chapter. In regard to posterior circulation TIA, classic teaching is that other brainstem symptoms are nearly always associated with dizziness, at least in patients presenting with episodes occurring over more than three weeks [40]. Others have reported that spells of dizziness (even over months) can herald a subsequent basilar stroke [41]. Several authors report that TIA can present with isolated dizziness [42–45].

Patients with PVS have a narrower differential diagnosis; BPPV is the most common benign cause. These patients have very brief episodes lasting about 15–30 seconds that are triggered by head movement. It is important to note that many episodes occur at night in bed, and therefore some patients have difficulty precisely fixing the duration of the spells. This is one instance in which a symptom waking a patient from sleep makes a benign diagnosis more likely. Patients with BPPV may feel an anticipation of dizziness and will sometimes report being dizzy constantly for days, but a careful history can tease out the true episodic nature of the dizziness. It is important to note that many patients with BPPV do not endorse true vertigo [28]. As well, BPPV may be less well recognized in elderly patients [46]. It bears re-emphasis that these patients may complain of vertigo or vague lightheadedness or dizziness that can easily be mistaken for orthostasis if symptoms occur on arising in the morning, as is often the case. The two can usually be distinguished, however, by inquiring whether the symptoms also occur on reclining or rolling over in bed, which should not occur in those with orthostatic hypotension.

More serious diagnoses that present as PVS include orthostatic hypotension of any cause and central positional vertigo. The former can be due to any dangerous cause of hypovolemia such as gastrointestinal bleeding, fluid losses from gastroenteritis, persistent vomiting, and others including medication side effects [47]. Abnormal orthostatic vital signs are very common in elderly patients, especially in those who live in extended care facilities [48]. This means that orthostasis is a common cause of dizziness, but also that the presence of an orthostatic blood pressure drop may be an incidental finding in an elderly patient with dizziness of another cause. Remember too that hypertensive elderly patients may be symptomatic at blood pressures that do not raise red flags (e.g., a systolic pressure of 110 mmHg could be very abnormal for someone whose brain is accustomed to a pressure of 150 mmHg).

Central positional vertigo is a very uncommon BPPV mimic that can be caused by tumors, strokes, and other CNS lesions [49–51]. Most of these patients will have physical examination clues during positional testing (Dix–Hallpike) that typical BPPV is not the correct diagnosis (persistent symptoms or signs lasting longer than one minute, downbeat nystagmus, lack of latency to nystagmus onset, and lack of therapeutic response to an Epley or other canal-repositioning maneuver) [52].

Patients with CVS, whose symptoms persist longer than weeks, most commonly have polysensory dizziness (sometimes called "presbylibrium"), bilateral vestibular failure, poorly compensated unilateral vestibular failure, degenerative neurologic disease, psychiatric syndromes, or drug side effects or drug-drug interactions, although specific data about the relative frequency for various causes are lacking. Occasionally, a patient with a slow-growing posterior fossa tumor can present with the CVS.

History

The history is nearly always the most important part of any diagnostic evaluation since it helps the physician begin forming a differential diagnosis, focus the physical examination, and direct any subsequent diagnostic testing. The steps that follow in this chapter are not meant to substitute for a complete and detailed history and chronology of the patient's symptoms, but rather to help focus and supply clues that may help pinpoint a diagnosis or at least help to narrow down a differential list of diagnoses.

Our approach is to use the ATTEST (see Table 14.1) mnemonic to gather the important elements of the history. Identifying associated symptoms that may be clues as to the underlying etiology (see Table 14.2) is important. Antecedent medication changes or head trauma may suggest a drug side effect or post-traumatic BPPV. The clinician's focus will be different with a patient who presents with severe abrupt-onset headache with dizziness than with a dizzy patient who reports abdominal pain and diarrhea as associated symptoms.

Distinguish between "triggering" the dizziness and "exacerbating" the dizziness. "Triggered" dizziness suggests that something made a patient dizzy when they started out not dizzy. An example is a patient who is lying on a stretcher completely asymptomatic and when a Dix–Hallpike is done, the patient becomes dizzy. "Exacerbated" suggests that something increased a dizzy patient's symptoms (but they were already dizzy to start with). An example of this would be a patient with vestibular neuritis who feels dizzy at baseline while lying still on the stretcher, but on head motion, the dizziness becomes more intense.

This is a very important distinction and highlights a common misconception about dizziness [53]. The misconception is that a patient whose dizziness worsens with head motion has a peripheral vestibular cause of their dizziness. This is not true. Dizzy patients, for example with stroke, multiple sclerosis, or a cerebellar tumor, will develop worse dizziness with head movement. A hypovolemic patient may also have worse dizziness upon changing position (standing up).

Next, to define a "timing and triggers" category, ask questions such as:

- When did the dizziness start?
- Did it begin suddenly or gradually?
- What were you doing when it started?
- How long does the dizziness last?
- Is it episodic or continuous?
- If it's episodic, how long do episodes last?

- Are the episodes triggered or do they occur without warning?
- If they are triggered, what seems to be the trigger?

Physical examination

Physical examination of the dizzy patient needs to be fairly comprehensive given the long list of possible causes, but always starts with considering the vital signs. Obviously, if the initial associated data suggest a particular problem or type of problem, the exam should focus on that issue. For example, if a patient has dizziness with a new fever, then the source of the fever should be sought. If the fever is associated with cough, then a chest X-ray is likely indicated. Dizziness and tachycardia should raise the suspicion of a gastrointestinal bleed or pulmonary embolism, or perhaps just dehydration from poor PO intake as a result of a vestibular disorder.

However, it is important not to pigeon-hole the patient too early in the evaluation and certainly not based on which word the patient uses to describe their dizziness. A patient endorsing true vertigo "like the room is spinning around" might have rapid atrial fibrillation whereas another patient complaining of "lightheadedness" might have BPPV. With the caveat that the physician has done relatively thorough general and cardiac examinations and that the vital signs do not suggest anything obvious or catastrophic, special care should be taken on the examination of the ears, eyes, and nervous system. Again, with the caveat that a thorough neurological exam should usually be done to look for new focal findings, the gait, cerebellar, and oculomotor exams are the most revealing components.

Examination of the tympanic membrane may show an otitis. Unilateral new hearing deficit plus dizziness suggests a peripheral cause, since hearing and balance end organs are co-located peripherally. However, in the appropriate setting (abrupt onset of symptoms in a patient with vascular risk factors), a stroke involving the AICA or its labyrinthine branch can cause acute hearing loss and dizziness.

The gait should be tested. Comparison to the baseline gait is important to establish since many elderly patients have a gait abnormality to start with. Patients who normally use a cane or a walker should be tested using those devices to allow for a meaningful comparison with their baseline. A new gait abnormality, especially the inability to walk without falling, should suggest a central cause of dizziness or severe volume depletion. In a patient who is vomiting, having the patient try to sit up on the stretcher without holding on to the side rails (e.g., with arms crossed across the chest) will test for truncal ataxia.

Data suggest that in patients with AVS, a brief battery of three specific bedside oculomotor tests can identify posterior circulation stroke more accurately than MRI, at least in the first 48 hours from symptom onset [29]. These three tests are the horizontal head impulse test (HIT), testing for direction-changing gaze-evoked nystagmus, and alternate cover test for skew deviation [29]. The reader is referred to this article for links to video clips that demonstrate these bedside tests. An important caveat to this study is that it was done by trained neuro-otologists. However, from the perspective of a practicing emergency physician, these tests are relatively easy to learn to perform and interpret. In patients presenting with AVS, the presence of any of the worrisome findings suggests stroke (or another central cause) whereas the absence of all the worrisome findings strongly suggests a peripheral problem.

The head impulse test was first described in 1988 [54]. Figure 14.1 shows how the test is performed and interpreted. The presence of a corrective saccade of the eyes back towards the examiner's nose is a positive test and means that the lesion is likely in the peripheral labyrinth. The maneuver tests the vestibulo-ocular reflex (VOR), which does not loop through the cerebellum or lower brainstem, which is why it is negative (no corrective saccade) in patients with cerebellar or medullary strokes. Pooled results across four studies identified as part of a systematic review showed that a normal HIT was found in 85% of patients with stroke ($n = 152$) and only 5% of patients with a peripheral vestibular problem ($n = 65$) [11]. However, because the reflex arc does loop through the brainstem, it will be positive in some patients with brainstem stroke that affects the vestibular nerve root entry zone in the pons. However, most patients with these brainstem strokes will have one of the other two eye findings on exam that indicates the central nature of the lesion [29]. The HIT is a safe test although a single case of transient complete heart block has been described [56].

There is one important issue with respect to the HIT that bears special emphasis. It should only be performed in patients presenting with AVS. This is because it is the "negative" or "normal" result (no corrective saccade) that is worrisome for a stroke etiology. For most elements of the physical examination, it is the abnormal result, which is cause for concern, but for the HIT, it is the opposite. If one were to perform the HIT on normal individuals (or patients with pneumonia or fractured wrists), the result would be "normal" (and thus "worrisome"). Therefore, if one were to do a HIT on a patient with EVS or PVS, it would also be falsely "normal" and incorrectly suggest a central cause.

Nystagmus can be the clinician's friend. Patients with both vestibular neuritis and cerebellar stroke may have nystagmus. Merely reporting the presence or absence of nystagmus is not particularly useful and certainly does not distinguish benign peripheral etiologies from serious central ones. It is the nature of the nystagmus that can help to differentiate the two groups.

Patients with vestibular neuritis will have predominantly horizontal nystagmus, sometimes with a very slight torsional component [30,57]. This will sometimes be present in primary (neutral) gaze, and nearly always be present on gaze towards one side. When these patients look to the other side, they may still have nystagmus, but, if they do, the direction of the fast movement will be in the same direction as with the first side tested. The intensity of the nystagmus diminishes with fixation [57]. In patients with CNS causes of dizziness, the nystagmus is usually still predominantly horizontal, but the direction of the fast component may "change direction." That is, when the patient looks to the left, the fast component beats to the left and when the patient looks to the right, the fast component beats to the right. Not very sensitive, this finding is found in approximately 20–50% of patients with central causes of dizziness; when present, however,

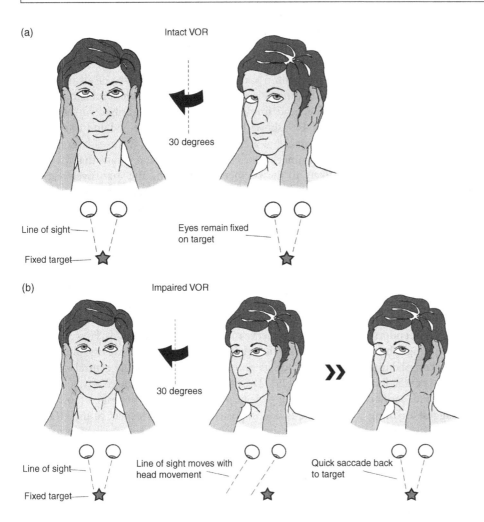

(a)

Intact VOR

30 degrees

Line of sight

Eyes remain fixed
on target

Fixed target

(b)

Impaired VOR

30 degrees

Line of sight

Line of sight moves with
head movement

Quick saccade back
to target

Fixed target

Figure 14.1. The head impulse test (HIT, sometimes referred to as the head thrust test) is a test of vestibular function that can be easily done during bedside examination. The HIT tests the vestibulo-ocular reflex (VOR), and can help to distinguish a peripheral process (vestibular neuritis) from a central one (cerebellar stroke). With the patient sitting on the stretcher, the physician instructs him/her to maintain their gaze on the examiner's nose. The physician holds the patient's head steady in the midline axis and then rapidly turns the head to about 20° off the midline.

(a) The normal response (intact VOR) is for the eyes to stay locked on the examiner's nose. (b) The abnormal response (impaired VOR) is for the eyes to move with the head, and then to snap back in one corrective saccade to the examiner's nose.

The HIT is usually "positive" (i.e., a corrective saccade is visible) with a peripheral lesion (vestibular neuritis), and the test is normal (no corrective saccade) in cerebellar stroke. This occurs because the VOR pathway does not loop through the cerebellum. Occasionally patients with small brainstem strokes may have a positive test because the VOR pathway does loop through the brainstem.

Because it is the "positive" test that is reassuring with the head impulse test and the "negative" test that is worrisome, it is very important only to use the test in patients with the AVS. If one were to use the HIT in patients with pneumonia or with a fractured wrist, the HIT would be "negative" (worrisome for a CNS event). Therefore it is critical that it only be applied to patients presenting with AVS.

Reproduced from Edlow et al. [68] with permission from Elsevier.

it is very specific. Of note, some normal patients will have slight direction-changing nystagmus on extreme end gaze both right and left that resolves after a few beats and is symmetric; this physiologic nystagmus is not helpful diagnostically.

Skew deviation is another relatively insensitive, but very specific finding indicating a CNS lesion in dizzy patients [29]. Skew deviation is tested by performing the "alternate cover" test. With the patient instructed to focus on a fixed point, each eye is alternately covered over and then uncovered sequentially. This forces the patient to take up visual fixation first with one eye and then the other, which allows the examiner to assess whether the eyes are completely aligned. The examiner looks at the eyes to see whether there is an upward or downward (hypertropia or hypotropia) correction as the eye is uncovered. This vertical misalignment of vestibular cause is termed skew deviation, assuming it is not the residuum of childhood strabismus, eye muscle surgery, or prior oculomotor palsy. Examiners should note that the presence of a horizontal misalignment (esophoria or exophoria) does not convey the same meaning.

Most patients with EVS will be asymptomatic by the time they present to the ED; however if they are not, these same tests as above may be useful. Note however that a central localization does not necessarily mean a serious diagnosis. Migraine

is a central phenomenon and patients with vestibular migraine may have findings that localize to the CNS.

In patients with PVS, the Dix–Hallpike should be performed to test for BPPV of the posterior semicircular canal (the most common form). If this is negative and the history is strongly suggestive of BPPV, then the horizontal canal should be tested by the supine roll test. Video clips of both of these tests are readily found by using the usual Internet search engines, although it is best if videos from approved practice parameters are used [10], since the techniques are not always demonstrated properly on all posted videos. The Dix–Hallpike test is considered positive when there is reproduction of symptoms after several seconds of latency, with a burst of upbeat-torsional nystagmus and spontaneous resolution within 45 seconds, usually less. It should generally be positive on one side and negative on the other. As above, patients with any cause of persistent dizziness, including CNS ones, will feel worse on head movements so tests producing only additional symptoms or exacerbating pre-existing horizontal nystagmus should not be interpreted as positive.

Diagnostic tests

Unless a diagnosis is totally clear based on history and physical examination, and many times it will be (such as a patient with

BPPV, vestibular neuritis, or hypovolemia), some basic testing probably makes sense. This is particularly true in elderly patients since the incidence of other diseases becomes increasingly common. Performing an electrocardiogram (ECG) may be useful in the geriatric patient with dizziness and no obvious cause by history or physical examination. Checking the hematocrit, a basic metabolic profile including creatinine, and a stool guaiac may also be helpful. Beyond these basics, diagnostic should be targeted rather than "shotgun." If pulmonary embolism is the suspect diagnosis, a CT angiogram of the chest might be the best first test. If drug toxicity in a heart failure patient taking digoxin is considered, then a serum digoxin level might be an appropriate first test.

If a patient is unable to communicate the details about their dizziness, the less well this system (or any other) will allow the physician to tailor their differential diagnosis and therefore, the subsequent testing. The important thing is to try to make a specific diagnosis. Because medication side effects are an important cause of chronic dizziness, an outpatient trial of stopping a medication might be the appropriate "test," but of course this should be coordinated with the primary care doctor.

Some of the important bedside diagnostic tests were discussed along with the physical examination since they can be easily incorporated into the clinical exam. It is very important to know the limitations of commonly used tests, especially CT of the head for posterior circulation stroke [58]. A recent study estimated the sensitivity of CT for acute posterior fossa stroke to be 42% [59], but studies with direct comparison to MRI scans suggest it could be as low as 16% in the first 24 hours [60]. If stroke is a serious consideration, MRI with diffusion-weighted imaging is needed. However the clinician must also be aware that even MRI is imperfect, and may miss up to 20% of posterior circulation strokes in the first 24–48 hours after symptom onset [11,29].

Treatment

As is usually the case, treatment flows from diagnosis, and given the long list of potential causes of dizziness, the list of potential treatments is equally long. This is probably even more so with dizziness, since some treatments for one cause of dizziness may worsen another cause; this is yet another reason why the "symptom quality" approach to dizziness performs less well than defining it by timing and triggers. We will only focus here on some of the treatments for a few selected vestibular and CNS causes.

The treatment for BPPV is a canal-repositioning maneuver, most commonly the Epley maneuver if the BPPV is of the posterior semicircular canal (~85% of cases). As with the diagnostic tests, the reader can rapidly access high-quality video clips and demonstrative cartoon-type drawings via the Internet. For someone who does not regularly perform the maneuver, it is probably wise to review how it is done just prior to doing it [10,61]. In elderly patients, one ought to make sure that the neck is sufficiently mobile to safely move the head and neck as needed; in these patients a different "side-lying" (Semont) maneuver may be used [62,63]. Some patients with a typical history of BPPV will have a negative Dix–Hallpike and will not respond to an Epley maneuver. Many of these patients will have horizontal (lateral) canal BPPV diagnosed by supine roll test and can be treated with a Lempert barbeque roll maneuver.

If a patient does not respond as expected (e.g., they have sustained nystagmus, downbeat nystagmus, no latency, bilateral positive positional test, or other new neurological signs), the clinician should consider a BPPV mimic, which can be due to various CNS lesions [50]. Even when maneuvers improve or resolve elderly patients' symptoms, follow-up is important as some patients have persistent dizzy symptoms not directly related to the BPPV [64].

Patients with vestibular neuritis who present within 72 hours of symptom onset should probably be treated with steroids unless there is a contraindication [57,65]. Some may benefit from vestibular rehabilitation after the ED visit. Although a vestibular "sedative" such as meclizine may be useful, its use should be limited to several days beyond which time it can impair vestibular compensation [57]. As well, meclizine *should not* be used for BPPV, for which it has no therapeutic effect and can only potentially worsen symptoms due to its sedating side effects. With any peripheral cause of dizziness, ensure that the patient is well hydrated as there is a tendency for them to have become dehydrated due to nausea and decreased oral intake.

Patients who have a posterior circulation stroke or high risk for one should be admitted to the hospital for further monitoring, vascular work-up, and treatment. Treatments should be applied to prevent secondary progression or complications such as obstructive hydrocephalus, as appropriate. Treatment for other specific diagnoses made are obviously based on the diagnosis made (heparin for PE, endoscopy and/or transfusion for a GI bleed, etc.).

Disposition

The disposition is a function of two issues – specific diagnosis and general environmental safety. The first factor is obvious. A patient with AVS due to an ischemic cerebellar stroke requires admission both to diagnose and treat the underlying vascular lesion as well as to observe for deterioration from posterior fossa edema. Another patient with the exact same presentation but which is due to vestibular neuritis can be sent home with oral steroids and meclizine for symptomatic control. Therefore, disposition is partly a function of the underlying diagnosis. Although vascular risk factors may help stratify those at highest risk for TIA and stroke (e.g., using the ABCD2 rule) [66], care should be taken not to rely too heavily on age or related risks to exclude vascular disease – it is well documented that younger patients with vertebral artery dissection may present with dizziness or vertigo due to TIA or stroke [11], and are most likely to be misdiagnosed with dangerous consequences [67,68].

Simultaneously, the second issue is ensuring environmental safety. This is especially important in elderly dizzy patients. Dizzy patients may become dehydrated, worsening their symptoms, whatever their initial cause. This can be compounded in elderly patients who have cardiovascular issues and often take multiple medications. Therefore, even the second patient (above) with AVS due to vestibular neuritis might require admission if they are dehydrated and still sufficiently symptomatic such that they cannot keep up with fluids. Most patients with BPPV can safely go home after canal-repositioning treatment. However an elderly BPPV patient who is somewhat dehydrated, volume sensitive, and lives alone may need to receive some slow intravenous fluids as an inpatient prior to safe discharge. A home safety evaluation (either formally or by questioning the patient and their family about the home situation) prior to discharge is important. A patient who has a few steps to get to the bathroom may need a different disposition than another who normally has to climb a flight of stairs to do the same. One who lives alone is different than another who lives with a healthy spouse or other family member.

Conclusions

Diagnosing the dizzy elderly patient can be frustrating. However, when using a systematic, algorithmic method, the physician can often confidently make a specific diagnosis and treat it accordingly. Knowing the common peripheral vestibular causes of dizziness well and learning a few bedside oculomotor physical findings and understanding the limitations of brain imaging will allow emergency physicians to make a specific diagnosis in many cases.

Pearls and pitfalls

- Use an algorithmic approach to patients with dizziness; identify timing and triggers to best define the category into which a patient falls.
- Use of the word "vertigo" or "near fainting" does not necessarily signify a vestibular or CNS cause in the first case or a cardiovascular one in the second.
- Dizzy patients in the ED often have significant co-chief complaints that help to narrow the differential diagnosis.
- Be aware that peripheral causes of the acute vestibular syndrome (vestibular neuritis) can closely mimic central causes (posterior circulation stroke).
- Learn to use bedside physical examination including gait testing and a focused oculomotor exam to differentiate peripheral from central causes of acute vestibular syndrome. The head impulse test will be falsely worrisome if it is performed in patients who do not have the acute vestibular syndrome.
- Learn to categorize nystagmus differently based on syndromic category. Direction-changing horizontal nystagmus on gaze testing or predominantly vertical or torsional nystagmus is due to CNS disease in the acute vestibular syndrome, but not necessarily in the peripheral vestibular syndrome.
- Focus more on the syndrome and exam findings than on the patient's age or vascular risk factors – young patients have strokes too, and these are most likely to be missed.
- Understand the limitations of CT scanning for cerebellar and brainstem infarction.
- Try to make a specific diagnosis as often as possible; learn the common peripheral vestibular causes well.
- Review the medication list of elderly patients with dizziness.

References

1. Neuhauser HK, Radtke A, von Brevern M, et al. Burden of dizziness and vertigo in the community. *Arch Intern Med.* 2008;168(19):2118–24.

2. Colledge NR, Wilson JA, Macintyre CC, MacLennan WJ. The prevalence and characteristics of dizziness in an elderly community. *Age Aging.* 1994;23(2):117–20.

3. Lammers W, Folmer W, Van Lieshout EM, et al. Demographic analysis of emergency department patients at the Ruijin Hospital, Shanghai. *Emerg Med Int.* 2011:748274.

4. Newman-Toker DE, Hsieh YH, Camargo CA, Jr, et al. Spectrum of dizziness visits to US emergency departments: cross-sectional analysis from a nationally representative sample. *Mayo Clin Proc.* 2008;83(7):765–75.

5. Royl G, Ploner CJ, Leithner C. Dizziness in the emergency room: diagnoses and misdiagnoses. *Eur Neurol.* 2011;66(5):256–63.

6. Yin M, Ishikawa K, Wong WH, Shibata Y. A clinical epidemiological study in 2169 patients with vertigo. *Auris Nasus Larynx.* 2009;36(1):30–5.

7. Cheung CS, Mak PS, Manley KV, et al. Predictors of important neurological causes of dizziness among patients presenting to the emergency department. *Emerg Med J.* 2010;27(7):517–21.

8. Herr RD, Zun L, Mathews JJ. A directed approach to the dizzy patient. *Ann Emerg Med.* 1989;18(6):664–72.

9. Kerber KA, Fendrick AM. The evidence base for the evaluation and management of dizziness. *J Eval Clin Pract.* 2010;16(1):186–91.

10. Fife TD, Iverson DJ, Lempert T, et al. Practice parameter: therapies for benign paroxysmal positional vertigo (an evidence-based review): report of the Quality Standards Subcommittee of the American Academy of Neurology. *Neurology.* 2008;70(22):2067–74.

11. Tarnutzer AA, Berkowitz AL, Robinson KA, Hsieh YH, Newman-Toker DE. Acute vestibular syndrome: does my patient have a stroke? A systematic and critical review of bedside diagnostic predictors. *Can Med Assoc J.* 2011;183(9):e571–92.

12. Baloh RW, Ying SH, Jacobson KM. A longitudinal study of gait and balance dysfunction in normal older people. *Arch Neurol.* 2003;60(6):835–9.

13. Ishiyama G. Imbalance and vertigo: the aging human vestibular periphery. *Semin Neurol.* 2009;29(5):491–9.

14. Kerber KA, Ishiyama GP, Baloh RW. A longitudinal study of oculomotor function in normal older people. *Neurobiol Aging.* 2006;27(9):1346–53.

15. Kerber K. Dizziness in older people. In *Vertigo and Imbalance: Clinical Neurophysiology of the Vestibular System*, ed. Eggers S, Zee D (Philadelphia, PA: Elsevier, 2010), pp. 491–501.

16. Tinetti ME, Williams CS, Gill TM. Dizziness among older adults: a possible geriatric syndrome. *Ann Intern Med.* 2000;132(5):337–44.

17. Kaufman DW, Kelly JP, Rosenberg L, Anderson TE, Mitchell AA. Recent patterns of medication use in the ambulatory adult population of the United States: the Slone survey. *JAMA.* 2002;287(3):337–44.

18. Shoair OA, Nyandege AN, Slattum PW. Medication-related dizziness in the older adult. *Otolaryngol Clin North Am.* 2011;44(2):455–71.

19. Newman-Toker DE, Camargo CA, Jr, Hsieh YH, Pelletier AJ, Edlow JA. Disconnect between charted vestibular diagnoses and emergency department management decisions: a cross-sectional analysis from a nationally representative sample. *Acad Emerg Med.* 2009;16(10):970–7.

20. Stevens JA, Corso PS, Finkelstein EA, Miller TR. The costs of fatal and non-fatal falls among older adults. *Inj Prev.* 2006;12(5):290–5.

21. Kannus P, Parkkari J, Koskinen S, et al. Fall-induced injuries and deaths among older adults. *JAMA.* 1999;281(20):1895–9.

22. Rubenstein LZ. Falls in older people: epidemiology, risk factors and strategies for prevention. *Age Aging.* 2006;35(Suppl. 2:ii37–41.

23. Drachman DA, Hart CW. An approach to the dizzy patient. *Neurology.* 1972;22(4):323–34.

24. Newman-Toker D. *Diagnosing Dizziness in the Emergency Department: Why "What do you mean by 'dizzy'?" Should Not be the First Question You Ask* (Baltimore, OH: Neurology & Otology, Johns Hopkins School of Medicine, 2007).

25. Newman-Toker DE, Cannon LM, Stofferahn ME, et al. Imprecision in patient reports of dizziness symptom quality: a cross-sectional study conducted in an acute care setting. *Mayo Clin Proc.* 2007;82(11):1329–40.

26. Newman-Toker DE, Dy FJ, Stanton VA, et al. How often is dizziness from primary cardiovascular disease true vertigo? A systematic review. *J Gen Intern Med.* 2008;23(12):2087–94.

27. Kerber KA, Brown DL, Lisabeth LD, Smith MA, Morgenstern LB. Stroke among patients with dizziness, vertigo, and imbalance in the emergency department: a population-based study. *Stroke.* 2006;37(10):2484–7.

28. Lawson J, Johnson I, Bamiou DE, Newton JL. Benign paroxysmal positional vertigo: clinical characteristics of dizzy patients referred to a Falls and Syncope Unit. *QJM.* 2005;98(5):357–64.

29. Kattah JC, Talkad AV, Wang DZ, Hsieh YH, Newman-Toker DE. HINTS to diagnose stroke in the acute vestibular syndrome: three-step bedside oculomotor examination more sensitive than early MRI diffusion-weighted imaging. *Stroke.* 2009;40(11):3504–10.

30. Baloh RW. Clinical practice. Vestibular neuritis. *N Engl J Med.* 2003;348(11):1027–32.

31. Schreiber BE, Agrup C, Haskard DO, Luxon LM. Sudden sensorineural hearing loss. *Lancet.* 2010;375(9721):1203–11.

32. Rauch SD. Clinical practice. Idiopathic sudden sensorineural hearing loss. *N Engl J Med.* 2008;359(8):833–40.

33. Lee H, Kim JS, Chung EJ, et al. Infarction in the territory of anterior inferior cerebellar artery: spectrum of audiovestibular loss. *Stroke.* 2009;40(12):3745–51.

34. Brandt T, Botzel K, Yousry T, Dieterich M, Schulze S. Rotational vertigo in embolic stroke of the vestibular and auditory cortices. *Neurology.* 1995;45(1):42–4.

35. Anagnostou E, Spengos K, Vassilopoulou S, et al. Incidence of rotational vertigo in supratentorial stroke: a prospective analysis of 112 consecutive patients. *J Neurol Sci.* 2010;290(1–2):33–6.

36. Lee H, Sohn SI, Cho YW, et al. Cerebellar infarction presenting isolated vertigo: frequency and vascular topographical patterns. *Neurology.* 2006;67(7):1178–83.

37. Uneri A, Polat S. Vertigo, dizziness and imbalance in the elderly. *J Laryngol Otol.* 2008;122(5):466–9.

38. Neuhauser H, Lempert T. Vestibular migraine. *Neurol Clin.* 2009;27(2):379–91.

39. Sajjadi H, Paparella MM. Meniere's disease. *Lancet.* 2008;372(9636):406–14.

40. Savitz SI, Caplan LR. Vertebrobasilar disease. *N Engl J Med.* 2005;352(25):2618–26.

41. Grad A, Baloh RW. Vertigo of vascular origin. Clinical and electronystagmographic features in 84 cases. *Arch Neurol.* 1989;46(3):281–4.

42. Karatas M. Vascular vertigo: epidemiology and clinical syndromes. *Neurologist.* 2011;17(1):1–10.

43. Moubayed SP, Saliba I. Vertebrobasilar insufficiency presenting as isolated positional vertigo or dizziness: a double-blind retrospective cohort study. *Laryngoscope.* 2009;119(10):2071–6.

44. Norrving B, Magnusson M, Holtas S. Isolated acute vertigo in the elderly: vestibular or vascular disease? *Acta Neurol Scand.* 1995;91(1):43–8.

45. Kerber KA, Rasmussen PA, Masaryk TJ, Baloh RW. Recurrent vertigo attacks cured by stenting a basilar artery stenosis. *Neurology.* 2005;65(6):962.

46. Oghalai JS, Manolidis S, Barth JL, Stewart MG, Jenkins HA. Unrecognized benign paroxysmal positional vertigo in elderly patients. *Otolaryngol Head Neck Surg.* 2000;122(5):630–4.

47. Gupta V, Lipsitz LA. Orthostatic hypotension in the elderly: diagnosis and treatment. *Am J Med.* 2007;120(10):841–7.

48. Freeman R. Clinical practice. Neurogenic orthostatic hypotension. *N Engl J Med.* 2008;358(6):615–24.

49. Carmona S, Nicenboim L, Castagnino D. Recurrent vertigo in extrinsic compression of the brain stem. *Ann N Y Acad Sci.* 2005;1039:513–16.

50. Dunniway HM, Welling DB. Intracranial tumors mimicking benign paroxysmal positional vertigo. *Otolaryngol Head Neck Surg.* 1998;118(4):429–36.

51. Johkura K. Central paroxysmal positional vertigo: isolated dizziness caused by small cerebellar hemorrhage. *Stroke.* 2007;38(6):e26–7; author reply, e28.

52. Buttner U, Helmchen C, Brandt T. Diagnostic criteria for central versus peripheral positioning nystagmus and vertigo: a review. *Acta Otolaryngol.* 1999;119(1):1–5.

53. Stanton VA, Hsieh YH, Camargo CA, Jr, et al. Overreliance on symptom quality in diagnosing dizziness: results of a multicenter survey of emergency physicians. *Mayo Clin Proc.* 2007;82(11):1319–28.

54. Halmagyi GM, Curthoys IS. A clinical sign of canal paresis. *Arch Neurol.* 1988;45(7):737–9.

55. Newman-Toker DE, Kattah JC, Alvernia JE, Wang DZ. Normal head impulse test differentiates acute cerebellar strokes from vestibular neuritis. *Neurology.* 2008;70(24 Pt 2):2378–85.

56. Ullman E, Edlow JA. Complete heart block complicating the head impulse test. *Arch Neurol.* 2010;67(10):1272–4.

57. Strupp M, Brandt T. Vestibular neuritis. *Semin Neurol.* 2009;29(5):509–19.

58. Edlow J. A physician's got to know his (test's) limitations. *J Emerg Med.* 2012;42(5):582–3.

59. Hwang DY, Silva GS, Furie KL, Greer DM. Comparative sensitivity of computed tomography versus magnetic resonance imaging for detecting acute posterior fossa infarct. *J Emerg Med.* 2012;42(5):559–65.

60. Chalela JA, Kidwell CS, Nentwich LM, et al. Magnetic resonance imaging and computed tomography in emergency assessment of patients with suspected acute stroke: a prospective comparison. *Lancet.* 2007;369(9558):293–8.

61. Bhattacharyya N, Baugh RF, Orvidas L, et al. Clinical practice guideline: benign paroxysmal positional vertigo. *Otolaryngol Head Neck Surg.* 2008;139(5 Suppl. 4):S47–81.

62. Lawson J, Bamiou DE, Cohen HS, Newton J. Positional vertigo in a Falls Service. *Age Aging.* 2008;37(5):585–9.

63. Cohen HS. Side-lying as an alternative to the Dix-Hallpike test of the posterior canal. *Otol Neurotol.* 2004;25(2):130–4.

64. Gamiz MJ, Lopez-Escamez JA. Health-related quality of life in patients over sixty years old with benign paroxysmal positional vertigo. *Gerontology.* 2004;50(2):82–6.

65. Strupp M, Zingler VC, Arbusow V, et al. Methylprednisolone, valacyclovir, or the combination for vestibular neuritis. *N Engl J Med.* 2004;351(4):354–61.

66. Navi BB, Kamel H, Shah MP, et al. Application of the ABCD2 Score to identify cerebrovascular causes of dizziness in the emergency department. *Stroke.* 2012;43(6):1484–9.

67. Savitz SI, Caplan LR, Edlow JA. Pitfalls in the diagnosis of cerebellar infarction. *Acad Emerg Med.* 2007;14(1):63–8.

68. Edlow JA, Newman-Toker DE, Savitz SI. Diagnosis and initial management of cerebellar infarction. *Lancet Neurol.* 2008;7(10):951–64.

Chapter

15

Headache in the elderly

Jolion McGreevy and Kerry K. McCabe

Background

Headache accounts for 2% of emergency department (ED) visits [1]. Although elderly patients are less likely to present to the ED with headache than younger patients, they are much more likely to have life-threatening illness [1,2]. When evaluating elderly patients with headache, clinicians should maintain a high index of suspicion for secondary (pathologic) causes – including malignancy, cerebrovascular emergencies, central nervous system (CNS) infection, ocular emergencies, and toxic-metabolic abnormalities – and have a low threshold for further work-up, especially of new-onset headache [2].

Headache prevalence decreases with age. A population-based study of elders in rural Italy found the 1-year headache prevalence to be 57% among 65–75-year-olds and 26% among those over 75 [3]. The likelihood of serious disease, on the other hand, increases dramatically with age. One percent of ED patients younger than age 50 presenting with headache have a secondary cause of their headache. After age 50, the risk jumps to 6%, then doubles after age 75 to 12% [1].

High-risk headache features and abnormal physical exam findings should prompt further evaluation, including in most cases a computed tomography (CT) scan. For many secondary causes of headache, prompt diagnosis is critical to reducing morbidity and mortality; therefore, EDs should have CT available 24 hours a day for the evaluation of elders with high-risk headache [1].

Given the marked increase in prevalence of pathologic diagnoses in elderly patients with headache, those without obvious high-risk features or abnormal physical exams should also be considered high risk and may warrant prompt and extensive work-up despite an overall benign appearance. As an example, consider subarachnoid hemorrhage (SAH), a frequently missed cause of headache in the elderly. The incidence of SAH doubles after age 55 and leads to significant morbidity and mortality. One in three patients with SAH is misdiagnosed [4]. Patients who present in good clinical condition and do not exhibit the classic "thunderclap" headache are the most likely to be misdiagnosed [5,6]. Twenty-five percent of patients with SAH develop headache gradually, and even more report only mild to moderate pain [7]. Failure to consider SAH in these patients has grave consequences: 20% will rebleed and 40% will

develop neurologic complications before their next visit to the doctor [5].

Emergency clinicians should recognize typical and atypical presentations of pathologic causes of headache in the elderly and maintain a low threshold for further evaluation. This chapter reviews serious causes of headache in elderly ED patients, first with an overview of high-risk features followed by a more detailed discussion of specific etiologies. Primary headache disorders are common in ED patients, including the elderly, and are also discussed. However, these diagnoses should be considered only after patients have been fully evaluated for pathologic causes of their headache.

High-risk headache features

Pathologic headache causes fit into five broad categories: malignancy, cerebrovascular emergencies, CNS infection, ocular emergencies, and toxic-metabolic abnormalities. Vigilance in assessment for high-risk historical features, signs, and symptoms is critical in recognizing a serious headache.

Since new-onset primary headache after age 65 is uncommon, occurring in only 5% of cases, any new-onset headache in an elderly patient should be considered secondary (pathologic) until proven otherwise [8]. In the elderly, a new headache alone warrants neuroimaging, as do the more obvious physical findings of seizure, mental status changes, and focal neurologic deficits. In elderly patients with a long history of headache, changes in headache timing, severity, or character are strong indications for a CT scan.

Fever raises concern for CNS infection, including encephalitis and meningitis, but may also be seen in SAH [7]. Hypertension is common in SAH and acute ischemic stroke but is not very specific for these diagnoses in the elderly [7]. Headache occurs in 22% of patients with hypertensive crisis [9].

Headache that develops suddenly and reaches maximum severity in a split second suggests SAH. The diagnostic significance of the "thunderclap" headache rests more on its rapid onset than its severity, but elderly patients may not recall how quickly the headache developed and instead may focus on the severity of the pain at the time of evaluation [7]. Patients should be asked about headaches in the previous days to weeks, since as many as 50% of patients with SAH report sentinel headaches [4].

Bilateral dull ache or pressure is seen in the majority of patients who have headache due to ischemic stroke [10]. Bifrontal pressure, though classically associated with tension-type headache, should also raise concern for an intracranial mass. Headache that is worse with bending over or associated with nausea and vomiting suggests an intracranial mass. Nausea and vomiting are also seen in the majority of patients with SAH and meningitis [11,12]. Temporal or occipital pain may point to giant cell arteritis, a sight-threatening vascular emergency. Half of these patients also experience pain with chewing from jaw claudication, which can serve as a diagnostic clue early in the evaluation of the headache [13].

Transient loss of consciousness is common in aneurysmal SAH [4]. Patients who regain consciousness at home and arrive at the ED in good condition are at highest risk for misdiagnosis [5]. Family members should be asked about transient loss of consciousness, and patients should be examined for signs of head trauma, which would suggest not only syncope associated with SAH but also additional intracranial injury associated with fall (e.g., subdural hemorrhage). Mental status changes that persist on arrival at the ED warrant further evaluation for cerebrovascular emergencies, CNS infection, and toxic-metabolic abnormalities.

Nuchal rigidity is present in nearly 90% of patients with meningitis; however, in SAH, it may take hours to develop and is absent half the time [12,14].

Headache plus nausea and dizziness, in addition to raising concern for cerebrovascular emergency, should prompt clinicians to ask about toxic exposure, such as carbon monoxide (CO). Elderly patients exposed to CO may develop signs of end-organ damage, such as altered mental status and myocardial ischemia or infarction [15]. Myocardial infarction (MI) by itself may cause headache, and electrocardiographic (ECG) changes that mimic MI have been associated with SAH [2,7].

Elderly patients with headache merit a basic eye exam. Vision loss may occur early in giant cell arteritis (GCA). Prompt treatment of GCA with corticosteroids aims to halt vision loss in the affected and contralateral eye but usually does not restore vision. On physical examination, the frontal or parietal branches of the superficial temporal artery may be tender to palpation and may feel thick or nodular; in some cases, there may be overlying erythema [13].

Blurred vision, nausea, and vomiting should raise concern for acute angle-closure glaucoma, as should focal eye pain. Since many patients experience pain around, rather than in, the eye, their symptoms are often misattributed to migraine [16]. A fixed pupil, cloudy cornea, and globe that is "rock hard" on palpation are sufficient to diagnose the ocular emergency [17].

Papilledema signals increased intracranial pressure, for example from a mass lesion, intracranial hemorrhage, or edema secondary to traumatic brain injury or cerebral infarction. Fundoscopic exam findings help narrow the diagnosis if flame-shaped retinal hemorrhages or large subhyaloid (pre-retinal) hemorrhages are seen. These are strongly associated with SAH

and would be an important diagnostic clue in an unconscious patient [4].

Secondary headache disorders

Headaches caused by an underlying pathologic process – such as infection or intracranial hemorrhage – are often called secondary headaches, in contrast with primary headaches (e.g., migraine and tension-type headache) in which the headache itself is the major symptom and consequence. Most secondary headaches are true emergencies that must be promptly recognized in the ED, but presentations may be subtle in elderly patients, especially those with CNS infections.

Cerebrovascular emergencies

Subarachnoid hemorrhage

One percent of patients who present to the ED with headache have SAH [18]. SAH incidence is 10% among ED patients with severe, acute-onset headache and a normal neurological exam, and 25% among those with neurological abnormalities [4,18]. SAH is common among the elderly, especially women, although the median age of SAH is lower than for other stroke types [19,20]. The incidence of SAH doubles between the fourth and fifth decades of life and then increases gradually, by an average of 2% per year [20,21]. Mortality from SAH is three times higher after age 60 [22].

Eighty-five percent of non-traumatic SAH cases are due to ruptured aneurysms. The majority of the remaining cases fit the pattern of non-aneurysmal perimesencephalic hemorrhage, a relatively benign condition in which extravasated blood is restricted to the cisterns around the midbrain [7,23]. Two-thirds of patients with SAH have modifiable risk factors, which include hypertension, smoking, and heavy alcohol use. Each of these roughly doubles SAH risk [7]. Patients with genetic risk factors, including a first-degree relative with SAH and a history of polycystic kidney disease, account for only 10% of cases [7].

Over the last two decades, improved management of SAH patients who reach the hospital in good condition has cut mortality in half [19]. Immediate aneurysm repair reduces rebleeding and subsequent death and may be indicated in many elderly patients who arrive at the ED neurologically intact. Since rebleeding risk is high in the first few days after the initial bleed, delayed diagnosis can be devastating [5].

The reported rate of misdiagnosis among SAH patients varies widely in the literature [4,5]. One study of 400 SAH patients admitted to a neurological intensive care unit found that 12% had been misdiagnosed on a previous visit to a health care professional. Patients who arrived with normal mental status and who were triaged as low acuity had a higher risk of misdiagnosis. Most commonly, no head CT was obtained, and the patient was diagnosed with migraine or tension-type headache. Twenty-one percent experienced a rebleed and 39% developed neurologic complications before SAH was diagnosed [5].

Subarachnoid hemorrhage classically presents as "thunderclap headache," a sudden, severe headache that patients describe as the worst headache of their lives. All patients with thunderclap headache merit evaluation for SAH. However, many patients do not report the classic features of headache from SAH. Twenty-five percent develop headache gradually, and an even greater proportion experience mild-to-moderate pain [7]. Therefore, clinicians must maintain a high index of suspicion for SAH, even among elders who arrive with mild symptoms, and learn to recognize a wide spectrum of presentations.

Up to 50% of patients experience sentinel headaches in the days or weeks leading up to the hemorrhage. These headaches are thought to be from small warning bleeds; they are often sudden and severe and may resolve spontaneously or after over-the-counter medication [4]. Failure to evaluate patients with warning headaches is a common reason for missing the diagnosis of SAH [4,5].

Two-thirds of patients admitted with SAH have a decreased level of consciousness. Patients with smaller hemorrhages are more likely to remain alert [5]. Elders who present with acute confusion are at risk for delayed diagnosis when the altered mental status is attributed to another etiology (e.g., infection). In these patients, transient loss of consciousness is an important clue pointing to SAH. Half of patients who arrive with a decreased level of consciousness are comatose [7]. Fundoscopic examination may be critical to early diagnosis in comatose patients [4]. Ocular hemorrhages – including flame-shaped retinal and large subhyaloid (pre-retinal) hemorrhages – occur in one in seven patients with SAH [7]. They are more common in patients with decreased consciousness because they result from increased intracranial pressure obstructing venous outflow from the eye. They may be especially helpful in early identification of SAH in comatose patients [7].

Other clinical features associated with SAH include seizure, vomiting, neck stiffness, and focal neurological deficits (e.g., third cranial nerve palsy). None of these is very sensitive or specific for SAH. Half of patients with thunderclap headache not due to SAH report vomiting [7]. Neck stiffness, caused by the inflammatory response to subarachnoid blood, may not develop for hours and is less reliable in patients both with minor hemorrhage and those in coma [7]. Neurologic deficits from ruptured aneurysms are often indistinguishable from those due to other stroke syndromes; seizure occurs in fewer than 10% of patients with SAH [7]. Three percent of patients with SAH go into cardiac arrest at the onset of hemorrhage; half of those who survive the cardiac arrest regain independence [7].

Computed tomography is the first diagnostic test for suspected SAH. In patients with headache as the presenting symptom, multi-row detector third-generation CT performed within six hours of onset and read by an experienced neuroradiologist is 100% sensitive for SAH [24]. Thus when third-generation CT performed within six hours of headache onset is negative, as read by an experienced neuroradiologist, lumbar puncture (LP) is not needed. The sensitivity declines to about 98% at 12 hours, 85% at 3 days, and 50% at 7 days as blood is cleared from the subarachnoid space [18,25,26]. Patients with suspected SAH and a normal CT performed more than 6 hours since headache onset should undergo LP. Ideally LP should be delayed until at least 12 hours from headache onset to allow erythrocytes in the subarachnoid space to break down to form bilirubin [7]; when performed earlier, LP can muddle the diagnosis as bilirubin may not have formed. Red blood cells present in the cerebral spinal fluid (CSF) could be due to a traumatic tap rather than SAH, and reduction in the number of red blood cells in consecutive tubes does not reliably distinguish traumatic tap from SAH [7]. A CT angiogram is not an appropriate follow-up test for SAH after a negative CT because it is more likely to reveal an asymptomatic aneurysm, which is common in the elderly [27].

Ischemic stroke and intracerebral hemorrhage

Headache is less common in ischemic stroke and intracerebral hemorrhage (ICH) than in subarachnoid hemorrhage. However, headache occurs in 27% of ischemic strokes and 50% of ICH [10,28]. Any elderly patient who presents with headache should have a careful neurologic examination. Non-contrast head CT is the initial test in the ED for suspected stroke as it provides rapid results to guide management. It is nearly 100% sensitive for hemorrhagic stroke and about 40–75% sensitive for ischemic stroke, depending on the time since symptom onset [29,30]. Diffusion-weighted MRI is more sensitive for acute ischemic stroke, especially in the first 12 hours, and can be used when ischemic stroke is still highly suspected after a normal head CT [30].

Headache from ischemic stroke is most commonly described as bilateral dull ache or pressure and is often associated with cerebellar infarct [10]. Headache from ICH may develop at stroke onset or over hours, along with vomiting and altered consciousness, as the hematoma expands.

Subdural hemorrhage

The elderly are at higher risk for subdural hemorrhage (SDH) as a result of cerebral atrophy, frequent falls, and antithrombotic/anticoagulant therapy [31]. Even an elder who presents after a minor injury with no external sign of trauma may have SDH. Headache is an important clue in an elderly patient who presents with a "lucid interval" after sustaining SDH from an acute injury. However, headache from SDH may not develop for weeks after an injury, until the slowly developing subdural hematoma raises the intracranial pressure enough to cause clinical findings. Patients with chronic subdural hemorrhage can present with headache, cognitive decline, altered consciousness, focal neurologic deficits, and/or seizure. Head CT is the most commonly used imaging study for an elder suspected of SDH from recent or remote trauma.

Brain tumor

Headache is the first complaint in half of patients diagnosed with brain tumors [11]. Most commonly, the headache mimics tension-type, with bifrontal pressure or dull ache. Headache associated with a brain tumor is worse with bending over in 30% of patients and associated with nausea and vomiting in 40% [32]. These features can help differentiate the patient with a mass lesion from the one with tension-type headache. The early morning headache classically associated with brain tumor is uncommon [32]. Headache as the only sign or symptom of a brain tumor is even less common. Patients may also present with syncope, seizures, or focal neurologic findings, including aphasia or motor or sensory deficits. MRI is the preferred imaging study in patients with suspected brain tumor; however, CT is often obtained in the emergency setting when other diagnoses are still high in the differential or the patient is unstable.

CNS infection

Two-thirds of patients with acute bacterial meningitis complain of headache [12]. The headache is typically severe and generalized. Only 44% of meningitis cases present with the classic triad of fever, neck stiffness, and altered mental status. Addition of headache significantly improves the classic definition: 95% of adult patients have at least two of the four symptoms of headache, fever, neck stiffness, and altered mental status [33]. Headache, fever, altered mental status, and seizure also raise suspicion for encephalitis and brain abscess, though none of these findings is very sensitive for either disease. Clinical features associated with brain parenchymal rather than meningeal inflammation, such as changes in behavior or speech and focal neurologic deficits, point toward encephalitis or brain abscess over meningitis; however, there may be significant overlap in the presentations of CNS infections [34]. Brain abscesses may be caused by direct spread from a dental or sinus infection or hematogenous spread from elsewhere in the body.

The presentation of CNS infection in the elderly may be subtle. Suspected meningitis and encephalitis cases require prompt lumbar puncture, followed immediately by empiric antibiotic and/or antiviral therapy. Patients who are immunocompromised, have a history of CNS disease or focal infection, or present with altered consciousness, new-onset seizure, papilledema, or focal neurologic deficit should have a head CT to exclude conditions that increase the theoretical risk of herniation after LP [35]. LP is contraindicated prior to CT in patients with focal neurologic deficits. Delay in antibiotic administration greater than six hours increases mortality in acute bacterial meningitis [36]. If the LP will be delayed, a blood culture should be drawn and the patient should be started on steroids and empiric antibiotics prior to LP [37]. Delay in antiviral treatment for herpes simplex virus (HSV) encephalitis also increases morbidity and mortality, though the critical time window in which to initiate treatment is less clear [34]. Empiric antibiotics for suspected meningitis in the elderly include vancomycin, ampicillin, and a third-generation cephalosporin [37]. Acyclovir should be added to cover HSV if the presentation suggests encephalitis [34]. Contrast head CT may be obtained in the emergency setting for suspected brain abscess, though MRI is more sensitive. Empiric therapy for a brain abscess should target organisms commonly associated with the presumed source.

GCA

Headache is the most common initial symptom of giant cell arteritis, but may be absent in one-third of patients [13]. Over the last few decades, improved disease recognition and corticosteroid treatment have reduced the incidence of permanent vision loss from ~60 to 15% [38]. Blindness is most often caused by optic nerve ischemia [13].

Increased risk for GCA begins after age 50 and peaks between 70 and 80. GCA most commonly affects individuals of Scandinavian descent who live at higher latitudes, indicating that multiple genetic and environmental factors contribute to disease susceptibility. Epidemiologic evidence suggests a link between GCA and parvovirus B19 [13,39]. About half of patients with GCA also have polymyalgia rheumatica, characterized by morning stiffness and persistent pain in the neck, shoulders, and pelvic girdle [13,39].

Although "temporal arteritis" is regularly used as a synonym for GCA, the headache does not always localize to the temporal region. It may instead be occipital or diffuse [13]. Other common cranial symptoms include jaw claudication, facial pain, scalp tenderness, odynophagia, and tongue pain [38]. Physical examination may reveal a thickened, nodular temporal artery that is tender to palpation. The temporal pulse may be diminished or absent. Fifteen percent of patients present with fever as the initial disease manifestation [40]. In two-thirds of cases, transient visual symptoms (amaurosis fugax, blurred vision, diplopia) precede blindness by an average of one week [38]. The cranial and visual symptoms associated with GCA often go unrecognized by clinicians, leading to delayed diagnosis and treatment and an increased risk of vision loss in one or both eyes [38,41]. Of note, patients aged 80 and older have a greater risk of complete blindness and are less likely to report premonitory visual symptoms than those under 80 [41]. Neurology and ophthalmology consultation should be obtained for patients with acute or transient blindness to assist in excluding other causes.

In patients with cranial or visual symptoms suggestive of GCA, an erythrocyte sedimentation rate (ESR) of greater than 50 mm/h supports the diagnosis. However, ESR may be normal in about 20% of patients with GCA as a result of localized arteritis or inability to mount an acute phase response [13,42]. Corticosteroids should be started promptly for patients highly suspected of having GCA, and these patients should be referred for temporal artery biopsy. Biopsy should be performed as soon as possible after treatment is initiated, although pathologic evidence of GCA may persist after two or more weeks of corticosteroids [13].

Acute glaucoma

The prevalence of angle-closure glaucoma rises exponentially after age 40. Three-quarters of patients with angle-closure glaucoma have an asymptomatic, chronic disorder similar to open-angle glaucoma; however, acute angle-closure glaucoma is an ocular emergency [43].

Acute glaucoma classically presents with sudden severe eye pain, decreased vision, nausea, and vomiting. Examination reveals a firm, red eye with an edematous, hazy cornea and a fixed, mid-dilated pupil [44]. These signs and symptoms suggest an acute rise in intraocular pressure and portend irreversible optic nerve damage. Left untreated, acute angle-closure glaucoma may lead to permanent blindness within hours [44].

The classic presentation is relatively straightforward to recognize, although significant delays in diagnosis have been attributed to easily correctable systems errors, such as lack of available Snellen charts to test visual acuity [16]. It is more difficult to recognize acute glaucoma in elderly patients who do not report ocular symptoms. Elders with acute glaucoma may instead report frontal or temporal headache, or they may be confused and unable to locate the pain at all [16]. Since delayed diagnosis of acute glaucoma has devastating consequences, elders with headache should have a basic eye examination prior to undergoing evaluation for intracranial pathology and common causes of the systemic symptoms associated with acute glaucoma (e.g., nausea and vomiting). There have been cases in which patients presented with headache, nausea, and vomiting and had exploratory laparotomies before the significance of their red eye was recognized [44].

Emergency department management of acute glaucoma consists of pressure-lowering eye drops (e.g., ophthalmic beta blockers and cholinergics) and emergent referral to an ophthalmologist for definitive diagnosis (gonioscopy) and treatment (laser iridotomy) [43].

Non-emergent secondary headache

Secondary causes of headache commonly identified in the headache clinic population include trigeminal neuralgia and cervicogenic headache [8]. In the ED, headache emergencies should first be excluded. Patients suspected of having one of these non-emergent conditions may then be referred to a neurologist or pain specialist for further evaluation and treatment.

Trigeminal neuralgia is characterized by intense electric shock-like pain in the distribution of the fifth cranial (trigeminal) nerve. The disorder typically develops after age 50 and is caused by demyelination of the nerve root secondary to compression by an aberrant overlying artery or vein. Most cases respond well to pharmacologic treatment (e.g., carbamazepine) [45].

Cervicogenic headache is pain referred from the cervical spine. The headache tends to be unilateral and associated with pain and limited range of motion in the neck. Patients may experience autonomic symptoms similar to those associated with migraine. No clinical or radiographic criteria have proven valid for diagnosis. Patients undergo fluoroscopically guided, controlled cervical nerve blocks aimed at identifying the pain source [46].

Primary headache disorders

Although headache incidence declines with age and new-onset primary headache is uncommon after age 50, 5–10% of elders experience severe, recurrent headaches [47]. The two most common benign headaches in the elderly are migraine and tension-type headache [8]. Two percent of migraine cases and 5% of tension-type headache cases begin after age 65 [8].

Adults with primary headaches often continue to have symptoms past age 65. However, headache patterns and characteristics change with age [47]. More than half of adults with life-long migraine continue to have attacks after age 65, but the proportion experiencing aura decreases [8,47]. Episodic migraine, chronic migraine, and tension-type headache each account for about 25–30% of the primary headache cases in elders. Cluster headache and hypnic headache account for the remaining cases [8].

Migraine in the elderly may be either unilateral or bilateral. The headache typically has a pulsating quality and is most frequently associated with photo- or phonophobia. One to two percent of elderly patients experience recurrent migraine-like visual symptoms (e.g., scintillating scotoma), as well as transient neurologic symptoms (e.g., vertigo, aphasia, weakness) in the absence of headache. These symptoms are thought to be from migraine-like activity in the brain. Elderly patients with these "late-life" acephalgic migraines do not have an increased risk of stroke, though clearly in the ED, this constellation of symptoms should be considered stroke until proven otherwise [47]. Acute migraine treatment options for the elderly include antiemetics, nonsteroidal anti-inflammatory drugs (NSAIDs), and opioids. Ergotamines and triptans are less desirable in elderly patients because of the risk of cerebral and coronary vasoconstriction [47].

Tension-type headache is typically bilateral, squeezing, and not associated with nausea, vomiting, or visual symptoms. NSAIDs and opioids should be limited to two or fewer days per week to avoid rebound headache and other adverse medication effects, particularly gastrointestinal bleeding [47].

Cluster headache presents as severe unilateral pain in or around the eye, associated with autonomic features (miosis and ptosis) [48]. Cluster headache often occurs at night and can lead to daytime sleepiness and cognitive impairment. Although cluster headaches do not typically develop after age 50, patients with a long history may continue to experience recurrent headache cycles throughout their lives [47]. Cluster headaches respond to inhaled oxygen (100% O_2 at 15 l/min via non-rebreather) and subcutaneous or intranasal sumatriptan; however, as with the treatment of migraine, triptans are contraindicated in elders with cardiovascular or cerebrovascular disorders [48].

Hypnic headache is a rare primary headache disorder that occurs only in the elderly. Patients awake from sleep, usually at the same time(s) each night, and experience bilateral throbbing headache and nausea [8,47]. Lithium is the treatment of choice.

Medication overuse is common among patients with migraine and chronic tension-type headache [8]. Elders who take analgesic medication frequently to treat primary headaches may develop constant, daily headache refractory to abortive therapy. Temporary withdrawal of the overused medication usually restores the effectiveness of abortive therapy for future episodes of headache [47]. Patients who chronically use an opioid, benzodiazepine, or barbiturate should taper, rather than abruptly stop, the medication.

Elders with migraine or chronic tension-type headache should be screened for depression. Headache seven or more days per month in the previous year is associated with depression [49]. One study conducted in an urban ED found that depression is present in one-third of geriatric patients but unrecognized most of the time by emergency physicians [50].

Conclusion

Elders who present to the ED with headache are much more likely than younger patients to have serious pathology. Prompt diagnosis of secondary headache is critical to reducing morbidity and mortality. Headache that is new or different, or associated with fever, altered consciousness, or focal neurologic deficit, should prompt further evaluation, which typically includes laboratory tests, ECG, and CT and/or LP.

Pearls and pitfalls

- Elders with headache have a high risk of serious pathology and, in most cases, warrant extensive evaluation, including computed tomography of the brain.
- New-onset headache is unusual in elders and suggests a secondary cause. Headache associated with fever, altered consciousness, or focal neurologic deficit likely represents serious disease.
- Subarachnoid hemorrhage is commonly misdiagnosed, especially in patients who appear well at presentation. Many of these patients have significant neurologic decline before returning to the hospital.
- Subdural hemorrhage (SDH) may develop in elders after relatively minor trauma. It is important to ask about both recent and remote trauma, as SDH may be either acute or chronic.
- Brain tumors may mimic tension-type headache. Headache that is worse when bending forward or associated with nausea and vomiting suggests brain tumor or other mass lesion rather than tension headache.
- Ninety-five percent of adult patients with meningitis have at least two of the four symptoms of headache, fever, neck stiffness, and altered mental status. Focal neurologic findings raise suspicion for other CNS infection (i.e., encephalitis or brain abscess).
- Headache from giant cell arteritis is not always temporal; it may instead be occipital or diffuse. Transient visual symptoms (amaurosis fugax, blurry vision, diplopia) often precede blindness by about one week and frequently go unnoticed by clinicians.
- Elders with headache should have a basic eye examination to exclude acute glaucoma.

References

1. Goldstein JN, Camargo CA, Pelletier AJ, et al. Headache in United States emergency departments: demographics, work-up and frequency of pathological diagnoses. *Cephalalgia.* 2006;26(6):684–90.

2. Tanganelli P. Secondary headaches in the elderly. *Neurol Sci.* 2010;31(Suppl. 1):S73–6.

3. Prencipe M. Prevalence of headache in an elderly population: attack frequency, disability, and use of medication. *J Neurol Neurosurg Psych.* 2001;70(3):377–81.

4. Edlow JA, Caplan LR. Avoiding pitfalls in the diagnosis of subarachnoid hemorrhage. *N Engl J Med.* 2000;342(1):29–36.

5. Kowalski RG, Claassen J, Kreiter KT, et al. Initial misdiagnosis and outcome after subarachnoid hemorrhage. *JAMA.* 2004;291(7):866–9.

6. Edlow JA. Diagnosis of subarachnoid hemorrhage: are we doing better? *Stroke.* 2007;38(4):1129–31.

7. van Gijn J, Kerr RS, Rinkel GJ. Subarachnoid haemorrhage. *Lancet.* 2007;369(9558):306–18.

8. Lisotto C, Mainardi F, Maggioni F, et al. Headache in the elderly: a clinical study. *J Headache Pain.* 2004;5(1):36–41.

9. Zampaglione B, Pascale C, Marchisio M, et al. Hypertensive urgencies and emergencies. Prevalence and clinical presentation. *Hypertension.* 1996;27(1):144–7.

10. Tentschert S, Wimmer R, Greisenegger S, et al. Headache at stroke onset in 2196 patients with ischemic stroke or transient ischemic attack. *Stroke.* 2005;36(2):e1–3.

11. Pfund Z, Szapáry L, Jászberényi O, et al. Headache in intracranial tumors. *Cephalalgia.* 1999;19(9):787–90; discussion, 765.

12. Hussein AS, Shafran SD. Acute bacterial meningitis in adults. A 12-year review. *Medicine (Baltimore).* 2000;79(6):360–8.

13. Salvarani C, Cantini F, Boiardi L, et al. Polymyalgia rheumatica and giant-cell arteritis. *N Engl J Med.* 2002;347(4):261–71.

14. Vannemreddy P, Nanda A, Kelley R, et al. Delayed diagnosis of intracranial aneurysms: confounding factors in clinical presentation and the influence of misdiagnosis on outcome. *South Med J.* 2001;94(11):1108–11.

15. Tomaszewski C. Carbon monoxide poisoning. Early awareness and intervention can save lives. *Postgrad Med.* 1999;105(1):39–40, 43–8, 50.

16. Siriwardena D, Arora AK, Fraser SG, et al. Misdiagnosis of acute angle closure glaucoma. *Age Aging.* 1996;25(6):421–3.

17. Walker RA, Wadman MC. Headache in the elderly. *Clin Geriatr Med.* 2007;23(2):291–305.

18. Edlow JA, Malek AM, Ogilvy CS. Aneurysmal subarachnoid hemorrhage: update for emergency physicians. *J Emerg Med.* 2008;34(3):237–51.

19. Lovelock CE, Rinkel GJ, Rothwell PM. Time trends in outcome of subarachnoid hemorrhage: Population-based study and systematic review. *Neurology.* 2010;74(19):1494–501.

20. Eden SV, Meurer WJ, Sánchez BN, et al. Gender and ethnic differences in subarachnoid hemorrhage. *Neurology.* 2008;71(10):731–5.

21. de Rooij NK, Linn FH, van der Plas JA, et al. Incidence of subarachnoid haemorrhage: a systematic review with emphasis on region, age, gender and time trends. *J Neurol Neurosurg Psychiatry.* 2007;78(12):1365–72.

22. Pobereskin H. Incidence and outcome of subarachnoid haemorrhage: a retrospective population based study. *J Neurol Neurosurg Psychiatry.* 2001;70(3):340–3.

23. van Gijn J, van Dongen KJ, Vermeulen M, et al. Perimesencephalic hemorrhage: a nonaneurysmal and benign form of subarachnoid hemorrhage. *Neurology.* 1985;35(4):493–7.

24. Backes D, Rinkel GJ, Kemperman H, et al. Time-dependent test characteristics of head computed tomography in patients suspected of nontraumatic subarachnoid hemorrhage. *Stroke.* 2012;43(8):2115–19.

25. van der Wee N, Rinkel GJ, Hasan D, et al. Detection of subarachnoid haemorrhage on early CT: is lumbar puncture still needed after a negative scan? *J Neurol Neurosurg Psychiatry*. 1995;58(3):357–9.

26. Morgenstern LB, Luna-Gonzales H, Huber JC, et al. Worst headache and subarachnoid hemorrhage: prospective, modern computed tomography and spinal fluid analysis. *Ann Emerg Med*. 1998;32(3 Pt 1):297–304.

27. Edlow JA. What are the unintended consequences of changing the diagnostic paradigm for subarachnoid hemorrhage after brain computed tomography to computed tomographic angiography in place of lumbar puncture? *Acad Emerg Med*. 2010;17(9):991–5; discussion, 996–7.

28. Gorelick PB, Hier DB, Caplan LR, et al. Headache in acute cerebrovascular disease. *Neurology*. 1986;36(11):1445–50.

29. Köhrmann M, Schellinger PD. Acute stroke triage to intravenous thrombolysis and other therapies with advanced CT or MR imaging: pro MR imaging. *Radiology*. 2009;251(3):627–33.

30. Mullins E, Schaefer W, Sorensen G, et al. CT and conventional and diffusion-weighted MR imaging in acute stroke: study in 691 patients at presentation to the emergency department. *Radiology*. 2002;224(2):353–60.

31. Baechli H, Nordmann A, Bucher HC, et al. Demographics and prevalent risk factors of chronic subdural haematoma: results of a large single-center cohort study. *Neurosurg Rev*. 2004;27(4):263–6.

32. Forsyth PA, Posner JB. Headaches in patients with brain tumors: a study of 111 patients. *Neurology*. 1993;43(9):1678–83.

33. van de Beek D, de Gans J, Spanjaard L, et al. Clinical features and prognostic factors in adults with bacterial meningitis. *N Engl J Med*. 2004;351(18):1849–59.

34. Whitley RJ. Viral encephalitis. *N Engl J Med*. 1990;323(4):242–50.

35. Hasbun R, Abrahams J, Jekel J, et al. Computed tomography of the head before lumbar puncture in adults with suspected meningitis. *N Engl J Med*. 2001;345(24):1727–33.

36. Proulx N, Fréchette D, Toye B, et al. Delays in the administration of antibiotics are associated with mortality from adult acute bacterial meningitis. *QJM*. 2005;98(4):291–8.

37. Tunkel AR, Hartman BJ, Kaplan SL, et al. Practice guidelines for the management of bacterial meningitis. *Clin Infect Dis*. 2004;39(9):1267–84.

38. Font C, Cid MC, Coll-Vinent B, et al. Clinical features in patients with permanent visual loss due to biopsy-proven giant cell arteritis. *Br J Rheumatol*. 1997;36(2):251–4.

39. Salvarani C, Gabriel SE, O'Fallon WM, et al. The incidence of giant cell arteritis in Olmsted County, Minnesota: apparent fluctuations in a cyclic pattern. *Ann Intern Med*. 1995;123(3):192–4.

40. Calamia KT, Hunder GG. Giant cell arteritis (temporal arteritis) presenting as fever of undetermined origin. *Arthritis Rheum*. 1981;24(11):1414–18.

41. Liozon E, Loustaud-Ratti V, Ly K, et al. Visual prognosis in extremely old patients with temporal (giant cell) arteritis. *J Am Geriatr Soc*. 2003;51(5):722–3.

42. Salvarani C, Hunder GG. Giant cell arteritis with low erythrocyte sedimentation rate: frequency of occurrence in a population-based study. *Arthritis Rheum*. 2001;45(2):140–5.

43. Quigley HA. Glaucoma. *Lancet*. 2011;377(9774):1367–77.

44. Leibowitz HM. The red eye. *N Engl J Med*. 2000;343(5):345–51.

45. Bennetto L, Patel NK, Fuller G. Trigeminal neuralgia and its management. *BMJ*. 2007;334(7586):201–5.

46. Bogduk N, Govind J. Cervicogenic headache: an assessment of the evidence on clinical diagnosis, invasive tests, and treatment. *Lancet Neurol*. 2009;8(10):959–68.

47. Biondi DM, Saper JR. Geriatric headache. How to make the diagnosis and manage the pain. *Geriatrics*. 2000;55(12):40, 43–5, 48–50.

48. May A. Cluster headache: pathogenesis, diagnosis, and management. *Lancet*. 2005;366(9488):843–55.

49. Wang S-J, Liu H-C, Fuh J-L, et al. Comorbidity of headaches and depression in the elderly. *Pain*. 1999;82(3):239–43.

50. Meldon SW, Emerman CL, Schubert DS, et al. Depression in geriatric ED patients: prevalence and recognition. *Ann Emerg Med*. 1997;302:141–5.

Chapter

16

Back pain in the elderly

Keli M. Kwok

Background

Back pain is a very common condition that will affect up to 90% of individuals at some point in their life [1–3]. It is the most frequent type of pain reported by adults in the US, and it accounts for approximately 1.5–3% of all emergency department (ED) visits [4–6]. Although back pain is seen most often in middle-aged individuals, restricting back pain among the elderly is also very common. It is the third most frequent cause of physician visits in patients over the age of 65 [7–9]. One prospective study reported that over a 10-year period, the cumulative incidence of restricting back pain among men and women more than 70 years old was 77.3% and 81.7%, respectively [10]. Most episodes of back pain are short lived and episodic; however, the prevalence of chronic back pain is increasing in all age groups, including those individuals age 65 and older [11].

Increasing age results in many changes in the lumbar spine and supporting structures. The nucleus pulposus, which is the center of the vertebral disk, decreases in size with age. This causes the vertebrae to move closer together, which leads to degeneration of the apophyseal joints and the formation of osteophytes. In addition, the vertebral bodies themselves show escalating osteoporosis as people get older, making them more susceptible to fractures and injury [12,13].

Frequently, a specific cause of back pain cannot be found in the ED. When this is the case, it is useful to seek to answer the following questions: Is there a serious systemic disease causing the pain? Is there neurologic compromise that might require surgical evaluation? Is there social or psychological distress that might amplify or prolong pain [14,15]?

History

Most episodes of back pain among the elderly are short lived and are not associated with significant pathology [10]. However, elderly patients are more likely than younger patients to have a serious cause of back pain, such as tumor, infection, fracture, or intra-abdominal process [3,15]. Elderly patients are also more likely to be admitted to the hospital if they present to the ED with back pain [5]. Using a thorough, systematic approach for all individuals who present with back pain aids in diagnosing those etiologies of back pain that are associated with high morbidity and mortality.

When collecting a history of back pain, it is important to ask about duration of symptoms. Back pain is considered acute if it has been present for 0–6 weeks, subacute if it has been present for 6–12 weeks, and chronic if it has been present for longer than 12 weeks. Back pain that has been present for more than 6 weeks should be considered particularly concerning because 80–90% of back pain with a benign cause will resolve within 4–6 weeks [1].

It is also vital to ask about the characteristics of back pain, such as nature, location, radiation, and alleviating and exacerbating factors. Thoracic pain, particularly in the absence of lumbar pain, should be further evaluated as it is more likely to be associated with serious pathology such as aortic dissection, osteomyelitis, malignancy, or perforated gastric ulcer. A trauma history is important, as even minor trauma can cause fractures in the elderly. Other important points in the history include bowel or bladder incontinence, systemic complaints, atypical features, associated neurologic complaints, and past medical history including recent procedures which have high risk for bacteremia [2,14].

Back pain due to mechanical causes is often intermittent, positional, and pain is maximal at onset. Back pain that is sudden in onset and severe may be indicative of an acute abdominal process such as a ruptured abdominal aortic aneurysm (AAA). Pain that is gradual in onset, constantly present including during rest, and progressive over a period of weeks to one month is concerning for cancer or an infectious process. A worsening neurologic deficit is particularly concerning for epidural abscess, hemorrhage, or neoplasm. Acute, severe midline back pain in a patient with a history of cancer should be considered a pathologic fracture until proven otherwise [2,7].

Historical features that should be considered in regard to patients with back pain include gradual onset of pain, pain located in the thoracic region, pain lasting longer than six weeks, history of trauma, and systemic symptoms such as fever, chills, night sweats, or unintentional weight loss. Other concerning features include pain that is worse at night or with recumbency, and unrelenting pain despite adequate analgesia. Patients who have a history of malignancy, immunosuppression, intravenous drug use, recent bacterial infection, or recent procedure that can cause bacteremia are considered high risk for critical causes of back pain [2,3].

Geriatric Emergency Medicine, ed. Joseph H. Kahn, Brendan G. Magauran Jr., and Jonathan S. Olshaker. Published by Cambridge University Press.
© Cambridge University Press 2014.

Table 16.1. Spinal nerve roots and functions

	Sensation	Motor	Deep tendon reflexes
L1	Anterior thigh	Hip flexors	
L2	Anterior thigh	Hip flexors, leg extension	Patellar reflex – minor
L3	Anterior thigh	Hip flexors, leg extension	Patellar reflex – minor
L4	Medial surface of leg and foot, including medial surface of great toe but not the first dorsal web space	Leg extension, ankle dorsiflexion, and ankle inversion	Patellar reflex – primary
L5	Lateral surface of leg and dorsum of the foot including the first web space	Great toe dorsiflexion	
S1	Lateral and plantar surfaces of the foot	Combines with S2 to plantarly flex the foot (toe walking)	Achilles reflex
S2	Perineal sensation	Combines with S1 to plantarly flex the foot, combines with S3 and S4 for intrinsic foot muscles, the bladder, the external anal sphincter, and the anal wink reflex	
S3	Perineal sensation	Combines with S2 and S4 for intrinsic foot muscles, the bladder, the external anal sphincter, and the anal wink reflex	
S4	Perineal sensation	Combines with S2 and S3 for intrinsic foot muscles, the bladder, the external anal sphincter, and the anal wink reflex	

Physical exam

The physical examination in patients who present with back pain can be accomplished quickly yet thoroughly. It should be directed toward signs of significant pathology, and it should include vital signs and general appearance. In general, patients who present with a benign cause of back pain will lie still and complain of pain that worsens with movement. Patients who are writhing and very uncomfortable are concerning for more serious causes of back pain such as aortic aneurysm, spinal infection, or nephrolithiasis [3]. A pulmonary and abdominal exam should be completed on all patients, evaluating for intra-thoracic or intra-abdominal causes for pain.

The back evaluation should begin with an inspection of the skin looking for signs of infection, trauma, or rashes. This is followed by palpation of the back, spine, and paraspinal muscles. Focal spinal tenderness is common in cases of fractures or infection, although absence of this sign does not rule these conditions out [1]. If the patient is able, they should perform four ranges of motion with the back. This would include side flexion to the right and left, flexion, and extension. Performing these motions will provide information about patient range of motion, symmetry, and reproduction of pain [12]. Hip joints should be carefully assessed as hip pathology can mimic low back pain [7].

Straight-leg and crossed straight-leg tests are also important tests in patients with back pain. To perform these tests, the patient lies supine with the knees fully extended. Each leg is individually raised to 70° elevation. A positive straight leg test occurs when the patient experiences radicular pain that radiates below the knee into one or both legs. This pain is improved by decreasing the elevation and worsened by ankle dorsiflexion. A positive crossed straight-leg test occurs when the patient experiences radicular pain below the knee in the affected leg while raising the asymptomatic leg [1,14].

Probably the most important aspect of a complete back pain physical exam is the neurologic evaluation. It is important to assess each of the spinal nerve roots. Sensation, motor function, and plantar and Achilles deep tendon reflexes should all be assessed. See Table 16.1 for a complete list of the lumbar and sacral nerve roots and their innervations.

The final aspect of a complete physical evaluation in elderly patients with back pain is a rectal exam. This will evaluate for rectal tone and sensation, for prostatic and rectal masses, and for perirectal abscesses. A rectal exam is not necessary in all patients who present with back pain, but should be performed in patients with severe pain or in those who have neurologic complaints or deficits [1,3].

Physical exam findings that should be red flags for serious causes of back pain include fever, hypotension or extreme hypertension, pale appearance, pulsatile abdominal mass, spinous process tenderness, focal neurologic signs, saddle anesthesia with decreased anal sphincter tone, and acute urinary retention [2,3].

Diagnostic tests

Diagnostic tests have a very high false positive rate in elderly patients, and interpretation of these tests in such patients can be challenging. Because of this, the history and physical examination remain the most helpful tools in the assessment of back pain in the elderly [12].

Nearly one in two patients who present to a US emergency department with back pain will have some sort of diagnostic testing done. In particular, the use of computed tomography (CT) or magnetic resonance imaging (MRI) in these patients has tripled from 2002 to 2006 [16]. However, most patients who present to the ED with back pain do not require further diagnostic testing. If there are any concerning features in their history or physical exam, or if they continue to have pain after 4–6 weeks of conservative management, further testing is warranted [3,17].

Laboratory testing

In patients who have concerning features for tumor or infection, a complete blood count (CBC), erythrocyte sedimentation rate (ESR), C-reactive protein (CRP), and urinalysis (UA) should be obtained [1,18]. Other tests such as blood cultures, calcium, and alkaline phosphatase may also be considered in the appropriate circumstances [3].

Plain spinal radiographs

Plain X-rays are rarely helpful in the emergent evaluation of back pain [3,19]. However, in the elderly patient, they can be more helpful than they are in younger patients as they can show some of the pathology more associated with older patients including vertebral compression fractures, advanced malignancy or infection, spondylolisthesis, or features associated with an unstable lumbar spine [6,12].

CT

Computed tomography is very useful for evaluating bony detail of the spine. It also can be used to identify infections, neoplasms, aortic pathology, renal calculi, and other abdominal pathology. However, CT does not visualize the subarachnoid space well, and cannot accurately diagnose spinal cord or nerve root impingement [17,18]. If MRI is unavailable or contraindicated, CT myelography can be used to visualize the subarachnoid space, but requires lumbar puncture for the injection of iodinated contrast [17].

MRI

Magnetic resonance imaging is the gold standard for most emergent causes of back pain [17]. It allows imaging of the spinal canal, the spinal cord, the disk space, and vertebral bodies. It can identify lesions within the bone marrow prior to any cortical destruction. However, MRI is limited in availability, time needed for exam, claustrophobia of patients, and its effects on metal or magnetic objects. This is particularly limiting in the elderly, who may have pacemakers, intra-cardiac wires, certain types of mechanical heart valves, certain types of intracranial aneurysm clips, or other metallic foreign bodies [1,3,20]. In addition, multiple studies have shown that a large percentage of patients who are asymptomatic will have signs of degenerative disk disease and disk herniation on MRI, making clinical correlation of MRI findings essential [12,15].

Differential diagnosis

Mechanical causes

Degenerative disk disease/unstable lumbar spine

Structural degeneration of the lumbar disks can begin in the third decade and is seen radiographically in the majority of patients

over the age of 65. The degree of degenerative disk changes seen on X-ray correlates poorly with patient symptoms [7].

Unstable lumbar spine is a term used to describe a syndrome of back pain frequently seen in older patients. It consists of sharp pain in the lumbar area which is worsened with bending movements and when going from the flexed to the erect position. On physical exam, these patients will often have asymmetric loss of range of motion in the lumbar spine, paraspinal muscle spasm, and weakness of the L4, L5, and S1 innervated muscles. They often have narrowed and sclerotic disk spaces in addition to spondylolisthesis [12].

Imaging or labs are generally not indicated in these patients, and in the absence of concerning findings, a trial of supportive care should be initiated before further diagnostic evaluation is pursued.

Lumbar spinal stenosis

Osteoarthritis in elderly patients can cause osteophytes to intrude centrally on the lumbar spinal canal in the region of the cauda equina and also laterally involving specific nerve roots [7]. While this is frequently seen on imaging, it is only considered clinically significant if the typical symptoms associated with lumbar spinal stenosis are also present [12].

The characteristic history is neurogenic claudication, or pain in the lower back or legs with occasional neurologic deficits after walking. Extension of the spine causes an increase in this pain due to a decreased volume of the spinal canal relative to nerve bulk. Conversely, flexion of the spine causes decreased pain due to an increase in the relative volume of the spinal canal [14]. Positions that extend the spine, such as standing, walking, or going downhill will exacerbate the symptoms. Positions that flex the spine, such as sitting, bending forward, or lying in a flexed position will improve the symptoms [7].

The symptom of pain in the calf muscles with walking is similar to the symptoms associated with arterial insufficiency, and is thus called "pseudoclaudication" [12].

Imaging to evaluate for spinal stenosis is indicated for patients who have the appropriate history and who have progressive neurologic impairment or evidence for systemic disease such as malignancy. CT and MRI will both show the bony margins of the spinal canal; MRI gives the added benefit of evaluation of the spinal cord and nerve roots [7].

In patients with a history consistent with lumbar spinal stenosis who do not have concerning associated neurologic or systemic symptoms, treatment should initially be supportive as up to 90% of patients improve with nonsurgical treatments. Surgical decompression is usually considered based on severity of patient symptoms and limitations in function [7].

Disk displacement causing sciatica

In younger patients with back pain, frequently the inner nucleus pulposus of the intervertebral disk herniates outside of the outer annulus fibrosis, which can produce pain and sciatic symptoms. However, with age comes decreased water content in the nucleus pulposus, and new herniation is infrequent in individuals over the age of 55 [12].

The classic patient who has disk herniation can identify the moment their pain started as a "tearing" or "giving" sensation in their lower back. Their pain is typically exacerbated by increased pressure in the intervertebral disk caused by various positions or movements such as sitting, sneezing, coughing, or straining [7]. Sciatica is very frequently present in these patients [14].

Cauda equina syndrome will occur in 1–2% of disk herniations [14]. The characteristic triad includes acute bowel or bladder sphincter dysfunction, saddle anesthesia, and motor deficits in the lower extremities [7]. The most consistent finding is urinary retention. Anal sphincter tone is diminished in 60–80% of cases [14]. MRI is the imaging modality of choice. Cauda equina syndrome is a surgical emergency and requires immediate surgical consultation.

Patients who have symptoms of a herniated intervertebral disk without symptoms of cauda equina syndrome should undergo at least a 1–2-month trial of conservative therapy prior to surgical referral [7,15].

Osteoporotic causes

Vertebral compression fractures

Compression fractures often occur in the elderly due to the increased prevalence of osteoporosis. It is estimated that there are approximately 500,000 new cases of vertebral compression fractures every year [7]. Often no specific trauma history can be identified. Patients who are white, female, or on long-term corticosteroid therapy are at higher risk for these fractures [14].

The presentation of compression fractures can be variable, and a history of a vertebral compression fracture is a risk factor for future fractures. Mid-thoracic fractures are usually asymptomatic and will result in a gradual thoracic kyphosis. In contrast, fractures in the lower thoracic and lumbar region can often be extremely painful, with constant, severe pain lasting at least two weeks. Generally pain is present in any position and is aggravated by movement [12]. Point tenderness is frequently present over the involved vertebra, as is paraspinal muscle spasm [7].

Patients who have new compression fractures should have a consult from a spine surgeon. In most cases without evidence of neurologic compromise, treatment is supportive. Pain from a compression fracture usually will be decreased 4 weeks post-fracture and resolved by 6–8 weeks [12].

Osteoporotic sacral fractures

Sacral insufficiency fractures occur in older individuals, most commonly women. Fifty percent of these patients will report a history of a fall. They present with dull, low back and buttock pain usually without neurologic deficits. The pain will often be sudden onset and they will be tender in the sacral region. Plain X-rays will often show old pelvic and vertebral compression fractures but no acute sacral fractures. CT scans of the sacrum will usually show a fracture of the anterior border of the sacrum. A spine surgeon should be consulted and treatment is usually supportive [12].

Systemic causes

Primary or metastatic cancer

Malignant neoplasm (either primary or metastatic) is the most common systemic disease affecting the spine, and the spine is the third most common site for cancer to metastasize [3,14]. Although it causes less than 1% of low back pain in the general population, 80% of these patients are over the age of 50, and one-third of them will have had a history of cancer. The most common sources of spinal metastases are the breast, lungs, and prostate [2,12,14].

The most common site of malignant spinal lesions is the thoracic spine (60%), although 30% are located in the lumbar region and 10% in the cervical spine [2]. Typically patients who have back pain from metastatic disease present with gradual onset of progressive pain over weeks or months. It is classically worse at night and when supine [7]. Patients who have had pain for longer than one month, have a history of unexplained weight loss, have an elevated ESR, and who fail to improve with conservative therapy are more likely to have this diagnosis [12,14].

Laboratory tests such as CBC, ESR, CRP, alkaline phosphatase, UA, and serum calcium may be helpful but are not specific. Although plain X-rays are not sensitive for the diagnosis of early metastatic lesions, they are typically the initial imaging test obtained [7,18]. CT can also be used, but MRI is the imaging modality of choice for spinal metastatic lesions, with a sensitivity ranging from 83 to 100% [2].

Patients who are found to have back pain due to malignancy should be treated based on their symptoms. Pain should be controlled with analgesics. Hypercalcemia should be treated with intravenous (IV) fluids and bisphosphonates. Those who have evidence of spinal cord compression or pathologic fractures need emergent oncologic and spine surgery consultation. In addition, those who have evidence of spinal cord compression should be treated with IV corticosteroids as they have been shown to delay neurologic deterioration [2,21].

Spinal infections

Patients who have a history of diabetes, long-term corticosteroid use, organ transplantation, HIV, intravenous drug use, or who are otherwise immunocompromised are at greater risk for an infectious cause of back pain [2].

Spinal infections are usually transmitted from other sites of the body through the blood. Positive blood cultures or a source of infection is only found in approximately 40–50% of cases [22]. Other sites include urinary tract infection, indwelling urinary catheters, skin infections, and injection sites for those who use IV drugs. The presence of fever is highly variable, and should not be used to rule in or rule out infection. Point spine tenderness is 86% sensitive but has low specificity [14]. *Staphylococcus aureus* and Gram-negative bacilli are the most common organisms responsible for infection [7].

Infection of the intervertebral disk can often mimic mechanical causes of back pain. Pain is usually gradual in onset. Patients may have associated fever, weight loss, and night sweats [7]. Spinal epidural abscess is often difficult to diagnose, as the classic triad of spinal pain, fever, and neurologic deficits is seen in less than 15% of patients [23]. Patients who have persistent back pain, especially in the setting of a risk factor for infection, should be evaluated further with blood cultures, ESR, CRP, and CBC. ESR and CRP are elevated in most patients with back infections; however, WBC can be variably elevated. ESR and CRP are often difficult to interpret in the elderly due to low specificity and multiple comorbidities. In addition, normal ESR and CRP do not completely rule out infection as there have been cases of spinal infection in the setting of normal inflammatory markers [2,12,24].

Spinal infections will not be detected on plain X-rays for several weeks to months after the onset of the infection. CT with IV contrast can be used but is limited by a low specificity and a high false-negative rate. MRI is the imaging modality of choice for suspected spinal infections, as even early on it can show signs of edema and inflammation [2,18,20]. In addition, MRI will show the extent of infection which is useful in determining which patients need emergent surgical intervention [25]. MRI should be obtained in patients who have significant risk of infection based on history, exam, and laboratory findings.

Vertebral osteomyelitis without neurologic symptoms can usually be successfully treated with IV antibiotics, spinal immobilization, and analgesics. If neurologic symptoms are present, a spine surgeon should emergently be consulted. Patients who have spinal epidural abscesses also require IV antibiotics, and all should have emergent surgical consultation as surgical decompression and drainage is the standard treatment and delay is associated with risk of permanent neurologic deficits. The prognosis of these patients is based on the degree of neurologic impairment at the time of surgery [2,18,26,27].

Visceral diseases unrelated to the spine

Abdominal aortic aneurysm or aortic dissection

An elderly patient who presents with back pain, abdominal pain, and hypotension should be considered to have an aortic catastrophe until proven otherwise. Risk factors include a history of hypertension, male sex, and a history of tobacco use [2].

The prevalence of AAA increases with age, and approximately 4–8% of individuals over the age of 65 will have an AAA. Most of these patients are asymptomatic with the AAA having been found incidentally. Patients who have a family history of AAA are 30% more likely to develop an AAA [2,28].

Ruptured AAA is the tenth leading cause of death in older men. On arrival these patients often complain of abdominal or back pain. They frequently will appear pale, ashen, or diaphoretic. The classic triad of hypotension, abdominal pain, and a pulsatile abdominal mass occurs in less than 50% of patients who have a ruptured AAA [2,28].

Aortic dissection (AD) is also a vascular emergency. Approximately 5–30 per million will have an AD each year. The classic description of AD is sudden onset of severe sharp pain that is maximal at the time of onset and which is described as

ripping or tearing. Neurologic symptoms are seen in 18–30% of patients with AD [2].

The prognosis for these patients is grim, and high mortality is associated with both conditions. All patients suspected of aortic pathology should be placed on a monitor and have large-bore IV access established. In most centers, CT with IV contrast is the diagnostic test of choice, although MRI and transesophageal echocardiogram can also be used. The location of the CT will depend on the suspected etiology; those with suspected thoracic aortic pathology should have CT with IV contrast of the thorax, those with suspected abdominal aortic pathology should have CT with IV contrast of the abdomen, and CT with IV contrast of the thorax, abdomen, and pelvis should be obtained in those who are suspected of having aortic pathology in multiple anatomic regions [2].

In patients suspected of ruptured AAA, hypotension should be treated with isotonic crystalloid fluids and blood transfusion. In patients suspected of AD, blood pressure should be tightly controlled using IV beta blockers and nitroprusside or another vasodilator. Emergent vascular surgical consultation is essential [2].

Other visceral causes

There are multiple other intra-abdominal diseases which can present with back pain, including pancreatic cancer, disorders of the kidneys such as renal colic or pyelonephritis, and disorders of the gastrointestinal tract. The history of these diseases is often different from mechanical causes of back pain in that they are usually not associated with position, are often progressive, and do not present with the neurologic findings associated with diseases of the lumbar spine.

Treatment

Individual treatments for specific causes of back pain are listed above. If a thorough history, physical exam, and the appropriate diagnostic studies do not indicate the presence of serious or systemic disease, back pain can most likely be attributed to musculoskeletal and nonspecific causes. The majority of these cases are self-limited and pain usually resolves within six weeks of symptom onset [17]. These patients can be reassured and managed with supportive care and close follow-up.

Supportive care includes analgesia, muscle relaxants, and anti-inflammatory medications. Polypharmacy is a frequent cause of morbidity and mortality in the elderly, and all medication decisions should be carefully considered based on patient symptoms, allergies, past medical history, and baseline medications. Acetaminophen is found in multiple combination medications and if taken in excess can be associated with hepatic toxicity [3]. Salicylates and nonsteroidal anti-inflammatory medications should be used with caution in patients with a history of or risks for peptic ulcer, gastrointestinal bleeding, or renal insufficiency. Sedatives and muscle relaxants should be used with caution and under supervision to ensure patient safety, as they have been associated with drowsiness, disequilibrium, and nausea. Narcotics should be used carefully and infrequently due to their association with constipation, fatigue, and altered mental status. They should be reserved for severe pain not relieved by other analgesics, or for severe pain caused by compression fractures or malignancy [3,7,29].

Bed rest does not increase the speed of recovery from back pain and can in fact delay recovery. If a patient receives symptomatic recovery from bed rest, it can be recommended for a few days (no more than two) while reassuring them that it is safe to get out of bed even if pain persists [15,29,30]. Low-level heat wrap therapy may help symptoms and side effects are mild and infrequent [29]. Physical therapy and exercise are not helpful in the acute phase of low back pain, but are frequently used for prevention of recurrent low back pain [15]. No studies have shown efficacy of these interventions in an elderly population [7].

Disposition

Following a complete history and physical examination and the appropriate diagnostic studies, patients can be divided into four main categories. The majority of patients will fall into the first category, which is nonspecific musculoskeletal low back pain. These patients should be managed supportively and can be discharged home with close primary care follow-up.

The second group of patients is those who have a specific mechanical cause of back pain, such as disk herniation or fracture. Those who do not have neurologic compromise will usually be treated supportively. In the case of a new fracture, a spine surgeon should be consulted.

The third category of patients is those who have emergent spinal pathology, including tumor, infection, or any cause of epidural compression. These patients require immediate spine surgery consultation and admission to the hospital, likely in an intensive care setting to ensure frequent serial neurologic evaluations.

The final group of patients is those who have back pain due to a visceral cause. If identified, these visceral causes should be evaluated and treatment and disposition determined on an individual case-by-case basis.

Summary

Back pain is a frequent cause of disability and pain in the elderly, and accounts for frequent physician visits to both EDs and primary care physicians in the US. The great majority of patients who present to the emergency department with back pain have benign causes, and laboratory testing and radiologic imaging are not indicated in most patients. Elderly patients are more likely to have a systemic or critical cause of back pain than younger patients. A thorough history and physical exam, focused on identifying concerning features, can help to identify critical causes of back pain in the elderly patient. If the history or physical exam elicits red flags for significant or emergent causes of back pain, the appropriate diagnostic tests should be obtained and acted upon. While some patients may require consultation and possible admission to the hospital, the majority of patients can be safely discharged home to follow-up with their primary care physicians.

Pearls and pitfalls

Pearls

- Back pain is the third most frequent cause of physician visits in individuals over the age of 65, and restricting back pain among the elderly is very common.
- The great majority of patients who present to the ED with back pain have musculoskeletal and benign causes.
- Elderly patients are much more likely to have a serious or systemic cause of back pain than younger patients.
- Using a thorough, systematic approach for all individuals who present with back pain aids in diagnosing those etiologies of back pain that are associated with high morbidity and mortality.

Pitfalls

- Neglecting to take a complete history can lead to missing red flags when evaluating back pain in the elderly. Historical red flags include gradual onset of pain, pain for more than 6 weeks, medical history of cancer or immunocompromised state, fever, night sweats, unintentional weight loss, isolated thoracic pain, recent infection, recent procedure associated with bacteremia, trauma (even minor), IV drug use, night pain, and unrelenting pain despite supratherapeutic analgesia.
- Neglecting to do a complete physical exam can lead to missing red flags when evaluating back pain in the elderly. Physical exam red flags include fever, pain which causes writhing, bowel or bladder incontinence, new urinary retention, saddle anesthesia, decreased anal sphincter tone, new or progressive neurologic deficit, new motor weakness, a pulsatile abdominal mass, pulse amplitude differences, and spinal process tenderness.
- Most patients who present to the ED with back pain do not require further diagnostic testing. Diagnostic tests have a very high false-positive rate in elderly patients, and interpretation of these tests in elderly patients can be challenging. However, in those who have red flags in their history or physical exam, appropriate diagnostic tests should be obtained.

References

1. Della-Giustina DA. Emergency department evaluation and treatment of back pain. *Emerg Med Clin North Am.* 1999;17:877–93.
2. Winters ME, Kluetz P, Zilberstein J. Back pain emergencies. *Med Clin North Am.* 2006;90:505–23.
3. Corwell BN. The emergency department evaluation, management, and treatment of back pain. *Emerg Med Clin North Am.* 2010;28:811–39.
4. Deyo RA, Mirza SK, Martin BI. Back pain prevalence and visit rates: Estimates from US national surveys, 2002. *Spine (Phila Pa 1976).* 2006;31:2724–7.
5. Waterman BR, Belmont PJ, Jr, Schoenfeld AJ. Low back pain in the United States: Incidence and risk factors for presentation in the emergency setting. *Spine J.* 2012;12:63–70.

6. Weiner AL, MacKenzie RS. Utilization of lumbosacral spine radiographs for the evaluation of low back pain in the emergency department. *J Emerg Med.* 1999;17:229–33.

7. Sauter S, Hadler NM. Back pain in elderly people. In *Oxford Textbook of Geriatric Medicine*, 2nd edn, ed. Evans JG, Williams TF, Beattie BL, et al. (Oxford, UK: University of Oxford Press, 2000), pp. 391–7.

8. Bressler HB, Keyes WJ, Rochon PA, et al. The prevalence of low back pain in the elderly. A systematic review of the literature. *Spine (Phila Pa 1976).* 1999;24:1813–19.

9. Hoy D, Brooks P, Blyth F, et al. The epidemiology of low back pain. *Best Pract Res Clin Rheumatol.* 2010;24:769–81.

10. Makris UE, Fraenkel L, Han L, et al. Epidemiology of restricting back pain in community-living older persons. *J Am Geriatr Soc.* 2011;59:610–14.

11. Freburger JK, Holmes GM, Agans RP, et al. The rising prevalence of chronic low back pain. *Arch Intern Med.* 2009;169:251–8.

12. Hazzard WR, Halter JB. *Hazzard's Geriatric Medicine and Gerontology* (New York: McGraw-Hill Medical, 2009), p. 1634.

13. Knauer SR, Freburger JK, Carey TS. Chronic low back pain among older adults: A population-based perspective. *J Aging Health.* 2010;22:1213–34.

14. Deyo RA, Rainville J, Kent DL. What can the history and physical examination tell us about low back pain? *JAMA.* 1992;268:760–5.

15. Deyo RA, Weinstein JN. Low back pain. *N Engl J Med.* 2001;344:363–70.

16. Friedman BW, Chilstrom M, Bijur PE, et al. Diagnostic testing and treatment of low back pain in US emergency departments. A national perspective. *Spine.* 2010;35:E1406.

17. Miller JC, Palmer WE, Mansfield FL, et al. When is imaging helpful for patients with back pain? *J Am Coll Radiol.* 2006;3:957–60.

18. Arce D, Sass P, Abul-Khoudoud H. Recognizing spinal cord emergencies. *Am Fam Physician.* 2001;64:631–8.

19. Isaacs DM, Marinac J, Sun C. Radiograph use in low back pain: A United States emergency department database analysis. *J Emerg Med.* 2004;26:37–45.

20. Broder J. *Diagnostic Imaging for the Emergency Physician* (London: W.B. Saunders, 2011).

21. Sun H, Nemecek AN. Optimal management of malignant epidural spinal cord compression. *Emerg Med Clin North Am.* 2009;27:195–208.

22. Nikkanen HE, Brown DF, Nadel ES. Low back pain. *J Emerg Med.* 2002;22:279–83.

23. Kulchycki LK, Edlow JA. Geriatric neurologic emergencies. *Emerg Med Clin North Am.* 2006;24:273–98, v–vi.

24. Chelsom J, Solberg CO. Vertebral osteomyelitis at a Norwegian university hospital 1987–97: Clinical features, laboratory findings and outcome. *Scand J Infect Dis.* 1998;30:147–51.

25. Jarvik JG, Deyo RA. Diagnostic evaluation of low back pain with emphasis on imaging. *Ann Intern Med.* 2002;137:586.

26. Davis DP, Wold RM, Patel RJ, et al. The clinical presentation and impact of diagnostic delays on emergency department patients with spinal epidural abscess. *J Emerg Med.* 2004;26:285–91.

27. Schmidt RD, Markovchick V. Nontraumatic spinal cord compression. *J Emerg Med.* 1992;10:189–99.

28. Salen P, Melanson S, Buro D. ED screening to identify abdominal aortic aneurysms in asymptomatic geriatric patients. *Am J Emerg Med.* 2003;21:133–5.

29. Linklater DR, Pemberton L, Taylor S, et al. Painful dilemmas: An evidence-based look at challenging clinical scenarios. *Emerg Med Clin North Am.* 2005;23:367–92.

30. Frymoyer JW. Back pain and sciatica. *N Engl J Med.* 1988;318:291–300.

Chapter

17

Eye, ear, nose, and throat emergencies in the elderly

Kara Iskyan Geren

Introduction

This chapter will cover geriatric eye, ear, nose, and throat emergencies. The topics covered include acute angle closure glaucoma, vitreous hemorrhage, retinal detachment, uveitis, conjunctivitis, central retinal artery occlusion, branch retinal artery occlusion, central retinal vein occlusion, branch retinal vein occlusion, giant cell arteritis, otitis externa, malignant otitis externa, epistaxis, dental abscess, Ludwig's angina, peritonsillar abscess, epiglottitis, retropharyngeal abscess, and angioedema from angiotensin-converting enzyme inhibitors.

Eye

Vision loss is one of the most feared complications of aging. Unfortunately it is very common, with visual impairment in 1 out of every 28 people older than the age of 40 years. In the US, adults older than 80 years account for only 8% of the population but 70% of the cases of severe visual impairment. The consequences of visual impairment in the elderly can be severe. These patients are more likely to be institutionalized and are at increased risk for depression, social isolation, and falls [1].

Acute angle closure glaucoma

Acute angle closure glaucoma (AACG) occurs when a blockage of aqueous humor flow produces increased intraocular pressure resulting in the loss of vision. In contrast to other glaucomas, such as chronic angle closure glaucoma and primary open angle glaucoma, symptoms are sudden, severe, and require immediate attention to prevent permanent vision loss.

As the US population ages, emergency medicine physicians will encounter AACG more frequently. The overall incidence of AACG is about 1 in 1000 people over the age of 40 [2]. It is primarily a disease of the elderly, with the peak incidence being between the ages of 55 and 70 [3]. Women are more commonly affected than men [4].

Normally the ciliary process of the eye, in the posterior chamber, produces the aqueous humor. The aqueous humor passes through the pupil, between the lens and the iris, and into the anterior chamber, where it is filtered through a trabecular meshwork. It drains into the canal of Schlemm [4]. In AACG, the pupil is partially dilated causing contact between the iris

and lens. This impedes the movement of the aqueous humor causing a build-up in the posterior chamber of the eye. As the aqueous humor collects, the pressure causes a forward bowing of the iris, closing the already narrow iridocorneal angle. Persistently elevated intraocular pressures cause rapidly progressive and potentially permanent vision loss [5,6].

The first pathologic step of AACG is partial pupillary dilation. Triggers of this mid-dilation include dim ambient lighting, accommodation (such as in reading), and medications. Topical mydriatics, especially in diabetics, may cause partial rather than full dilation of the pupil due to autonomic neuropathy. Systemic anticholinergics, tricyclic antidepressants, selective serotonin reuptake inhibitors, and adrenergic agonists can also cause pupillary dilation resulting in AACG [3,6].

The elderly are at risk for AACG because of lens enlargement that occurs with age. The bigger lens pushes the iris against the cornea, constricting the iridocorneal angle even further. Other anatomic conditions, such as myopia, a shallow anterior chamber, and a narrow iridocorneal angle, also increase the likelihood of aqueous humor blockage. Additional risk factors for AACG include Asian descent, female gender, diabetes, hypertension, pre-existing elevated intraocular pressure, and a family history of a first-degree relative with glaucoma [5,7,8].

The typical AACG presentation is a severe, sudden, unilateral, frontal headache with abdominal pain, nausea, and vomiting. The red eye is acutely painful with blurry and decreased vision. There are often halos around lights due to corneal edema [3,4,6]. Symptoms are unilateral unless the cause of pupillary dilation is a systemic medication [3].

About half of patients have preceding, intermittent episodes of headache from partial or temporary AACG. These headaches often occur at night, when light is dim, and are aborted by pupillary constriction from bright light or sleep [3,5]. Unfortunately AACG, especially in the elderly, is often misdiagnosed because systemic symptoms are more prominent than the ocular complaint [3].

Physical examination of AACG uncovers a partially dilated, fixed pupil with a cloudy or steamy cornea. There is prominent conjunctival injection, especially around the limbus, from vascular congestion. On palpation the globe is "rock hard" and tender. Measured intraocular pressure is greater than 30 mmHg. Fundoscopic examination may show optic nerve cupping. Slit lamp examination may uncover keratitic precipitates, anterior chamber cells and flare, posterior synechiae, and a shallow anterior chamber [3–6].

Given the systemic symptoms of AACG, many other conditions may be on the differential diagnosis. These include migraine headaches, temporal arteritis, subarachnoid hemorrhage, and intra-abdominal emergency [4]. Increased intraocular pressure of AACG should not be confused with glaucomatocyclitic crisis, inflammatory open-angle glaucoma, and pigmentary glaucoma [6].

The goals of treatment of AACG are to reduce intraocular pressure and preserve vision [3]. Vision loss associated with AACG occurs within hours so timely treatment is key. Prompt consultation with an ophthalmologist helps guide immediate treatment and arrange for definitive surgery such as an iridotomy, iridectomy, or trabeculectomy [3,5].

Analgesics and antiemetics make the patient more comfortable but should not delay medications to decrease intraocular pressure [9].

There are five main medication groups used to treat AACG. Topical beta blockers, such as timolol, lower intraocular pressure by reducing aqueous humor production by as much as 40% within 30–60 minutes. As with systemic beta blockers, caution is suggested if the patient has a history of reactive airway disease or cardiac disease. Carbonic anhydrase inhibitors also decrease aqueous humor production by preventing bicarbonate, produced by the ciliary epithelium, from entering the posterior chamber. Before the carbonic anhydrase inhibitor is effective, however, 99% of the enzyme must be inhibited. Topical carbonic anhydrase inhibitors, such as dorzolamide and brinzolamide, are optimal because they have fewer systemic side effects. If topical carbonic anhydrase inhibitors are not effective, an oral preparation, such as acetazolamide, can be used. The third medication used to treat AACG is a miotic drug such as pilocarpine. Increased pupillary constriction widens the anterior chamber angles and restores aqueous outflow. Results may not be seen until the intraocular pressure is below 50 mmHg, when the ischemic paralysis of the iris is relieved. Fourth, topical steroids reduce intraocular inflammation. In the event that the previous medications do not adequately decrease intraocular pressure, hyperosmotic agents, such as intravenous mannitol or oral glycerol, should be used. The blood–ocular barrier prevents the hyperosmotic agents from entering the aqueous fluid. As a result, the osmolality of the intravascular fluid causes a shift of fluid from the aqueous humor into the vasculature. Unfortunately the effects of hyperosmotic medications are systemic so there must be vigilance for complications such as fluid overload in patients with impaired cardiac function, electrolyte abnormalities in renal patients, and hyperglycemia in diabetics receiving glycerol [6,9,10].

Medications should be instilled into the eye concurrently. Repeat the intraocular pressure one hour after initial treatment to confirm an improvement. Continue medical therapy until the intraocular pressure decreases or definitive surgical treatment occurs [3].

Vitreous hemorrhage

Vitreous humor is a clear, gelatinous substance that fills the center of the eye. It attaches to the retina along the course of major retinal vessels and does not regenerate. When blood enters the vitreous fluid it is called vitreous hemorrhage (VH). Although it is not common, with an incidence of 7 cases per 100,000 people, VH is largely a disease of the elderly [2,11].

In younger people the cause of VH is generally trauma. In contrast, VH in the geriatric population is commonly due to posterior vitreous detachment, proliferative diabetic retinopathy, and retinal vein occlusion. These are further discussed below because the cause of VH determines the treatment. There are other causes of VH that are far less frequent, examples being retinal arterial macroaneurysm (in elderly women with hypertension), Terson's syndrome (which occurs after a subarachnoid hemorrhage), and age-related macular degeneration (producing a subretinal hemorrhage that spreads) [11–13].

Posterior vitreous detachment occurs when the vitreous body undergoes syneresis, a normal age-related change that renders the vitreous body more like liquid than gel. As a result, the posterior vitreous cortex separates from the retina causing VH. Most of these cases involve retinal tears that, if left untreated, may develop into retinal detachment. Proliferative diabetic retinopathy and retinal vein occlusion produce VH through retinal ischemia. In proliferative diabetic retinopathy, ischemia produces angiogenic factors that stimulate new, fragile blood vessels. When tugged on, due to vitreous shrinkage or movement of the globe, the weak blood vessels bleed. Proliferative diabetic retinopathy accounts for most VHs in diabetics. The first sign of a retinal vein occlusion may be VH [11,12].

The pathognomonic presentation of VH is "hundreds of tiny black specks appearing before the eye" [2]. There is a sudden appearance of floaters that progresses to painless loss of vision. The degree of vision loss depends on the amount of hemorrhage and may change with head position. If posterior vitreous detachment occurs, there may be a sensation of flashing lights, or photopsia [2,11].

Usually the vitreous body is clear and transparent. In VH there may be a reddish haze that makes fundoscopy difficult or impossible. Measurement of the intraocular pressure of the affected eye and inspection of the unaffected eye may provide clues to the underlying cause of VH. As the retina is often obscured by blood, ultrasound can determine whether there is an underlying retinal tear or retinal detachment. It can also help determine whether the blood of the VH is old or new [11,13].

Management of VH is tailored to the underlying cause. A timely consultation with an ophthalmologist should determine the course of action. If there is a concern for retinal detachment or the emergency medicine physician can not adequately evaluate for retinal detachment, the ophthalmologic evaluation is emergent. Early surgery for patients with retinal tears and detachment improves outcomes. If there is no retinal tear or detachment, the VH may be allowed to clear spontaneously. This is a slow, constant process that takes weeks and is used in diseases that will not cause rebleeding. The patient's head should remain elevated. If, despite thorough evaluation, there is a chance that a retinal tear or detachment was missed, the patient should undergo serial ultrasound.

Patients with proliferative diabetic retinopathy should undergo laser photocoagulation when the retina becomes visible. Tight sugar and blood pressure control should also be established. In the event that VH recurs, a vitrectomy may be needed. Complications such as ghost cell glaucoma (degenerating red blood cells blocking the trabecular meshwork) and blurring of the vision due to slow clearing of the blood can also be managed through vitrectomy [11,13].

Retinal detachment

Retinal detachment (RD) is the separation of the neurosensory layer of the retina from the underlying choroid and retinal pigment epithelium [14]. While it afflicts all age groups, RD is most common in the elderly. Over half of people in their 8th decade of life have experienced RD. It is relatively uncommon affecting 1–2 people in 10,000 people per year or 1 in 300 over a lifetime. RD causes irreversible blindness much less frequently compared with other retinal diseases like diabetic retinopathy and macular degeneration [15,16].

There are three main mechanisms that result in RD. Exudative, or serous, RD results from hydrostatic factors (such as severe acute hypertension) or inflammation (such as HLA-B27-associated uveitis). This causes an accumulation of serous and/or hemorrhagic fluid in the subretinal space. Tractional RD occurs when a centripetal mechanical force pulls on fibroid tissue attached to the retina. The fibrotic tissue is from previous damage to the retina. The most common form of RD is rhegmatogenous. With age, the vitreous humor undergoes liquefaction. This causes the vitreous trabecular network to pull on the retina. The posterior vitreous detachment creates a retinal tear that allows vitreous fluid to enter the subretinal space, causing further dissection. The severity of rhegmatogenous RD depends on the amount of retina that has detached from the underlying components. It usually begins in the periphery and travels towards the macula. If untreated, rhegmatogenous RD eventually reaches the macula, causing central vision loss [15–17].

The most common risk factors for RD are age, myopia, and previous cataract surgery. With age the vitreous humor shrinks, making detachment more likely. Patients with myopia, or nearsightedness, have a thinner retina that is more susceptible to centripetal forces. Myopics suffer RD earlier in adulthood. Previous cataract surgery accelerates the shrinkage and detachment of the vitreous humor, causing about 1% of patients with that surgical history to develop RD [14,15].

The initial symptom of RD is usually unilateral photopsia. If vitreous hemorrhage is involved, there are floaters in the vision. Vision loss starts in the periphery where the retina is the thinnest. Patients may not notice the visual field defect for hours to weeks. When the RD begins to involve the macula, the vision loss may be described as curtain-like or cloudy. The retina does not have any pain receptors so there is no sensation of pain or tearing associated with RD [14–17].

On physical examination, a patient with RD may have an abnormal red reflex. Fundoscopic examination may reveal a billowing retina described as ballooning, flapping, or fluttering waves. If there is vitreous hemorrhage or posterior vitreous detachment, there may be floaters in the vitreous humor making it difficult to see the retina. A normal direct ophthalmoscope examination, however, cannot exclude the diagnosis of RD because the narrow view may miss the peripheral retina [2,16,18]. Ultrasound is sensitive for retinal detachment; the few false positives are usually vitreous hemorrhage. On ultrasound, RD will appear as an echogenic band suspended in the vitreous of the eye [19].

The definitive treatment for RD is surgery. Without surgery, every eye with RD will become blind [17]. The surgical procedures performed by retinal specialists to fix RD include laser photocoagulation, cryotherapy, scleral buckle, pneumatic retinopexy, expanding gases, air injection, silicone oil injections, and vitrectomy. If definitive treatment for RD occurs prior to macular involvement, the visual acuity often returns to predetachment levels. If the macula is already involved, final visual acuity varies from complete recovery to blindness. As a result, surgery is most urgent in those with preserved central vision at the time of diagnosis [15–17].

In the emergency department (ED) an ophthalmologist should be consulted, even if the diagnosis is not confirmed. Depending on the patient's symptoms, definitive treatment may be immediate or delayed. There should be restriction of physical activity and reduction of eye movement. Bilateral eye patching can help decrease eye movements. When lying down, the patient should lie with their face on the side of the detachment to the pillow to prevent extension to the macula [17,18].

Uveitis

Uveitis is the inflammation of the uveal tissues, which includes the iris, ciliary body, and choroid. It can be further categorized by the location of inflammation: anterior uveitis (involving the iris and/or ciliary body), intermediate uveitis (involving the vitreous humor, peripheral retina, and/or posterior ciliary body), posterior uveitis (involving the choroid), and panuveitis. Anterior uveitis accounts for the vast majority of all uveitis cases and will be the main focus of this section [20–22].

Uveitic diseases are significant as they account for 10% of blindness in the Western world [23,24]. Previously thought to be a disease of the young and middle aged [3,20], recent studies concluded that uveitis in the elderly is more common than expected. The incidence is 341 cases per 100,000 Medicare beneficiaries [22,24].

The traditional teaching was that uveitis in an elderly patient was a masquerade for a malignant disease, namely ocular lymphoma. However as uveitis in the geriatric population was further studied, malignant disease accounted for a very small fraction of total cases [20,21]. Similar to younger adults, about half of all geriatric anterior uveitis cases remain idiopathic [21,23]. The causes of anterior uveitis are classified as nongranulomatous or granulomatous. Nongranulomatous causes of anterior uveitis are mainly autoimmune disorders such as HLA-B27 ankylosing spondylitis and inflammatory bowel disease. Reiter's syndrome or reactive arthritis is rare in the elderly [20,21]. Granulomatous anterior uveitis causes include syphilis, tuberculosis, herpes, varicella zoster, sarcoidosis, toxoplasmosis, and lens-induced [25].

Anterior uveitis presents with unilateral deep, dull, aching, or throbbing eye pain from ciliary muscle spasm. The pain often radiates to the periorbital or temple area. Blurring of the vision, one of the most common symptoms, is due to the turbidity of the aqueous humor. Photophobia and tearing or watering of the eye is often present. Nongranulomatous anterior uveitis is usually acute while the granulomatous conditions have a more insidious onset [6,25,26].

The hallmarks of an anterior uveitis physical examination are erythema throughout the cornea, with a focus on the limbus, and inflammatory cells and flare (protein extravasation from inflamed blood vessels) in the anterior chamber. The affected pupil is often constricted, irregular, and may be slow to respond to light compared with the other eye. There is both direct and consensual photophobia. Severe or HLA-B27-related cases may have hypopyons. Intraocular pressure varies but is more likely to be elevated in a chronic uveitis. Keratic precipitates, cellular deposits on the corneal endothelium, are small and fine with nongranulomatous uveitis. In comparison, granulomatous uveitis has large, yellow (or mutton fat), keratic precipitates with iris nodules at the pupillary margin [6,20,25,26].

The work-up of the geriatric patient with anterior uveitis in the ED is dictated by the presentation. If the disease is mild without visual disturbance, referral to ophthalmology is appropriate [26]. The first episode of nongranulomatous anterior uveitis or herpes zoster associated uveitis does not require further investigation. If symptoms are acute and severe, further investigation in the ED is warranted. Evaluation for syphilis, viruses (specifically herpes, cytomegalovirus (CMV), and Epstein–Barr virus), toxoplasmosis, and tuberculosis should be started [25,27].

Anterior uveitis can be managed medically, reserving surgical intervention for later complications. The general goals for anterior uveitis treatment are to preserve visual acuity, decrease ocular pain, and prevent later complications. Treatment decisions should be made in conjunction with an ophthalmologist given the broad differential and need for timely follow-up. If the cause for anterior uveitis is not considered to be infectious, topical steroids decrease inflammation. Mydriatics and cycloplegics relieve the ciliary spasm, which improves the eye pain and avoids adhesions between the pupil and the lens (synechiae). Nonsteroidal anti-inflammatories (NSAIDs) should be used for pain control [6,25].

The complications of anterior uveitis are cataracts, secondary glaucoma, posterior synechiae, retinal detachment, and chronic uveitis [6]. Despite these long-term complications, about half of patients maintain normal visual acuity. Others will progress to near complete blindness [21].

Intermediate uveitis is rare compared with anterior uveitis. The major site of inflammation is the vitreous humor although the posterior retina and posterior ciliary body can be involved. Patients may have minimal symptoms, floaters, and/or blurred vision. The anterior chamber may not have signs of inflammation. Vitreous snowballs, yellow–white inflammatory aggregates, and snowbanks, exudates on the pars plana, are common. Causes and treatment of intermediate uveitis are similar to those of anterior uveitis [28].

Posterior uveitis involves inflammation of the vitreous humor, optic nerve head, retinal vessels, and/or choroid. While there are numerous non-infective causes of posterior uveitis, toxoplasmosis accounts for nearly 25% of posterior uveitis cases in immunocompetent patients. Immunosuppressed patients are at risk for herpes, CMV, and tuberculous posterior uveitis. Symptoms and physical findings depend on the area of greatest inflammation and the cause of posterior uveitis. Thorough investigation of the cause of posterior uveitis often uncovers a serious underlying problem that provides the basis of treatment [29].

Conjunctivitis

Conjunctivitis is the inflammation of the membrane that lines both the outer aspect of the globe (known as the bulbar conjunctiva) and the palpebral conjunctiva, which reflects back to line the inner eyelid [6]. The most common causes of acute conjunctivitis are allergic and infectious while mechanical, irritative, and immune-mediated mechanisms are more likely to cause subacute and chronic conjunctivitis [6]. Underlying ophthalmologic conditions, such as chronic dry eyes and senile entropion, as well as a decrease in the amount and quality of tear film (which contains numerous immune defense mechanisms) puts geriatric patients at risk for conjunctivitis [30]. Nearly 30% of all eye complaints presenting to the ED are conjunctivitis [6].

Infectious conjunctivitis is viral or bacterial. Viral conjunctivitis is overwhelmingly due to adenovirus, however herpes simplex and varicella are noteworthy causes with potentially significant complications. In adults, bacterial conjunctivitis is usually due to *Haemophilus influenzae* or *Staphylococcus aureus* [30–32].

The hallmark signs and symptoms of acute infective conjunctivitis are a red eye with discharge and minimal to no visual disturbance [30,33]. Infectious conjunctivitis starts unilateral but within a few days is usually bilateral [26]. An upper respiratory tract infection prodrome, a known sick contact, and preauricular lymphadenopathy are common for viral conjunctivitis [31]. No history of previous conjunctivitis and a lack of pruritis point to a bacterial cause. A bacterial cause is also more likely, by an odds ratio of 15:1, if both eyes are glued shut with discharge in the morning [30]. Beyond these, there are few other clinical predictors to help differentiate between viral and bacterial conjunctivitis [33]. As a result, multiple studies have shown that clinicians are accurate only 40–75% of the time in distinguishing between viral and bacterial conjunctivitis [31].

The physical examination of infectious conjunctivitis reveals chemosis and eye discharge of varying colors and quantities. There may be large subconjunctival hemorrhages and significant soft tissue swelling. Complaints or findings of severe pain, decreased vision, or a hazy cornea are not consistent with infectious conjunctivitis and should prompt a different diagnosis [30,33].

The mainstay of treatment for infectious conjunctivitis is eye care, preventing transmission and, potentially, antibiotics. Patients should cleanse the eyes frequently with sterile water and cotton balls. Warm water compresses may help symptoms. All eye drop bottles, whether over-the-counter lubricant or prescription, should be replaced in case of contamination. Contacts should be disposed of or thoroughly cleaned as described by the manufacturer. A new contact lens case should be used [30,34].

Conjunctivitis, especially that caused by adenovirus, is extremely contagious as it is transmitted through hands, medical instruments, and even swimming pools [6]. Patients and their families should be counseled to wash hands frequently, use separate towels, and avoid close contact with others while contagious. When patients can return to school or work is unclear. Adequately treated bacterial conjunctivitis may no longer be infectious after 24 hours while viral conjunctivitis may be contagious for 7–14 days. This decision is best made on an individual basis depending on patient circumstances (compliance with avoiding eye contact and performing hand hygiene, contact with immunosuppressed), duration of symptoms, use of antibiotics, and apparent infectivity of strain (current outbreak) [33].

The use of topical antibiotics to treat infectious conjunctivitis is a source of debate. Secondary bacterial infections as a consequence of viral conjunctivitis are infrequent so antibiotics are not needed for viral conjunctivitis [31]. About 70% of cases of bacterial conjunctivitis resolve spontaneously within 8 days without major complications. Antibiotics reduce the duration of clinical illness by 0.5 to 1.5 days [33]. Additionally, antibiotics reduce the risk of relapse, prevent complications (such as orbital cellulitis, keratitis, and panophthalmitis), and reduce transmission to others [30,32]. On the other hand, treatment with antibiotics produces further antibiotic resistance, is expensive, may delay a non-infective diagnosis, and may cause antibiotic-associated complications such as an allergic reaction [34].

A middle ground on this debate may be a strategy of delayed antibiotic use, similar to that of treating children with acute otitis media. After providing conjunctivitis education, a prescription for topical antibiotics can be provided to be filled 2–3 days after the diagnosis. The patient is to fill the prescription for worsening or persistent symptoms. Clinically this reduces antibiotic use and reduces future visits for conjunctivitis [34]. The key to this strategy is education. A study in the United Kingdom outlined that patients did not know that conjunctivitis was self-limited and welcomed the potential of avoiding antibiotics [33].

There are many choices for a topical antibiotic to treat infectious conjunctivitis. No significant differences have been found in clinical outcomes with different agents. The options range from an aminoglycoside to a fluoroquinolone. Cost, local resistance patterns, and side effects should be considered when choosing an antibiotic [30]. Drops are generally recommended for adults as they are easier to apply and do not blur vision [6].

Patients should follow up in 3–4 days if there is not improvement in symptoms. In addition to another evaluation and examination, a conjunctival culture may be required at that time.

Allergic conjunctivitis, also known as hay fever conjunctivitis, is often seasonal or in response to allergens such as dust or pet dander. It is common, with nearly a fifth of the US population suffering from allergic ophthalmologic symptoms. In addition to itchy, watery, red eyes, near half of patients with allergic conjunctivitis complain of allergic rhinitis as well. Treatment consists of avoiding allergy triggers, cold compresses, over-the-counter vasoconstrictors, ocular NSAIDs, and oral antihistamines [6,35].

Central retinal artery occlusion

An interruption of blood flow to the retina, or central retinal artery occlusion (CRAO), is a painless, ocular stroke that can cause permanent, severe vision loss. Unfortunately even with early recognition, the treatment for CRAO remains unclear with variable outcomes [14].

The retina is perfused by the retinal artery, which is a branch of the ophthalmic artery. The ophthalmic artery branches off from the internal carotid artery. Interruption of blood flow through the ophthalmic artery occurs from embolic, thrombotic, and rheumatologic disorders. Patients less than 40 years old are more likely to have a systemic disorder, such as cardiac valvular disease, collagen vascular disease, or hypercoagulable disorder as the cause of CRAO. In older patients, atherosclerotic disease of the ipsilateral carotid artery is a common cause of CRAO. Giant cell arteritis (GCA) is thought to account for 5–10% of cases in the elderly. Given these causes, risk factors for CRAO include age greater than 70 years old, hypertension, hypercholesterolemia, diabetes, elevated homocysteine levels, and tobacco use. CRAO is usually unilateral. The incidence of acute CRAO is thought to be about 1 per 100,000 people [2,14,16,36].

Patients with CRAO have a dramatic, sudden onset of painless monocular vision loss that is nearly complete. Sometimes there is a history of amaurosis fugax (transient unilateral vision loss) or "stuttering" vision loss as the embolus moves along the vascular tree. Some patients have additional perfusion of the retina through the cilioretinal artery. This anatomic variant preserves central vision in CRAO [2,14,16].

On examination, CRAO produces a complete or relative afferent papillary defect due to ischemia of the ganglion cells. The pupil may be dilated and react sluggishly to light. Fundoscopic exam may reveal a cherry red spot on a ground glass retina with boxcarring. In 90% of patients with permanent CRAO, the cherry red spot is the fovea which maintains its bright red appearance as its blood supply, from the choroidal or ciliary circulation, is still intact. About half of patients will have an opacified retina as it turns to a pale yellow–white hue due to ischemia and eventually necrosis. Boxcarring occurs in about 20% of patients; this is due to Rouleau stacking of red blood cells as the serum separates in the retinal artery. Lastly, in patients with an embolus as the cause of CRAO, the clot may be visible as a shiny iridescent cholesterol plaque, gray platelet deposit, or bright white calcium fragment [2,14,16].

Central retinal artery occlusion can be confused with many conditions. Other conditions of ocular origin, such as central retinal vein occlusion, vitreous hemorrhage, and retinal detachment have monocular vision loss with different physical examination findings. Systemic conditions, such as heart failure and hypertensive emergencies, may cause a low flow state, decreasing retinal artery perfusion. Migraines may also be blamed for CRAO symptoms [14].

A true ocular emergency, retinal ischemia from CRAO for more than 4 hours can lead to massive, irreversible vision loss. Restoring blood flow to the retina in the first 100 minutes may preserve vision, however, treatment remains beneficial up to 48 hours after the beginning of symptoms [36]. After identification of CRAO, ophthalmology should be consulted. Unfortunately even with prompt recognition and consultation, there is no standard medical therapy for CRAO that has proven clinical benefit. Without any treatment about 1–8% of patients with CRAO will have spontaneous improvement of vision. Many treatments for CRAO have been proposed and are used despite lack of clear evidence. These include: dilation of the retinal artery (through sublingual isosorbide dinitrate, rebreathing expired carbon dioxide, or breathing a fixed mixture of 95% oxygen and 5% carbon dioxide), physical removal of the obstruction (through massage of the eyeball over a closed lid), increased perfusion pressure by decreasing intraocular pressure (by anterior chamber paracentesis, trabeculectomy, or IV acetazolamide or mannitol), thrombolysis (local or systemic), antiplatelet medications, decreasing red blood cell rigidity (with pentoxifylline), systemic steroids, and enhanced external counter pulsation (EECP) [2,14,16,36]. Systemic steroids are thought to work at times because a portion of CRAO is due to GCA [2]. EECP involves inflating and deflating pneumonic cuffs on the lower extremities in order to change systemic hemodynamics. A Cochrane Review found only two randomized controlled trials and concluded that neither provided sufficient evidence for routine use of pentoxifylline or EECP [36]. Ultimately the visual acuity at presentation of CRAO is most predictive of the eventual vision changes [16].

After the acute management of CRAO, an evaluation to determine the underlying cause may include carotid ultrasonography, cardiac echocardiography, and hypercoagulable blood work [14]. The 5-year mortality for patients with CRAO is 5.5 years compared with that of 15.4 years for age-matched controls without CRAO [2]. This underscores the importance of diet and lifestyle modifications and treatment of hypercholesterolemia, hypertension, and diabetes to prevent CRAO and further ischemic events [14].

Branch retinal artery occlusion

Branch retinal artery occlusion (BRAO) occurs after the bifurcation of the central retinal artery. It is not mentioned as often as CRAO as it is less prevalent. Despite the difference in occlusion location, BRAO and CRAO have many similarities [37].

The pathophysiology between BRAO and CRAO is nearly identical with BRAO usually due to embolism. Unlike CRAO, however, BRAO is not associated with GCA because branch retinal arteries are actually arterioles. By definition, GCA is a disease of medium and large arteries, not arterioles [38].

Like CRAO, BRAO can be transient or permanent. On fundoscopic examination there is often boxcarring [38]. There is no proven treatment for BRAO. A thorough work-up for an underlying cause of BRAO is like that of CRAO. This may help prevent the development of recurrent BRAO, CRAO, or strokes [37,38]. Unless the fovea is involved in the area of ischemia, BRAO has a better visual prognosis than that of CRAO. Without treatment, 80–90% of patients with BRAO have a visual acuity better than 20/40 [37,38].

Recurrent BRAO is rare. One cause receiving increased attention is Susac's syndrome. Susac's syndrome, an autoimmune microangiopathy of the precapillary arterioles of the brain, retina, and inner ear, affects mainly young women with the triad of encephalopathy, BRAO, and hearing loss. On fundoscopic examination there are Gass plaques, yellow–white deposits in the midsegments of the arteriole. On magnetic resonance imaging (MRI) there are microinfarcts of the corpus callosum. Diagnosis often remains elusive and treatment is immunosuppression [37].

Central retinal vein occlusion

Retinal vein occlusion is the second most common retinal vascular disorder after diabetic retinopathy. The retinal vein system can be divided into multiple branches including the central vein, hemicentral vein, major branch vein, and macular branch vein. Occlusion can occur at any of these locations, however the most common sites are the central and branch veins [16,39,40].

About 2.5 million adults worldwide were affected by CRVO in 2008 [40], with a prevalence of about 5.2 per 1000 people in the US [41]. CRVO occurs mainly in middle-aged and elderly patients with a history of hypertension, diabetes, atherosclerotic disease, dyslipidemia, high body mass index, and smoking [39,41]. Only 10–15% of patients with CRVO are under the age of 40 [40].

The central retinal artery and vein share an adventitial sheath as they exit the optic nerve head. The opening in the lamina cribrosa through which the sheath travels is narrow [2]. The collagen tissue of the lamina cribrosa becomes thicker and stiffer with age. This, along with degenerative changes in the central retinal artery, causes compression of the retinal vein. The turbulent flow from venous compression increases the risk of endoluminal thrombus formation [40,41]. As a result, CRVO can be divided into non-ischemic and ischemic subtypes. The emergency physician does not need to differentiate between the two CRVO subtypes. Ophthalmology will determine whether the CVRO is ischemic or non-ischemic as prognosis and management differs. Patients may also progress from non-ischemic to ischemic CRVO [2,16,41].

Non-ischemic CRVO, also known as venous stasis retinopathy, presents with vague blurring of the central vision with sparing of peripheral vision. It is worse in the morning and gradually improves throughout the day. The lesion is more proximal, so some patients are relatively asymptomatic due to collateral retinal circulation. Visual acuity is often around

20/30 and nearly always better than 20/200 [2,16,41]. In contrast, ischemic CRVO is a dramatic loss of vision, often upon awakening in the morning. It can be preceded by episodes of amaurosis fugax. Visual acuity is much worse than in non-ischemic CRVO, with the end result often being worse than 20/400 [2,16].

The fundoscopic examination of CRVO is key to diagnosis as it is very dramatic. Early on, the classic findings are "blood and thunder" with "cotton wool spots." Flame-shaped "blood and thunder" retinal hemorrhages are visible in all four quadrants. An ischemic retina is yellow–white producing "cotton wool spots." Macular edema is an early finding while tortuous, congested vessels around the optic disk are a later finding [39–41].

The diagnosis of CRVO is made based on symptoms and observation of the ocular fundus. Ophthalmologists may perform fluorescein angiography to confirm the diagnosis. When considering CRVO as a diagnosis, CRAO, diabetic retinopathy, and occlusion from a systemic vasculitis should also be considered [41].

Central retinal vein occlusion is generally self-limited but the natural history is highly variable. In some patients, the retinal hemorrhages and macular edema resolve, while in others the associated complications of CRVO produce long-term vision loss. Macular edema and ischemia as well as vitreous hemorrhages, retinal detachment, and neovascular glaucoma are the most common vision-reducing complications of CRVO [16,40,41].

In the acute phase of CRVO, management focuses on identification and treatment of the underlying vascular risk factors, prevention of secondary ocular complications, and prevention of another episode. About 7% of patients have an episode of CRVO in the other eye within 4 years [40,41]. Urgent referral to ophthalmology is important. Similar to CRAO, there is no proven treatment for CRVO. Treatment options include anticoagulation, fibrinolytics, hemodilution, hyperbaric oxygen, steroids, and surgical procedures such as laser photocoagulation, radial optic neurotomy, vitrectomy, and chorioretinal venous anastomosis [2,16].

Branch retinal vein occlusion

The differences between CRVO and branch retinal vein occlusion (BRVO) are often unclear as literature frequently refers to them as a single entity. BRVO is 3–5 times more common than CRVO. More than 90% of patients with BRVO are over the age of 50. It is usually unilateral but 9% of cases are bilateral [39–41].

Branch retinal vein occlusion typically occurs where the artery passes anterior to the vein in the adventitial sheath. The number of these crossings partially determines the severity of the disease [41]. Risk factors of BRVO are similar to those for CRVO and include cardiovascular disease, hypertension, diabetes, dyslipidemia, hypercoagulability, and glaucoma [16,39].

As only a portion of the retinal blood supply is affected in BRVO, symptoms are often less severe and involve certain visual fields. Vision is usually misty and mildly worse. The superotemporal and inferotemporal quadrants of vision are most affected. The examination findings are similar to those of CRVO, but less in quantity and severity. Complications and treatment of BRVO are the same as CRVO. BRVO has a better prognosis, with over half of patients reporting a final visual acuity of 20/40 or better, even without treatment [41].

GCA

Giant cell arteritis (GCA), or temporal arteritis, is an immune-mediated vasculitis of the medium and large arteries. It is the most common vasculitis among the elderly. Annual incidence jumps from 15–25 cases per 100,000 individuals more than 50 years old to 45 cases per 100,000 patients older than 80 years old. Peak incidence is between 70 and 80 years old. It is much more common in those of Northern European descent and women [16,42–44].

An elderly woman with a new headache should always raise GCA as a possible diagnosis. The classic symptoms of GCA are temporal headache, sudden vision loss, jaw claudication, and scalp tenderness [16,43–45]. Vision loss at initial presentation occurs only in one-quarter to one-half of patients. The vision loss occurs within a few days and is often irreversible. Transient vision loss due to hypoperfusion of the optic nerve, retina, or choroid often precedes anterior ischemic optic neuropathy, a true infarct of the optic nerve. Given GCA is systemic, there are often generalized symptoms such as low-grade fever, anorexia, weight loss, and malaise. Polymyalgia rheumatica, characterized by proximal upper and lower extremity weakness, is found in nearly one-third of patients at the time of GCA diagnosis [16,43].

Physical examination of GCA often reveals firm, tender temporal and occipital arteries with overlying erythema. Findings on fundoscopic examination vary depending on the flow to the optic nerve, retina, and choroid. As the disease progresses, there may be a pale, swollen, "chalky white" optic nerve with scattered cotton wool spots and small hemorrhages. The physical examination, however, may also be completely normal [16,42].

The gold standard for the diagnosis of GCA is a temporal artery biopsy, although a negative biopsy is found in nearly 10–15% of patients. Treatment with steroids should not be delayed for the biopsy. The patient should undergo a 2 cm temporal artery biopsy within 2 weeks of starting treatment, although histopathologic evidence of GCA can be detected for up to 6 weeks [16,43,44]. In 1990 the American College of Rheumatology determined, with 92% specificity and nearly 94% sensitivity, that GCA is an appropriate diagnosis if a patient has three or more of the following criteria: age greater than 50 years, onset of new headache, temporal artery abnormality (i.e., tenderness or reduced pulsation), elevated erythrocyte sedimentation rate (ESR) >50 mm/h, and positive temporal artery biopsy [16,43].

Prior to a definitive diagnosis, treatment with high-dose steroids (60–100 mg/day of prednisone, 1.0–1.5 mg/kg/day of methylprednisolone) should be started. It is unclear whether oral or intravenous steroids are superior, however intravenous are more appropriate for patients with vision loss or neurologic symptoms [16,44]. Urgent consultation or next-day follow-up

159

with a physician who can complete a temporal artery biopsy should occur. Depending on the institution, this may be ophthalmology, general surgery, or vascular surgery. Within a few days the patient should be seen by ophthalmology and neurology.

Vision loss associated with GCA is usually irreversible and remains at the level of presentation. Severe visual loss occurs in one-fifth of patients [43]. The headache and constitutional symptoms, however, begin to improve within hours to days of steroid treatment. Symptoms may wax and wane but as laboratory markers improve, most patients are tapered off steroids in 1–2 years [43]. Failure to rapidly respond to steroids should raise the possibility of an alternate diagnosis [45].

While the main initial presentation of GCA occurs in the temporal arteries, the subclavian, axillary, ophthalmic, and vertebral arteries and aorta can become inflamed, resulting in limb claudication, tissue gangrene, neuropathies, transient ischemic attacks and aortic dilation, aneurysm formation, and dissection [42,43].

Ears

Otitis externa

Otitis externa is mainly a disease of children. It can occur in the elderly as a complication of ear care and hearing aids. Also known as "swimmer's ear" or "tropical ear" [46], otitis externa is the diffuse inflammation of the external ear canal. Acute otitis externa (AOE) is present for less than 6 weeks, usually unilateral and peaks at the age of 7–12. The incidence declines after 50 years of age [47]. Lifetime incidence is 10% [46].

The apocrine glands of the ear produce acidic cerumen which provides protection from microbial growth. A change in this cerumen, prolonged moisture in the ear (swimming, humid environment), trauma to the ear canal (wax removal, use of hearing aids), dermatologic conditions (eczema, psoriasis), anatomic abnormalities (narrow canal), and an immunocompromised state predispose patients to AOE. Nearly all AOE in North America is bacterial. The common pathogens are *Pseudomonas aeruginosa* and *Staphylococcus aureus* [46,47].

Symptoms of AOE range from pruritis and mild discomfort in the ear canal to severe otalgia with purulent ear discharge, hearing loss, and headache. The pain with manipulation of the tragus and pinna may be out of proportion to the erythema seen in the ear canal. The tympanic membrane is often erythematous, causing a concomitant but incorrect diagnosis of otitis media. The best way to differentiate between AOE and otitis media is pneumatic otoscopy. The tympanic membrane in AOE will be mobile while mobility is absent or limited with otitis media. It is possible that the ear canal is so edematous that the tympanic membrane is not visible [46–48].

Acute otitis externa can be confused with furunculosis (infected hair follicles of the lateral ear canal), contact dermatitis of the ear canal (possibly from a hearing aid), sensitization to otic treatments (especially neomycin), viral infection, and middle ear disease (which may produce discharge in the ear canal) [46].

The mainstays of treatment for AOE are clearing debris from the ear canal, topical otic drops, and avoidance of precipitating factors. Prior to clearing debris from the ear canal, patients may require pain control with oral medications [46]. The otorrhea hydrates the cerumen well so it can be removed with a small suction tip or ear curette. Lavage should be avoided until the integrity of the tympanic membrane is confirmed [48].

There has been much debate about the best topical otic drop to treat AOE. A meta-analysis found no significant difference in clinical outcomes of AOE between antiseptic versus antimicrobial drops and quinolone versus nonquinolone antibiotics. Regardless of the topical agent used, 65–90% of patients had clinical resolution of symptoms in 7–10 days. Recent studies, however, have shown that concomitant use of steroids with antimicrobials likely hastens the time to resolution. Fluoroquinolones and aminoglycosides are topical antimicrobial options for treating AOE. Aminoglycosides are ototoxic and should be used only if an intact tympanic membrane has been confirmed [46].

Drug delivery must be adequate for topical medications to work. The otic drops should be warmed to body temperature before application to avoid dizziness from caloric stimulation [48]. The patient should lie down with the affected ear upward. Self-administration has been proven to be inadequate, so another person should place the amount required to fill the canal and pump the tragus to eliminate trapped air. The patient should remain lying down for 3–5 minutes [46].

If the ear canal is more than 50% narrowed, a wick should be placed to ensure the medial canal receives medication. There are commercially produced wicks, however compressed cellulose or ribbon gauze are alternatives. Topical otic drops should be used for a least a week or for 3 days after the resolution of symptoms, whichever occurs last [48].

Oral antibiotics may be needed if the patient is immunocompromised (diabetes, HIV, elderly), the infection has spread beyond the confines of the ear canal, there is a co-existing otitis media, or otic drops can not be used effectively [46,48]. Nearly 20–40% of AOE patients receive oral antibiotics. This number is thought to be high and puts those who do not need oral antibiotics at risk for bacterial resistance. Additionally, otic drops deliver significantly higher antibiotic concentrations at the site of infection than oral antibiotics [47].

Malignant otitis externa

Malignant otitis externa (MOE) is better described by its other names – necrotizing otitis externa and skull base osteomyelitis [48,49]. A rare complication of otitis externa [50], this infection travels through small perforations in the external auditory canal to the skull base. The bone of the skull base is replaced with granulation tissue. The infection can also spread medially to the tympanomastoid suture and along venous canals and fascial planes [49].

While other immunosuppressed patients are at risk, diabetics account for nearly 90% of those affected by MOE. Diabetes is thought to produce a poor vascular supply to the ear and impair the immune function of ear cerumen by increasing the pH. Many diabetics who acquire MOE are also elderly. Although a relatively rare disease, the incidence may be increasing due to growing geriatric and diabetic populations [49,51,52].

Virtually all cases of MOE are due to *Pseudomonas*, which is ubiquitous in water. When combined with suppressed host defenses and local aural trauma, *Pseudomonas* is able to penetrate the ear canal. A common iatrogenic cause of MOE is ear irrigation with tap water, generally for the purpose of disimpacting cerumen [51,52].

Severe, unrelenting otalgia is the main complaint associated with MOE. The pain is worse than that of otitis externa and often extends to the temporomandibular joint causing trimus. Otorrhea, a sensation of aural fullness, hearing loss, and headache also occurs with MOE. Fever, however, may be absent. In addition to recent aural trauma, many patients have a recent history of otic drops for otitis externa [49,52].

Similar to simple otitis externa, the physical examination of a patient with MOE includes pain with manipulation of the ear, purulent otorrhea, and an erythematous, edematous external auditory canal. The tympanic membrane and middle ear are usually healthy and uninvolved. Granulation tissue or exposed bone on the floor of the auditory canal at the bony–cartilaginous junction is pathognomonic for MOE [49,52]. As the infection of MOE spreads within the cranium, cranial nerve palsies occur. These occur only with MOE. The facial nerve is the most commonly involved cranial nerve. Vertigo and meningeal signs indicate late infection [48].

The work-up of MOE often includes imaging to evaluate the extent of the infection. Bone scans are considered the mainstay of diagnosis and follow-up because of their sensitivity. In addition to being unavailable in most EDs, they can not distinguish between infection, trauma, and neoplasm and do not differentiate between new and recurrent MOE [49,51]. A computed tomography (CT) scan can detect the change in bone density as the minerals are eroded and replaced with granulation tissue. However, one-third of the bone must be lost before CT can detect the infection and bone remineralization continues long after acute MOE has resolved. Similar difficulties apply to magnetic resonance imaging (MRI) [49,52].

Cultures for aerobic, anaerobic, and fungal organisms should be done from the otorrhea of MOE, even if the patient has been on antibiotics. If *Pseudomonas* is not isolated from the otorrhea, a bone biopsy should be performed to evaluate for malignancy. If the patient does not have a known history of an immunocompromised state, a search for diabetes or other immunosuppressive diseases should be done [49,52].

Treatment for MOE includes antibiotics, ear care, and control of the disease causing immunosuppression. The introduction of penicillins decreased MOE mortality from 50 to 20%. Until the introduction of fluoroquinolones, MOE treatment involved multiple intravenous antibiotics and extensive hospital admissions. High-dose ciprofloxacin (750 mg orally twice a day), the current antibiotic of choice, has good activity against *Pseudomonas*, penetrates bone well, and has excellent oral bioavailability. The cure rate for MOE is 90% with few adverse side effects. Despite the relief of symptoms, antibiotics should be continued for 6–8 weeks. As with many other infections, ciprofloxacin-resistant *Pseudomonas* has been isolated and is

becoming more common. Cleaning of the external auditory canal should be done. It is unclear whether topical otic drops are of use. Lastly, diabetes and other immune-suppressing conditions should be aggressively managed [51,52].

Despite these treatment measures the recurrence rate of MOE is about 15%. Treatment failures are often elderly diabetic patients with inadequate antibiotic treatment. Mortality from MOE is now below 15% [49].

Nose

Epistaxis

Epistaxis is very common, with a lifetime incidence of 60% [53]. It accounts for about 1 in every 200 ED visits in the US [54]. Most episodes are minor and do not require medical evaluation or intervention. Severe nosebleeds are most often in those older than age 50 [53].

Geriatric epistaxis has many local and systemic contributing factors. Common local factors include digital trauma, nasal septal deviation, chemical irritants (especially from steroid nasal sprays), and mucosal dryness (from non-humidified oxygen or low humidity) [53,54]. The main systemic factor associated with epistaxis in the elderly is coagulopathy. Aspirin, clopidogrel, and warfarin are independent risk factors for epistaxis through platelet inhibition [55]. Comorbidities such as renal failure, liver disease, and alcoholism affect platelet function despite normal platelet counts [53]. The association between hypertension and epistaxis is debated. While there is no firm cause and effect, elevated blood pressure does make bleeding more difficult to control. Controlling hypertension may not help epistaxis, but it will unlikely be detrimental [54,55].

Epistaxis is classified as anterior or posterior. The vast majority of epistaxis cases are anterior and occur at Kieselbach's plexus. These bleeds are controlled with anterior rhinoscopy or anterior nasal packing. In comparison, posterior nasal bleeds are rare, originate from Woodruff's plexus, and require posterior packing for control [53,54,56].

Evaluation and treatment of epistaxis occur at the same time. Vital signs are important. Geriatric patients with already tenuous hemodynamics may have unstable vital signs from the loss of blood and require a blood transfusion. Next the focus should move towards stopping the bleeding. Depending on the severity, the bleeding may be controlled by simple direct pressure. The patient should pinch the anterior aspect of the nose for a full, uninterrupted 15 minutes. The patient should watch the clock because time perception feels altered during this wait. A cold compress and sucking on ice may help patient comfort. Leaning forward is best as this decreases the amount of blood entering the stomach, a common cause of vomiting. This can be done while preparing for a nose examination. If the bleeding stops with direct pressure, a thorough examination should still be done [54,56].

If direct pressure does not stop the bleeding, the patient should forcefully blow the nose to expel clots. Then topical vasoconstrictors (phenylephrine 1% or oxymetazoline 0.05%) and local anesthetics (lidocaine) should be applied to slow the bleeding and improve patient comfort. Caution should be exercised when vasoconstrictors are used on the nasal mucosa of patients with severe hypertension or cardiovascular disease. Small doses for short periods of time are generally considered safe but there have been reports of cardiac ischemia after intranasal vasoconstrictors [57,58]. After adequate time for the medications to work, a thorough nose examination with the use of adequate personal protective equipment, light, suction, and a nasal speculum often uncovers the source of anterior epistaxis [53,56]. The use of silver nitrate sticks around the bleeding site decreases blood flow to the offending site. Then the bleeding vessel can be cauterized. In the event of bleeding from both nostrils, the nasal septum should only be cauterized on one side to avoid ischemia causing septal perforation. Silver nitrate may not work on brisk, large bleeds because the chemicals wash away before they are able to act [53,54].

If epistaxis continues despite cautery or if there is no obvious source of bleeding, an anterior pack should be placed. Traditional nasal packing, nasal sponges, epistaxis balloons, and absorbable materials are options for anterior packing. Directions for placing premade nasal sponges and balloons should be read as they vary greatly. Although coating the pack with antibiotic ointment is often suggested, it has not demonstrated a reduction in infectious complications. The anterior pack is left in for 1–5 days. Although some question the practice, prophylactic antibiotics to prevent sinusitis and toxic shock syndrome are often used with anterior nasal packing. Hemodynamically stable patients without airway impairment can be discharged home [53,55,56].

If epistaxis continues despite bilateral anterior packing, the bleeding may originate from Woodruff's plexus. Posterior packing relies on direct pressure and accumulation of blood within the nasal cavity to tamponade the bleeding vessel. If a commercially prepared posterior pack is not available, a Foley catheter with anterior packing can be used. If placed improperly, posterior packing can cause airway compromise or pressure necrosis of nasal tissues. Posterior packing requires an otolaryngology consultation and admission to the hospital. In addition to being uncomfortable, posterior packing may cause apnea, hypoxia, and dysrhythmias, especially in those with comorbidities [53,54,56].

Patients with epistaxis who are on anticoagulation, particularly warfarin, deserve particular mention. Clotting studies, particularly an international normalized ratio (INR), should be checked as about one-third of patients will be above their target INR [59]. A prospective controlled study of patients with epistaxis showed that, when the INR is within the target range, warfarin can be continued without increased bleeding risk [60]. In patients with an INR above goal, however, the degree of overanticoagulation and the indication for anticoagulation should be considered. Patients with an INR <4 may only require warfarin to be withheld for a few days, while patients with an INR >8 may require fresh frozen plasma or vitamin K. Patients with mechanical heart valves, recurrent deep vein thrombosis, or pulmonary embolisms are at high risk for clots when anticoagulation is stopped or reversed [59]. Decisions about when and how to reverse anticoagulation with epistaxis

should be made on a case-by-case basis with the assistance of a pharmacist.

Throat

Dental abscess

The face of US geriatric dentistry has changed dramatically in the past half century. In the 1950s, nearly three-fourths of adults more than 75 years old had no natural teeth. Since then the prevalence of decayed and missing teeth has dropped by half, resulting in about 35% of elderly Americans missing all teeth [61]. Despite this impressive transition, nearly one-third of Americans older than 65 years of age have untreated dental caries. In 1997 only about half of the non-institutionalized elderly reported a dental visit in the previous year [62].

Improving US geriatric dental health has numerous societal barriers and physiological challenges. The lack of perceived need is often cited as the most important hurdle for the elderly receiving dental care. The belief that dental deterioration is a normal part of the aging process prevents active engagement of patients with the dental system [62,63]. If dental care is desired, the cost may be prohibitive. Only 10% of American seniors have dental insurance, leaving the remainder to pay expenses out of their own pocket [61,63].

Lastly, many seniors have difficulty performing routine dental care and little help exists. As manual dexterity, tactile acuity, and visual ability decline, efforts at personal oral care are often inadequate. Whether due to lack of knowledge about the importance of dental hygiene or an aversion to cleaning another's mouth, caregivers often do not step in to fill the gap [61].

Age-related changes to the mouth and teeth make dental caries and abscesses more common but less noticed in the elderly. Diminished salivary flow, often due to medications, and modified saliva composition allow an alteration of the oral pH, spurring bacterial growth [61]. At the same time, tooth enamel becomes less hydrated and thinner. In response to continued use, secondary dentin causes an overall expansion of dentin volume that encroaches on the pulp chamber. The blood vessels and nerves in the pulp atrophy. These changes produce more brittle and less resilient teeth that are much less sensitive [63,64]. As a result, the same pathologic dental infection that would cause dramatic symptoms in a younger patient may not be noticed by an older patient [63].

While dental caries in the elderly is common, the rate of acute dental abscesses is unknown. Acute dental abscesses usually occur due to dental caries, trauma, or failed root treatment. After bacteria breach the pulp chamber, the root canal becomes colonized. Asymptomatic necrosis is common but when the bacteria enter the periapical tissue they induce acute inflammation and pus formation [65]. The most common bacteria associated with dental infections are *Streptococcus mutans*, *Lactobacillus* and *Actinomyces* [64].

The pain associated with an acute apical abscess often occurs rapidly and ranges from slight discomfort to intense, throbbing pain. The source of the pain is easy to identify and tender to touch. On physical examination, swelling, erythema, and suppuration are usually localized to the affected tooth but can spread, causing a deeper infection [65].

The best treatment for an acute apical tooth abscess is removal of the necrotic tissue. This is best done by draining the infection through trephination of the tooth, pulpectomy, or extraction of the offending tooth. These are not procedures done by emergency medicine physicians or carried out in the ED. Incision and drainage of the abscessed area is the next best treatment. If drainage is not possible, antibiotics may be prescribed. While antibiotics are thought to be overused in this localized infection, the elderly have a higher risk of worsening and spreading infection. Penicillin is the antibiotic of choice, however clindamycin should be substituted for patients with a true penicillin allergy. NSAIDs are recommended for pain control, although recent studies have shown a dramatic increase in narcotic prescriptions for dental pain and dental infections [66]. Elderly patients, however, are less likely to receive prescriptions for analgesia [67].

Acute apical abscesses should be referred to a dentist for definitive management. Although usually uncomplicated, hematogenous seeding can cause systemic complications such as bacterial endocarditis and late prosthetic joint infections [61].

Ludwig's angina

Ludwig's angina is an infection of the sublingual, submandibular, and submental spaces of the head and neck [68]. Its name derives from the German physician Wilhelm Friedrich von Ludwig who first described the condition in 1836 [69] and the Latin verb *angere*, to strangle [70]. The infection starts as a rapidly spreading cellulitis that turns into a true abscess [71]. The vast majority of Ludwig's angina cases begin with a periapical abscess of the second or third molars [69,72]. Because of this origin, the most common causative organisms are *Staphylococcus*, *Streptococcus*, and *Bacteroides* species. Many infections are polymicrobial [69]. Less common causes of Ludwig's angina are mandibular fractures, oral lacerations, tongue piercing, neoplasms, salivary calculi, inferior alveolar nerve blocks, and peritonsillar abscesses [70,73,74].

Since the advent of antibiotics and improved dental care, the incidence of Ludwig's angina has dropped significantly. It is most common in men between the ages of 20 and 60 [73]. Geriatric patients are at risk for Ludwig's angina due to underlying predisposing factors (such as diabetes mellitus and immunosuppression) and lack of dental care (discussed in the Dental Abscess section) [72,75].

The presenting symptoms of Ludwig's angina depend on the degree of infection. The most common complaints are tooth pain, dysphagia, dyspnea, fever, and malaise. As the disease progresses, patients complain of pain with tongue movement, dysarthria, neck swelling, neck stiffness, and a protruding tongue [73,75].

The main features of the physical examination of a patient with Ludwig's angina focus on the edematous, "woody" neck and protruding tongue. The swelling of the deep tissues forces the tongue out of its contained area of the mouth [74]. Stridor, trismus, difficulty managing secretions, anxiety, and cyanosis are signs of impending airway collapse [75].

The diagnostic sensitivity of clinical exam alone is only 55%. Assuming the patient's airway is stable, a CT scan with contrast increases the diagnostic sensitivity significantly and provides information about the extent of the infection [69,76]. When CT can not be used, ultrasound is a reliable, accurate alternative to distinguish edema from fluid collection [69].

The treatment for Ludwig's angina includes airway management, antibiotics, and possible surgical drainage [77]. The plan, developed with the immediate involvement of an otolaryngologist and anesthesiologist, should be individualized based on the stage of disease, comorbid conditions, physician experience, and available resources and personnel [72,75]. It is unclear how many patients with Ludwig's angina require airway intervention, however it may be as high as 35–50% [77]. Airway compromise is the leading cause of death in patients with Ludwig's angina [75]. Ideally, airway control should occur in the operating room with a surgeon at bedside in case a surgical airway is needed. The optimal technique for obtaining an airway is an awake, fiberoptic nasotracheal intubation with the patient sitting up [68,70]. The posterior pharynx is variably involved so this technique provides the best opportunity for successful intubation. If this fails, a cricothyrotomy or tracheostomy is often needed [70,72]. Oral intubation is generally not an option because the elevation of the tongue prevents sufficient space for laryngoscopy and trismus is often present. Blind nasal intubation can cause hemorrhage and abscess rupture [78].

Even if the patient does not require an emergent airway, the team should discuss the plan for airway management. Traditionally, airway management for Ludwig's angina was aggressive by securing an airway early. There has been recent support for a "wait and see" approach as this maintains low mortality rates, decreases morbidity associated with tracheotomy, shortens hospital stays, and may lead to faster recovery. This approach is best suited for young, healthy patients who do not have rapid progression of disease. Comorbidities, as those frequently found with geriatric patients, are associated with a greater risk of airway obstruction [77].

Antibiotic coverage for Ludwig's angina should include Gram-positive cocci, Gram-negative bacilli, and anaerobes. The combination of high-dose penicillin, clindamycin, and metronidazole is the most common cocktail [69]. If an incision and drainage is done, a culture can help customize antibiotic need [71]. Although not proven in a randomized controlled trial, intravenous steroids are thought to reduce the soft tissue swelling and edema associated with Ludwig's angina [69,72].

If airway management is required or medical therapy fails, patients with Ludwig's angina require a surgical incision and drainage [72,74]. Patients with Ludwig's angina, whether intubated or not, are admitted to the intensive care unit. Until the infection is improving, airway compromise is possible [69].

Prior to antibiotics the mortality of Ludwig's angina was over 50% [76], but with antibiotics and airway management, mortality is now less than 10% [70]. The leading cause of death is airway compromise, but there are many other complications caused by spreading infection. These include mediastinitis, empyema, pericardial or pleural effusion, jugular vein thrombosis, and osteomyelitis of the mandible or cervical spine [70,72].

Peritonsillar abscess

A peritonsillar abscess (PTA) forms between the palatine tonsil and its capsule. It is most often near the superior pole of the tonsil. Other structures, such as Weber's glands, also play a role in PTAs as they can still occur after a tonsillectomy. The infection leading to a PTA starts as an acute exudative tonsillitis that develops into a cellulitis and then into tissue necrosis and pus formation. It is not considered a "deep" neck space infection although it is anatomically contiguous with several deep spaces [70,79,80].

The incidence of PTA is estimated to be 30 cases per 100,000 people per year in the US. Although it occurs in all age groups, the highest incidence occurs in adults 20–40 years old. Elderly patients are at higher risk due to periodontal disease. PTAs occur most commonly in November, December, April, and May, which coincides with the highest incidence of streptococcal pharyngitis and exudative tonsillitis [80].

Prior to presentation with a PTA, patients may have had an acute pharyngotonsillitis or a viral illness like mononucleosis. The symptoms of a PTA are fever, sore throat, dysphagia, odynophagia, and otalgia. The sore throat can often be identified as unilateral [70,79–81].

Often the first features noticed on physical examination of a patient with a PTA are a muffled "hot potato" voice, drooling or spitting of secretions, and foul-smelling breath. On further investigation there is bulging of the superior pole of the tonsil, pushing the uvula away from the affected side. Mucopurulent tonsillar exudate and ipsilateral cervical lymphadenopathy are common. Examination may be limited due to trismus [70,79,81].

Intracavity ultrasound is reliable in distinguishing between cellulitis and an abscess but a CT scan is required if there is severe trismus or concern for extension into deep neck spaces [70,79]. Ultrasound and CT can also help differentiate a PTA from neoplasia, foreign body, and infection of other deep spaces [80,81].

If left untreated, the PTA will slowly leak or burst, potentially causing aspiration and pneumonia [79]. In addition to pain control and antibiotics, the treatment of a PTA requires drainage of the pus. Needle aspiration, incision, and drainage or abscess drainage with simultaneous tonsillectomy are choices. The traditional abscess drainage with simultaneous tonsillectomy is now reserved for refractory and complicated cases. Needle aspiration and incision and drainage of the abscess have very similar success rates, with incision and drainage being more painful. Needle aspiration has the benefits of being easy to perform, being well tolerated, confirming the diagnosis, and avoiding injury to adjacent structures. In the 10–15% of cases where needle aspiration fails, an incision and drainage or tonsillectomy can be performed [80,81].

Antibiotics should be effective against Group A *Streptococcus* and oral anaerobes. With the emergence of resistant organisms, ten days of penicillin with metronidazole, clindamycin, a second- or third-generation cephalosporin, or amoxicillin

clavulanate are good choices. It is unclear whether steroids speed recovery but they have been more commonly used in the past few years [80].

Few patients require airway management or admission. In a case series of PTA patients requiring intubation, awake fiberoptic bronchoscopy was the method of choice but nearly all patients could have been orally intubated with standard technique. After observation and the ability to tolerate liquids and pain medications, patients can usually be discharged home. Follow-up should occur within 24–36 hours. Tonsillectomy after PTA is not required in patients older than 40 years [80,81].

Epiglottitis

Since the widespread use of the *Haemophilus influenzae* vaccine in the early 1990s, pediatric epiglottitis has been on the decline. At the same time, adult epiglottitis has been on the rise. Only 20% of adult epiglottitis is due to *Haemophilus influenzae*; other common bacterial causes are *Haemophilus parainfluenzae*, *Streptococcus pneumoniae*, and group A *Streptococcus*. Trauma by a foreign body, burns, drug inhalation, and reactions to chemotherapy can also cause epiglottitis. Supraglottitis is an alternate name for epiglottitis as the inflammation is not confined to only the epiglottis. Usually supraglottic structures such as the pharynx, uvula, base of the tongue, and false vocal cords are also involved. The peak incidence of adult epiglottitis is 35–39 years old with an annual incidence of about 1–1.5 per 100,000 people. This incidence is more than double that of children. Epiglottitis in adults strikes those with underlying medical conditions such as hypertension, diabetes, and alcohol abuse [82,83].

The main features of adult epiglottitis are sore throat, dysphagia, odynophagia, muffled voice, drooling, stridor, and dyspnea [83,84]. Unfortunately, physical examination does not add much to the diagnosis of epiglottitis. Most cases have tenderness to the anterior hyoid with an only mildly erythematous oropharynx. The pain of epiglottitis is often out of proportion to the benign findings on physical examination [83,84]. Similar to children, the tripoding position, which moves the edematous epiglottic structures forward, is a sign of impending airway obstruction [85].

The gold standard to diagnose epiglottitis is direct or indirect visualization of the inflamed epiglottis and supraglottic structures. While this is dangerous in children, laryngospasm and airway compromise have not been described during laryngoscopic examination of adults [83]. X-rays can be an adjunct to diagnosis. The classic "thumb sign," a rounded mass shadow of a thickened and edematous epiglottis, is present about 75% of the time while the "vallecula sign," partial or complete obliteration of the airpocket around the base of the tongue and epiglottis, is rarely found. The use of X-rays is controversial as the sensitivity and specificity are widely debated [86]. CT or MRI are suggested to exclude complications, like PTA, ingested foreign body, laryngitis, tonsillitis, and deep-space neck abscess, rather than diagnose epiglottitis. Acute epiglottitis on CT will appear as swelling of the supraglottic structures, loss of fat planes, and thickening of the platysma muscle and prevertebral fascia [82,83].

Treatment for epiglottitis should be started immediately. A second- or third-generation cephalosporin provides coverage for the most common bacterial causes [82]. Steroids are often recommended but have not been proven to decrease the need for intubation or duration of illness [83]. Nebulized epinephrine can be used but may have rebound edema causing airway obstruction [85].

Both otolaryngology and anesthesiology should be included early in the management of a patient with epiglottitis. The cornerstone of acute epiglottitis treatment is airway management. It is a controversial topic with the aggressive approach of "intubate on presentation" against the conservative "wait and see" approach. Advocates of early intubation point out that there are no clear criteria discriminating between patients who develop sudden airway obstruction and those with a benign course [86]. Additionally, the mortality of children with epiglottitis dropped significantly when the prophylactic use of intubation started [83]. On the other hand, less than 20% of adults with epiglottitis require an airway intervention [82]. Stridor, drooling, dyspnea, chest wall retractions, sitting erect, and rapid progression of epiglottitis indicate the need for intubation [83,84,86]. Ideally, intubation for acute epiglottitis is done as an elective procedure with a conscious patient in the operating room in case a tracheostomy is required. It should be regarded as a potentially difficult airway [87]. Unsuccessful intubation attempts produce swelling and bleeding, complicating further airway management [85]. Whether intubated or not, adults with epiglottitis require constant observation in the intensive care unit because the loose mucosa and rich vascularity of the supraglottic region can cause sudden airway obstruction [82,85].

The most common complications of epiglottitis are epiglottic and vallecular abscesses, uvulitis, and pneumonia [83]. Mortality of adults with epiglottitis is 1.2–7.1% [85] Misdiagnosis and inadequate treatment are thought to contribute to this high figure. Using standardized management, like that in children, may help decrease mortality [83]. Practitioners should have a high level of suspicion for epiglottitis and treat it aggressively.

Retropharyngeal abscess

The retropharyngeal space, also known as the retrovisceral or retroesophageal space, is a potential space between the posterior pharynx, esophagus, and prevertebral fascia. It extends from the base of the skull to the area of the first thoracic vertebrae [70,74].

The space is fused down the midline by two chains of lymph nodes that disappear by puberty [79]. A retropharyngeal abscess (RPA) usually occurs in children as drainage from nasal, sinus, and pharyngeal infections travels to the lymph nodes of the retropharyngeal space [70]. In adults a RPA is usually due to trauma to the posterior pharynx or esophagus from instrumentation (e.g., endoscopy, nasogastric tube, frequent suctioning, intubation attempts), foreign body, traumatic esophageal rupture, or extension of an infection from a communicating space (often pharyngitis, rarely vertebral osteomyelitis) [70,74,79]. RPA infections are often polymicrobial with organisms such as *Streptococcus viridans*, beta-hemolytic *Streptococcus*, *S. aureus*, *Bacteroides*, *Veillonella*, and *H. influenzae* [70].

Adults with RPA present with an abrupt onset of fever, sore throat, dysphagia, odynophagia, neck pain, drooling, and dyspnea. The patient with a RPA may have unilateral bulging of the posterior pharynx. Unfortunately this edema is often not apparent on physical examination. Palpation of the pharynx should be avoided as the pressure can precipitate abscess rupture. Cervical lymphadenopathy, nuchal rigidity, and head tilting to the contralateral side can also be seen with a RPA [70,74,79,88].

A lateral soft tissue neck X-ray is concerning when the retropharyngeal space is more than half the width of the adjacent vertebral body. Air is a very specific finding for a RPA, while air–fluid levels and foreign bodies may also be seen [79,88]. A CT scan can be used to distinguish between cellulitis and abscess, to confirm the diagnosis of RPA, and to delineate the extension of the infection into adjacent spaces [70,79]. The signs and symptoms of RPA can mimic cervical osteomyelitis, meningitis, Pott's disease, and calcified tendinitis of the longus colli muscle [79].

Treatment for RPA requires airway management, antibiotics, and incision and drainage [79]. If a patient has signs of airway compromise, immediate transfer to the operating room prior to examination is indicated. In addition to the catastrophe of airway obstruction, the abscess may rupture precipitating massive aspiration or asphyxiation. Intubation should occur on the opposite side to the pharyngeal edema [70,79].

Complications from a RPA increase the mortality rate significantly. Mediastinal extension of the RPA requires surgical debridement. Even with effective treatment, the mortality rate of RPA with mediastinal extension is 25–40% [74]. Other complications include epidural abscess, jugular venous thrombosis, necrotizing fasciitis, and erosion into the carotid artery. The most common cause of death related to a RPA is multi-organ failure from sepsis [88].

Angioedema due to angiotensin-converting enzyme inhibitors

Angioedema is a transient and localized epidermal swelling due to permeable submucosal or subcutaneous capillaries and venules [89,90]. It has multiple causes, including allergens, medications, and decreased C1-inhibitor function or production. As angiotensin-converting enzyme inhibitors (ACE inhibitors) have become more popular, the epidemiology of angioedema has changed [91]. ACE inhibitor angioedema has become an important topic in geriatric emergency medicine.

Angiotensin-converting enzyme inhibitors reduce mortality in patients with hypertension, congestive heart failure, and diabetic nephropathy [92]. Given their success, ACE inhibitors are prescribed to nearly 40 million people worldwide [91]. Known side effects of ACE inhibitors include cough, hypotension, hyperkalemia, and renal failure [90]. Angioedema was previously thought to be a rare complication of ACE inhibitors, but as both awareness of this side effect and the population taking the medications grew, so did the incidence. In the 1990s,

ACE inhibitors accounted for 10–25% of all angioedema cases. This is now thought to be nearly 80% [89].

Generally ACE inhibitor angioedema is a self-limited, non-pitting swelling of the head, neck, lips, mouth, tongue, larynx, pharynx, and subglottal areas [90,91]. In contrast to allergic angioedema, there is minimal or no urticaria. Allergic angioedema is mediated by mast cell degranulation and histamine release, causing urticaria, while ACE inhibitor angioedema is thought to be related to the levels of bradykinin. This results in vasodilation and increased vascular permeability, causing interstitial fluid accumulation and angioedema [89,90]. While the mechanism of ACE inhibitor angioedema is not completely understood, there are a number of clear risk factors including previous episodes of angioedema, history of inherited or acquired C1 inhibitor deficiency, African ancestry, smoking, older age, and female gender [89,92].

Unlike allergic angioedema, ACE inhibitor angioedema is unrelated to the dose or duration of treatment of the offending medication. Although the risk for angioedema is greatest in the first month of taking an ACE inhibitor, most cases occur well after the first month. Given the unclear time pattern, ACE inhibitor angioedema may be misdiagnosed, causing a delay in effective care, and the true incidence, thought to be from 0.1% to 6%, is likely higher [89,91,92].

The severity of ACE inhibitor angioedema ranges from very mild to life threatening. Patients often have preceding episodes of insignificant angioedema that are not noticed or reported [89,90]. Patients have swelling to the lips, tongue, eyes, and posterior pharynx. About 20% of patients complain of more severe symptoms such as dyspnea, dysphagia, and stridor [90]. Rarely, ACE inhibitor angioedema can occur in the bowel wall causing nausea, vomiting, abdominal pain, diarrhea, and ascites. Given it is uncommon and the symptoms overlap with many other conditions, ACE inhibitor angioedema of the bowel wall is often misdiagnosed [89,90,92].

Diagnosis of ACE inhibitor angioedema is made through history and physical. Given the unclear time frame between the ACE inhibitor and symptoms, emergency medicine physicians should think of this in all cases of head and neck edema.

The treatment for ACE inhibitor angioedema is mainly supportive through airway management and discontinuation of the ACE inhibitor. Anesthesiology and otolaryngology should be involved early if there is concern for airway compromise. Airway obstruction is thought to occur in 10–22% of patients with ACE inhibitor angioedema. Because the tongue edema is not pitting, oral intubation may be impossible. Nasotracheal intubation is preferred. Few require a cricothyroidotomy or tracheostomy [89,90,92].

Patients with ACE inhibitor angioedema are often given antihistamines and corticosteroids in the event that there is an allergic component to the symptoms. This treatment, however, has not been proven to be effective for ACE inhibitor angioedema. Anecdotally, C1-inhibitor concentrate, fresh frozen plasma, and bradykinin antagonists have improved ACE inhibitor angioedema [89,90,92].

Cessation of the ACE inhibitor is key to treatment for ACE inhibitor angioedema. Angiotensin receptor blockers (ARBs) are generally considered safe substitutes as they do not potentiate the response to bradykinin, but some believe there should be a reasonable justification for the use of ARBs after ACE inhibitor angioedema [90–92].

If there is concern about airway compromise, patients with ACE inhibitor angioedema should be hospitalized. The swelling usually resolves in 24–48 hours. The overall mortality rate of 11% has declined significantly over the past decade with improved recognition of and earlier intervention for ACE inhibitor angioedema [89,90].

Summary

Eye, ear, nose, and throat emergencies of the elderly may resemble those of their younger counterparts. Geriatric pathophysiology and comorbid conditions make such emergencies more complicated. Certain conditions such as acute angle closure glaucoma, vitreous hemorrhage, retinal detachment, and uveitis are more common due to aging of the body. Other conditions such as central retinal artery occlusion, branch retinal artery occlusion, central retinal vein occlusion, branch retinal vein occlusion, and malignant otitis externa should prompt a search for an underlying condition causing the disease. Comorbid conditions make the management of epistaxis, dental abscess, Ludwig's angina, peritonsillar abscess, epiglottitis, retropharyngeal abscess, and angioedema due to ACE inhibitors increasingly complicated.

Pearls and pitfalls

- Patients with acute angle closure glaucoma often present with headache, abdominal pain and vomiting. Do not miss the eye complaint.
- Medical therapy for acute angle closure glaucoma should be aggressive but is only a stop gap measure; definitive treatment is surgical.
- A thorough evaluation for retinal tears and retinal detachment in vitreous hemorrhage is key as it alters the urgency of treatment.
- Vision loss due to retinal detachment can be progressive, starting in the periphery and becoming severe only when the macula is involved.
- Acute, severe uveitis in a geriatric patient should prompt a search for an underlying infectious disease.
- Central retinal artery occlusion and branch retinal artery occlusion are ocular strokes. Although treatment is unclear, it requires a timely, thorough evaluation for the underlying cause.
- Consider giant cell arteritis on the differential diagnosis for elderly women with a headache.
- Start steroids for giant cell arteritis immediately; visual loss is usually permanent and temporal artery biopsy will not be altered for at least two weeks.
- Do not diagnosis an elderly, diabetic patient with otitis externa without great consideration that the disease may be osteomyelitis of the skull base, or malignant otitis externa.

- Geriatric patients with epistaxis require admission if there is hemodynamic instability, posterior packing, or potential airway compromise.
- Adequate dental care in the elderly is difficult; discuss these barriers with geriatric patients who present with a dental complaint.
- Airway compromise can occur quickly in Ludwig's angina, epiglottitis, and retropharyngeal abscess; have airway adjuncts available and consult anesthesiology and otolaryngology early.
- Do not let a normal examination in patients with epiglottitis and retropharyngeal abscesses lull you into a false sense of security; lack of physical findings does not correlate with severity of disease.
- In contrast to those with deep-space infections, most patients who receive definitive treatment for a peritonsillar abscess can be discharged home.
- Think of ACE inhibitors as a cause of any head and neck edema.

References

1. Pelletier AL, Thomas J, Shaw FR. Vision loss in older persons. *Am Fam Physician.* 2009;79:963–70.
2. Beran DI, Murphy-Lavoie H. Acute, painless vision loss. *J La State Med Soc.* 2009;161:214–16, 218–23.
3. Dargin JM, Lowenstein RA. The painful eye. *Emerg Med Clin N Am.* 2008;26:199–216, viii.
4. Walker RA, Wadman MC. Headache in the elderly. *Clin Geriatr Med.* 2007;23:291–305, v–vi.
5. Gandhewar RR, Kamath GG. Acute glaucoma presentations in the elderly. *Emerg Med J.* 2005;22:306–7.
6. Mahmood AR, Narang AT. Diagnosis and management of the acute red eye. *Emerg Med Clin N Am.* 2008;26:35–55, vi.
7. Koch J, Sikes K. Getting the red out: Primary angle-closure glaucoma. *Nurse Pract.* 2009;34:6–9.
8. Volfson D, Barnett B. Bilateral acute angle-closure glaucoma after bronchodilator therapy. *Am J Emerg Med.* 2009;27:257.e5–257, e6.
9. See JL, Aquino MC, Aduan J, et al. Management of angle closure glaucoma. *Indian J Ophthalmol.* 2011;59(Suppl.):S82–7.
10. Singh A. Medical therapy of glaucoma. *Ophthalmol Clin N Am.* 2005;18:397–408.
11. Manuchehri K, Kirkby G. Vitreous haemorrhage in elderly patients: Management and prevention. *Drugs Aging.* 2003;20:655–61.
12. Lindgren G, Lindblom B. Causes of vitreous hemorrhage. *Curr Opin Ophthalmol.* 1996;7:13–19.
13. Saxena S, Jalali S, Verma L, et al. Management of vitreous haemorrhage. *Indian J Ophthalmol.* 2003;51:189–96.
14. Pokhrel PK, Loftus SA. Ocular emergencies. *Am Fam Physician.* 2007;76:829–36.
15. Gariano RF, Kim CH. Evaluation and management of suspected retinal detachment. *Am Fam Physician.* 2004;69:1691–8.
16. Vortmann M, Schneider JI. Acute monocular visual loss. *Emerg Med Clin N Am.* 2008;26:73–96, vi.
17. Jones W, Cavallerano A, Morgan K, et al. Optometric clinical practice guideline: Care of the patient with retinal detachment and related peripheral vitreoretinal disease. *Am Optometr Assoc.* 2004 (www.aoa.org/documents/CPG-13.pdf).
18. Kang HK, Luff AJ. Management of retinal detachment: A guide for non-ophthalmologists. *BMJ.* 2008;336:1235–40.
19. Yoonessi R, Hussain A, Jang TB. Bedside ocular ultrasound for the detection of retinal detachment in the emergency department. *Acad Emerg Med.* 2010;17:913–17.
20. Barton K, Pavesio CE, Towler HM, et al. Uveitis presenting de novo in the elderly. *Eye (Lond).* 1994;8(Pt 3):288–91.
21. Chatzistefanou K, Markomichelakis NN, Christen W, et al. Characteristics of uveitis presenting for the first time in the elderly. *Ophthalmology.* 1998;105:347–52.
22. Reeves SW, Sloan FA, Lee PP, et al. Uveitis in the elderly: Epidemiological data from the National Long-term Care Survey Medicare Cohort. *Ophthalmology.* 2006;113:307.e1.
23. Hunter RS, Lobo AM. Current diagnostic approaches to infectious anterior uveitis. *Int Ophthalmol Clin.* 2011;51:145–56.
24. Gregoire MA, Kodjikian L, Varron L, et al. Characteristics of uveitis presenting for the first time in the elderly: Analysis of 91 patients in a tertiary center. *Ocul Immunol Inflamm.* 2011;19:219–26.
25. Agrawal RV, Murthy S, Sangwan V, et al. Current approach in diagnosis and management of anterior uveitis. *Indian J Ophthalmol.* 2010;58:11–19.
26. Mueller JB, McStay CM. Ocular infection and inflammation. *Emerg Med Clin N Am.* 2008;26:57–72, vi.
27. Herbort CP. Appraisal, work-up and diagnosis of anterior uveitis: A practical approach. *Middle East Afr J Ophthalmol.* 2009;16:159–67.
28. Babu BM, Rathinam SR. Intermediate uveitis. *Indian J Ophthalmol.* 2010;58:21–7.
29. Sudharshan S, Ganesh SK, Biswas J. Current approach in the diagnosis and management of posterior uveitis. *Indian J Ophthalmol.* 2010;58:29–43.
30. Tarabishy AB, Jeng BH. Bacterial conjunctivitis: A review for internists. *Cleve Clin J Med.* 2008;75:507–12.
31. O'Brien TP, Jeng BH, McDonald M, et al. Acute conjunctivitis: Truth and misconceptions. *Curr Med Res Opin.* 2009;25:1953–61.
32. Sheikh A, Hurwitz B. Antibiotics versus placebo for acute bacterial conjunctivitis. *Cochrane Database Syst Rev.* 2006;(2):CD001211.
33. Oliver GF, Wilson GA, Everts RJ. Acute infective conjunctivitis: Evidence review and management advice for New Zealand practitioners. *N Z Med J.* 2009;122:69–75.
34. Visscher KL, Hutnik CM, Thomas M. Evidence-based treatment of acute infective conjunctivitis: Breaking the cycle of antibiotic prescribing. *Can Fam Physician.* 2009;55:1071–5.
35. Rosario N, Bielory L. Epidemiology of allergic conjunctivitis. *Curr Opin Allergy Clin Immunol.* 2011;11:471–6.
36. Fraser SG, Adams W. Interventions for acute non-arteritic central retinal artery occlusion. *Cochrane Database Syst Rev.* 2009;(1):CD001989.
37. Haymore JG, Mejico LJ. Retinal vascular occlusion syndromes. *Int Ophthalmol Clin.* 2009;49:63–79.
38. Hayreh SS. Acute retinal arterial occlusive disorders. *Prog Retin Eye Res.* 2011;30:359–94.

39. Hamid S, Mirza SA, Shokh I. Branch retinal vein occlusion. *J Ayub Med Coll Abbottabad.* 2008;20:128–32.

40. Marcucci R, Sofi F, Grifoni E, et al. Retinal vein occlusions: A review for the internist. *Intern Emerg Med.* 2011;6:307–14.

41. Rehak M, Wiedemann P. Retinal vein thrombosis: Pathogenesis and management. *J Thromb Haemost.* 2010;8:1886–94.

42. Kale N, Eggenberger E. Diagnosis and management of giant cell arteritis: A review. *Curr Opin Ophthalmol.* 2010;21:417–22.

43. Falardeau J. Giant cell arteritis. *Neurol Clin.* 2010;28:581–91.

44. Graves JS, Galetta SL. Acute visual loss and other neuro-ophthalmologic emergencies: Management. *Neurol Clin.* 2012;30:75–99, viii.

45. Kesten F, Aschwanden M, Gubser P, et al. Giant cell arteritis – a changing entity. *Swiss Med Wkly.* 2011;141:w13272.

46. Rosenfeld RM, Brown L, Cannon CR, et al. Clinical practice guideline: Acute otitis externa. *Otolaryngol Head Neck Surg.* 2006;134:S4–23.

47. Kaushik V, Malik T, Saeed SR. Interventions for acute otitis externa. *Cochrane Database Syst Rev.* 2010;(1):CD004740.

48. Osguthorpe JD, Nielsen DR. Otitis externa: Review and clinical update. *Am Fam Physician.* 2006;74:1510–1516.

49. Carfrae MJ, Kesser BW. Malignant otitis externa. *Otolaryngol Clin N Am.* 2008;41:537–49, viii-ix.

50. Omran AA, El Garem HF, Al Alem RK. Recurrent malignant otitis externa: Management and outcome. *Eur Arch Otorhinolaryngol.* 2012;269:807–11.

51. Handzel O, Halperin D. Necrotizing (malignant) external otitis. *Am Fam Physician.* 2003;68:309–12.

52. Rubin Grandis J, Branstetter B, Yu V. The changing face of malignant (necrotising) otitis externa: Clinical, radiological and anatomical correlations. *Lancet Infect Dis.* 2004;4:34–9.

53. Gifford TO, Orlandi RR. Epistaxis. *Otolaryngol Clin N Am.* 2008;41:525–36, viii.

54. Manes RP. Evaluating and managing the patient with nosebleed. *Med Clin N Am.* 2010;94:903–12.

55. Melia L, McGarry GW. Epistaxis: Update on management. *Curr Opin Otolaryngol Head Neck Surg.* 2011;19:30–5.

56. Pope L, Hobbs C. Epistaxis: An update on current management. *Postgrad Med J.* 2005;81:309–14.

57. Bader JD, Bonito AJ, Shugars DA. A systematic review of cardiovascular effects of epinephrine on hypertensive dental patients. *Oral Surg Oral Med Oral Pathol Oral Radiol Endod.* 2002;93:647–53.

58. Hecker RB, Hays JV, Champ JD, et al. Myocardial ischemia and stunning induced by topical intranasal phenylephrine pledgets. *Mil Med.* 1997;162:832–5.

59. Choudhury N, Sharp H, Mir N, et al. Epistaxis and oral anticoagulation therapy. *Rhinology.* 2004;42(2):92–7.

60. Srinivasan V, Patel H, John DG, et al. Warfarin and epistaxis: Should warfarin always be discontinued? *Clin Otolaryngol Allied Sci.* 1997;22:542–4.

61. Shay K. Infectious complications of dental and periodontal diseases in the elderly population. *Clin Infect Dis.* 2002;34(9):1215–23.

62. Vargas CM, Kramarow EA, Yellowitz JA. *The oral health of older Americans.* (Centers for Disease Control, National Center for Health Statistics, 2001)3.

63. Helgeson MJ, Smith BJ, Johnsen M, et al. Dental considerations for the frail elderly. *Spec Care Dentist.* 2002;22:40–55S.

64. MacDonald DE. Principles of geriatric dentistry and their application to the older adult with a physical disability. *Clin Geriatr Med.* 2006;22:413–34, x.

65. Robertson D, Smith AJ. The microbiologyof the acute dental abscess. *J Med Microbiol.* 2009;58(Pt 2):155–62.

66. Emergency management of an acute apical abscess in adult. In *Canadian Collaboration on Clinical Practice Guidelines in Dentistry,* 2003 (www.cda-adc.ca/_files/dental_profession/practising/clinical_practice_guidelines/acute_apical_abcesses.pdf).

67. Okunseri C, Okunseri E, Thorpe JM, et al. Medications prescribed in emergency departments for nontraumatic dental condition visits in the United States. *Med Care.* 2012;50:508–12.

68. Shockley WW. Ludwig angina: A review of current airway management. *Arch Otolaryngol Head Neck Surg.* 1999;125:600.

69. Hasan W, Leonard D, Russell J. Ludwig's angina – A controversial surgical emergency: How we do it. *Int J Otolaryngol.* 2011;2011:231816.

70. Vieira F, Allen SM, Stocks RM, et al. Deep neck infection. *Otolaryngol Clin N Am.* 2008;41:459–83, vii.

71. Quinn FB, Jr. Ludwig angina. *Arch Otolaryngol Head Neck Surg.* 1999;125:599.

72. Buckley MF, O'Connor K. Ludwig's angina in a 76-year-old man. *Emerg Med J.* 2009;26:679–80.

73. Costain N, Marrie TJ. Ludwig's angina. *Am J Med.* 2011;124:115–17.

74. Reynolds SC, Chow AW. Severe soft tissue infections of the head and neck: A primer for critical care physicians. *Lung.* 2009;187:271–9.

75. Saifeldeen K, Evans R. Ludwig's angina. *Emerg Med J.* 2004;21:242–3.

76. Duprey K, Rose J, Fromm C. Ludwig's angina. *Int J Emerg Med.* 2010;3:201–2.

77. Marple BF. Ludwig angina: A review of current airway management. *Arch Otolaryngol Head Neck Surg.* 1999;125:596–9.

78. Barton ED, Bair AE. Ludwig's angina. *J Emerg Med.* 2008;34:163–9.

79. Brook I. Non-odontogenic abscesses in the head and neck region. *Periodontol 2000.* 2009;49:106–25.

80. Galioto NJ. Peritonsillar abscess. *Am Fam Physician.* 2008;77:199–202.

81. Khayr W, Taepke J. Management of peritonsillar abscess: Needle aspiration versus incision and drainage versus tonsillectomy. *Am J Ther.* 2005;12:344–50.

82. Bizaki AJ, Numminen J, Vasama JP, et al. Acute supraglottitis in adults in Finland: Review and analysis of 308 cases. *Laryngoscope.* 2011;121:2107–13.

83. Wick F, Ballmer PE, Haller A. Acute epiglottis in adults. *Swiss Med Wkly.* 2002;132:541–7.

84. Ehara H. Tenderness over the hyoid bone can indicate epiglottitis in adults. *J Am Board Fam Med.* 2006;19:517–20.

85. Shepherd M, Kidney E. Adult epiglottitis. *Accid Emerg Nurs.* 2004;12:28–30.

86. Ng HL, Sin LM, Li MF, et al. Acute epiglottitis in adults: A retrospective review of 106 patients in Hong Kong. *Emerg Med J.* 2008;25:253–5.

87. Mathoera RB, Wever PC, van Dorsten FR, et al. Epiglottitis in the adult patient. *Neth J Med.* 2008;66:373–7.

88. Harkani A, Hassani R, Ziad T, et al. Retropharyngeal abscess in adults: Five case reports and review of the literature. *Scient World J.* 2011;11:1623–9.

89. Andrew N, Gabb G, Del Fante M. ACEI associated angioedema – a case study and review. *Aust Fam Physician.* 2011;40:985–8.

90. Flattery MP, Sica DA. Angiotensin-converting enzyme inhibitor-related angioedema: Recognition and treatment. *Prog Cardiovasc Nurs.* 2007;22:47–51.

91. Beltrami L, Zingale LC, Carugo S, et al. Angiotensin-converting enzyme inhibitor-related angioedema: How to deal with it. *Expert Opin Drug Saf.* 2006;5:643–9.

92. Byrd JB, Adam A, Brown NJ. Angiotensin-converting enzyme inhibitor-associated angioedema. *Immunol Allergy Clin N Am.* 2006;26:725–37.

Chapter 18

Neurological emergencies in the elderly

Lauren M. Nentwich

Introduction

Neurological diseases are a major cause of disability and death in the elderly, with many elderly adults presenting to the emergency department (ED) with a neurological emergency. Due to physiological effects of aging as well as increased comorbidities in older adults, neurological diseases often have more complex clinical presentations and difficult work-ups and treatment decisions in geriatric patients than in the younger patient population. This chapter will focus specifically on neurological emergencies that occur frequently in elderly patients, such as: acute stroke, traumatic brain injury, meningitis, spinal epidural abscess, and seizures. It will present the differing clinical presentations of these diseases in the elderly as well as factors complicating diagnosis, clinical work-up, treatment, and prognosis.

Ischemic stroke

Acute ischemic stroke

Stroke is the fourth leading cause of death and the leading cause of long-term disability in the US, and approximately 795,000 Americans suffer an acute stroke annually [1]. Acute ischemic stroke (AIS) occurs when there is loss of blood supply to a region of the brain due to a thrombotic or embolic event, with resulting focal neurological deficits dependent on the area and size of the affected brain [2]. AIS tends to be a disease of the elderly, with an average age of first stroke being 75 years for women and 71 years for men. Compared with younger patients, AIS in elderly patients is associated with higher morbidity and increased disability in stroke survivors. Additionally, many risk factors for AIS are diseases of the elderly, including: hypertension, atrial fibrillation, diabetes, and kidney disease. In fact the percentage of AIS caused by atrial fibrillation increases with age, accounting for approximately 23.5% of AIS in patients aged 80–89 years [1]. Given the high incidence, morbidity, and mortality of AIS in the geriatric population, it is important that elderly patients with AIS be rapidly diagnosed and treated in order to offer them the best chance for a good outcome.

The diagnosis of AIS is made using a combination of patient history, clinical exam, and imaging procedures. Patients

suffering an acute ischemic stroke present with any number of focal neurological deficits, including: motor weakness or hemiparesis, sensory loss, aphasia or dysarthria, neglect, vertigo, ataxia, or visual field deficits [2]. Though elderly patients suffering an acute stroke will commonly present with these typical stroke symptoms, due to their advanced age and multiple comorbidities, geriatric patients suffering an AIS also tend to present with atypical symptoms, such as: falls, reduced mobility [3], and altered mental status. Certain symptoms occur more frequently in the elderly, such as: paralysis, language deficits, swallowing problems, and urinary incontinence [4]. In addition to presenting with atypical symptoms, elderly patients are less likely to know signs or symptoms of AIS [1] and are more likely to present to the hospital late [3]. As such, a high degree of suspicion and rapid work-up is necessary in elderly patients presenting with possible AIS in order to provide them optimal care.

Acute ischemic stroke should be immediately considered in all elderly patients presenting with acute focal neurological deficits, as well as in elderly patients presenting with falls or altered mental status. Elderly patients presenting with suspected stroke should be triaged with the highest priority and should undergo immediate evaluation by an emergency physician with subsequent urgent consultation and assessment by the stroke team or neurology service. If a neurologist is not readily available, urgent neurological consultation should be obtained via telemedicine services or transfer to a hospital with stroke neurology expertise and services.

The initial evaluation of an older patient with suspected acute stroke is similar to any other critically ill patient, with immediate stabilization of the patient's airway, breathing, and circulation followed quickly by a secondary assessment of neurological deficits and possible comorbidities. A precise history should be obtained from either the patient or his/her close family members or caregivers. The most important piece of necessary history is the time of symptom onset, defined specifically as the time the patient was last seen without new symptoms, as this information will often guide treatment in the patient with AIS. Additional history includes circumstances around the development of neurological symptoms as well as prior medical history, including prior strokes and risk factors

Geriatric Emergency Medicine, ed. Joseph H. Kahn, Brendan G. Magauran Jr., and Jonathan S. Olshaker. Published by Cambridge University Press.
© Cambridge University Press 2014.

for arteriosclerosis and cardiac disease, and current medications, especially anticoagulants such as warfarin or dabigatran. In elderly patients presenting with fall and suspected stroke, it is important to obtain a history of trauma to the head, significant injury, or witnessed seizure.

A rapid and thorough physical exam should be performed, including full vital signs, evaluation for any evidence of trauma or comorbidities, and a cardiac examination focusing on identifying concurrent myocardial ischemia, valvular conditions, irregular rhythm, or possible aortic dissection. A brief but thorough neurological examination should be performed and is enhanced by the use of a formal stroke score or scale, such as the National Institutes of Health Stroke Scale (NIHSS) (Table 18.1). The NIHSS ensures that the major components of a neurological examination are performed in a timely fashion, allows for rapid reassessment of the patient's clinical status, and aids in facilitating communication between health care professionals.

Routine laboratory tests should be obtained in all patients presenting with suspected AIS. A fingerstick blood glucose should be obtained on arrival, as hypoglycemia may cause focal neurological signs and symptoms that mimic stroke. Coagulation studies and platelets, especially in patients with concern for bleeding abnormality, thrombocytopenia, or coagulation use, are important as abnormal results will limit treatment. Given the increased incidence of cardiac arrhythmias and ischemia in the elderly, a 12-lead electrocardiogram (ECG), cardiac monitoring, and cardiac enzyme tests should be performed in elderly patients with suspected AIS [5].

An essential component in diagnosing AIS and differentiating ischemic from hemorrhagic stroke is brain imaging with either computed tomography (CT) or magnetic resonance imaging (MRI) (Figure 18.1). Imaging by CT or MRI is necessary to exclude the presence of hemorrhage and may help to guide therapy in patients with AIS. Non-contrast brain CT is typically the first choice in imaging patients with suspected acute stroke due to its accuracy in excluding hemorrhage, speed in acquisition, and general availability in most US EDs. Additionally, many elderly patients have cardiac pacemakers or certain ferromagnetic metallic implanted substances which are absolute contraindications to undergoing MRI [6]. A full review of neuroimaging in AIS is beyond the scope of this chapter, but the American Heart Association (AHA) Guidelines recommend that neuroimaging by CT or MRI in all patients with suspected AIS should be completed within 25 minutes of the patient's arrival to the ED and undergo expert interpretation within 45 minutes of ED arrival [7].

Intravenous (IV) thrombolysis with recombinant tissue plasminogen activator (rt-PA) is currently the only treatment approved by the Food and Drug Administration for patients presenting with AIS [8]. The benefit, safety, and frequency of use of IV rt-PA in the elderly are uncertain. Elderly patients are at higher risk for stroke-related death and disability, which makes them an important target group for acute treatment, but they may also be at increased risk for hemorrhagic complications from IV rt-PA [9]. The 1995 NINDS IV rt-PA trial, which treated patients with symptoms of AIS less than 3 hours with

IV rt-PA, enrolled 44 patients with baseline age more than 80 (19 placebo and 25 IV rt-PA) [8,10]. Of the 25 patients randomized to IV rt-PA in this study, 4 experienced symptomatic intracranial hemorrhages within 36 hours of treatment, and these older patients were 2.87 times more likely to experience a symptomatic intracranial hemorrhage within 36 hours when compared with younger patients [10]. A follow-up study to the 1995 NINDS IV rt-PA trial that attempted to expand the hours for treatment in AIS is the European Cooperative Acute Stroke Study III (ECASS III), which treated patients with AIS with IV rt-PA within 3–4.5 hours after the onset of stroke. Due to concern for increased risk of hemorrhagic complications, elderly patients of age greater than 80 years were excluded from enrollment in ECASS III [11]. Despite these apparent contradictions to treatment with IV rt-PA in elderly patients with AIS, multiple studies have shown a benefit to thrombolysis with IV rt-PA in patients older than 80 years who are treated within 3 hours of symptom onset [9,12–14]. Given the current data, there is no compelling reason to exclude elderly patients from receiving treatment with IV rt-PA if therapy can be started within 3 hours of symptom onset. However, given the facts of increased morbidity and mortality in elderly patients with AIS and the increased risk of hemorrhagic complications, detailed discussions should be held with the patient and family when deciding the proper course of treatment for older patients. Though IV rt-PA within 3 hours of symptom onset in elderly patients is accepted treatment, current AHA guidelines do not recommend expanding the treatment window to 4.5 hours for elderly patients and do not endorse administering IV rt-PA to patients older than 80 years outside of 3 hours of symptom onset [15].

Transient ischemic attack

A transient ischemic attack (TIA) is defined as a transient episode of neurological dysfunction caused by focal brain, spinal cord, or retinal ischemia, without acute infarction [16]. Though, by definition, the neurological dysfunction in patients suffering a TIA is temporary, the risk of AIS after TIA is high, particularly in the first few days. Up to 23% of all AIS are preceded by a TIA [17], and the pooled early risk of stroke after TIA has been reported as 3.1–3.5% at 2 days, 5.2% at 7 days, 8.0% at 30 days, and 9.2% at 90 days [18,19]. TIA incidence markedly increases with increasing age, from 1–3 cases per 100,000 in those younger than 35 years up to 600–1500 cases per 100,000 in those patients older than 85 years, making TIA an important disease in the geriatric population [16,20]. In addition to an increased stroke risk after TIA, the risk of cardiac events is also elevated after TIA, and equal numbers of patients with TIA will suffer a myocardial infarction or sudden cardiac death as will have a cerebral infarction in the 5 years after a TIA [21].

Given the high risk for early AIS after TIA, elderly patients presenting with symptoms suggestive of TIA should undergo urgent triage and rapid evaluation by a physician. The diagnosis of TIA is clinical, and the history should focus on whether patients have abrupt onset of focal neurological deficits and the duration of those symptoms [22]. Historical information may be difficult to obtain from elderly patients, and family members or witnesses to the event should be interviewed to provide

Table 18.1. National Institutes of Health Stroke scale

1a. Level of consciousness	0 – Alert; keenly responsive
	1 – Not alert, but arousable by minor stimuli
	2 – Not alert, requires repeated or strong stimuli to attend
	3 – Unresponsive or responds only with reflex or autonomic effects
1b. Level of consciousness questions: Current month Patient's age	0 – Answers both questions correctly 1 – Answers one question correctly, or patient unable to speak for reasons not due to aphasia 2 – Answers neither question correctly, or aphasic
1c. Level of consciousness Commands: Open and close eyes Grip and release hand	0 – Performs both tasks correctly 1 – Performs one task correctly 2 – Performs neither task correctly
2. Best gaze	0 – Normal 1 – Partial gaze palsy 2 – Forced deviation, or total gaze paresis that is not overcome by oculocephalic maneuver
3. Visual fields	0 – No visual loss 1 – Partial hemianopia 2 – Complete hemianopia 3 – Bilateral hemianopia
4. Facial palsy	0 – Normal symmetrical movements 1 – Minor paralysis 2 – Partial paralysis 3 – Complete paralysis of one or both sides
5. Motor arm 5a. Left arm 5b. Right arm	0 – No drift 1 – Drift, but does not hit bed or other support 2 – Some effort against gravity, but drifts to bed 3 – No movement against gravity 4 – No movement UN – Amputation
6. Motor leg 6a. Left leg 6b. Right leg	0 – No drift 1 – Drift, but does not hit bed or other support 2 – Some effort against gravity, but drifts to bed 3 – No movement against gravity 4 – No movement UN – Amputation or joint fusion
7. Limb ataxia	0 – Absent 1 – Present in one limb 2 – Present in two limbs UN – Amputation or joint fusion
8. Sensory	0 – Normal 1 – Mild to moderate sensory loss 2 – Severe to total sensory loss
9. Best language	0 – No aphasia 1 – Mild to moderate aphasia 2 – Severe aphasia 3 – Mute, global aphasia
10. Dysarthria	0 – Normal 1 – Mild to moderate dysarthria 2 – Severe dysarthria UN – Intubated or other physical barrier
11. Extinction and inattention	0 – No abnormality 1 – Visual, tactile, auditory, spatial, or personal inattention 2 – Profound hemi-inattention or extinction to more than one modality

Adapted from National Institutes of Health, National Institute of Neurological Disorders and Stroke (accessed from http://stroke.nih.gov/resources/scale.htm).

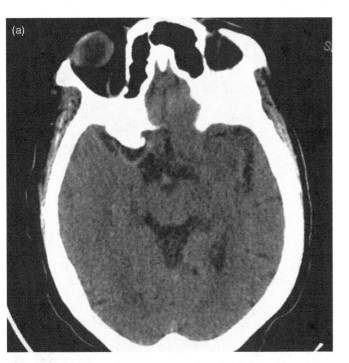

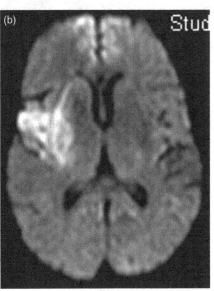

Figure 18.1. (a) Non-contrast brain CT of a patient suffering an acute ischemic stroke. A hyperdense right middle cerebral artery is apparent, concerning for thrombus. (b) Corresponding right middle cerebral artery territory shows acute ischemic stroke on MRI. Acute ischemic strokes appear hyperintense on diffusion-weighted imaging.

clarifying or collaborating details. An accurate and full neurological exam should be performed to determine whether baseline neurological function has been restored, as a recent study showed that one-quarter of patients referred to a same-day TIA clinic with reportedly resolved symptoms had persistent neurological deficits on the neurologist's exam [23]. Auscultation of the neck for carotid bruits and the heart for arrhythmias and valvular or structural heart lesions is also important. Routine laboratory testing, including a complete blood count, chemistry panel, and basic coagulation studies, is reasonable, though often low yield [16,22]. As the heart is a common source of emboli, cardiac evaluation is important in patients with TIA

[22]. ECG should be performed as soon as possible after TIA to assess for atrial fibrillation, left ventricular aneurysm, or recent myocardial infarction. Prolonged monitoring with inpatient telemetry or Holter monitor is useful in patients with unclear origin after initial evaluation [16,22].

The AHA currently recommends that all patients with TIA should preferably undergo neuroimaging evaluation within 24 hours of symptoms onset, and MRI, including diffusion-weighted imaging (DWI), is the preferred brain diagnostic imaging modality [16]. In addition to brain imaging, the AHA also recommends routine noninvasive imaging of the cervicocephalic vessels as part of the evaluation of patients with suspected TIA [16]. Nearly half of patients with TIA with DWI lesions have stenosis or occlusion of either extracranial or intracranial larger arteries, and imaging of the cervicocephalic vessels can be performed noninvasively using carotid duplex with transcranial doppler, CT angiography, or MR angiography [16,22]. Work-up should be performed under consultation with a stroke expert, for if abnormalities are found on imaging, carotid endarterectomy is highly beneficial in reducing stroke risk in patients with 70% or more stenosis without near-occlusion [17]. Additionally, a similar benefit has been shown in patients with 50–70% stenosis, especially in men, elderly patients older than 75 years, and within 2 weeks of the previous ischemic event [24].

Determining which patients suffering a TIA should be hospitalized versus admitted to an observation unit versus discharged with rapid follow-up is a subject of great uncertainty and controversy. The National Stroke Association Guidelines for the management of TIA recommend the consideration of hospitalization for patients with their first TIA within the past 24–48 hours, as well as patients with multiple and increasingly frequent symptoms, to facilitate possible early lytic therapy or other medical management if symptoms were to recur as well as to expedite the work-up for definitive secondary prevention [25]. It is generally recommended that the best care is to evaluate patients suffering a TIA immediately on diagnosis via an inpatient hospitalization, an observation unit, or in an outpatient 24-hour specialty TIA clinic [22]. Though no specific guidelines exist, given the increased morbidity and mortality of geriatric patients who suffer a TIA, it is prudent to consider hospitalization or admission to an observational unit to facilitate rapid work-up as well as close monitoring in this patient population.

Non-traumatic intracranial hemorrhage

Intracerebral hemorrhage

Intracerebral hemorrhage (ICH) is defined as spontaneous, non-traumatic bleeding into the brain parenchyma [26]. ICH constitutes 10–15% of all first-ever strokes and is a medical emergency with a 30-day mortality rate of 35–52% and a high morbidity rate, with only 20% of patients functionally independent at six months [27]. The incidence of ICH increases with increasing age, and the rate doubles each decade of life after 35 years of age [28]. Older age is an important risk factor for ICH; additionally, other risk factors for ICH are often seen in elderly patients, including: presence of cerebral amyloid angiopathy (CAA), hypertension, previous ischemic or hemorrhagic stroke, and oral anticoagulation use [29]. ICH is classified as primary or secondary dependent on whether there is not or is an underlying congenital lesion, respectively. Chronic hypertension causes 75% of all primary ICH, and CAA is the second most common cause of primary ICH and accounts for more than 20% of ICH in patients of age greater than 70 [28]. Additionally, elderly patients suffering an ICH tend to have a substantially worse prognosis than older patients with AIS, and 1-year mortality rates in patients older than 65 years diagnosed with ICH are around 50% [30].

The presentation of ICH depends on its location, size, and speed of development [31]. Like AIS, ICH causes sudden dysfunction of neural tissue in a specific territory of the brain resulting in focal neurologic deficits. In patients presenting with focal neurologic deficits, initial findings more likely to be associated with ICH include loss of consciousness, coma, neck stiffness, seizure accompanying the onset of neurologic deficits, diastolic blood pressure greater than 110 mmHg, vomiting, and headache. However, many patients with ICH lack any of these distinctive clinical findings and the diagnosis of ICH, as well as its differentiation from AIS, cannot be made clinically but requires definitive neuroimaging [32].

Both the AHA and the European Stroke Initiative (EUSI) recommend rapid neuroimaging to distinguish ischemic stroke from ICH [31,33].

Elderly patients presenting with concern for ICH should undergo rapid neuroimaging by non-contrast CT or MRI. Non-contrast CT is considered the gold standard for the diagnosis of ICH and is thought to be 100% sensitive [33] (Figure 18.2). Gradient-echo (GRE) and T2* susceptibility-weighted MRI are as sensitive as CT for the detection of acute ICH with the added benefit of being more sensitive in diagnosing AIS and chronic ICH [34,35]. However, CT is typically more readily available in US EDs, and many elderly patients suffering an ICH may be too medically unstable or have contraindications for MRI [36,37]. Once ICH is diagnosed, additional neuroimaging such as CT angiography/venography or MR angiography/venography may be performed in select patients to identify secondary causes of ICH amenable to intervention, such as: aneurysms, arteriovenous malformations, fistulas, tumors, or cerebral vein thrombosis [33].

Given the high incidence of hypertension as well as oral anticoagulation treatment in the elderly, elderly patients diagnosed with ICH should have rapid vital signs and rapid serum laboratory tests, including an international normalized ratio (INR)/prothrombin time, as part of their initial work-up. Acutely elevated blood pressure (BP) is common in patients with ICH and may lead to adverse outcomes via hematoma expansion or perihematomal edema formation, though it is unclear whether reducing the BP improves clinical outcomes [33]. Presently, the AHA Stroke Council recommends aggressive reduction of BP with continuous intravenous infusion and frequent BP monitoring for systolic BP (SBP) >200 mmHg or mean arterial pressure (MAP) >150 mmHg. If SBP >180 mmHg or MAP >130 mmHg, the AHA recommends more modest reductions in BP, and in

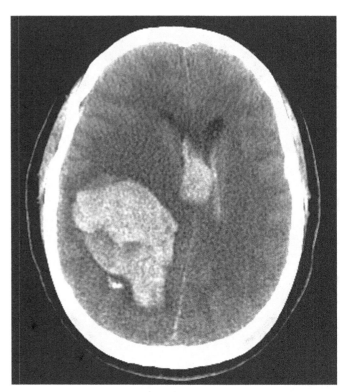

Figure 18.2. Non-contrast brain CT of a large acute intracerebral hemorrhage within the right parietal lobe with associated intraventricular hemorrhage and midline shift.

cases of possible elevated intracranial pressure (ICP), the AHA recommends monitoring ICP and maintaining cerebral perfusion pressure (CPP) ≥60 mmHg. Currently recommended antihypertensive medications for patients with ICH include IV labetalol, nicardipine, esmolol, enalapril, hydralazine, sodium nitroprusside, or nitroglycerin [27,33]. Many elderly patients are on oral anticoagulation treatment, and warfarin-associated ICH is a devastating complication of this treatment with high mortality rate and poor neurologic outcome in survivors. Elderly patients with ICH who are known to be on warfarin or have an elevated INR should undergo urgent correction of their coagulopathy to prevent continued bleeding. These patients should have the warfarin held, be given IV vitamin K, and undergo normalizing of the INR with fresh frozen plasma (FFP) or prothrombin complex concentrates (PCCs) [29].

All elderly patients diagnosed with ICH should undergo urgent neurology and neurosurgical consultation, or be transferred to a hospital with full neurology, neuroradiology, and neurosurgical capabilities. Patients may need specialty consultation for evaluation and management of many possible complications of ICH, including: elevated ICP, hydrocephalus, brainstem compression, or brain herniation. Given that they are medically and neurologically unstable, patients with ICH should be admitted to an intensive care unit (ICU) for frequent monitoring of vital signs and neurologic status as well as to receive intensive treatments as needed [29]. ICH is associated with high mortality rate and significant morbidity among survivors, especially in the elderly. However, studies have shown that the most important prognostic variable in determining outcome after ICH is the level of medical support provided, and patients who are initially predicted to have a poor outcome can achieve reasonable recovery if they are treated aggressively [38]. Limiting care in response to early Do Not Resuscitate (DNR) orders, withdrawal of care, or deferral of life-sustaining interventions is independently associated with both short- and long-term mortality after ICH, independent of other predictors of death [39]. New DNR orders or withdrawal of care are generally not recommended in the ED, and the AHA recommends aggressive full care early after ICH onset with postponement of new DNR orders until at least the second full day of hospitalization [33]. This recommendation does not apply to elderly patients with established DNR orders prior to developing an ICH.

Aneurysmal subarachnoid hemorrhage

Aneurysmal subarachnoid hemorrhage (aSAH) is a neurological emergency characterized by extravasation of blood into the cerebrospinal fluid covering the central nervous system (CNS), caused by the rupture of an intracranial aneurysm. It accounts for approximately 2–5% of all new strokes and has high morbidity and mortality with an average case fatality rate of 51%, and approximately one-third of survivors requiring lifelong care. aSAH is an important disease of the elderly as the incidence increases with age [40]. There is a higher prevalence of intracranial aneurysms in patients over 60 years of age, and age-related risk factors such as increased atherosclerosis and hypertension likely compound both the risk of aneurysm formation and aneurysm rupture in the elderly [41]. Additionally, advanced age, as well as the patient's level of consciousness on admission and amount of blood on initial head CT, are the major factors associated with poor outcome [40].

aSAH should always be suspected in patients who present with the typical presentation of sudden-onset severe headache with associated nausea and/or vomiting and brief loss of consciousness. The physical exam may show retinal hemorrhages, restlessness, diminished level of consciousness, nuchal rigidity, photophobia, and focal neurological signs. Patients with a "typical" presentation present little diagnostic difficulty, but patients without these signs and symptoms are often misdiagnosed [42]. Disorders of consciousness are more frequently seen in geriatric patients than in the general population [41], and often the diagnosis of aSAH is overlooked in elderly patients. Misdiagnosis of aSAH is most commonly due to failure to obtain a non-contrast head CT. Non-contrast head CT remains the cornerstone of diagnosis of aSAH and should be performed in all patients with suspected aSAH [40] (Figure 18.3). SAH is often more abundant on CT in elderly patients than in younger people due to the presence of parenchymal atrophy in the geriatric patient population, which allows for a larger quantity of blood to collect after aneurysmal rupture; this more abundant hemorrhage may partly explain the generally worsened neurologic status in the elderly population at admission and resulting worsened clinical outcome [41]. The sensitivity of CT decreases over time from onset of symptoms, as the dynamics of cerebral spinal fluid and spontaneous lysis can result in rapid clearing of subarachnoid blood [42]. As such, lumbar puncture should be performed in any patient with suspected aSAH and negative

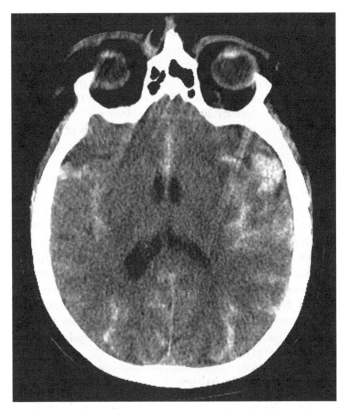

Figure 18.3. Non-contrast brain CT of extensive subarachnoid hemorrhage within the bilateral cerebral sulci.

CT results; findings consistent with SAH include: elevated opening pressure, elevated red cell count that does not diminish from tube 1 to tube 4, and xanthochromia [40]. If SAH is diagnosed by CT or lumbar puncture (LP), a CT angiography (CTA) should be considered to investigate for an aneurysm and to help guide decisions regarding the type of aneurysm repair; if the CTA is inconclusive, digital subtraction angiography is recommended to identify small aneurysms not detected by CTA [43].

All patients with aSAH should be emergently evaluated and treated with maintenance of the airway and cardiovascular function as needed. Neurology and neurosurgery should be rapidly consulted or the patient should be transferred to a center with neurovascular expertise. The main goals of treatment are the prevention of rebleeding, the prevention and management of vasospasm, and the treatment of other medical neurologic complications [40]. Risk of rebleeding is maximal in the first 2–12 hours and is associated with poor outcome and high mortality [43], and the rebleeding rate in elderly patients is higher and earlier than in younger patients [41]. Acute hypertension should be controlled from the time of diagnosis of aSAH until aneurysm obliteration using a titratable IV antihypertensive to balance the risk of stroke, hypertension-related rebleeding, and maintenance of cerebral perfusion pressure; parameters for blood pressure control have not been clearly defined, but AHA guidelines recommend a decrease in SBP <160 mmHg as reasonable.

Early obliteration of the aneurysm is required to prevent rebleeding, and experienced cerebrovascular surgeons and endovascular specialists should be consulted to determine proper treatment of the aneurysm by either microsurgical clipping or endovascular coiling depending on the characteristics of both the patient and aneurysm. Though the data are conflicting, some suggest that elderly patients older than 70 years of age are ideal candidates for coiling rather than clipping [43]. Though approximately 20 years ago, elderly patients suffering an aSAH were treated conservatively on the basis of advanced age alone and subsequently suffered a poor outcome, the management of aSAH has considerably changed in recent years with a more aggressive approach for elderly patients with improved results. If elderly patients are carefully selected, endovascular coiling or microsurgical clipping can lead to a positive outcome [41]. All patients with aSAH should be admitted to an ICU, preferentially a neurologic critical care unit, to optimize care and monitor closely for common complications. Neurologic complications are common after aSAH and include symptomatic vasospasm, hydrocephalus, rebleeding, and seizures [40]. Due to their advanced age and resulting comorbidities, elderly patients suffering an aSAH are at increased risk for both neurologic and general complications and should be monitored closely [41].

Traumatic brain injury

Traumatic brain injury (TBI) is an important health problem in the US affecting about 1.5 million people per year with high morbidity, accounting for approximately 1.2 million ED visits and 220–290 thousand hospitalizations per year, and high mortality with approximately 50 thousand deaths per year. Though TBI rates are highest among infants and young children, TBI hospitalizations and death rates are highest among older adults 65 years of age and older, making TBI an important disease state in the elderly population [44]. Falls are the leading cause of TBI for older adults, accounting for 51% of all geriatric TBI patients, and motor vehicle accidents (both driver/passenger and pedestrians struck) are the second leading cause accounting for 9% [45]. Additionally, older age is associated with worsening outcome after TBI [46].

TBI is caused by a high-energy acceleration or deceleration of the brain within the cranium or with penetration of the brain. It is classified as either focal or diffuse; focal injuries tend to occur at the site of impact with resulting focal neurologic deficits in those areas, whereas diffuse shearing of axons may occur in the cerebral white matter, gray–white junction, corpus callosum, and/or brainstem causing both nonlateralizing neurologic deficits and/or focal deficits. TBI is often classified by severity, which is usually based on the Glasgow Coma Scale (GCS) (Table 18.2). GCS evaluates best motor response, verbal response, and eye opening in patients who have suffered acute trauma. Mild TBI is defined as an isolated head injury with a GCS score of 13–15. Patients with moderate TBI have a GCS score of 9–12. Severe TBI is defined as a patient who presents acutely with a GCS of 8 or less or any patient with an intracranial contusion, hematoma, or laceration [47].

Many young patients with TBI may have normal head imaging with no acute abnormalities found on CT. Abnormalities on brain imaging are much more common in

Table 18.2. Glasgow Coma Scale [87]

		Score
Best eye response (E)	Spontaneous eye opening	4
	Eye opening to verbal stimuli or command	3
	Eye opening to pain	2
	No eye opening	1
Best verbal response (V)	Oriented	5
	Confused	4
	Inappropriate words	3
	Incomprehensible speech	2
	No verbal response	1
	Intubated	T
Best motor response (M)	Obeys commands	6
	Localizing response to pain	5
	Withdrawal response to pain	4
	Flexion to pain (decorticate posture)	3
	Extension to pain (decerebrate posture)	2
	No motor response	1
Total score		3–15 (T)

elderly patients as well as in those who have suffered moderate to severe TBI. Abnormalities found on imaging of patients who have suffered a TBI may include: skull fractures, diastasis of the skull, intracranial hemorrhage (epidural hematoma, subdural hematoma, intracerebral hematoma, intraventricular hemorrhage, brain contusion, traumatic subarachnoid hemorrhage), cerebral edema, pneumocephalus, traumatic infarction, and diffuse axonal injury [47,48]. All patients with moderate to severe TBI (GCS <13) should undergo immediate head CT given a higher likelihood of abnormal findings on neuroimaging studies [47]. In adult patients with minor TBI (GCS 13–15), neuroimaging is generally recommended only for patients who meet certain criteria, with older age being one of the most important for ordering brain imaging. Three decision rules: the Canadian CT Head Rule, the New Orleans Criteria, and the National Emergency X-Radiography Utilizations Study-II have been derived to indicate which patients suffering a minor TBI should undergo CT to most efficiently identify acute abnormalities on CT; elderly patients, age >60 or >65, are excluded from these decision rules due to a higher rate of acute intracranial abnormalities in such patients [49–51]. Geriatric patients with blunt minor TBI are more likely to have an acute abnormality on head CT which may require neurosurgical intervention, and liberal use of head CT is recommended in this patient population [48,52]. It is generally recommended to obtain neuroimaging in all elderly patients who suffer acute head trauma and sustain a TBI, regardless of the severity of the injury or the initial clinical presentation.

After sustaining a TBI, elderly patients tend to suffer worse outcomes with higher mortality and worsened neurologic outcomes [53]. Elderly patients have twice the mortality of younger patients (30 versus 14%) and increased poor functional outcome in survivors (13 versus 5%) [54]. The mechanism by which advanced age is an independent predictor of worse outcome is largely unknown, but factors that likely contribute include: increased incidence of pre-existing medical comorbidities (particularly diabetes mellitus, hypertension, coronary disease, and prior stroke) in elderly patients, increased use of anticoagulants or antiplatelet drugs in elderly patients for management of chronic medical conditions, and age-related changes in the brain (i.e., the dura becoming more adherent to the skull, decreased elasticity and increased fragility of cerebral vessels, increased stress placed on venous structures due to cerebral atrophy, cerebrovascular atherosclerosis, and decreased free radical clearance) [45,52,55]. While subdural hematoma (SDH) and epidural hematoma (EDH) may both be identified on initial CT in patients suffering a TBI (Figure 18.4), SDH is much more common in elderly adults and EDH is rare in the elderly due to the close attachment of the dura to the skull. When a SDH is diagnosed as a component of TBI, mortality is increased and neurologic outcomes are worsened. Factors associated with worsening prognosis in patients with acute SDH are large hematoma size, midline shift, and concurrent parenchymal lesions. Time to neurosurgical management appears to be critical in these patients, and elderly patients with SDH should undergo urgent neurosurgical evaluation [47,53,55,56].

With some exceptions, the general management of elderly patients presenting to the ED who have suffered a severe TBI is similar to that in younger patients. Many recommendations on the treatment of patients with severe TBI are derived from guidelines developed and maintained by the Brain Trauma Foundation (www.braintrauma.org).

An initial GCS should be measured and repeatedly monitored to watch for clinical improvement or deterioration. Airway, breathing, and circulation should be emergently evaluated and stabilized. Hypoxemia (SpO_2 <90%) should be avoided and rapidly corrected if identified. An airway should be established in those patients with a GCS <9, who are unable to maintain an adequate airway, or if hypoxemia is not corrected by supplemental oxygen. After intubation, patients should be maintained with normal breathing rates (end-tidal CO_2 [$ETCO_2$] 35–40 mmHg) and hyperventilation avoided unless the patient shows signs of cerebral herniation [57]. Once the airway is secured, vital signs should be noted and continuously monitored. Hypotension, defined as a single systolic BP (SBP) <90 mmHg, causes poor outcomes in patients who suffer a TBI and should be avoided and rapidly corrected if it occurs [58]. A secondary survey should be performed and the patient should be assessed for secondary trauma.

Patients should be frequently assessed for clinical signs of cerebral herniation, including: dilated and unreactive pupils, asymmetric pupils, motor exam that identifies extensor posturing or no response, or progressive neurological deterioration [57]. In cases of suspected elevated ICP, simple techniques can be instituted to prevent and treat elevated ICP, such as: elevating head of bed to 30°, optimizing venous drainage by keeping the neck in neutral position and loosening neck braces if too tight, monitoring central venous pressure, and avoiding excess hypervolemia. Additionally, doses of mannitol or infusions of hypertonic saline can be effective for control of raised ICP [58].

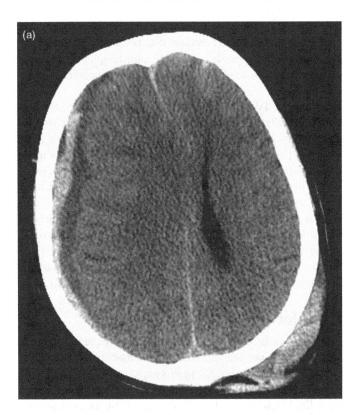

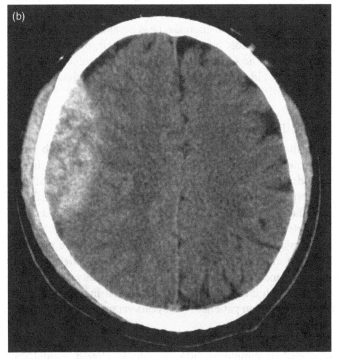

Figure 18.4. (a) Non-contrast brain CT of an acute large right subdural hematoma with associated midline shift. (b) Non-contrast brain CT of a large epidural hematoma with mass effect and associated midline shift.

Trauma surgery and neurosurgery should be immediately consulted on patient arrival for further management of patients suffering a severe TBI, including necessity of ICP monitoring as well as possible surgical management as dictated by the patient's clinical status and neuroimaging. Due to age-related differences in biology and concomitant comorbidities, a lower threshold for trauma activation should be used for elderly trauma patients who are evaluated at trauma centers and for transferring older patients at acute care hospitals without a dedicated trauma service to designated trauma centers for their care [59].

Adequate IV access should be obtained and proper labs sent, especially a complete blood count and coagulation parameters, to assess for any potential coagulopathy that needs to be reversed [57]. Warfarin-related coagulopathy, which is more common in the geriatric population, increases the risks of post-injury hemorrhage. All elderly patients with suspected head injury on anticoagulants should be evaluated by head CT as soon as possible after ED arrival. In elderly patients on warfarin with intracranial bleeding, the INR should be rapidly corrected to a value of less than 1.6 with IV vitamin K and FFP or PCCs. Depending on their injuries and clinical status, patients should be admitted to the intensive care unit or trauma service [59].

CNS infections

Infections in the elderly are typically more frequent and more severe than in younger patients and are associated with worsened outcome. Additionally, in this population, infection tends to have a more subtle presentation with fewer symptoms. Fever, a cardinal sign of infection in younger patients, is absent or blunted in 20–30% of severe infections in the elderly. The most common signs of infection in the elderly are very nonspecific, such as falls, delirium, anorexia, or generalized weakness [60]. This is true of most infections in the elderly, but particularly infections of the CNS. Two important CNS infections to be aware of in elderly adults are meningitis and spinal epidural abscess.

Community-acquired bacterial meningitis

With the success of the *Haemophilus influenzae* type b (Hib) and pneumococcal vaccines, the rates of bacterial meningitis have decreased over the past 15 years. The age group with the highest incidence of bacterial meningitis in the US is children less than 2 years, but elderly patients aged 65 years and above comprise the group with the second highest incidence of bacterial meningitis with 1.92 cases per 100,000 people in 2006–2007. In addition to being more common in older patients, bacterial meningitis causes increased mortality in geriatric patients with an overall mortality rate that increases linearly with age (8.9% in patients 18–34 years versus 22.7% in patients over 65 years) [61].

Elderly patients with bacterial meningitis may present with a myriad of symptoms, including: fever, altered mental status, neck stiffness, headache, seizure, shock, or focal neurologic abnormalities. Neck stiffness and headache are found to occur less frequently in older people, and a much larger proportion of elderly patients presented with altered mental status or focal neurological abnormalities [62–64]. If bacterial meningitis is suspected, LP is indicated. Due to the risk of brain herniation as a complication of diagnostic LP in select patients with bacterial meningitis, neuroimaging by CT or MRI prior to LP is recommended in selected patients to detect

brain shift. Neuroimaging should precede LP in patients with: new-onset seizures, immunocompromised state, signs suspicious for space-occupying lesions including papilledema, or moderate-to-severe alteration in level of consciousness. Best practice dictates that if neuroimaging is performed before LP, antibiotic therapy should be initiated before the patient is sent for neuroimaging [65].

The predominant bacterial organisms found in elderly patients with community-acquired bacterial meningitis include: *Streptococcus pneumoniae*, *Neisseria meningitidis*, and *Listeria monocytogenes*. As such, empiric antibiotic therapy that should be started in elderly patients prior to knowing the organism from Gram stain or culture is vancomycin plus a third-generation cephalosporin plus ampicillin. Additionally, due to a proven mortality benefit, adjunctive dexamethasone therapy should be initiated in patients with suspected bacterial meningitis before or with the first dose of antibiotics [65,66]. Admission to the hospital is recommended for all patients with suspected bacterial meningitis, and respiratory isolation for 24 hours is indicated for patients with suspected meningococcal infection [65].

Advanced age is associated with unfavorable outcome in patients with bacterial meningitis [67], and complications are more likely to occur in older patients than younger patients [64]. Early recognition and treatment are important to reduce the high morbidity and mortality of infectious diseases in older adults, and bacterial meningitis is always a medical emergency [63]. In addition, although this section addresses community-acquired bacterial meningitis in older patients, nosocomial meningitis is a distinct disease that should also be considered in the elderly patient, especially those presenting with fever and altered level of consciousness with a history of neurosurgery, a distant focus of infection, or following penetrating trauma or basilar skull fracture [62,66].

Spinal epidural abscess

Spinal epidural abscess (SEA) represents the accumulation of purulent material in the space between the dura mater and the osseo-ligamentous confines of the vertebral canal. It is an uncommon disease with a relatively high rate of morbidity and mortality and prognosis that is often determined by early diagnosis and initiation of appropriate therapy [68]. SEA is a difficult diagnosis to make in general as most patients do not present with the classic triad of back pain, fever, and neurological deficit, and misdiagnosis and delayed diagnosis is common [69]. A dangerous infection that is more common in elderly patients, diagnosis of SEA in the geriatric population is further complicated by the fact that elderly patients frequently present to the ED with back pain from degenerative disease [70]. Most patients with SEA have one or more predisposing conditions, and many of these conditions are common in elderly patients, including: underlying diabetes mellitus or alcoholism, a spinal abnormality such as degenerative joint disease or trauma, spinal intervention such as surgery, placement of stimulators or catheters, or a potential source of infection such as skin and soft-tissue infections, osteomyelitis, urinary tract infection, sepsis, indwelling vascular access, epidural analgesia, or nerve block [71]. Additionally, though the disease can affect any age group, SEA seems to have increased in incidence over the past 25 years and one of the potential reasons is thought to be aging of the general population [68].

In SEA, the spinal cord is injured by the infection either directly by mechanical compression or indirectly as a result of vascular occlusion caused by septic thrombophlebitis. An established staging system by Heusner outlines the progression of symptoms of SEA: stage 1, back pain at the level of the affected spine; stage 2, nerve root pain radiating from the involved spinal area; stage 3, motor weakness, sensory deficit, and bladder and bowel dysfunction; and stage 4, paralysis [71,72]. The most common presenting symptoms include back pain (present in about 70–90% of patients), fever (documented in 60–70% of patients), and neurological dysfunction (noted in approximately 33–70% of patients). Other complaints in patients presenting with SEA may include paravertebral muscle spasm, limited spinal motion, paresthesias, weakness, and difficulty ambulating [68,71].

Diagnosis of SEA is suspected on the basis of clinical findings and supported by laboratory data and imaging studies. Leukocytosis is only detected in about two-thirds of patients, but inflammatory markers (erythrocyte sedimentation rate and C-reactive protein) are almost uniformly elevated. Bacteremia as the cause of or arising from SEA is detected in about 60% of patients, and can provide identification of the causative pathogen [71]. When SEA is suspected, gadolinium-enhanced MRI of the spine should be obtained emergently (Figure 18.5), as this imaging modality is highly sensitive and highly specific and can accurately delineate the extent and location of

the abscess. Myelography followed by CT is useful when MRI is contraindicated, but it is less specific than MRI and cannot distinguish SEA from other lesions that compress the thecal sac [68].

Emergent surgical depression and drainage of the abscess, together with systemic antibiotics is the treatment of choice for the vast majority of patients diagnosed with SEA. Since the preoperative neurologic function is the most important predictor of final outcome and the rate of progression of neurologic impairment is difficult to predict, decompressive surgery and debridement of infected tissues should be performed as soon as possible after diagnosis. Immediate consultation with a spine surgeon is necessary, and hospitals without qualified spine surgeons should immediately transfer the patient to an appropriate spine center. Pending results of the cultures, empiric antibiotic therapy should provide coverage of the most common causative organisms (i.e., *Staphylococcus* and *Streptococcus* spp.), with additional coverage for Gram-negative organisms especially in patients who are immunocompromised, have a history of IV drug abuse, or have had recent infection or manipulation of the genitourinary tract [68,70,71].

Of patients diagnosed with SEA, 10–23% die due to the disease process [68]. Of those who survive, irreversible paralysis is the most feared complication of SEA affecting 4–22% of all patients. The single most important predictor of the final neurologic outcome is the patient's pre-surgical neurologic status [71]. Diagnostic delays often lead to irreversible neurologic deficits [73], and a high index of suspicion is required to make the diagnosis, especially in elderly patients.

Seizures

New seizures

Nearly 25% of first epileptic seizures occur in patients who are 60 years of age or older [74], and the geriatric population has a higher incidence of new-onset seizures and epilepsy than any other age group [75]. The causes, clinical presentations, and prognosis of first seizures in elderly patients differ from those in younger patients, affecting the acute work-up and management in older patients. New seizures may be either the result of acute symptomatic seizures (defined as provoked seizures occurring at the time of a systemic insult or in close temporal association with a documented brain insult) or unprovoked seizures (defined as seizures occurring in the absence of precipitating factors and may be caused by a static or progressing injury). Unprovoked seizures may be single or recurrent, and epilepsy is defined as at least one unprovoked seizure in the presence of an enduring predisposition to further seizures. Both types of new seizures predominate in the very young (less than 1 year of age) and the elderly [76,77]. However, there is usually a cause for seizure found in elderly patients, and almost no idiopathic epilepsies start in patients over 60 years of age [78].

Approximately 25% of elderly patients who suffer a seizure have seizures of unknown etiology. Known etiological factors of seizures in elderly patients include: stroke and cerebrovascular disease, intracranial hemorrhage, head injury, infection, brain tumor or vascular malformation, neurodegenerative disorders

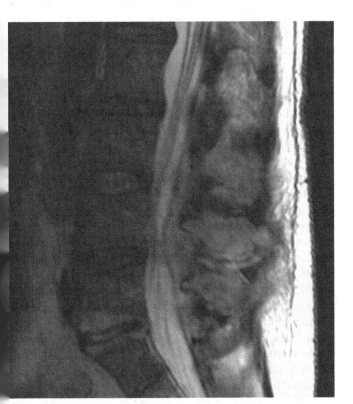

Figure 18.5. T2-weighted MRI of a spinal epidural abscess within the posterior spinal canal centered at L4–L5.

(i.e., Alzheimer's dementia), neuropsychiatric disorders (i.e., depression, anxiety), toxic and metabolic abnormalities, and normal aging [75,76,79]. Diagnosing seizures and epilepsy in the elderly is difficult due to the subtle manifestations of partial seizures, as well as the presence of age-related cognition difficulties, comorbid conditions, and medications. Though generalized tonic–clonic seizures are more easily diagnosed, complex partial seizures in the elderly are a more elusive diagnosis [76]. Most new seizures in elderly patients are partial in onset, with or without secondary generalization [80]. Complex partial seizures in the elderly may manifest as simple motor or sensory symptoms, memory lapses, episodes of confusion, periods of inattention, apparent syncope, or a blank stare with transient disturbance of consciousness [76,81]. Often seizures in the elderly are misdiagnosed as altered mental status, confusion, or syncope, and a high degree of suspicion for seizure should be maintained in elderly patients presenting with these symptoms [76]. In almost half of all elderly patients who are ultimately diagnosed with epilepsy, epilepsy is not the initial suspected diagnosis [78].

Work-up of first seizures in the elderly can be difficult and time intensive. A reliable history and a witnessed event by an observer are invaluable in making the diagnosis, but may not always be available as many elderly live alone and may remember little or nothing about the event. In the elderly, many disorders may mimic or co-exist with seizure activity, and the differential diagnosis is broad, including: cardiac arrhythmias, transient global amnesia, transient ischemic attacks, migraine, hypoglycemia, hyperglycemic non-ketotic states, hyponatremia, orthostatic hypotension, carotid sinus sensitivity, adverse drug effects, and vasovagal episodes. Electrocardiogram with cardiac monitoring, full vital signs including orthostatic vital signs, and full laboratory testing including thyroid-stimulating hormone can help to differentiate these disorders from seizure [78,81]. Brain imaging with head CT or MRI is recommended in elderly patients presenting with new seizure, as there is a high rate of abnormalities found in this patient population and an identified intracranial lesion may elucidate the etiology of the seizure [78,82]. MRI is more sensitive than CT for detection of relevant anatomical abnormalities [81], but may be difficult to obtain in elderly patients especially if they are unstable or have altered mental status. Abnormalities found on brain imaging more commonly in elderly patients can include: strokes, small vessel disease, cerebral atrophy, encephalomalacia, or tumor [78,82]. Electroencephalography (EEG) is less specific and sensitive than neuroimaging in the evaluation of elderly people with seizure. With advancing age, 12–38% of patients develop EEG abnormalities in the absence of a seizure and fewer elderly patients with seizures have abnormal interictal EEGs [78].

Treatment for provoked seizures should be directed toward the underlying cause [81]. In general, a first, single unprovoked seizure is not considered epilepsy and treatment with an anti-epileptic medication is usually not recommended. However, in the older patient, a first, unprovoked seizure carries a higher risk for recurrent seizures than in younger adults, and any elderly patient with a new-onset seizure should be rapidly referred to an epilepsy specialist for evaluation and initiation of treatment as indicated [76,81]. Due to frequent comorbidities, the changed physiology of elderly patients, and the interactions with concomitant medications, the decision on whether to start anti-epileptic drug treatment in the elderly patient is complicated and should be made only after consultation with a neurologist and an extensive discussion with the patient and family about the risks and benefits. Anti-epileptic medications with a more favorable profile in elderly patients include: levetiracetam, pregabalin, lamotrigine, and oxcarazepine [78,82]. Many elderly patients require smaller doses than younger patients, and adverse effects may be minimized by starting with a lower dose and titrating slowly [78]. Elderly patients seem to respond better to treatment with anti-epileptic medications than younger patients, and up to 80% of patients with seizure onset in old age remain seizure free on anti-epileptic medication, though treatment is generally lifelong [82].

Status epilepticus

Although exact definitions vary, status epilepticus (SE) is typically defined as seizures that persist for 20–30 minutes, which is the estimated time to cause injury to CNS neurons. However, given that physicians should not wait 20–30 minutes prior to treating a patient with seizure, an operational definition of SE is continuous seizures persisting for at least five minutes or two or more discrete seizures between which there is incomplete recovery of consciousness. SE is a medical emergency with a high mortality rate of approximately 20% and should be intervened upon rapidly [83]. SE can be classified according to clinical spectrum, type of seizure (convulsive versus nonconvulsive), or on the basis of EEG features (partial versus generalized) [84]. Up to 30% of acute seizures in elderly patients present as SE, with an associated higher mortality rate of up to 50% [78,82,84]. Additionally, in the elderly, partial SE with secondary generalization is the most common presentation, followed by partial, and then generalized tonic–clonic [84].

In older patients, SE is usually caused by stroke, hypoxia, metabolic insults, and low anticonvulsant drug concentrations. When an elderly patient presents in SE, general acute treatment actions should be taken, including: monitoring and/or establishing an airway, monitoring vital signs and oxygenation, obtaining IV access, measuring blood glucose levels, and checking basic laboratory studies including anti-epileptic drug levels. There is no established protocol for the management of SE in elderly patients, but treatment generally follows the widely accepted guidelines for all adults presenting with SE. Benzodiazepines (e.g., lorazepam, diazepam) are typically first-line agents for aborting SE as they have rapid onset and are effective for all seizure types. Phenytoin or fosphenytoin should be administered immediately after benzodiazepines when seizures persist or even when they have been aborted; it is important to monitor the ECG and BP in the elderly when giving these medications [84]. Valproate or levitiracetam may also be considered as an alternative to IV phenytoin/fosphenytoin or in addition to phenytoin/fosphenytoin if the seizure is not halted by the initial medications.

If SE continues despite treatment with benzodiazepines and one anti-epileptic drug, it is considered refractory status epilepticus (RSE), and mortality for RSE is about three times higher than for non-refractory SE. In general, anesthetic agents such as pentobarbital, midazolam, or propofol are recommended for patients in RSE. Patients in RSE who receive these agents will require intubation. These patients should also undergo an urgent neurology consult for further management and treatment for continued seizures [84–86].

Non-convulsive status epilepticus (NCSE) is characterized by a clinically evident alteration in mental status or behavior from baseline, without signs of convulsions, lasting at least 30 minutes, with a pattern of seizure activity on the EEG that disappears with the treatment and recovery of consciousness. Elderly patients in NCSE often present with no convulsive activity or less apparent clinical manifestations that go unrecognized [84]. NCSE is particularly difficult to diagnose in elderly patients and should be considered in patients with unexplained coma or prolonged confusional state, even if there is no past history of epilepsy. Due to the lack of motor findings, diagnosis is often delayed. Altered mental status is a key feature of NCSE, and an early high degree of suspicion and early EEG is required for prompt recognition, especially in elderly patients [82]. It is important to consider an EEG in the evaluation of acute mental and behavioral changes in the geriatric population [78,84].

Conclusion

Neurological emergencies are common in the geriatric population. Due to the physiologic changes of aging as well as increased comorbidities in elderly patients, neurological diseases in geriatric patients are generally more difficult to diagnosis and manage and are associated with increased morbidity and mortality than in younger patients. When caring for older patients with suspected neurological emergencies, it is important to maintain a high degree of suspicion and obtain urgent expert consultation in order to provide geriatric patients with the best possible care and offer them the best chance for a positive outcome.

Pearls and pitfalls

Pearls

- Due to the physiological effects of aging and multiple comorbidities, many elderly patients suffering neurological emergencies present with atypical symptoms, and a high degree of suspicion is necessary when evaluating older patients with potential neurological emergencies.
- Acute ischemic stroke and transient ischemic attack tend to be diseases of the elderly with increased morbidity and mortality in the geriatric population, and a rapid evaluation is necessary in elderly patients presenting with neurologic symptoms.
- Geriatric trauma patients suffering a traumatic brain injury often have higher morbidity and mortality. A lower threshold for trauma activation at a designated trauma center or transfer to a designated trauma center should exist for elderly patients suffering a traumatic brain injury.
- Central nervous system infections in the elderly may present with nonspecific symptoms, and fever is blunted

or absent in 20–30% of geriatric patients with severe infection.
- New-onset idiopathic epilepsy in patients over 60 years of age is extremely rare, and all elderly patients with new seizure should undergo a thorough evaluation to identify a cause.

Pitfalls

- Delaying immediate work-up, including neuroimaging and neurology consultation, of a patient suffering a transient ischemic attack, given the high risk of acute ischemic stroke in the days and months following a transient ischemic attack.
- Failure to rapidly reverse warfarin-associated coagulopathy and treat severe hypertension in patients suffering an intracerebral hemorrhage.
- Failure to obtain expert consultation regarding the consideration of endovascular coiling or microsurgical clipping in elderly patients suffering an aneurysmal subarachnoid hemorrhage.
- Failing to consider intravenous recombinant tissue plasminogen activator in elderly ischemic stroke patients within 3 hours of symptom onset simply due to advanced age.
- Not obtaining neuroimaging in elderly patients greater than 60 years of age who suffered a minor traumatic brain injury and potentially missing an acute intracranial abnormality.
- Failure to consider spinal epidural abscess in elderly patients presenting with back pain, especially if these patients have a fever, potential infectious source or comorbid diabetes, spinal abnormality, or prior spinal intervention.

References

1. Roger VL, Go AS, Lloyd-Jones DM, et al. Heart disease and stroke statistics – 2012 update: a report from the American Heart Association. *Circulation*. 2012;125(1):e2–220.

2. Pare JR, Kahn JH. Basic neuroanatomy and stroke syndromes. *Emerg Med Clin North Am*. 2012;30(3):601–15.

3. Muangpaisan W, Hinkle JL, Westwood M, Kennedy J, Buchan AM. Stroke in the very old: clinical presentations and outcomes. *Age Aging*. 2008;37(4):473–5.

4. Di Carlo A, Lamassa M, Pracucci G, et al. Stroke in the very old: clinical presentation and determinants of 3-month functional outcome: A European perspective. European BIOMED Study of Stroke Care Group. *Stroke*. 1999;30(11):2313–19.

5. Adams HP Jr, del Zoppo G, Alberts MJ, et al. Guidelines for the early management of adults with ischemic stroke: a guideline from the American Heart Association/American Stroke Association Stroke Council, Clinical Cardiology Council, Cardiovascular Radiology and Intervention Council, and the Atherosclerotic Peripheral Vascular Disease and Quality of Care Outcomes in Research Interdisciplinary Working Groups: the American Academy of Neurology affirms the value of this guideline as an educational tool for neurologists. *Stroke*. 2007;38(5):1655–711.

6. Nentwich LM, Veloz W. Neuroimaging in acute stroke. *Emerg Med Clin North Am.* 2012;30(3):659–80.

7. Jauch EC, Cucchiara B, Adeoye O, et al. Part 11: adult stroke: 2010 American Heart Association Guidelines for Cardiopulmonary Resuscitation and Emergency Cardiovascular Care. *Circulation.* 2010;122(18 Suppl. 3):S818–28.

8. Tissue plasminogen activator for acute ischemic stroke. The National Institute of Neurological Disorders and Stroke rt-PA Stroke Study Group. *N Engl J Med.* 1995;333(24):1581–7.

9. Hemphill JC, 3rd, Lyden P. Stroke thrombolysis in the elderly: risk or benefit? *Neurology.* 2005;65(11):1690–1.

10. Longstreth WT, Jr, Katz R, Tirschwell DL, Cushman M, Psaty BM. Intravenous tissue plasminogen activator and stroke in the elderly. *Am J Emerg Med.* 2010;28(3):359–63.

11. Hacke W, Kaste M, Bluhmki E, et al. Thrombolysis with alteplase 3 to 4.5 hours after acute ischemic stroke. *N Engl J Med.* 2008;359(13):1317–29.

12. Sylaja PN, Cote R, Buchan AM, Hill MD. Thrombolysis in patients older than 80 years with acute ischaemic stroke: Canadian Alteplase for Stroke Effectiveness Study. *J Neurol Neurosurg Psychiatr.* 2006;77(7):826–9.

13. Mishra NK, Ahmed N, Andersen G, et al. Thrombolysis in very elderly people: controlled comparison of SITS International Stroke Thrombolysis Registry and Virtual International Stroke Trials Archive. *BMJ.* 2010;341:c6046.

14. Pundik S, McWilliams-Dunnigan L, Blackham KL, et al. Older age does not increase risk of hemorrhagic complications after intravenous and/or intra-arterial thrombolysis for acute stroke. *J Stroke Cerebrovasc Dis.* 2008;17(5):266–72.

15. Del Zoppo GJ, Saver JL, Jauch EC, Adams HP, Jr. Expansion of the time window for treatment of acute ischemic stroke with intravenous tissue plasminogen activator: a science advisory from the American Heart Association/American Stroke Association. *Stroke.* 2009;40(8):2945–8.

16. Easton JD, Saver JL, Albers GW, et al. Definition and evaluation of transient ischemic attack: a scientific statement for health care professionals from the American Heart Association/American Stroke Association Stroke Council; Council on Cardiovascular Surgery and Anesthesia; Council on Cardiovascular Radiology and Intervention; Council on Cardiovascular Nursing; and the Interdisciplinary Council on Peripheral Vascular Disease. The American Academy of Neurology affirms the value of this statement as an educational tool for neurologists. *Stroke.* 2009;40(6):2276–93.

17. Rothwell PM, Warlow CP. Timing of TIAs preceding stroke: time window for prevention is very short. *Neurology.* 2005;64(5):817–20.

18. Giles MF, Rothwell PM. Risk of stroke early after transient ischaemic attack: a systematic review and meta-analysis. *Lancet Neurol.* 2007;6(12):1063–72.

19. Wu CM, McLaughlin K, Lorenzetti DL, et al. Early risk of stroke after transient ischemic attack: a systematic review and meta-analysis. *Arch Intern Med.* 2007;167(22):2417–22.

20. Kleindorfer D, Panagos P, Pancioli A, et al. Incidence and short-term prognosis of transient ischemic attack in a population-based study. *Stroke.* 2005;36(4):720–3.

21. Heyman A, Wilkinson WE, Hurwitz BJ, et al. Risk of ischemic heart disease in patients with TIA. *Neurology.* 1984;34(5):626–30.

22. Siket MS, Edlow JA. Transient ischemic attack: reviewing the evolution of the definition, diagnosis, risk stratification, and management for the emergency physician. *Emerg Med Clin North Am.* 2012;30(3):745–70.

23. Moreau F, Jeerakathil T, Coutts SB, FRCPC for the ASPIRE Investigators. Patients referred for TIA may still have persisting neurological deficits. *Can J Neurol Sci.* 2012;39(2):170–3.

24. Rothwell PM, Eliasziw M, Gutnikov SA, Warlow CP, Barnett HJ. Endarterectomy for symptomatic carotid stenosis in relation to clinical subgroups and timing of surgery. *Lancet.* 2004;363(9413):915–24.

25. Johnston SC, Nguyen-Huynh MN, Schwarz ME, et al. National Stroke Association guidelines for the management of transient ischemic attacks. *Ann Neurol.* 2006;60(3):301–13.

26. Qureshi AI, Tuhrim S, Broderick JP, Batjer HH, Hondo H, Hanley DF. Spontaneous intracerebral hemorrhage. *N Engl J Med.* 2001;344(19):1450–60.

27. Broderick J, Connolly S, Feldmann E, et al. Guidelines for the management of spontaneous intracerebral hemorrhage in adults: 2007 update: a guideline from the American Heart Association/American Stroke Association Stroke Council, High Blood Pressure Research Council, and the Quality of Care and Outcomes in Research Interdisciplinary Working Group. *Stroke.* 2007;38(6):2001–23.

28. Weigele JB, Hurst RW. Neurovascular emergencies in the elderly. *Radiol Clin North Am.* 2008;46(4):819–36, vii.

29. Nentwich LM, Goldstein JN. Intracerebral hemorrhage. In *Vascular Emergencies,* ed. Rogers RL, Scalea T, Wallis L, Geduld H (Cambridge: Cambridge University Press, 2013), pp. 18–29.

30. Lee WC, Joshi AV, Wang Q, Pashos CL, Christensen MC. Morbidity and mortality among elderly Americans with different stroke subtypes. *Adv Ther.* 2007;24(2):258–68.

31. Steiner T, Kaste M, Forsting M, et al. Recommendations for the management of intracranial haemorrhage – part I: spontaneous intracerebral haemorrhage. The European Stroke Initiative Writing Committee and the Writing Committee for the EUSI Executive Committee. *Cerebrovasc Dis.* 2006;22(4):294–316.

32. Runchey S, McGee S. Does this patient have a hemorrhagic stroke? Clinical findings distinguishing hemorrhagic stroke from ischemic stroke. *JAMA.* 2010;303(22):2280–6.

33. Morgenstern LB, Hemphill JC, 3rd, Anderson C, et al. Guidelines for the management of spontaneous intracerebral hemorrhage: a guideline for health care professionals from the American Heart Association/American Stroke Association. *Stroke.* 2010;41(9):2108–29.

34. Chalela JA, Kidwell CS, Nentwich LM, et al. Magnetic resonance imaging and computed tomography in emergency assessment of patients with suspected acute stroke: a prospective comparison. *Lancet.* 2007;369(9558):293–8.

35. Kidwell CS, Chalela JA, Saver JL, et al. Comparison of MRI and CT for detection of acute intracerebral hemorrhage. *JAMA.* 2004;292(15):1823–30.

36. Ginde AA, Foianini A, Renner DM, Valley M, Camargo CA, Jr. Availability and quality of computed tomography and magnetic resonance imaging equipment in US emergency departments. *Acad Emerg Med.* 2008;15(8):780–3.

37. Singer OC, Sitzer M, du Mesnil de Rochemont R, Neumann-Haefelin T. Practical limitations of acute stroke MRI due to patient-related problems. *Neurology.* 2004;62(10):1848–9.

38. Becker KJ, Baxter AB, Cohen WA, et al. Withdrawal of support in intracerebral hemorrhage may lead to self-fulfilling prophecies. *Neurology.* 2001;56(6):766–72.

39. Zahuranec DB, Brown DL, Lisabeth LD, et al. Early care limitations independently predict mortality after intracerebral hemorrhage. *Neurology.* 2007;68(20):1651–7.

40. Suarez JI, Tarr RW, Selman WR. Aneurysmal subarachnoid hemorrhage. *N Engl J Med.* 2006;354(4):387–96.

41. Sedat J, Dib M, Rasendrarijao D, et al. Ruptured intracranial aneurysms in the elderly: epidemiology, diagnosis, and management. *Neurocrit Care.* 2005;2(2):119–23.

42. Edlow JA, Caplan LR. Avoiding pitfalls in the diagnosis of subarachnoid hemorrhage. *N Engl J Med.* 2000;342(1):29–36.

43. Connolly ES, Jr, Rabinstein AA, Carhuapoma JR, et al. Guidelines for the management of aneurysmal subarachnoid hemorrhage: a guideline for health care professionals from the American Heart Association/American Stroke Association. *Stroke.* 2012;43(6):1711–37.

44. Rutland-Brown W, Langlois JA, Thomas KE, Xi YL. Incidence of traumatic brain injury in the United States, 2003. *J Head Trauma Rehabil.* 2006;21(6):544–8.

45. Thompson HJ, McCormick WC, Kagan SH. Traumatic brain injury in older adults: epidemiology, outcomes, and future implications. *J Am Geriatr Soc.* 2006;54(10):1590–5.

46. Hukkelhoven CW, Steyerberg EW, Rampen AJ, et al. Patient age and outcome following severe traumatic brain injury: an analysis of 5600 patients. *J Neurosurg.* 2003;99(4):666–73.

47. Decuypere M, Klimo P Jr. Spectrum of traumatic brain injury from mild to severe. *Surg Clin North Am.* 2012;92(4):939–57, ix.

48. Holmes JF, Hendey GW, Oman JA, et al. Epidemiology of blunt head injury victims undergoing ED cranial computed tomographic scanning. *Am J Emerg Med.* 2006;24(2):167–73.

49. Stiell IG, Wells GA, Vandemheen K, et al. The Canadian CT Head Rule for patients with minor head injury. *Lancet.* 2001;357(9266):1391–6.

50. Haydel MJ, Preston CA, Mills TJ, et al. Indications for computed tomography in patients with minor head injury. *N Engl J Med.* 2000;343(2):100–5.

51. Mower WR, Hoffman JR, Herbert M, et al. Developing a decision instrument to guide computed tomographic imaging of blunt head injury patients. *J Trauma.* 2005;59(4):954–9.

52. Mack LR, Chan SB, Silva JC, Hogan TM. The use of head computed tomography in elderly patients sustaining minor head trauma. *J Emerg Med.* 2003;24(2):157–62.

53. Zink BJ. Traumatic brain injury outcome: concepts for emergency care. *Ann Emerg Med.* 2001;37(3):318–32.

54. Mosenthal AC, Lavery RF, Addis M, et al. Isolated traumatic brain injury: age is an independent predictor of mortality and early outcome. *J Trauma.* 2002;52(5):907–11.

55. Gaetani P, Revay M, Sciacca S, et al. Traumatic brain injury in the elderly: considerations in a series of 103 patients older than 70. *J Neurosurg Sci.* 2012;56(3):231–7.

56. Rakier A, Guilburd JN, Soustiel JF, Zaaroor M, Feinsod M. Head injuries in the elderly. *Brain Inj.* 1995;9(2):187–93.

57. Badjatia N, Carney N, Crocco TJ, et al. Guidelines for pre-hospital management of traumatic brain injury, 2nd ed. *Prehosp Emerg Care.* 2008;12(Suppl. 1):S1–52.

58. Brain Trauma Foundation; American Association of Neurological Surgeons; Congress of Neurological Surgeons. Guidelines for the management of severe traumatic brain injury. *J Neurotrauma.* 2007;24(Suppl. 1):S1–106.

59. Calland JF, Ingraham AM, Martin N, et al. Evaluation and management of geriatric trauma: an Eastern Association for the Surgery of Trauma practice management guideline. *J Trauma Acute Care Surg.* 2012;73(5 Suppl. 4):S345–50.

60. Gavazzi G, Krause KH. Aging and infection. *Lancet Infect Dis.* 2002;2(11):659–66.

61. Thigpen MC, Whitney CG, Messonnier NE, et al. Bacterial meningitis in the United States, 1998–2007. *N Engl J Med.* 2011;364(21):2016–25.

62. Lai WA, Chen SF, Tsai NW, et al. Clinical characteristics and prognosis of acute bacterial meningitis in elderly patients over 65: a hospital-based study. *BMC Geriatr.* 2011;11:91.

63. Cabellos C, Verdaguer R, Olmo M, et al. Community-acquired bacterial meningitis in elderly patients: experience over 30 years. *Medicine (Baltimore).* 2009;88(2):115–19.

64. Weisfelt M, van de Beek D, Spanjaard L, Reitsma JB, de Gans J. Community-acquired bacterial meningitis in older people. *J Am Geriatr Soc.* 2006;54(10):1500–7.

65. van de Beek D, de Gans J, Tunkel AR, Wijdicks EF. Community-acquired bacterial meningitis in adults. *N Engl J Med.* 2006;354(1):44–53.

66. Brouwer MC, Tunkel AR, van de Beek D. Epidemiology, diagnosis, and antimicrobial treatment of acute bacterial meningitis. *Clin Microbiol Rev.* 2010;23(3):467–92.

67. van de Beek D, de Gans J, Spanjaard L, et al. Clinical features and prognostic factors in adults with bacterial meningitis. *N Engl J Med.* 2004;351(18):1849–59.

68. Tompkins M, Panuncialman I, Lucas P, Palumbo M. Spinal epidural abscess. *J Emerg Med.* 2010;39(3):384–90.

69. Pope JV, Edlow JA. Avoiding misdiagnosis in patients with neurological emergencies. *Emerg Med Int.* 2012;2012:949275.

70. Kulchycki LK, Edlow JA. Geriatric neurologic emergencies. *Emerg Med Clin North Am.* 2006;24(2):273–98, v–vi.

71. Darouiche RO. Spinal epidural abscess. *N Engl J Med.* 2006;355(19):2012–20.

72. Heusner AP. Nontuberculous spinal epidural infections. *N Engl J Med.* 1948;239(23):845–54.

73. Davis DP, Wold RM, Patel RJ, et al. The clinical presentation and impact of diagnostic delays on emergency department patients with spinal epidural abscess. *J Emerg Med.* 2004;26(3):285–91.

74. Sander JW, Hart YM, Johnson AL, Shorvon SD. National General Practice Study of Epilepsy: newly diagnosed epileptic seizures in a general population. *Lancet.* 1990;336(8726):1267–71.

75. Hauser WA. Seizure disorders: the changes with age. *Epilepsia.* 1992;33(Suppl. 4):S6–14.

76. Verellen RM, Cavazos JE. Pathophysiological considerations of seizures, epilepsy, and status epilepticus in the elderly. *Aging Dis.* 2011;2(4):278–85.

77. Hauser WA, Beghi E. First seizure definitions and worldwide incidence and mortality. *Epilepsia.* 2008;49(Suppl. 1):8–12.

78. Poza JJ. Management of epilepsy in the elderly. *Neuropsychiatr Dis Treat.* 2007;3(6):723–8.

79. Ramsay RE, Rowan AJ, Pryor FM. Special considerations in treating the elderly patient with epilepsy. *Neurology.* 2004;62(5 Suppl. 2):S24–9.

80. Stephen LJ, Brodie MJ. Epilepsy in elderly people. *Lancet.* 2000;355(9213):1441–6.

81. Brodie MJ, Kwan P. Epilepsy in elderly people. *BMJ.* 2005;331(7528):1317–22.

82. Brodie MJ, Elder AT, Kwan P. Epilepsy in later life. *Lancet Neurol.* 2009;8(11):1019–30.

83. Lowenstein DH, Alldredge BK. Status epilepticus. *N Engl J Med.* 1998;338(14):970–6.

84. de Assis TM, Costa G, Bacellar A, Orsini M, Nascimento OJ. Status epilepticus in the elderly: epidemiology, clinical aspects and treatment. *Neurol Int.* 2012;4(3):e17.

85. Rossetti AO, Lowenstein DH. Management of refractory status epilepticus in adults: still more questions than answers. *Lancet Neurol.* 2011;10(10):922–30.

86. Lowenstein DH. The management of refractory status epilepticus: an update. *Epilepsia.* 2006;47(Suppl. 1):35–40.

87. Teasdale G, Jennett B. Assessment of coma and impaired consciousness. A practical scale. *Lancet.* 1974;2(7872):81–4.

Chapter
19
Pulmonary emergencies in the elderly

Thomas Perera

Introduction

Pulmonary disease in the elderly is a significant cause of morbidity in the elderly and a frequent cause of emergency department (ED) visits. Pulmonary disease represents a total of 9.47 million deaths each year and makes up four of the CDC's top ten causes of death for 2008 (lower respiratory infections, chronic obstructive pulmonary disease [COPD], respiratory cancers, and tuberculosis). Advanced age can increase or complicate each of these diseases.

The effect of smoking and its clinical manifestations on geriatric respiratory illness cannot be overstated. Even in the absence of smoking, the physiological processes of aging cause changes in the lung and chest wall which predictably alter the way in which elderly patients handle pulmonary disease processes. In this section we will review the physiologic changes of aging and summarize the changes in pulmonary function tests (PFTs). The additional effects of smoking on pulmonary physiology will be discussed at the end of the section.

Pathophysiology

The lung reaches maturity at age 20–25. After this age it slowly deteriorates. Age alone has been shown to cause dilatation of alveoli, enlargement of airspaces, decrease in exchange surface area, and loss of supporting tissue for peripheral airways. These changes together have been called "senile emphysema" [1]. These changes result in loss of lung elasticity and increased deadspace. Replacement of elastase with more fibrous connective tissue causes the lung to expand more readily during a deep breath but recoil less easily. This adds to the lung's ability to expand, increasing the total lung capacity (TLC) but decreasing the lung's ability to contract. The work of breathing is increased with this loss of elasticity.

Another important change is stiffening of the chest wall. As with many jointed muscular structures, with aging the chest wall muscles and joints stiffen. Stiffening of the thoracic spine and age-related kyphosis also physically increase the work of breathing. This loss of chest wall compliance means that the chest wall expands and contracts less, which on its own would decrease TLC and cause an increase in residual volume (RV), the air left in the lung after forced exhalation.

These physiological changes lead to predictable changes in pulmonary function tests. The opposing changes of decreased lung compliance, which increases volumes, and stiffening of the chest wall, which decreases maximum volumes, usually results in a relatively stable TLC. These same changes act together to increase RV. The total volume of air that can be moved in and out of the lung is called vital capacity (VC). Vital capacity is a function of total lung capacity minus residual volume: $VC = TLC - RV$, so vital capacity decreases with age.

Over time, respiratory muscles including the diaphragm and chest wall muscles lose strength and endurance. The increased work of breathing associated with loss of compliance leaves the elderly with less functional reserve. These changes can impair an effective cough. This loss of muscle endurance is one of the factors which leads to more elderly patients needing intubation in the ED. All flow-related PFTs are dependent on the balance between muscle strength, lung and chest wall compliance, and airway diameter. In the acute setting we are most familiar with the value of forced expiratory volume in one second (FEV_1). FEV_1 decreases with age.

Increased fibrosis of lung tissues, increased ventilation/perfusion (V/Q) mismatch, and increased deadspace are some of the factors that lead to impaired oxygen exchange (diffusion capacity) and age-dependent decrease in PO_2. Conversely there is little or no predictable change in PCO_2. There is an age-related decrease in respiratory drive, partially due to a decreased response by the elderly to hypoxia and hypercarbia. It has also been shown that older adults have a decreased sensation of dyspnea and may wait longer before seeking help [2].

Another change in the geriatric lung is that the airways, particularly the mid-sized airways, have increased airway reactivity. This can lead to increased extrinsic asthma and increased respiratory difficulties in response to many upper and lower respiratory processes. Unfortunately, studies have shown that there is no corresponding change in bronchodilator responsiveness to balance this change [3]. The resultant increased disease with no increase in therapeutic response is a setup for respiratory distress.

Smoking and secondary smoke exposure have many detrimental effects on the pulmonary system. Decreased lung compliance, increased deadspace, increased work of breathing, and

Geriatric Emergency Medicine, ed. Joseph H. Kahn, Brendan G. Magauran Jr., and Jonathan S. Olshaker. Published by Cambridge University Press.
© Cambridge University Press 2014.

Table 19.1. How common pulmonary function tests are affected by age, COPD, and restrictive lung disease

Pulmonary function test	Aging	COPD	Restrictive lung disease
Forced expiratory volume in 1 s (FEV_1)	↓	↓	↓ or =
Forced vital capacity (FVC)	↓	↓ or =	↓
FEV_1/ FVC	↓	↓	=
Total lung capacity (TLC)	=	= or ↑	↓
Residual volume (RV)	↑	↑	↓
Functional residual capacity (FRC)	↑	=	↓

decreased ventilator response to hypoxia and hypercarbia are seen with both aging and smoking. Decreased ciliary function, increased mucus production, and direct tissue injury are more associated with smoking than aging. These processes work together to increase the susceptibility of the geriatric population to a multitude of disease processes. As with aging, certain pulmonary function tests worsen with the physiologic changes caused by smoking. In chronic smokers, VC and FEV_1 both decrease.

Summary: The aging lung undergoes predictable changes which overall decrease its oxygen exchange and deplete its reserve. Changes to the chest wall and diaphragm also contribute to this. Table 19.1 summarizes these changes.

History

Taking a pulmonary history should focus on diseases that affect lung or cardiac function and lifetime exposures. As with many patients, simply asking generalized questions about past medical history may miss important facts. A patient may state that they have no lung problems or medical history but still use inhalers daily. It is important in a complete pulmonary history to ask detailed questions about occupational as well as secondary exposures.

Dyspnea is the typical pulmonary complaint. The usual historical questions about duration and rate of onset should be supplemented with questions about baseline exercise tolerance and activities of daily living (ADL). The history of home oxygen use tells the clinician a lot about the baseline severity of disease and will be an early guide to therapy. Aggravating or alleviating factors should include whether nitroglycerin or inhalers affect the disease. Associated symptoms should include questions about chest pain, palpitations, diaphoresis, paroxysmal nocturnal dyspnea, orthopnea, leg swelling (bilateral or unilateral), fever, changes in sputum, or hemoptysis. Elderly patients are known to present in many disease processes with complicated, atypical, and sometimes vague complaints. Taking a complete and accurate history can drastically affect the quality of the care given.

The past medical history is essential and should start with an assessment of severity of previous disease. Questions should include number of hospitalizations, use of home oxygen, and intubation history. Previous pneumonias, malignancy, deep

vein thrombosis (DVT), diabetes, and other immunosuppressive processes should all be explored. An accurate list of medications and allergies will allow for a more thorough evaluation of the patient's past medical history. Also be cognizant that just because a patient has a list of medication does not mean that the list accurately reflects medications taken that day. A smoking history is essential, and it is important to ask about the smoking habits of all members of the household. Occupational exposures to pulmonary irritants are common and may increase risk of cancer and other lung diseases. A family history of cardiac, thromboembolic, malignant, or metabolic disease will often reveal important clues to help in the emergency management of these patients. Finally, assessing the patient's wishes in terms of a living will or do not resuscitate (DNR) or intubate orders is helpful, especially in the geriatric population.

Physical

In the stable patient, it is important to focus the physical exam on the common, dangerous, and treatable pulmonary disorders. If the patient is able to converse normally, then begin with a general impression of breathing. Observe the work of breathing looking specifically at body posture and whether there is a prolonged expiratory phase of breathing. Move on to inspection of the oral cavity including soft tissues, dentition, mandibular range of motion, and calculation of a Mallampati score. A general inspection of the neck should be followed by palpation for nodes, masses, crepitus, and a thorough evaluation of the thyroid. Auscultate for stridor, bruit, and upper airway rhonchi. Inquire about whether the patient has noticed a change in their voice. The patient will be much more aware of fremitus changes than a clinician who does not know what the patient's voice usually sounds like. Inspection, palpation, auscultation, and percussion of the chest are the next steps. Chest wall movement and spine curvature often affect the air movement in the elderly. Occult rib fractures and crepitus may be elicited especially in patients whose mental status is altered for any reason. Auscultation and percussion for effusion may help guide imaging or suggest the diagnosis even in patients with vague complaints. Unfortunately, no physical exam finding can reliably rule out pneumonia. Differentiating between COPD and congestive heart failure (CHF) may be difficult in patients with some aspects of both diseases. Wheezing, prolonged expiratory phase, and tubular breath sounds may point the clinician toward COPD, but these findings and rales can occur in both CHF and COPD.

It is essential to include a cardiac exam as well as an abdominal exam in even the most focused exam of the geriatric pulmonary system. The heart and lung are so interrelated in many disease processes that even small changes in cardiac function may have profound effects on the pulmonary system, and vice versa. A distended abdomen may increase the work of breathing significantly.

Diagnostic tests

Many diagnostic tests are used in the ED to evaluate pulmonary disease. Oxygen saturation from a pulse oximeter has almost become a standard vital sign. Because of the decreased ability of patients to perceive hypoxia and hypercarbia, and the aging body's decreased response to these stimuli, it is important to have these data in the elderly. The minimal variance of oxygen saturation associated with age alone in the absence of lung pathology is not detectable by pulse oximetry. At any age a low pulse oximetry value should prompt an evaluation for pulmonary pathology. Peripheral vascular disease and other circulatory issues may make obtaining an oxygen saturation more difficult. If it cannot be obtained in another way, a blood gas may be necessary to evaluate oxygen saturation. The blood gas values for elderly patients may vary for an individual over a lifetime, but the reference values for PaO_2 and SaO_2 in an elderly population are sex specific but age independent [4].

Concern about hypoventilation and hypercarbia in the elderly and in those patients with COPD often prompts the clinician to check the PCO_2 with an arterial or venous blood gas. The advent of end-tidal CO_2 monitors has decreased the need for blood gas testing. One study of elderly patients found the result of end-tidal CO_2 monitor to be on average within 6 mmHg when compared to standard blood gas sampling [5].

Some institutions use B-type natriuretic peptide (BNP) to differentiate COPD from CHF when other studies have not proven definitive. BNP can be positive in myocardial ischemia (MI), pulmonary embolism (PE), COPD, and in those patients with baseline right-sided heart failure. The test is most useful when a baseline BNP is known. Despite the lack of specificity of BNP, it can be very helpful in some elderly patients, especially when very high values are recorded.

Vital signs are an essential part of the evaluation. In the elderly, vital signs may not respond in the usual way because of medications and the presence of comorbidities. The perception of dyspnea can be blunted in the geriatric population. Disease processes which present in an insidious manner will often present with nonspecific complaints. For these and other reasons, the chest X-ray is often used as a screening tool in the elderly. In one study, 37% of geriatric patients presenting to an ED had a chest X-ray [6]. The literature on preoperative or routine admission chest X-rays in the geriatric population found abnormalities in 65–85% overall; 10–15% of these positive studies were in patients with no discernible indication for chest X-ray. Even though only a small percent of these resulted in a change in management, these findings seem to support a low threshold in the elderly for obtaining a chest X-ray. The chest radiograph is a vital component of making the diagnosis of lung disease, and should be obtained from all patients in whom lung pathology is suspected. It is, however, not always definitive – the sensitivity and specificity of the chest X-ray varies by disease. Underlying diseases such as COPD, CHF, and malignancy often obscure findings.

The use of ED ultrasound in pulmonary diseases is increasing. Pneumothorax and CHF can be quickly and accurately identified. Ultrasound is often used in the setting of known or suspected PE to look at the lower extremities for DVT and to assess the severity of the disease by evaluating the right atrium. In addition, ultrasound has the advantage of diagnosis without interrupting resuscitation.

Computed tomography (CT) is the most sensitive test for many lung pathologies – it can be used when the diagnosis cannot be definitively made by other modalities. In one study of patients with clinical findings consistent with pneumonia but with a negative chest radiograph, 26% were shown to have abnormalities consistent with the diagnosis of pneumonia on high-resolution chest CT [7]. Although chest CT is not suggested for routine use in the work-up of patients with pneumonia, it may be useful in certain settings.

Asthma/COPD

Chronic obstructive pulmonary disease, asthma, and CHF make up the three most common causes of intermittent dyspnea in older adults. Similarities in the ED treatment of COPD and asthma make this distinction less important than ruling out CHF.

Asthma is a disease of narrowed airways due to muscular constriction and inflammation, with 4–8% of elderly patients affected. One report showed that older patients with asthma were twice as likely as young adults with asthma to be hospitalized during one year of follow-up (14 versus 7%) [8]. A previous history of asthma will usually be present in those patients presenting with an asthma exacerbation. Although a new diagnosis of asthma in elderly patients is always looked at skeptically, the onset of new cases is reported relatively equally over all decades of life. Also suggestive of asthma is the presence of atopic symptoms like seasonal allergies and intermittent or chronic urticaria. These symptoms are often found in younger asthmatics and are part of the syndrome that causes increased response to bronchial stimulation due to higher levels of immunoglobulin E (IgE). The prevalence of this hyperreactivity decreases with age. The vast majority of older asthmatics, however, will have at least one positive allergen test to a common outdoor allergen. If asthma triggers can be identified and avoided, this may represent the simplest way to avoid emergency department visits.

Chronic obstructive pulmonary disease is a disease of airflow obstruction and loss of gas exchange surface. It is a progressive disorder that is punctuated in its later stages with acute exacerbations, and has a disproportionate impact on older patients. Physiologic changes in the aging lung cause many of the same pulmonary function test changes that are found in COPD. This fact, as well as a general trend of underreporting, makes an estimate of the prevalence of COPD in the elderly population difficult. The incidence of a new diagnosis after age 55 has been estimated at about 1% per year and the overall prevalence in the geriatric population may be as high as 11%. About 75% of exacerbations are caused by viral or bacterial infections while the rest are attributed to environmental exposure or do not have an identifiable cause.

The typical presentation of asthma and COPD, with intermittent chest tightness, shortness of breath, wheezing, cough, and increased sputum, is no different in older persons than in younger persons. Tachypnea, a variable decrease in pulmonary function, constitutional symptoms, and an unchanged chest radiograph are typical of acute exacerbations. The problem is that older individuals are more likely to have a poor perception of dyspnea related to airway obstruction. Elder patients may have moderate to severe airway obstruction yet may not complain of dyspnea. Older patients have often been found to have a limited understanding of their COPD or asthma, undertake less self-care, and are less likely to recognize symptoms of exacerbation prior to hospitalization. Because of this, it is more likely that older patients will present later and have more severe exacerbations of their disease.

On presentation, a good history and physical may confirm the diagnosis, assess the severity, and identify possible triggers. A history of new medications should be elicited, including new topical or ophthalmologic medications. Beta blockers may be well tolerated and decrease mortality in patients with asthma or COPD, but a small portion of patients will have bronchoconstriction and decreased response to inhaled beta-receptor agonists when started on beta blockers. An early FEV_1 helps assess the level of bronchial obstruction and serves as a baseline to evaluate the response to therapy. It has been shown that >90% of elderly patients can give an accurate FEV_1.

The ED treatment of asthma or COPD exacerbations in the elderly does not differ much from that used in younger adults. However, it may be complicated by comorbidities and decreased functional reserve. Oxygen therapy should be initiated to alleviate symptoms. There is some concern that high-flow oxygen may harm patients with COPD who are prone to retain carbon dioxide. Patients with severe COPD may be dependent on hypoxia for respiratory drive and when put on higher levels of oxygen may exhibit increased hypercarbia. It is still recommended that oxygen be given to increase the oxygen saturation to around 90%. An arterial blood gas or end-tidal CO_2 can be used to monitor the patient's respiratory status.

The mainstay of therapy for asthma and COPD in an acute exacerbation is short-acting beta-adrenergic agonists such as albuterol. The onset is about 5–15 minutes and the duration is 3–4 hours. In the ED, albuterol may be delivered by metered dose inhaler (MDI) or nebulizer. Although studies have shown the use of the MDI is equivalent to the nebulizer, many EDs still use the nebulizer because of patient and clinician preference. Continuous nebulized albuterol may be initiated and no maximum dose has been established. In the elderly, the tachycardia and sympathomimetic response may not be well tolerated especially in those patients with significant heart disease. Patients' symptoms often limit the continuous use of albuterol. It should be noted that the mechanism of tachycardia from the use of beta-adrenergic agonists is caused by a reflex in response to vasodilation from stimulation of receptors on peripheral vasculature and also by direct stimulation of beta-adrenergic receptors located in both the left ventricle and right atrium. The use of levalbuterol has not been fully evaluated in the elderly but has not been shown to provide a benefit in the acute setting in this population.

Anticholinergic agents such as ipratropium bromide are also frequently used in the treatment of asthma and COPD exacerbations in the ED. Ipratropium bromide, like albuterol, has an onset of 5–15 minutes, a peak effect of 2 hours, and a duration of 3–4 hours. The bronchodilatary effects of ipratropium are about the same as a dose of albuterol [9]. Several studies have shown in asthma and COPD that anticholinergic agents when combined with albuterol produce more bronchodilation than either agent alone [10]. This combined use has also been shown to decrease the rate of hospitalization [11]. Studies on the use of ipratropium bromide in asthma have shown some variability in its effectiveness. Among these studies, however, older patients with long-standing disease tend to show the most benefit [12,13]. The usual dose in the ED is 500 μg in the first two nebulizers in combination with albuterol. Higher doses and repeated doses have not shown added benefit [14].

Subcutaneous or intramuscular injection of the short-acting beta-adrenergic agonists epinephrine or terbutaline should be considered in severe exacerbations that significantly limit airflow or when inhaled administration is not possible for other reasons. Several studies have investigated this issue and found no significant difference between these two drugs in terms of bronchodilatory effects or side effects. The parenteral use of these agents causes significantly greater systemic symptoms, resulting in increased heart rate and increased myocardial oxygen demands and may result in arrhythmias or myocardial ischemia in susceptible individuals.

Methylxanthines such as theophylline were once used for their bronchodilatory effects as well as the strengthening effect on the diaphragm, but studies have not shown a benefit over standard treatment with the short-acting beta-adrenergic agonists. Theophylline is no longer recommended because of its limited benefit and narrow therapeutic window.

Glucocorticoids have been shown to be effective in both asthma and COPD. In asthma they are thought to increase beta-adrenergic responsiveness and reduce or delay the inflammatory effects of these diseases. Hospitalizations and relapse have both been shown to decrease with the use of glucocorticoids. The typical dose of 60 mg of oral prednisone or 125 mg of IV methylprednisolone should be given early, as the peak effect takes 1–2 hours. The biological half-life of prednisone is 18 hours. The route of administration does not seem to change the onset or effect. Higher-dose steroids have not proven more effective. Discharged patients should stay on prednisone at a non-tapering dose of 40–60 mg per day for 5–14 days. In the appropriate patient, the clinician may consider starting an inhaled steroid as the systemic steroids are stopped.

Magnesium at a dose of 1–2 g IV over 30 minutes has been shown to affect the course of moderate to severe asthmatics (FEV_1 <25% predicted). Magnesium has bronchodilatory properties although it is not very long acting. It should always be given in conjunction with short-acting beta-adrenergic agonists and anticholinergics. Its benefit in mild asthma has not been proven.

Antibiotics are currently recommended for COPD exacerbations, as several studies have shown decreased hospital length of stay and decreased rate of relapse in patients thus treated [15,16]. Finding an inciting infection and treating it specifically is the best option. Since that information is often not available in the ED, treatment is aimed at typical respiratory flora with some modification depending on the patient's history.

In the setting of impending respiratory failure, noninvasive ventilation (NIV) and mechanical ventilation should be considered. Indications include evidence of fatigue, acidosis, altered mental status, hypercarbia, and hypoxia not responsive to treatment. Patients with COPD and hypercapnic respiratory distress or respiratory failure are the group most likely to be successfully treated with NIV. One large study in patients with COPD showed that NIV decreased the intubation rate by 28%, the in-hospital mortality rate by 10%, and had an absolute reduction in length of stay by 4 days [17]. Smaller studies have also shown success with NIV in asthmatics. Although generally used with cooperative patients, noninvasive respiration has been successfully used in patients who are obtunded with a GCS of 8 or less. Configure the NIV to a spontaneously triggered mode with a backup respiratory rate. Typical initial settings are an inspiratory pressure of 8–12 cmH$_2$O and an expiratory pressure of 3–5 cmH$_2$O. The inspiratory pressure can then be increased slowly to desired effect.

In patients who are not candidates for NIV or those who fail to improve, mechanical ventilation is used to support patients in the setting of severe asthma or COPD exacerbations. High pressures and the removal of the body's compensatory mechanisms make this a last resort in most cases. The underlying airway constriction and air trapping does not abate with intubation. Special attention needs to be paid to continuing medication therapy and using ventilator settings to minimize air trapping and high airway pressures.

Most patients will be treated in the ED, show significant improvement, and eventually be discharged back to their usual living environment. The choice of delivery devices for inhaled medications is important in the elderly, and patients should be properly trained to correct inhaler use and their dexterity should be assessed.

There are four major components of advanced COPD management: 1) assessment and monitoring of the disease, 2) reduction of risk factors, 3) education, pharmacologic and non-pharmacologic treatment, and 4) management of exacerbations. Although the ED mostly focuses on the management of exacerbations, making every effort to get patients to stop smoking and receive annual influenza and pneumococcal vaccines and/or assuring primary care follow-up should be part of each encounter. Smoking cessation is one of the most effective interventions in COPD and is strongly associated with improved survival. It is also important to be aware that COPD patients are likely to experience anxiety and depression. The rate of depression in patients with advanced COPD may be as high as 79% and anxiety rates are similarly high [18]. These comorbidities have been associated with a substantial decrease in psychological and physical functional status and increases in hospitalization rates.

Summary: Physiologic changes in the aging lung cause many of the same pulmonary function test changes that are found in COPD. Elderly patients are more likely to have a poor perception of dyspnea related to airway obstruction and thus present with more severe disease. Be aware that high-flow oxygen may harm patients with COPD who are prone to retain carbon dioxide. The ED treatment of asthma or COPD exacerbations in the elderly does not differ significantly from that used in younger adults. However, COPD exacerbations in the elderly may be complicated by comorbidities and decreased functional reserve.

Bronchiectasis

Bronchiectasis can be considered a type of COPD. Its prevalence increases with age. It is defined as abnormal dilation of the proximal bronchi caused by weakening or fibrosis of the muscular and elastic components of the bronchial walls. The consequence of this altered airway anatomy is severely impaired clearance of secretions from the bronchial tree and transmural inflammation. The presentation resembles many respiratory illnesses and includes cough, daily mucopurulent sputum production, with occasional hemoptysis, often lasting months to years. Other symptoms may include dyspnea, pleuritic chest pain, wheezing, fever, weakness, and weight loss.

Bronchiectasis is usually diagnosed on radiologic exam. Chest X-rays are usually abnormal, but are often inadequate to diagnosis or assess bronchiectasis. The gold standard study for bronchiectasis is high-resolution CT. Bronchiectasis can have many causes. The congenital causes, such as cystic fibrosis, alpha-1-antitrypsin deficiency, or Kartagener's syndrome would be readily apparent or already known by age 65. The acquired causes of bronchiectasis include recurrent infection, aspiration of foreign bodies or other materials, inhalation of toxic gases such as ammonia, alcohol and drug abuse, tuberculosis, and inflammatory bowel disease. A mnemonic of the causes of bronchiectasis is listed in Table 19.2.

The anatomical location can help identify the cause. Bronchiectasis as a result of infection is usually found in the lower lobes, right middle lobe, or lingula. Right middle lobe involvement alone suggests an anatomic abnormality or neoplastic lesion. Upper lobe involvement may suggest *Mycobacterium tuberculosis*, chronic fungal infections, or cystic fibrosis. Allergic bronchopulmonary aspergillosis can also affect the upper lobe but usually involves the central bronchi, which is not seen in other forms of the disease.

The treatment of bronchiectasis is determined by the suspected cause. Because the underlying process is often

Table 19.2. Mnemonic for bronchiectasis

A SICK AIRWAY
Airway lesion, chronic obstruction
Sequestration
Infection, inflammation
Cystic fibrosis
Kartagener's syndrome
Allergic brochopulmonary aspergillosis
Immunodeficiencies (hypogammaglobulinemia, myeloma, lymphoma)
Reflux, inhalation injury
William Campbell syndrome (and other congenitals)
Aspiration
Yellow nail syndrome/**Y**oung syndrome

chronic inflammation, respiratory antibiotics are usually part of this treatment, including coverage for *Pseudomonas aeruginosa*. Inhalers and corticosteroids are also often part of therapy.

Summary: Although the pathophysiology of bronchiectasis is different to that of COPD, it can be considered a type of COPD. It is sometimes seen on chest X-ray but is usually diagnosed by CT scan. Treatment is similar to COPD initially but should be guided by the suspected underlying cause.

Pneumonia

The seriousness of pneumonia cannot be overestimated in the geriatric population. Pneumonia is the third leading cause of death in patients 65 and older [19]. It is the second most common infection in nursing home residents and the leading infectious cause of death in the US [20]. Pneumonia is the third leading cause of hospitalization in patients 65 and older [21]. Complications such as empyema, bacteremia, and even meningitis are more common in patients with pneumonia. The incidence of pneumonia increases with age, with patients 85 years old having more than twice the rate of those at age 65.

Multiple factors appear to have a role in the pathogenesis of pneumonia in the older population. The aging lung undergoes a number of changes which lead to an increased work of breathing. Decrease in elastic recoil, decrease in expiratory flow, and increase in air trapping as well as decreased lung compliance all contribute. Respiratory muscles also undergo a loss of mass and efficiency. Mucociliary clearance of potentially pathogenic organisms is an important host defense which has been shown to be slower and less efficient in older patients. There is also a decrease in cell-mediated and humeral immunity as well as a decrease in phagocytosis. Elderly patients have been shown to have significant colonization of the upper respiratory tract by bacteria. Bacterial colonization of the stomach is also more common in old age and can be exacerbated by antacids or H2 blockers. Although there is significant individual variation in many of these factors, it is felt that together they constitute part of the reason for the increased rate of pneumonia in the elderly population. Certain comorbidities have a strong association with pneumonia in the elderly. These include COPD and asthma, diabetes, cancer, heart failure, renal failure, alcoholism, and immune suppression.

The presentation of pneumonia may be as subtle as a change in mental status but in most cases involves dyspnea (75%), cough (75%), increased sputum (52%), pleuritic chest pain (31%), and hemoptysis (10%). Systemic symptoms often include fatigue (86%), anorexia (61%), sweats (50%), chills (35%), and change in mental status (28%). Signs include fever (59%), tachypnea (66%), tachycardia (39%), and rales (81%) [22]. Many of these finding are quite nonspecific and in some studies up to 35% of elderly pneumonia patients lacked physical findings of pneumonia, so a high level of suspicion should be maintained. Compared with younger populations with pneumonia, the symptoms in the elderly are usually present 1–3 days longer before ED presentation.

Pneumonia can be separated into many different categories. In the ED we tend to categorize pneumonia by its treatment. Community-acquired (CAP), health care-associated, and aspiration pneumonia are important distinctions because the common pathogens differ in these groups. It is tempting to assign all elderly patients or patients with significant comorbidities to the health care-associated group but the definition remains: 1) Hospitalization for 2 days or more in the preceding 90 days; 2) residence in a nursing home or extended care facility; 3) home infusion therapy (including antibiotics); 4) chronic dialysis within 30 days; 5) home wound care; and 6) family member with multidrug-resistant pathogen. Community- and health care-acquired pneumonia pathogens are listed in Table 19.3. Drug-resistant organisms have been found in up to 19% of this group. Patients with drug-resistant pathogens (DRP) have more comorbidities and a baseline of lower functional status. *Staphylococcus aureus* was identified as the most common drug-resistant pathogen (31%), followed by Gram-negative bacilli (including *P. aeruginosa*) (28%), and *Streptococcus pneumoniae* (25%) [23].

As in the younger patient who presents with CAP, in the elderly *S. pneumoniae* is the predominant organism accounting for more than 50% of cases. For other organisms see Table 19.3. Aspiration pneumonia should be suspected in patients with voice or swallowing disorders, those with seizures, those provided tube feeding, or those with altered mental status. The characteristic right lower lobe infiltrate may or may not be present. Organisms responsible for aspiration pneumonia are listed in Table 19.3. *Staphylococcus aureus* pneumonia has been called "post-viral pneumonia" because both methicillin-

Table 19.3. Organisms causing pneumonia

Type of pneumonia	Community-acquired (CAP)	Hospital-acquired (HAP)	Aspiration findings
Common pathogens in the elderly	*Streptococcus pneumoniae*	*S. aureus*	*S. pneumoniae*
	Haemophilus influenzae	*P. aeruginosa*	*S. aureus*
	Staphylococcus aureus	*Klebsiella* spp.	*H. influenzae*
	Chlamydia pneumoniae	*Escherichia coli*	*P. aeruginosa*
	Enterobacteriaceae	*Acinetobacter* spp.	Often in combination with
	Group B Streptococci	*Enterobacter* spp.	anaerobic bacteria:
	Moraxella catarrhalis	Also, a small percent of CAP	*Bacteroides*
	Legionella	organisms	*Prevotella*
	Pseudomonas aeruginosa		*Fusobacterium*
			Peptostreptococcus

Table 19.4. Antibiotic treatment for different types of pneumonia

Type of pneumonia	Community-acquired (CAP)	Hospital-acquired (HAP)	Aspiration findings
Outpatient	Azithromycin or		Clindamycin or
	Clarithromycin or		Amoxicillin/clavulanate
	Doxycycline or		
	Moxifloxacin or		
	Levofloxacin		
	With comorbidity add:		
	Amoxicillin/clavulanate or		
	2nd or 3rd generation cephalosporin		
Inpatient	Moxifloxacin or	Piperacillin-tazobactam or	Clindamycin or
	Levofloxacin or	Cefepime or	Piperacillin-tazobactam or
	Ceftriaxone and azithromycin	Meropenem	Ampicillin-sulbactam or
		If MRSA suspected add vancomycin	Ceftriaxone and clindamycin

sensitive and -resistant *S. aureus* pneumonias have been found in patients who develop pneumonia 1–4 days after influenza infection [24].

Treatment should be initiated early and be aimed at the suspected organism. Two sets of blood cultures are sometimes recommended although studies have shown only a small percent (1–16) of these identify the organism or lead to a change in therapy. Getting a sputum sample often proves difficult. Some elderly patients have a nonproductive cough or are too weak to give an adequate sputum sample. Suctioning to get a specimen can cause discomfort to the patient and does not have significant overall benefit. It is important not to delay resuscitation or therapy for sputum collection. Depending on the population and the season it may be appropriate to get rapid testing for *Legionella*, *S. pneumoniae*, and influenza and respiratory syncytial viruses to help guide therapy.

The chest X-ray is obviously the tool used most often to make the diagnosis of pneumonia and should be obtained in all patients with suspected pneumonia. The radiographic appearance of the pneumonia may be helpful in deciding the appropriate treatment. Chest X-ray is not always definitive. The presence of CHF, COPD, or effusions may make further imaging necessary. It is also believed by some that some patients with an initially negative X-ray may later develop pneumonia following resuscitation, but it is unclear how often this occurs.

Suggested antibiotics are listed in Table 19.4.

Other important tools for the emergency physician in treating patients with pneumonia are the pneumonia severity scores (see Table 19.5). The PORT study gave us a tool with parameters to place patients in one of five risk groups with varying associated mortalities. Patients falling into the lowest two groups with the lowest potential mortalities are considered safe to be treated as outpatients, whereas those in the highest groups with the highest potential mortality risks are usually treated as inpatients. The CURB score is also used, but the CURB-65 rule is not as helpful in the elderly because 1 point is given simply for age over 65. Additional factors such as social situation and ability to ambulate and call for help should all be considered in the decision to treat a patient with pneumonia in the hospital.

A discussion about the patient's wishes in terms of invasive procedures, intubation, and resuscitation should be initiated when possible even in elderly patients who do not immediately require ventilator assistance. Noninvasive ventilation can be used in pneumonia patients with impending respiratory failure. In patients with impending respiratory failure who tolerate NIV, there is a significant reduction in intubation (50 to 21%), as well as length of intensive care unit (ICU) stay [25]. There is a significant failure rate in this group depending on factors that include comorbidities and altered mental status. If NIV fails or cannot be used, intubation may be necessary in severe cases of pneumonia.

Summary: Pneumonia is more common in the elderly population for a variety of reasons including aging changes in the lung and prevalent comorbidities. The presentation may be more subtle in this population. It is important to have a high level of suspicion. Treatment should be started early and guided by the type of pneumonia suspected.

Pulmonary embolism

Pulmonary embolism is a common and often underdiagnosed clinical entity. It is one of the most common causes of unexpected death with over 300,000 deaths annually in the US, most often diagnosed during autopsy. It accounts for 10% of hospital deaths. Studies have shown that the prevalence of venous thomboembolic disease (VTE) and PE increases markedly with age. There is a mild increase in patients over 45 years old which becomes a much steeper increase after age 65. Survival after VTE is highest in patients who are less than 40 years old and lowest in those older than 70 [26].

The elderly are susceptible to all three parts of Virchow's triad and thus at higher risk for VTE. The predisposing factors for VTE are stasis, vascular injury, and hypercoagulability. Venous stasis is felt to contribute to VTE by decreased flow, which leads to local hypoxia and thus increased conversion of factor X to Xa in the coagulation pathway. Stasis in the elderly can be caused by immobilization, injury, stroke, heart failure, and peripheral vascular insufficiency. Vascular injury can trigger injured endothelial cells to synthesize tissue

Table 19.5. Pneumonia severity index

Criterion	Points scoring	Class	Points	30-day mortality (%)	Disposition
Age	1 point per year	I	<51	0.1	Discharge
Female	−10	II	51–70	0.6	Discharge
Nursing home resident	+10	III	71–90	0.9	Discharge or Admit
Neoplastic disease history	+30	IV	91–130	9.3	Admit
Liver disease	+20	V	>130	27	Admit
Congestive heart failure	+10				
Cerebrovascular disease	+10				
Renal disease	+10				
Altered mental status	+20				
Respiratory rate >29	+20				
Systolic blood pressure <90	+20				
Pulse >124	+10				
Temp. >103.8°F or <95°F	+15				
pH <7.35	+30				
Blood urea nitrogen >29	+20				
Sodium <130	+20				
Glucose >249	+10				
Hematocrit <30%	+10				
PO_2 <60	+10				
Pleural effusion on X-ray	+10				

PSI index/PORT SCORE [43].
Dispositions are suggested and should be modified based on clinical judgment and social situation.

factor and plasminogen activator inhibitor-1, which promote thrombogenesis as well as the activation of platelets and clot formation. The elderly are susceptible to vascular injury from trauma, surgery, chemotherapy, and sepsis, among other causes. Hypercoagulable states cause a shift in the delicate balance between thrombus formation and the fibrinolytic systems promoting clot breakdown. The elderly develop hypercoagulable states including malignancy, joint replacement surgeries, trauma, systemic infections, and decreased mobility.

The diagnosis of pulmonary embolism in elderly people is difficult because many cardiopulmonary conditions have a similar clinical presentation. The presentation of pulmonary embolism in the elderly does not differ significantly from that in the young. Presentation includes dyspnea, tachypnea, tachycardia, and pleuritic chest pain. The major risk factors for pulmonary embolism in the geriatric population are bed rest and venous stasis [27,28]. Sinus tachycardia, new or changed right bundle branch block, and ST-T wave abnormalities are the most common ECG findings. The classic S1Q3T3 pattern is found in less than 15% of ECGs in elderly patients with proven pulmonary embolism. Chest X-ray has abnormalities in 50–70% of elderly patients with PE. The most common abnormalities include cardiomegaly (22–64%), pulmonary edema (13–30%), pleural effusion (15–50%), atelectasis (9–70%), and elevated hemidiaphragm (5–28%), all of which are too nonspecific to be helpful in the diagnosis of PE [29]. In fact many of these findings are misleading and contribute to the high misdiagnosis rate. Studies that looked at arterial blood gas results in the elderly with PE found hypoxia, low arterial carbon dioxide partial pressure, and an increased A–a gradient, but these findings had a very low specificity [30].

The Patient Education Research Center decision rule for PE cannot be used in the elderly since age less than 50 is one of the criteria. The Geneva score starts by allotting 1 point for age over 60 and another for age over 80. The Wells criteria for PE do not include age as a variable, but these have not been specifically validated in this population. Emergency physicians often use D-dimer tests to assess the probability of PE. In younger patients this will be negative in up to 60% of cases but in patients 80 years or older it is only negative in 5%. Some studies have invesigated whether an age-dependent cutoff for D-dimers would increase the test's usefulness, and have shown an increased specificity but at the cost of decreased sensitivity [31].

The sensitivity of lower extremity ultrasound in investigating DVT increases with age without loss of specificity. A positive result is helpful, but absence of DVT does not rule out PE.

The ventilation–perfusion scan is also a test that becomes less helpful with age. Because any pre-existing lung diseases can make the test non-diagnostic, its usefulness decreases with age and comorbidity. V/Q scanning of lung is diagnostic in 68% of patients less than 40 years old but in only 42% of patients 80 years and older [32].

Studies have shown that even with increasing age, CT angiogram is a useful test for pulmonary embolism. The diagnostic yield remains high and often identifies an alternative diagnosis in patients without evidence of pulmonary embolism. CT angiogram is most sensitive when clots are present in the main, lobar, or proximal (segmental) pulmonary vasculature and less sensitive when clots are present in the distal (subsegmental) pulmonary vasculature.

MRI has been shown useful in the diagnosis of DVT, and some small studies have looked at its use in PE. Small studies have shown this modality to be both sensitive and specific for the diagnosis of PE, although the ability of MRI to detect small clots in vessels at or beyond segmental branches is even more limited than with CT.

Although pulmonary angiogram remains the "gold standard," it is rarely used because of the higher risk of renal damage and other complications. It is not 100% sensitive or specific and, because of its complication rate, its diagnostic accuracy in the elderly has not been specifically studied.

Age and comorbidities affect survival of patients with PE. The simplified PESI scoring system for risk stratification in PE uses age over 80 as one of its criteria. Elevated troponins have been shown to have predictive value in elderly patients with PE. Cardiac ultrasound in patients with PE will often show signs of right heart strain, which has been shown to predict increased morbidity and mortality.

Anticoagulation remains the treatment of choice in pulmonary embolism. It has been shown to significantly decrease thrombus formation and extension, and decrease the rate of recurrent and fatal PE. Practice guidelines recommend anticoagulation for the treatment of PE in all patients, including the elderly. It should also be considered in those patients with at least moderate risk for VTE in whom studies may be delayed. The exceptions are those patients with active bleeding, major trauma, stroke, and certain neoplasms. The elderly are at increased risk of bleeding when anticoagulated compared with younger patients, even when comorbid factors are controlled for. Unfractionated heparin and low-molecular weight heparin (LMWH) have both been shown to be safe and effective. Difficulty getting activated partial thromboplastin time (PTT) values to stay within the therapeutic range has always been an issue with the use of unfractionated heparin. Subtherapeutic PTT values may lead to recurrent venous thromboembolism, but the association of supratherapeutic PTT values and bleeding is not so well documented. The use of LMWH often requires adjustment to a patient's creatinine clearance, which can be an issue in the elderly. Long-term use of heparin has been associated with increased osteopenia in the elderly. Oral anticoagulation with warfarin should be initiated after initial anticoagulation. Other oral anticoagulants are now entering the market but their safety and efficacy in the elderly is still being investigated. The optimal duration of anticoagulation therapy is unknown: 6 months has been shown to have a lower recurrence rate than 6 weeks in first-time PE patients, but this should be individualized. Patients with recurrent VTE or known hypercoagulable states may be on lifelong anticoagulation.

Thrombolytic therapy for PE has been used in cases of hemodynamic instability. Urokinase, streptokinase, and recombinant tissue plasminogen activator (rt-PA) have been shown to be similarly effective in accelerating the lysis of an embolus. These agents have been shown to decrease pulmonary arterial pressure and decrease the incidence of subsequent pulmonary hypertension, but have not been shown to decrease mortality or the incidence of recurrent PE. Thrombolytic agents show a threefold increase in the risk of major bleeding compared with conventional heparin therapy. Major bleeding (fatal hemorrhage, intracranial hemorrhage, or bleeding that requires surgery or blood transfusion) occurs in approximately 12% of patients with PE treated with thrombolytics regardless of which thrombolytic agent is used.

When anticoagulation cannot be used or has failed to prevent recurrent PE, it is appropriate to admit the patient for placement of an inferior vena cava (IVC) filter. Patients thus treated are prone to having it fail (about 5%) or migrate. The long-term benefits of this device have not been demonstrated, and it does not significantly reduce the incidence of rehospitalization for PE after 1 year. In elderly patients who underwent IVC filter insertion, 2-year mortality was found to be almost 50% but this may be because of the underlying conditions which led to filter placement [33].

Open surgical embolectomy and catheter thrombectomy have been used in patients with massive PE and have both shown reasonable success; one study on open thrombectomy showed an 89% survival rate [34]. These interventions have not been compared to standard therapy and are used when other options are not available and require a willing surgeon or interventional radiologist.

Summary: Pulmonary embolism becomes more common with increasing age. Although the presentation does not differ significantly with age, the diagnosis of pulmonary embolism in the elderly is more difficult because its presentation is similar to many cardiopulmonary conditions. Many of the studies looking for PE lose specificity in older patients with comorbid diseases. CT angiogram remains the modality of choice. Anticoagulation should be started early in patients without contraindications. Thrombolysis should be considered in the most severe cases.

Pneumothorax

Pneumothorax can be defined as a collection of air in the pleural space that causes part or all of a lung to collapse. Pneumothorax can be divided into traumatic and spontaneous. In geriatric trauma, the increased brittleness of the bones as well as changes in chest wall and lung compliance combine with an increase in pre-existing lung pathology such as emphysema to increase the incidence of pneumothorax. Geriatric patients have an increase in complication rates and a higher mortality associated with traumatic pneumothorax. In the elderly who have lower pulmonary reserve, the presence of pneumothorax in the setting of significant pulmonary contusion, flail chest, or multiple rib fractures may warrant ICU admission. Iatrogenic traumatic pneumothorax secondary to lung procedures such as bronchoscopy or lung biopsy also increases in the geriatric population.

Spontaneous pneumothorax has been shown to occur in a bimodal distribution. The first peak is in young adults aged 20–24, while a second peak occurs in patients in the geriatric population aged 80–84. The acute presentation of pneumothorax appears to differ with age – more elderly patients presented with a complaint only of dyspnea. Chest pain was present in less than 20% of the elderly population with spontaneous pneumothorax, whereas it was present in two-thirds of the younger population [35]. Pneumothorax must be immediately considered in elderly patients with COPD or asthma who acutely decompensate. The most common physical finding is a nonspecific tachycardia. As with many diseases, a previous history of pneumothorax increases the probability that a given patient has pneumothorax. The recurrence rate approaches 45%.

Another difference in regard to pneumothorax in the older population concerns the presence of comorbid diseases such as asthma, COPD, pulmonary hypertension, and cancer. In the presence of lung scarring, bullous changes, and fibrosis of the lung, pneumothorax may be occult on chest X-ray. If there is a reasonable level of suspicion for pneumothorax with a negative chest X-ray, a chest CT may be needed to confirm or exclude the diagnosis.

True tension pneumothorax is relatively rare in any population, but because this condition may require urgent intervention and the elderly population have less pulmonary reserve one must remain vigilant. Even in the absence of tension pneumothorax, the changes caused by a relatively small pneumothorax may be sufficient to markedly affect the ventilatory status of older patients. Those patients who cannot compensate adequately require thoracostomy tube placement in the ED. In patients who do not require immediate decompression, 100% oxygen is the first-line therapy. Oxygen increases pleural air absorption by a factor of three or four. In the population with COPD or other reasons for CO_2 retention, care should be taken to avoid the hypoventilation associated with 100% oxygen. (In the stable patient, defining the presence of cavitary lesions, scarring of the chest wall, or other sources of complications may guide the clinician to arrange for chest tube placement in the operating room or under direct visualization.) In the elderly, the complication of persistent air leak is seen in 85% of patients receiving a thoracostomy tube. There is some suggestion that intraoperative pleurodesis during thoracostomy placement may be warranted to prevent this complication [36].

Summary: Pneumothorax occurs in the elderly population in both the trauma and non-trauma setting. Pneumothorax should be considered in older patients with COPD or asthma who acutely decompensate. Pre-existing lung pathology may make the placement of chest tubes more difficult. The complication rate of tube thoracostomy increases in the geriatric population.

Tuberculosis

Mycobacterium tuberculosis infection remains a significant concern in the elderly. *Mycobacterium tuberculosis* is a slow-growing aerobic rod with an acid-fast cell wall. Several studies have shown that elderly patients have the highest case rate of any subgroup in the US population for tuberculosis. Nursing home patients are particularly at risk, and the longer the

patient has been in a nursing home the higher the prevalence of TB. Reactivation of a dormant infection is the predominant mechanism of disease in the elderly, with a lifetime risk of reactivation of 10%. Geriatric patients still have a significant rate of primary infection and patients with a history of TB are vulnerable to exogenous reinfection. The elderly also represent a disproportionate number of TB deaths.

Hemoptysis often leads the emergency physician to suspect TB, but this finding is neither sensitive nor specific. The clinical presentation of TB can be atypical and subtle in the elderly. The diagnosis must be considered in a variety of clinical scenarios. Symptoms such as unexplained weight loss, "failure to thrive," fever, weakness, or a change in mental status may be the only manifestation of the disease. Several papers have looked at the differences in presentation in elderly patients but have failed to show consistent findings. The use of corticosteroids for more than 1 month at a dose equivalent to 15 mg of prednisone per day has been shown to decrease tuberculin activity [37]. Patients with a history of previous TB infection, contact with known TB cases, HIV infection, as well as those from nursing homes who have not been recently tested should be isolated in the ED until *M. tuberculosis* infection can be ruled out.

Testing for *M. tuberculosis* in the geriatric population presents certain challenges. In the US more than 5% of cases of TB are diagnosed by autopsy. The tuberculin skin test of purified protein derivative (PPD) has long been the standard mechanism for testing, but it is neither perfectly sensitive nor specific. Sensitivity of PPD compared with ELISA assay ranged from 83 to 98%, depending on the study. False-positive skin tests occur in patients who have non-tuberculous mycobacteria or have received Bacille–Calmette–Guérin (BCG) vaccine. False-negative PPD results can occur as a result of immunosuppression, known as "anergy," and are seen in patients with severe febrile illness, HIV, and other viral infections, or following the administration of corticosteroids or other immunosuppressive drugs. Skin tests may also be negative in up to 28% of patients with active TB. These tests usually become positive 2–3 weeks after treatment is initiated. Although the rate of anergy is difficult to assess, it is more common in the geriatric population and has been attributed to an age-dependent decline in cellularly mediated immunity [38]. In the ED, these failings of PPD make skin testing a poor choice for investigation of the sickest patients.

The gold standard test for tuberculosis is the culture and smear of sputum, but culture may take up to 6 weeks to show positive. Collection of sputum in the ED often yields unsatisfactory samples, and thus collection by someone trained to induce sputum is preferred. Gastric and pleural fluid aspirates and tissue samples can also be cultured for TB. Bronchial washes or biopsies are used when available. Staining for acid-fast bacilli will be present in up to 60% of culture-positive cases of *M. tuberculosis*. Three negative smears is often enough to remove suspected cases from isolation. Some hospitals have access to direct amplified tests for tuberculosis RNA which take 1–3 days, others provide ELISA blood testing for TB, and recently a bedside immunoassay has been tested. These may prove helpful in future in the ED, but currently a high level of suspicion for TB should prompt the emergency physician to isolate the patient.

The chest X-ray findings in TB are different between those in primary cases and reactivation TB. In primary TB infections the findings are often nonspecific and may include infiltrates in any lobe, pleural effusions, hilar or mediastinal fullness, or adenopathy. Reactivation TB is likely to show the classic cavitary and noncavitary lesions in the upper lobe or the upper segment of the lower lobe. These cavitary lesions are associated with a higher rate of infectivity. Calcified and non-calcified nodules can be found in patients with old treated disease as well as in those who have reactivation of their tuberculosis. The chest X-ray of a patient with miliary TB may show diffuse nodules (1–3 mm) throughout the lung or be completely negative. In an immunocompromised host the presentation may not be classic: TB has long been known as one of the "great imitators." The overall sensitivity for TB on chest X-ray when compared with a sputum sample is 86–92% [39].

In the US, extrapulmonary TB comprises a little under 20% of the cases diagnosed, with lymphatic and pleural TB being the two most common such manifestations. Hematologic spread may occur at any stage of the disease. Diagnosis is often delayed because clinicians are less familiar with these manifestations and invasive procedures are often required to obtain samples to confirm the diagnosis.

Although therapy is usually started long after patients with suspected TB leave the ED, there are some important facts for the emergency physician to be aware of. Moxifloxacin, often use as part of therapy in CAP, has activity against *M. tuberculosis* and its use may lead to subsequent false-negative testing for TB. When treatment is started for TB, three or four drugs are usually required and used for 8 weeks, followed by a two-drug regimen for up to 31 weeks. Drugs used include isoniazid, rifampin, and pyrazinamide, all of which have potential hepatotoxicity, so obtaining baseline liver function tests (LFTs) may be indicated.

Patients with tuberculosis or those with suspected tuberculosis are often kept in the hospital for confirmatory testing, initiation of treatment, and for public health protection. *Mycobacterium tuberculosis* is one of the reasons for which patients may be kept in the hospital against their will to protect the public. It is important to involve hospital administration and risk management personnel if this situation arises. Tuberculosis can be managed in an outpatient setting, but this requires adequate linkage to primary care physicians or the appropriate public health organizations.

Summary: Initial infection and reactivation of *M. tuberculosis* remain of significant concern in the elderly. Presentation of this disease may be subtle and yet the consequences may be more severe. PPD is a good screening test but is not perfectly sensitive or specific. Sputum smear and culture is the gold standard. Isolating patients suspected of having TB from other susceptible patients is an important step in the ED. Therapy should be tailored to the patient's pre-existing conditions.

Pulmonary hypertension

Pulmonary hypertension (PH) is the disease caused by elevation of pulmonary vascular pressure. In most cases it is characterized by vascular proliferation and remodeling of the small pulmonary arteries or veins, vasoconstriction, and thrombosis in situ, which cause increased pulmonary vascular resistance ultimately resulting in RV failure. Hemodynamically it is defined as mean pulmonary artery pressure ($\overline{P}_{pa}$) >25 mmHg at rest or >30 mmHg during exercise in the presence of pulmonary capillary wedge pressure (P_{pcw}) ≤15 mmHg.

Pulmonary hypertension is a severe progressive disease, and prognosis can be tied to its severity. Patients who are classes I and II have a mean survival of 6 years, class III 2.6 years, and class IV 6 months [40]. Pulmonary hypertension is an increasingly recognized cause of dyspnea in elderly patients and should be added to the differential diagnosis when common causes of dyspnea are absent. The exact incidence is difficult to estimate, as many processes lead to PH: 25–50% of patients with severe heart failure have PH while only about 5% of patients with COPD develop the disease. In patients 60 years and older, the most common cause of PH is diastolic heart failure (31%), while connective tissue disease (15%) and pulmonary disease (13%) are less common [41]. The cause of pulmonary hypertension is important to identify, as treatment in many cases needs to be aimed at the underlying diagnosis. For patients with PH caused by thromboembolic disease, treatment needs to include anticoagulation, while PH caused by other conditions such as sclerodema or lupus will respond well to steroids or other immunosuppressive agents. Many of the causes and classifications are listed in Table 19.6.

Pulmonary hypertension may be suspected in patients with dyspnea, angina, syncope, edema, and Reynaud's disease. Signs of right ventricular strain or failure such as jugular venous distension (JVD), hepatosplenomegaly, edema, or ascites may be present. On cardiac exam there may be a loud P2, evidence of S3 or S4 gallop, as well as tricuspid or pulmonic regurgitation.

Table 19.6. Causes of pulmonary hypertension

Group	Cause	Diseases
I	Small pulmonary muscular arterioles	Connective tissue diseases, HIV infection, portal hypertension, schistosomiasis
II	Left-sided heart disease	Systolic or diastolic dysfunction, or valvular heart disease
III	Lung disease or hypoxia	Interstitial lung disease, COPD, sleep-disordered breathing, causes of hypoxemia
IV	Thromboembolic occlusion of the pulmonary vasculature	Pulmonary embolus
V	Idiopathic	Hematologic (myeloproliferative dx), metabolic (glycogen storage dx), or systemic (sarcoidosis)

On chest X-ray there may be prominent hilar pulmonary arteries with marked peripheral hypovascularity (pruning), as well as RV enlargement into the retrosternal clear space. ECG may show right atrial (RA) enlargement, RV enlargement, and RV strain.

In the acute setting, treatment of PH is relatively straightforward. Giving oxygen to maintain a saturation of about 90% will give symptomatic relief. Diuretics such as furosemide are used to diminish hepatic congestion and peripheral edema. Caution needs to be taken to avoid decreased right and/or left ventricular preload, which may decrease cardiac output. In patients who cannot tolerate diuresis, fluid can be removed by dialysis or ultrafiltration. Digoxin may improve the RV ejection fraction of some patients but should be used with caution in the elderly because of its narrow therapeutic window. Vasodilators such as nitroglycerin will often drop the preload precipitously, so early inotropic support with dopamine or norepinephrine may be needed. Atrial arrhythmias are not uncommon during acute decompensation, and these are not well tolerated because of poor cardiac reserves. The standard treatment with calcium channel blockers or beta blockers may lead to profound hypotension or cardiogenic shock in the setting of PH. Use these agents cautiously and consider the alternatives of amiodarone or direct current cardioversion.

After the acute treatment these patients are usually admitted to the hospital, where stabilization and diuresis may take several days. Long-term therapies may be started or continued. Typically patients undergo a vasoreactivity test, and those showing positive may be given oral calcium channel blocker therapy; patients showing negative require advanced therapy with a prostanoid, endothelin receptor antagonist, or phosphodiesterase-5 inhibitor. It is important for emergency physicians to be aware that some of these medications (e.g., treprostinil or epoprostenol) may be given by continual infusion and therefore interruption of the infusion may be the cause of the acute exacerbation of disease. Restoring flow may be the most important step in treating the patient. In the appropriate patient on these agents it may be worthwhile to check LFTs, as the main adverse effect of certain endothelin receptor antagonists is hepatotoxicity.

Summary: Pulmonary hypertension is a severe, progressive disease which mimics and accompanies many cardiopulmonary conditions. Treatment includes oxygen and diuretic treatment while care should be taken to avoid decreasing preload. Vasoconstrictor medication may be needed in the most severe cases.

Restrictive lung disease

Restrictive lung disease can be defined as a disease that decreases lung expansion, resulting in a decreased lung volume, an increased work of breathing, and inadequate ventilation. Restrictive lung disease causes a decrease in FEV_1 and forced vital capacity (FVC). One suggested criterion for restrictive lung disease is an FVC of less than 80% predicted. Restrictive lung diseases can be divided into extrinsic and intrinsic. Extrinsic causes include diseases of the chest and spine which decrease chest volume, such as kyphosis and extreme obesity, as well as pleural thickening. Neuromuscular diseases such as

Table 19.7. Causes of restrictive lung disease

Idiopathic pulmonary fibrosis
Sarcoidosis
Asbestosis
Radiation fibrosis
Drugs: amiodarone, methotrexate, bleomycin
Hypersensitivity pneumonitis
Acute respiratory distress syndrome
Idiopathic interstitial pneumonia
Eosinophilic pneumonia
Lymphangioleiomyomatosis
Neuromuscular diseases
Nonmuscular diseases of chest wall
Pulmonary Langerhans cell histiocytosis

Guillain–Barré syndrome, poliomyelitis, or myasthenia gravis are also considered extrinsic causes of restrictive lung disease. Intrinsic causes include asbestosis, radiation fibrosis, rheumatoid arthritis, hypersensitivity pneumonitis, certain drugs such as amiodarone, and pulmonary fibrosis from many causes. Cases of restrictive lung disease are labeled idiopathic when no cause can be found (see Table 19.7).

The presentation of restrictive lung disease is usually a slow to moderate progression of shortness of breath (SOB). Cough and hemoptysis may also be present. Because the elderly do not perceive dyspnea as early as younger patients they may have severe disease by the time they present to the ED. The length of time that a patient suffers SOB has some diagnostic value for the etiology of restrictive lung disease. Shortness of breath over a period of years points toward more chronic syndromes like idiopathic pulmonary fibrosis (IPF), sarcoidosis, and pulmonary histiocytosis X. Weeks to months of symptoms may be caused by hypersensitivity pneumonitis, drug-induced interstitial lung disease, and connective tissue diseases. Acute presentations include acute interstitial pneumonitis, eosinophilic pneumonia, and diffuse alveolar hemorrhage.

Treatment of restrictive lung disease includes treating the underlying cause if one is found or suspected. Supplemental oxygen for acute exacerbations is helpful. Steroids and bronchial dilators can be used and have been shown to be effective for certain causes. Pulmonary hygiene has been helpful in some cases. Typically, extrinsic disease does not respond well to these interventions. In severe cases, NIV has been used successfully to treat patients with restrictive lung disease. Patients in whom these devices fail may require endotracheal intubation. When intubation is required, the largest-diameter tube possible should be used to allow lower peak pressures and better pulmonary toilet.

Summary: Restrictive lung disease has a variety of causes which should be considered in the geriatric population. Supplemental oxygen and treatment of the underlying cause comprise most of the emergency department treatment of these diseases.

Lung cancer

There are two reasons that lung cancer is discovered in the ED. The first is that a patient has a complication associated with the cancer. The most urgent of these include: superior vena cava syndrome, acute tumor lysis syndrome, hypercalcemia of malignancy, malignant pericardial disease, and spinal cord compression by cancer. The second reason is when a cancer or something suggestive of it is found unexpectedly in a patient under evaluation for something else. Lung cancer is the leading cause of cancer death in the US, and the average age at which it is diagnosed is 71 years. Smoking is considered the cause of lung cancer in 90% of men and 80% of women diagnosed with the disease; 16% of cases are diagnosed at the earliest stage, 25% after spread to lymph nodes, and 51% after metastasis beyond the lymph nodes. The overall 5-year survival rate for lung cancer is 16.3%, which is much lower than that of the three next most common cancers: colon (65.2%), breast (90.0%), and prostate (99.9%) [42].

When lung cancer is discovered, emergency care needs to focus on the urgent conditions listed above. It is important to perform a complete neurologic exam, a full set of labs, as well as other tests driven by presentation to rule out emergent conditions associated with the cancer. Patients in most cases do not need admission for an incidentally found tumor but they should not be lost to the system. A frank discussion with the patient in the presence of whatever support system can be mustered in the acute setting is important. It is best not to over- or understate what has been discovered in the ED. The disposition decision should include the patient's social and physical condition as well as how they appear to be understanding and coping with what they are being told. If discharge seems safe, ensuring follow-up with redundant systems is advisable. Because denial and misunderstandings are common, it is important to write out explicit instructions regarding when and where to follow up and when to return to the ED.

Summary: Lung cancer is occasionally discovered in the ED. Once the dangerous sequelae are excluded, care should be based on the patient's needs and the hospital's resources.

Pearls and pitfalls

Pearls

- Changes in the geriatric lung, poor perception of dyspnea, and comorbidities make older patients more likely to have more severe lung disease by the time they present to the ED.
- When a geriatric patient with pulmonary disease decompensates, consider pneumothorax and pulmonary embolism as two possible causes.
- Noninvasive ventilatory support can be used in a variety of clinical situations to postpone or avoid the morbidity of orotracheal intubation.

Pitfalls

- Simply because the diagnosis of COPD is in the patient's medical history does not mean that *this* ED visit for shortness of breath is caused by COPD. Keep an open mind, as many pulmonary emergencies have similar presentations.

- A chest X-ray is a good screening test but do not be fooled by an initially negative chest X-ray in the right clinical scenario.
- Be careful putting patients with a history of advanced lung disease on 100% O_2 as this may cause some to retain CO_2.

References

1. Janssens JP, Pache JC, Nicod LP. Physiological changes in respiratory function associated with aging. *Eur Respir J.* 1999;13(1):197–205.
2. Sharma G, Goodwin J. Effect of aging on respiratory system physiology and immunology. *Clin Interv Aging.* 2006;1(3):253–60.
3. Parker AL. Aging does not affect beta-agonist responsiveness after methacholine-induced bronchoconstriction. *J Am Geriatr Soc.* 2004;52(3):388–92.
4. Hardie JA, Vollmer WM, et al. Reference values for arterial blood gases in the elderly. *Chest.* 2004;125(6):2053–60.
5. Casati A, et al. Transcutaneous monitoring of partial pressure of carbon dioxide in the elderly patient: a prospective, clinical comparison with end-tidal monitoring. *J Clin Anesth.* 2006;18(6):436–40.
6. HJ Lim, KB Yap. Presentation of elderly people at an emergency department in Singapore. *Singapore Med J.* 1999;40(12):742–4.
7. Syrjala H, Broas M, Suramo I, et al. High resolution computed tomography for the diagnosis of community-acquired pneumonia. *Clin Infect Dis.* 1998;27:358–63.
8. Diette GB, Krishnan JA, Dominici F, et al. Asthma in older patients: factors associated with hostipalization. *Arch Intern Med.* 2002;162:1123.
9. Easton P, Jadue C, et al. A comparison of the bronchodilating effects of a beta-2 adrenergic agent (albuterol) and an anticholinergic agent (ipratropium bromide), given by aerosol alone or in sequence. *N Engl J Med.* 1986;315:735–9.
10. Gross N, Tashkin D, et al. Inhalation by nebulization of albuterol-ipratropium combination is superior to either agent alone in the treatment of chronic obstructive pulmonary disease. Dey Combination Solution Study Group. *Respiration.* 1998;65(5):354–62.
11. Lin RY, Pesola GR, Bakalchuk L, et al. Superiority of ipratropium plus albuterol over albuterol alone in the emergency department management of adult asthma: A randomized clinical trial. *Ann Emerg Med.* 1998;31:208–13.
12. Ullah MI, Newman GB, Saunders KB. Influence of age on response to ipratropium and salbutamol in asthma. *Thorax.* 1981;36:523–9.
13. Kradjan WA, Driesner NK, Abuan TH, Emmick G, Schoene RB. Effect of age on bronchodilator response. *Chest.* 1992;101(6):1545–51.
14. Whyte KF, Gould GA, Jeffrey AA, et al. Dose of nebulized ipratropium bromide in acute severe asthma. *Respir Med.* 1991;85(6):517–20.
15. Saint S, Bent S, Vittinghoff E, Grady D. Antibiotics in chronic obstructive pulmonary disease exacerbations. A meta-analysis. *JAMA.* 1995;273:957–60.
16. Adams SG, Melo J, Luther M, Anzueto A. Antibiotics are associated with lower relapse rates in outpatients with acute exacerbations of COPD. *Chest.* 2000;117(5):1345–52.

17. Keenan SP, Sinuff T, et al. Which patients with acute exacerbation of chronic obstructive pulmonary disease benefit from noninvasive positive-pressure ventilation? A systematic review of the literature. *Ann Intern Med.* 2003;138(11):861–70.

18. Yohannes AM, Baldwin RC, Connolly MJ. Depression and anxiety in elderly outpatients with chronic obstructive pulmonary disease: prevalence, and validation of the BASDEC screening questionnaire. *Int J Geriatr Psychiatry* 2000;15:1090–6.

19. *10 Leading Causes of Death by Age Group, United States – 2010,* Data Source: National Vital Statistics System, National Center for Health Statistics, CDC. Produced by: Office of Statistics and Programming, National Center for Injury Prevention and Control, CDC using WISQARS™.

20. Mills K, Graham AC, Winslow BT, Springer KL. Treatment of nursing home-acquired pneumonia. *Am Fam Physician.* 2009;79(11):976–82.

21. May DS, Kelly JJ, Mendlein JM, et al. Surveillance of major causes of hospitalization among the elderly 1988. *MMWR CDC Surveill Summ.* 1991;40:7–21.

22. Donowitz GR, Cox HL. Bacterial community-acquired pneumonia in older patients. *Clin Geriatr Med.* 2007;23:515–34.

23. Jamshed N, Woods C, et al. Pneumonia in the long-term resident. *Clin Geriatr Med.* 2011;27:117–33.

24. Mohan SS, Nair V, Cunha BA. Post-viral influenza *Streptococcus pneumoniae* pneumonia in an intravenous drug abuser. *Heart Lung.* 2005;34(3):222–6.

25. Carrillo A, Gonzalez-Diaz G et al. Non-invasive ventilation in community-acquired pneumonia and severe acute respiratory failure. *Intensive Care Med.* 2012;38(3):458–66.

26. Heit JA, Silverstein MD, Mohr DN, et al. Predictors of survival after deep vein thrombosis and pulmonary embolism: A population-based cohort study. *Arch Intern Med.* 1999;159(5):445–53.

27. Busby W, Bayer A, Pathy J. Pulmonary embolism in the elderly. *Age Aging.* 1988;17:205–9.

28. Masotti L, Ceccarelli E, Cappelli R, et al. Pulmonary embolism in the elderly: clinical, instrumental and laboratory aspects. *Gerontology.* 2000;46:205–11.

29. Masotti L, Ray P, et al. Pulmonary embolism in the elderly: a review on clinical, instrumental and laboratory presentation. *Vasc Health Risk Manag.* 2008;4(3):629–36.

30. Hardie JA, Vollmer WM, Buist S, et al. Reference values for arterial blood gases in the elderly. *Chest.* 2004;125:2053–60.

31. Righini M, Goehring C, et al. Effect of age on the performance of common diagnostic tests for pulmonary embolism. *Am J Med.* 2000;109:357–61.

32. Stein PD, Henry JW, et al. Elderly patients with no prior cardiopulmonary disease show ventilation/perfusion lung scan characteristics that are sensitive and specific. *Am J Ger Card.* 1996;5:36–40.

33. Goldhaber SZ, Visani L, De Rosa M. Acute pulmonary embolism: clinical outcomes in the International Cooperative Pulmonary Embolism Registry. *Lancet.* 1999;353:1386–9.

34. Aklog L, Williams C, et al. Acute pulmonary embolectomy: A contemporary approach. *Circulation.* 2002;105:1416–19.

35. Liston R, McLoughlin R. Acute pneumothorax: A comparison of elderly with younger patients. *Age Aging.* 1994;23(5):393–5.

36. Zhang Y, Jiang G, et al. Surgical management of secondary spontaneous pneumothorax in elderly patients with chronic obstructive pulmonary disease: Retrospective study of 107 cases. *Thorac Cardiovasc Surg.* 2009;57(6):347–52.

37. Vassilopoulos B et al. Usefulness of enzyme-linked immunospot assay (Elispot) compared to tuberculin skin testing for latent tuberculosis screening in rheumatic patients scheduled for anti-tumor necrosis factor treatment. *J Rheumatol.* 2008;35(7):1271–6.

38. Zevallos M, Justman JE. Tuberculosis in the elderly. *Clin Geriatr Med.* 2003;19:121–38.

39. van Cleeff MR, Kivihya-Ndugga LE, Meme H, Odhiambo JA, Klatser PR. The role and performance of chest X-ray for the diagnosis of tuberculosis: a cost-effectiveness analysis in Nairobi, Kenya. *BMC Infect Dis.* 2005;5:111.

40. D'Alonzo GE, et al. PAH Prognosis: Functional class correlates with survival. *Ann Intern Med.* 1991;115:343–9.

41. Bone-Larson C, Chan KM. Pulmonary hypertension in the elderly, part 1: Evaluation. *J Respir Dis.* 2008;29(11):443–50.

42. McCurdy MT, Shanholtz CB. Oncologic emergencies. *Crit Care Med.* 2012;40:2212–22.

43. Fine MJ, Auble TE, Yealy DM, et al. A prediction rule to identify low-risk patients with community-acquired pneumonia. *N Engl J Med.* 1997;336(4):243–50.

Chapter
20

Cardiovascular emergencies in the elderly

Aileen McCabe and Abel Wakai

Introduction

An aging population is one of the major challenges to health care systems worldwide. For example, in the European Union, the proportion of people aged 65 years or over in the total population is projected to increase from 17.1 to 30.0% and the number is projected to rise from 84.6 million in 2008 to 151.5 million in 2030 [1]. In the US, the number of people over the age of 65 will double from 35 million in 2000 to more than 70 million in 2030 [2]. Consequently, older patients comprise a large and growing subset of patients attending emergency departments (EDs). Meanwhile, the most important determinant of cardiovascular health is a person's age [3]. In patients aged 65 or older, cardiovascular diseases (CVD) will result in 40% of all deaths and rank as the leading cause [3]. This chapter discusses the identification and treatment of the following cardiovascular emergencies in elderly patients: acute coronary syndrome (ACS), dysrhythmia, acute heart failure syndromes, syncope, and acute thoracic aortic syndromes.

Acute coronary syndrome

"Acute coronary syndrome" has evolved as a useful operational term to refer to any constellation of clinical symptoms that are compatible with acute myocardial ischemia [4]. It encompasses myocardial infarction (ST-segment elevation and depression, Q wave and non-Q wave) and unstable angina (UA) [4]. In the context of ACS, although the precise definition of "elderly" or "older patients" has not been established in the medical literature, many studies have used this term to refer to those who are 75 years or older [4]. Elderly patients have a high relative frequency among patients presenting with UA/non-ST-segment elevation myocardial infarction (NSTEMI), with 35% older than 75 years and 11% aged more than 85 years [5].

Identification

Elderly patients may have atypical ACS symptoms such as generalized weakness, stroke, syncope, or a change in mental status [4]. Approximately 33% of elderly patients with ACS do not have chest pain on presentation to the hospital [6]. This group of myocardial infarction (MI) patients are, on average, 7 years older than those with chest pain (74.2 versus 66.9 years) [6]. The dominant presenting symptoms associated with increased hospital mortality rates in patients without chest pain are dyspnea, diaphoresis, nausea or vomiting, and presyncope/syncope [7]. The diagnostic challenge of ACS in the elderly is further complicated by the fact that non-cardiac comorbidities such as chronic obstructive pulmonary disease, gastro-esophageal reflux disease, upper body musculoskeletal symptoms, pulmonary embolism, and pneumonia are also more frequent and may be associated with chest pain at rest that can mimic classic symptoms of UA/NSTEMI [4]. A high index of suspicion is therefore required to diagnose ACS in this patient subset.

Although physical examination in younger patients with ACS is frequently normal, the elderly are more likely to have signs of altered or abnormal cardiovascular anatomy and physiology, including diminished beta-sympathetic response, increased cardiac afterload due to decreased arterial compliance and arterial hypertension, orthostatic hypotension, cardiac hypertrophy, and ventricular dysfunction, especially diastolic dysfunction [4].

Treatment

Although elderly patients with ACS have a higher baseline risk of adverse outcomes and have more comorbidities, they derive equivalent or greater benefit (for example, invasive versus conservative strategy) compared with younger patients [4,8]. Despite the fact that the elderly have been generally underrepresented in the relevant randomized controlled trials (RCTs), older patient subgroups appear to have similar relative risk reductions and similar or greater absolute risk reductions in many endpoints as younger patients for commonly used treatments in the management of UA/NSTEMI.

Despite the generally low rates of serious adverse events associated with the use of evidence-based treatment for UA/NSTEMI in elderly patients, precautions need to be taken to personalize these therapies (that is, beginning with lower doses than in younger patients, whenever appropriate, and providing careful observation for toxicity) [4]. The elderly are particularly vulnerable to adverse events from cardiovascular drugs due to altered drug metabolism and distribution, as well as to exaggerated drug effects [4]. For example, in the elderly, drugs such

Geriatric Emergency Medicine, ed. Joseph H. Kahn, Brendan G. Magauran Jr., and Jonathan S. Olshaker. Published by Cambridge University Press.
© Cambridge University Press 2014.

as beta blockers that undergo first-pass metabolism exhibit increased bioavailability [4,9].

Percutaneous coronary intervention (PCI) has a demonstrably clear benefit in the elderly. The majority of the benefits from an invasive strategy in the elderly have accrued from contemporary strategies used in clinical trials published after 1999 and in patients with positive troponins or cardiac biomarkers [4,10]. These trials indicate that compared with younger patients, the elderly gain important absolute benefits from an early invasive strategy but at a cost of increased bleeding. Finding the appropriate balance between benefit and risk of aggressive therapies to maximize net clinical outcome remains a challenge in the elderly [4].

Dysrhythmias

Dysrhythmias occur frequently in elderly patients with or without cardiac disease (e.g., coronary artery disease) or other comorbidities (e.g., hypertension) [11]. This is because aging is associated with decreases in myocardial cell density within the sinus node, loss of atrial myocardial fibers in approaches to the sinus node and internodal myocardium, and deposition of amyloid and interstitial fibrosis in the atria and specialized conduction system [12]. Such abnormalities can lead to sinus node exit block, sinus arrest, or transient or persistent atrioventricular (AV) block [12]. Fibrosis in the atria may result in areas of slow conduction, one of the factors associated with the maintenance of atrial fibrillation (AF) [12]. The high incidence of annular calcification, hypertension, and ischemic heart disease in the elderly also contributes to the development of electrophysiological abnormalities that predispose to the development of conduction system disease or ventricular tachyarrhythmias [12].

Atrial fibrillation is the most common cardiac dysrhythmia managed by emergency physicians [13]. It is a supraventricular tachydysrhythmia characterized electrocardiographically by replacement of consistent P waves by rapid, irregular, fibrillatory waves that vary in size, shape, and timing. It is associated with an irregular, frequently rapid, ventricular response when AV node conduction is intact. AF affects up to 4% of those over 60 years of age and may be an independent risk factor for death. After adjustment for known risk factors, the relative risk of mortality is 1.5 for men and 1.9 for women [14,15].

Identification

Specific diagnosis of dysrhythmias requires a high-quality electrocardiographic printout. However, successful management of dysrhythmias mandates clinical assessment of the whole patient, not just the dysrhythmia. The elderly patient with dysrhythmia may present with palpitations, presyncope, unexplained falls, intermittent confusion, thromboembolic events, syncope, or cardiac arrest [12]. Some elderly patients are asymptomatic and the dysrhythmia may be detected as an incidental finding on physical examination or during electrocardiographic monitoring. If AF is suspected, clinical assessment for hypertension is recommended because about half of

elderly patients with AF have hypertension [16]. Furthermore, in patients older than 75 years of age, independent of other cardiovascular risk factors, hypertension is associated with an increased risk of thromboembolism [17].

Management

In all patients presenting with an acute dysrhythmia, immediate provision of supplementary oxygen or ventilatory support as clinically indicated, establishment of intravenous access, and continuous electrocardiographic monitoring are mandatory. The principles of the definitive management of an acute dysrhythmia in the emergency care setting are prevention of immediate complications and symptom relief. As an illustrative example, these goals are achieved in the emergency management of AF by a three-part approach.

First, to prevent the risk of embolic stroke associated with restoration of sinus rhythm (cardioversion), anticoagulation is required. Although the risk of thromboembolism is low (0.8%) if AF is of less than 48 hours' duration, ED patients should not be assumed to be free of left atrial thrombus because 15% of those with acute AF (i.e., <3 days) have evidence of atrial thrombi [18,19]. As an alternative to anticoagulation prior to cardioversion for AF, current guidelines state that it is reasonable to perform transesophageal echocardiography (TEE) to investigate the presence of thrombus in the left atrium (LA) or left atrial appendage (LAA) [17]. Current guidelines also state that in patients with AF undergoing cardioversion (electrical or pharmacological) to restore normal sinus rhythm, anticoagulation therapy should be administered [17].

Second, ventricular rate should be appropriately controlled. The rate is generally considered controlled when the ventricular response ranges between 60 and 80 beats per minute at rest [20], although it may not be necessary to achieve such tight rate control in the ED setting.

Patients who are symptomatic with rapid ventricular rates during AF require prompt medical management, and cardioversion should be considered if symptomatic hypotension, angina, or heart failure (HF) is present [17]. Amelioration of symptoms by rate control in elderly patients may steer the clinician away from attempts to restore sinus rhythm with its attendant increased risk of thromboembolic events (due to atrial stunning) [21]. In the absence of pre-excitation, intravenous administration of beta blockers (esmolol, metoprolol, or propranolol) or non-dihyropyridine calcium channel antagonists (verapamil, diltiazem) is recommended to slow the ventricular response to AF in the acute setting, exercising caution in patients with hypotension or heart failure [17]. Intravenous digoxin or amiodarone is recommended to control the heart rate in patients with AF and HF who do not have an accessory pathway [17]. A combination of digoxin and either a beta blocker or non-dihydropyridine calcium channel antagonist is reasonable to control the heart rate in patients with AF [17]. The choice of medication should be individualized and the dose modulated to avoid bradycardia. Intravenous amiodarone can be useful to control the heart rate in patients with AF when other measures are unsuccessful or contraindicated [17].

Third, the need for, the proper timing of, and the appropriate method of cardioversion should be assessed. Cardioversion, theoretically, relieves symptoms, prevents thromboembolism, and prevents tachycardia-related cardiomyopathy (deterioration of ventricular function due to a sustained, uncontrolled tachycardia) [17]. It also improves cardiac output and exercise capacity, particularly in patients with heart failure [17]. It has recently been demonstrated that an aggressive ED strategy to treat recent-onset episodes of AF is safe [22].

Although cardioversion may be performed in the ED, it is also acceptable to admit hemodynamically stable patients with new-onset AF for delayed cardioversion.

Acute HF syndromes

Heart failure is a complex clinical syndrome that can result from any structural or functional cardiac disorder that impairs the ability of the ventricle to fill with or eject blood [23]. The annual incidence is about one new case per 1000 population, and is increasing by about 10% every year [24]. The incidence increases with age to more than 10 cases per 1000 population in those 85 years and over. The prevalence of HF differs little worldwide, with population prevalence rates estimated between 11,000 and 19,000 per million population [25]. Premature vascular and valve disease lead to a high prevalence in younger age groups in developing countries. Aging populations and improved post-infarction survival lead to a high number of older patients with HF in more developed countries [25]. Annual mortality for those with HF ranges from 10 to 50% depending on severity [26]. In the US, it is estimated that HF accounts for more than 1 million hospital admissions annually, and it is the leading discharge diagnosis for all patients older than 65 years. Meanwhile, acute HF syndrome (AHFS) is defined as a gradual or rapid change in HF signs and symptoms resulting in the need for urgent therapy [27].

Identification

In general, patients with HF present in one of three ways: with a syndrome of decreased exercise tolerance, with a syndrome of fluid retention, or with no symptoms or symptoms of another cardiac or non-cardiac disorder [28]. The diagnosis of AHFS is primarily based on signs and symptoms derived from a thorough history and physical examination aimed at determining the following: adequacy of systemic perfusion, volume status, the contribution of precipitating factors and/or comorbidities, whether the AHFS is new onset or an exacerbation of chronic disease, and whether it is associated with preserved ejection fraction [28]. Chest radiographs, electrocardiography, and echocardiography are key tests in the identification of AHFS.

Measurement of natriuretic peptides (BNP and NT-proBNP) can be useful in the evaluation of elderly patients in whom the clinical diagnosis of HF is uncertain [29]. In elderly patients with severe dyspnea, a single BNP measurement is useful in the diagnosis of cardiogenic pulmonary edema with an area under the curve (AUC) of 0.87 [29]. Although age may influence BNP and NT-proBNP measurements, post hoc analyses have shown that BNP measurements may retain discriminatory power in

the elderly [30]. However, more research is necessary to better understand the direction and magnitude of these effects to provide further specific guidance in the interpretation of results [27].

Management

The main principles of management of AHFS are symptom relief, reversal of acute hemodynamic abnormalities, and search for underlying precipitants of HF decompensation [31]. For patients with pre-existing chronic HF the following may be responsible for exacerbation of the underlying condition: lack of compliance with diet or drug regimen, acute MI, uncontrolled hypertension, cardiac arrhythmia (e.g., atrial fibrillation), recent addition of negative inotropic drugs (e.g., verapamil, nifedipine, diltiazem, beta blockers), pulmonary embolus, nonsteroidal anti-inflammatory drugs, excessive alcohol or illicit drug use, endocrine abnormalities (e.g., diabetes mellitus, hyperthyroidism, hypothyroidism), or concurrent infection (e.g., pneumonia, viral illnesses) [28].

Intravenous loop diuretics (e.g., furosemide) are the recommended first-line drugs for patients with AHFS with evidence of significant fluid overload [28]. High-dose, continuous IV infusion of furosemide has been shown to be safe and cost-effective in the elderly [32]. If AHFS patients are already receiving loop diuretic therapy, the initial IV dose should equal or exceed their chronic oral daily dose [28]. Acute reduction in high left ventricular filling pressure with IV vasodilators corresponds most closely with symptomatic relief of dyspnea at rest, and is the only significant hemodynamic predictor of subsequent mortality [33]. Thus, using intravenous vasodilators to reverse acute heart failure decompensation is more physiologically rational in that it primarily targets elevated ventricular filling pressures and elevated systemic vascular resistance. In addition, IV vasodilators reduce myocardial oxygen consumption and are not associated with worsening of myocardial ischemia or precipitation of ventricular arrhythmias [34]. However, the role of IV vasodilators for patients with AHFS cannot be generalized [28]. The principles of treating AHFS with vasodilators, in the absence of definitive data, include a more rapid resolution of congestive symptoms; relief of angina symptoms while awaiting coronary intervention; control of hypertension complicating HF; and, in conjunction with ongoing hemodynamic monitoring while IV drugs are administered, improvement of hemodynamic abnormalities prior to instituting oral HF drugs [28]. Current guidelines recommend vasodilators such as intravenous nitroglycerin or nitroprusside in patients with evidence of severely symptomatic fluid overload in the absence of systemic hypotension [28].

Regarding noninvasive ventilatory assistance in AHFS, there is good evidence supporting the use of face mask continuous positive airway pressure (CPAP) or biphasic positive airway pressure (BiPAP) over standard mask oxygen for elderly patients with acute hypoxemic respiratory failure (i.e., $PaO_2/FiO_2 \leq 300$) resulting from cardiogenic pulmonary edema [35]. Compared with standard mask oxygen, patients receiving face mask CPAP at 7.5 mmHg have significantly less need for BiPAP or endotracheal ventilatory assistance, as well as lower 48-hour mortality

[35]. The use of 5–10 mmHg CPAP by nasal or face mask is now recommended as therapy for dyspneic patients with AHFS without hypotension or the need for emergent intubation to improve heart rate, respiratory rate, blood pressure, and reduce the need for intubation, and possibly in-hospital mortality [27].

Syncope

Syncope, defined as transient loss of consciousness, is estimated to account for 1–3% of ED visits [36]. The incidence of syncope is 11 per 1000 person-years for both men and women aged 70–79, and 17 per 1000 person-years for men and 19 per 1000 person-years for women aged 80 years and older [37]. The most common causes of syncope in the elderly are orthostatic hypotension (OH), reflex syncope – especially carotid sinus syndrome (CSS), and cardiac arrhythmias [38]. Different forms may co-exist in a patient making diagnosis difficult [39]. In symptomatic patients, 25% have "age-related" OH; in the remainder, OH is predominantly due to medication and primary or secondary atrial fibrillation [39]. Supine systolic hypertension is often present in older patients with OH and complicates treatment, given that most agents used for the treatment of OH exacerbate supine hypertension and vice versa [39]. Meanwhile, cardioinhibitory CSS is the recognized cause of symptoms in up to 20% of elderly patients with syncope [39]. Carotid sinus hypersensitivity (CSH) of predominantly vasodepressor form is equally prevalent, but its role in syncope is less clear [39].

Identification

A definitive diagnosis may be reached in more than 90% of older patients with syncope based on specific early symptoms [38]. Symptoms such as nausea, blurred vision, and sweating are predictive of non-cardiac syncope, whereas only dyspnea is predictive of cardiac syncope in older persons [38]. Some aspects of the history, which may be difficult to obtain during clinical assessment, are pertinent in older patients [39]. For example, syncope occurring in the morning favors OH [39]. Drug history is also important, and should include the temporal relationship with onset of syncope. A witness account of syncopal episodes is an important aspect of the history, although it is not available in up to 60% of cases [40].

On physical examination, evaluation of cardiac, neurological, and locomotor systems, including observation of gait and balance, is useful [40]. If cognitive impairment is suspected, the Mini-Mental State Examination should be performed [40].

Management

Clinical decision rules may aid decision making regarding the disposition of elderly patients presenting to the ED with syncope [41]. The primary reason for admitting patients with syncope to an inpatient unit, observation unit, or other monitored area should be that the physician's [2] risk assessment indicates that a patient may be at risk for significant dysrrhythmia or sudden death and that observation might detect that event and enable an intervention [36]. Current recommendations are for the admission of patients with syncope and evidence

of HF or structural heart disease or other factors that lead to stratification as high-risk of adverse outcome [36].

The principles of managing patients with syncope are to prolong survival, limit physical injuries, and prevent recurrences [40]. For example, in elderly patients with malignant bradyarrhythmias, cardiac pacemaker therapy is indicated [40]. Although permanent pacing frequently relieves symptoms, it may not affect survival [40]. Elimination of drugs that may exacerbate or unmask underlying susceptibility to bradycardia is an important element in preventing syncope recurrence [40].

Guidelines with risk criteria which require hospitalization have been published by the European Society of Cardiology (Box 20.1). However, the threshold for admitting elderly patients with syncope should be low as the clinician must factor the social circumstances of the patient (e.g., living alone and available home supports) and comorbidities such as cognitive impairment and poor mobility.

Acute thoracic aortic syndromes

Acute thoracic aortic syndromes can be traumatic or atraumatic in origin.

Traumatic rupture of the aorta (TRA) is an autopsy finding in approximately 20% of motor vehicle crash fatalities [42]. It is estimated that only 9–14% of patients with TRA reach a hospital alive and only 2% ultimately survive [42].

Atraumatic acute aortic syndromes consist of three interrelated conditions with similar clinical characteristics and

---

Box 20.1. Short-term risk criteria which require prompt hospitalization or intensive evaluation

Severe structural or coronary artery disease (heart failure, low left ventricular ejection fraction (LVEF)), or previous myocardial infarction: clinical or ECG features suggesting arrhythmic syncope. Adopted from the European Society of Cardiology's Guidelines for the diagnosis and management of syncope [39].

- Syncope during exertion or supine
- Palpitations at the time of syncope
- Family history of sudden cardiac death
- Non-sustained ventricular tachycardia (VT)
- Prolonged or short QT interval
- Inadequate sinus bradycardia <50 beats per minute (bpm) or sinoatrial block in absence of negative chronotropic medications or physical training
- Pre-excited QRS complex
- Negative T-waves in right precordial leads, epsilon waves, and ventricular late potentials suggestive of arrhythmogenic right ventricular cardiomyopathy (ARVC)
- Bifascicular-block: left and right bundle branch block (LBBB and RBBB, respectively) combined with left anterior or left posterior fascicular block or other intraventricular conduction abnormalities with QRS ≥120 ms
- RBBB pattern with ST-elevation in leads V1–3 (Brugada pattern)
- Severe anemia
- Electrolyte disturbance

include aortic dissection (AoD), intramural hematoma (IMH), and penetrating atherosclerotic ulcer (PAU) [43,44]. AoD is defined as disruption of the media layer of the aorta with bleeding within and along its wall resulting in separation of its layers [43]. Among acute aortic syndromes, acute dissection is the most common, but approximately 10–20% of patients with a clinical picture of dissection exhibit an IMH via imaging without identification of blood flow in a false lumen or an intimal lesion [43,45]. PAU is defined as an atherosclerotic lesion with ulceration that penetrates the internal elastic lamina and allows hematoma formation within the media of the aortic wall [43]. PAU sets the stage for development of IMH, AoD, or frank vessel rupture [43]. Anatomically PAUs develop in aortic segments where atherosclerotic changes are most common and are therefore localized to the descending thoracic aorta in over 90% of cases [43,46].

The mean age at presentation of AoD is 63 years, with significant male predominance (65%) [47]. The prevalence of AoD appears to be increasing, independent of aging of the population [48]. In the majority of patients with AoD (90%), an intimal disruption is present that results in tracking of the blood in a dissection plane within the media. This may rupture through the adventitia or back through the intima into the aortic lumen. This classic dissection results in a septum, or "flap," between the two lumina [43]. The false lumen may thrombose over time [43]. Meanwhile, 15% of patients with aortic dissection syndromes have an apparent IMH on noninvasive imaging without evidence of an intimal tear. Occasionally, AoD originates from a small atheromatous ulcer that is difficult to identify [43]. On the other hand, extensive atheromatous disease of the aorta may lead to PAU or a localized IMH [43].

Anatomically, acute thoracic AoD can be classified according to either the origin of the intimal tear or whether the dissection involves the ascending aorta (regardless of the site of origin) [43]. Accurate classification is important as it drives decisions regarding surgical versus nonsurgical management [43]. For purposes of classification, the ascending aorta refers to the aorta proximal to the brachiocephalic artery, and the descending aorta refers to the aorta distal to the left subclavian artery. The two most commonly used classification schemes are the DeBakey and the Stanford systems (Box 20.2).

At this time, there is no unanimity regarding which classification system is the ideal one to use [43].

Identification

In TRA, evidence of polytrauma is common and examination of the patient usually reveals signs similar to those of coarctation of the aorta (arm blood pressure higher than leg blood pressure, delay between radial versus femoral artery pulsation, and a harsh interscapular murmur) [43]. The best method for detection of a TRA is debated [43]. A chest X-ray with a nasogastric tube in position has 80% sensitivity for suggesting TRA by showing displacement of the nasogastric tube by the hematoma [43]. However, signs of hemomediastinum are more often false positive than true positive [43,49]. Even when present, mediastinal blood is less likely to be due to arterial/aortic injury than to less consequential venous bleeding [43]. A biplane contrast

Box 20.2. Classification schemes for acute thoracic aortic dissection

DeBakey Classification

- Type I: Dissection originates in the ascending aorta and propagates distally to include at least the aortic arch and typically the descending aorta (surgery usually recommended)
- Type II: Dissection originates in and is confined to the ascending aorta (surgery usually recommended)
- Type III: Dissection originates in the descending aorta and propagates most often distally (nonsurgical treatment usually recommended)
- Type IIIa: Limited to the descending thoracic aorta
- Type IIIb: Extending below the diaphragm

Stanford Classification

- Type A: All dissections involving the ascending aorta regardless of the site of origin (surgery usually recommended)
- Type B: All dissections that do not involve the ascending aorta (nonsurgical treatment usually recommended). Note: Involvement of the aortic arch without involvement of the ascending aorta in the Stanford Classification is labeled as Type B.

aortogram may fail to detect the tear until the development of a pseudoaneurysm. Transesophageal echocardiography may be used, but if dilatation has not occurred the diagnosis may still be in doubt [43]. CT is used but is not absolutely certain to establish the diagnosis. In questionable cases, intravascular ultrasound can also be used [49–53]. Realistically, the imaging sequence often depends on the stability of the patient and the need for the diagnosis of concomitant injuries [43]. Sometimes, this may even fail to detect the tear, and the study may have to be repeated at a later date to detect the tear [43].

In atraumatic acute aortic syndromes, time from onset of initial symptoms to time of presentation in acute AoD is defined as occurring within 2 weeks of onset of pain; in subacute, between 2 and 6 weeks from onset of pain; and in chronic, more than 6 weeks from onset of pain [43]. Patients with acute aortic syndromes often present in a similar fashion, regardless of whether the underlying condition is AoD, IMH, PAU, or contained aortic rupture. Pain is the most commonly reported presenting symptom of acute AoD regardless of patient age, gender, or other associated clinical complaint [43].

A high index of suspicion is required to identify acute AoD in elderly patients [43]. One study with 550 patients with type A dissection found that among patients older than 70 years of age (32% of total), typical symptoms (abrupt onset of pain) and signs (murmur of aortic regurgitation or pulse deficits) were significantly less common [51]. Meanwhile, the typical patient with PAU is elderly (usually over 65 years of age) and has hypertension and diffuse atherosclerosis, having presented with chest or back pain but without signs of aortic regurgitation or malperfusion. Less commonly, patients presented only with signs of distal embolization [43].

Any clinical suspicion of dissection mandates an indication for CT imaging. These include the typical symptoms (abrupt onset of pain), but the clinician must have a low threshold for ordering an appropriate scan as atypical presentations are not unusual in the elderly. In atraumatic acute aortic syndromes, routine chest X-ray may occasionally detect abnormalities of aortic contour or size that require definitive aortic imaging. Chest X-ray often serves as a part of the evaluation of a patient with potential acute AoD, primarily to identify other causes of the patient's symptoms, but also as a screening test to identify findings due to a dilated aorta or bleeding [43]. However, chest X-ray is inadequately sensitive to definitively exclude the presence of AoD in all except the lowest-risk patients and therefore rarely excludes the disease. Imaging of the thoracic aorta with CT imaging, MRI, or in some cases, echocardiographic examination is the only method to detect thoracic aortic diseases and determine risk for future complications [43]. Selection of the most appropriate imaging study may depend on patient-related factors (i.e., hemodynamic stability, renal function, contrast allergy) and institutional capabilities (i.e., rapid availability of individual imaging modalities, state of the technology, and imaging specialist expertise) [43].

Management

The 2010 joint guidelines of the American Association for Thoracic Surgery and American Heart Association give a detailed current evidence base for management of acute thoracic aorta syndromes [43]. Emergency surgery is the preferred treatment for Stanford type A, as such patients are at risk for life-threatening complications including cardiac tamponade from hemopericardium, aortic rupture, stroke, visceral ischemia, and HF due to severe aortic regurgitation.

Generally medical therapy is the preferred approach to acute type B dissection, and surgery or endovascular therapy is reserved for patients with acute complications [43].

Summary

The most important determinant of cardiovascular health is a person's age. Therefore, as health care systems around the world face the challenge of aging populations, identification and treatment of cardiovascular emergencies will become a significant health care issue. Elderly patients have a high relative frequency of patients presenting with unstable angina/non-ST segment elevation myocardial infarction. Meanwhile, dysrhythmias are also common in the elderly due to the development of conduction system disease and electrophysiological abnormalities as part of the aging process. The elderly patient with dysrhythmia may present with palpitations, presyncope, unexplained falls, intermittent confusion, thromboembolic events, syncope, or cardiac arrest. Heart failure is also increasing in prevalence due to the aging populations in many health care systems. Measurement of natriuretic peptides (BNP and NT-proBNP) can be useful in the evaluation of elderly patients in whom the clinical diagnosis of heart failure is uncertain. Clinical decision rules may aid decision making regarding the disposition of elderly patients

presenting to the ED with syncope. The principles of managing the older patient with syncope are to prolong life, limit physical injuries, and prevent recurrences. Among atraumatic acute aortic syndromes, acute aortic dissection is the most common. A high index of suspicion is required to identify acute aortic dissection in elderly patients. However, approximately 10–20% of patients with a clinical picture of acute aortic dissection exhibit an intramural hematoma.

Pearls and pitfalls
Pearls

- Whenever possible in the drug treatment of unstable angina/non-ST elevation myocardial infarction in the elderly, begin with lower drug doses than in younger patients and carefully observe for features of drug toxicity.
- If atrial fibrillation (AF) is suspected, clinical assessment for hypertension is recommended because half of elderly patients with AF have hypertension.
- Compared with standard mask oxygen, patients receiving face mask continuous positive airway pressure at 7.5 mmHg have significantly less need for biphasic positive airway pressure or endotracheal ventilatory assistance, as well as lower 48-hour mortality.
- Clinical suspicion of aortic dissection is an indication for computed tomographic imaging.

Pitfalls

- Elderly patients with ACS may present with atypical symptoms, such as generalized weakness, stroke, syncope, or a change in mental status.
- Supine systolic hypertension is often present in older patients with orthostatic hypotension.
- In patients older than 70 years with Stanford type A aortic dissection, typical symptoms (abrupt onset of pain) and signs (murmur of aortic regurgitation or pulse deficits) are significantly less common.

References

1. Giannakouris K. *Population and Social Conditions. Eurostat Statistics in Focus 72/2008* (accessed July 27, 2012 from http://epp.eurostat.ec.europa.eu/cache/ITY_OFFPUB/KS-SF-08-072/EN/KS-SF-08-072-EN.PDF).

2. Gupta R, Kaufman S. Cardiovascular emergencies in the elderly. *Emerg Med Clin N Am.* 2006;24:339–70.

3. North BJ, Sinclair DA. The intersection between aging and cardiovascular disease. *Circ Res.* 2012;110:1097–108.

4. Anderson JL, Adams CD, Antman EM, et al. 2011 ACCF/AHA focused update incorporated into the ACC/AHA 2007 guidelines for the management of patients with unstable angina/non-ST-elevation myocardial infarction: a report of the American College of Cardiology Foundation/American Heart Association Task Force on Practice Guideline. *Circulation.* 2011;123:e426–579.

5. Alexander KP, Roe MT, Chen AY, et al. Evolution in cardiovascular care for elderly patients with non-ST-segment elevation acute coronary syndromes: results from CRUSADE National Quality Improvement Initiative. *J Am Coll Cardiol.* 2005;46:1479–87.

6. Canto JG, Shlipak MG, Rogers WJ, et al. Prevalence, clinical characteristics, and mortality among patients with myocardial infarction presenting without chest pain. *JAMA.* 2000;283(24):3223–9.

7. Brieger D, Eagle KA, Goodman SG, et al. Acute coronary syndromes without chest pain, an underdiagnosed and undertreated high-risk group: insights from the Global Registry of Acute Coronary Events. *Chest.* 2004;126:461–9.

8. Avezum A, Makdisse M, Spencer F, et al. Impact of age on management and outcome of acute coronary syndrome: observations from the Global Registry of Acute Coronary Events (GRACE). *Am Heart J.* 2005;149:67–73.

9. Stein B, Kupersmith J. Principles and practice of pharmacotherapy. In *The Pharmacologic Management of Heart Disease,* ed. Kupersmith J, Deedwania PC (Baltimore, MD: Williams and Wilkins, 1997), pp. 3–38.

10. Mehta SR, Cannon CP, Fox KA, et al. Routine vs selective invasive strategies in patients with acute coronary syndromes: a collaborative meta-analysis of randomized trials. *JAMA.* 2005;293:2908–17.

11. Manolio TA, Furberg CD, Rautaharju PM, et al. Cardiac arrhythmias on 24-hr ambulatory electrocardiography in older women and men: The Cardiovascular Health Study. *J Am Coll Cardiol.* 1994;23:916–25.

12. Gillis AM. Sinus node disease. In *Clinical Cardiac Pacing,* 2nd edn, Ellenbogen KA, Kay GN, Wilkoff BL (Philadelphia, PA: WB Saunders & Co, 2000), pp. 405–25.

13. Wakai A, O'Neill J. Emergency management of atrial fibrillation. *Postgrad Med J.* 2003;79:313–19.

14. Benjamin EJ, Levy D, Vaziri SM. Independent risk factors for atrial fibrillation in a population-based cohort: the Framingham Heart Study. *JAMA.* 1994;271:840–4.

15. Benjamin EJ, Wolf PA, D'Agostino RB, *et al.* Impact of atrial fibrillation on the risk of death: the Framingham Heart Study. *Circulation* 1998;98:946–52.

16. Fuster V, Rydén LE, Asinger RW, et al. ACC/AHA/ESC Guidelines for the Management of Patients With Atrial Fibrillation: Executive Summary A Report of the American College of Cardiology/American Heart Association Task Force on Practice Guidelines and the European Society of Cardiology Committee for Practice Guidelines and Policy Conferences (Committee to Develop Guidelines for the Management of Patients With Atrial Fibrillation) Developed in Collaboration With the North American Society of Pacing and Electrophysiology. *Circulation.* 2001;104:2118–50.

17. Hart RG, Pearce LA, Rothbart RM, et al. Stroke with intermittent atrial fibrillation: incidence and predictors during aspirin therapy. Stroke Prevention in Atrial Fibrillation Investigators. *J Am Coll Cardiol.* 2000;35:183–7.

18. Weigner MJ, Caulfield TA. Risk of clinical thromboembolism associated with conversion to sinus rhythm in patients with atrial fibrillation lasting less than 48 hours. *Ann Intern Med.* 1997;126:615–20.

19. Stoddard MF, Dawkins PR, Prince CR, *et al.* Left atrial appendage thrombus is not uncommon in patients with acute atrial fibrillation and a recent embolic event: a transesophageal echocardiographic study. *J Am Coll Cardiol.* 1995;25:452–9.

20. Rawles JM. What is meant by a "controlled" ventricular rate in atrial fibrillation? *Br Heart J.* 1990;63:157–61.

21. Khan IA. Atrial stunning: determinants and cellular mechanisms. *Am Heart J.* 2003;145:787–94.

22. Stiell IG, Clement CM, Perry JJ, et al. Association of the Ottawa Aggressive Protocol with rapid discharge of emergency department patients with recent-onset atrial fibrillation or flutter. *CJEM.* 2010;12(3):181–91.

23. Hunt SA, Baker DW, Chin MH, et al. ACC/AHA guidelines for the evaluation and management of chronic heart failure in the adult. *J Am Coll Cardiol.* 2001;38:2101–13.

24. Department of Health. *Heart failure.* In *National Service Framework for Coronary Heart Disease* (accessed September 17, 2012 from www.doh.gov.uk/nsf/coronary.htm).

25. Cleland JGF, Khand A, Clark A. The heart failure epidemic: exactly how big is it? *Eur Heart J.* 2001;22:623–6.

26. The CONSENSUS Trial Study Group. Effects of enalapril on mortality in severe congestive heart failure. Results of the Cooperative North Scandinavian Enalapril Survival Study (CONSENSUS). *N Engl J Med.* 1987;316:1429–35.

27. Silvers SM, Howell JM, Kosowsky JM, et al. Clinical policy: Critical issues in the evaluation and management of adult patients presenting to the emergency department with acute heart failure syndromes. *Ann Emerg Med.* 2007;49:627–69.

28. Jessup M, Abraham WT, Casey DE, et al. ACCF/AHA guidelines for the diagnosis and management of heart failure in adults: a report of the American College of Cardiology/American Heart Association Task Force on Practice Guidelines. *J Am Coll Cardiol.* 2009;53:1343–82.

29. Ray P, Arthaud M, Birolleau S, et al. Comparison of brain natriuretic peptide and probrain natriuretic peptide in the diagnosis of cardiogenic pulmonary edema in patients aged 65 and older. *J Am Geriatr Soc.* 2005;53:643–8.

30. Maisel AS, Clopton P, Krishnaswamy P, et al. Impact of age, race, and sex on the ability of B-type natriuretic peptide to aid in the emergency diagnosis of heart failure: results from the breathing not properly (BNP) multinational study. *Am Heart J.* 2004;147:1078–84.

31. Niemen MS and the Task Force on Acute Heart Failure of the European Society of Cardiology. Executive summary of the guidelines on the diagnosis and treatment of acute heart failure: the Task Force on Acute Heart Failure of the European Society of Cardiology. *Eur Heart J.* 2005;26(4):384–416.

32. Howard PA, Dunn MI. Aggressive dieresis for severe heart failure in the elderly. *Chest.* 2001;119:807–10.

33. Lucas C, Johnson W, Hamilton MA, et al. Freedom from congestion predicts good survival despite previous class IV symptoms of heart failure. *Am Heart J.* 2000;140:840–7.

34. Nohria A, Lewis E, Stevenson LW. Medical management of advanced heart failure. *JAMA.* 2002;287:628–40.

35. L'Her E, Duquesne F, Girou E, et al. Noninvasive continuous positive airway pressure in elderly cardiogenic pulmonary edema patients. *Intensive Care Med.* 2004;30:882–8.

36. Huff JS, Decker WW, Quinn JV, et al. Clinical policy: critical issues in the evaluation and management of adult patients presenting to the emergency department with syncope. *Ann Emerg Med.* 2007;49(4):431–44.

37. Soteriades ES, Evans JC, Larson MG, et al. Incidence and prognosis of syncope. *N Engl J Med.* 2002;347:878–85.

38. Galizia A, Abete P, Mussi C, et al. Role of the early symptoms in assessment of syncope in elderly people. Results from the Italian Group for the Study of Syncope in the elderly (GIS STUDY). *J Am Geriatr Soc.* 2009;57:18–23.

39. The Task Force for the Diagnosis and Management of Syncope of the European Society of Cardiology (ESC) developed in collaboration with the European Heart Rhythm Association (EHRA), Heart Failure Association (HFA), and Heart Rhythm Society (HRS). Guidelines for the diagnosis and management of syncope (version 2009). *Eur Heart J.* 2009;30:2631–71.

40. Van der Velde N, van den Meiracker AH, Pols HA, Stricker BH, van der Cammen TJ. Withdrawal of fall-risk-increasing drugs in older persons: effect on tilt-table test outcomes. *J Am Geriatr Soc.* 2007;55:734–9.

41. Reed MJ, Newby DE, Coull AJ, et al. The ROSE (risk stratification of syncope in the emergency department) study. *J Am Coll Cardiol.* 2010;55(8):713–21.

42. Richens D, Kotidis K, Neale M, et al. Rupture of the aorta following road traffic accidents in the United Kingdom 1992–1999. The results of the co-operative crash injury study. *Eur J Cardiothorac Surg.* 2003;23:143–8.

43. Hiratzka LF et al. 2010 ACCF/AHA/AATS/ACR/ASA/SCA/SCAI/SIR/STS/SVM Guidelines for the diagnosis and management of patients with thoracic aortic disease: a report of the American College of Cardiology Foundation/American Heart Association Task Force on Practice Guidelines, American Association for Thoracic Surgery, American College of Radiology, American Stroke Association, Society of Cardiovascular Anesthesiologists, Society for Cardiovascular Angiography and Interventions, Society of Interventional Radiology, Society of Thoracic Surgeons, and Society for Vascular Medicine. *Circulation.* 2010;121:e266–369.

44. Vilacosta I, Roman JA. Acute aortic syndrome. *Heart.* 2001;85:365–8.

45. Evangelista A, Mukherjee D, Mehta RH, et al. Acute intramural hematoma of the aorta: a mystery in evolution. *Circulation.* 2005;111:1063–70.

46. Cho KR, Stanson AW, Potter DD, et al. Penetrating atherosclerotic ulcer of the descending thoracic aorta and arch. *J Thorac Cardiovasc Surg.* 2004;127:1393–9.

47. Hagan PG, Nienaber CA, Isselbacher EM, et al. The International Registry of Acute Aortic Dissection (IRAD): new insights into an old disease. *JAMA.* 2000;283:897–903.

48. Olsson C, Thelin S, Stahle E, et al. Thoracic aortic aneurysm and dissection: increasing prevalence and improved outcomes reported in a nationwide population-based study of more than 14,000 cases from 1987 to 2002. *Circulation.* 2006;114:2611–18.

49. Mirvis SE, Bidwell JK, Buddemeyer EU, et al. Value of chest radiography in excluding traumatic aortic rupture. *Radiology.* 1987;163:487–93.

50. Antman EM, Anbe DT, Armstrong PW, et al. ACC/AHA guidelines for the management of patients with ST-elevation myocardial infarction: executive summary. *J Am Coll Cardiol.* 2004;44:671–719.

51. Svensson LG, Crawford ES. *Cardiovascular and Vascular Disease of the Aorta* (Philadelphia, PA: WB Saunders Co, 1997).

52. Bruckner BA, DiBardino DJ, Cumbie TC, et al. Critical evaluation of chest computed tomography scans for blunt descending thoracic aortic injury. *Ann Thorac Surg.* 2006;81:1339–46.

53. Fabian TC, Davis KA, Gavant ML, et al. Prospective study of blunt aortic injury: helical CT is diagnostic and antihypertensive therapy reduces rupture. *Ann Surg.* 1998;227:666–76.

54. Mehta RH, O'Gara PT, Bossone E, et al. Acute type A aortic dissection in the elderly: clinical characteristics, management, and outcomes in the current era. *J Am Coll Cardiol.* 2002;40:685–92.

Chapter

21

Gastrointestinal emergencies in the elderly

Maura Dickinson and Megan M. Leo

Background

The evaluation of the elderly patient who presents with an abdominal complaint can be very challenging for emergency physicians due to the subtle presentations of potentially serious gastrointestinal (GI) emergencies. Abdominal pain is a common chief complaint in the elderly who present to the emergency department (ED). The majority of elderly patients, defined as those aged 65 and older, who present with abdominal pain have a serious etiology for their symptoms including infection, mechanical obstruction, gallbladder disease, or urinary tract infection. There are a number of variables that lead to challenges in assessing geriatric patients, including the lack of reliability of the physical exam to identify dangerous pathology [1]. The chief complaint of abdominal pain has been shown to consume more time and resources than other acute presentations, because the emergency physician feels the need to do more of a diagnostic work-up to rule out dangerous and deadly etiologies [2].

This chapter will review several important GI emergencies that are present in the geriatric patient population and will discuss diagnostic work-up, the proper use of imaging, and treatment.

History

Adequate history taking can be a challenge in the elderly, making the usual clinical approach to diagnostic work-up based on history and physical exam sometimes unreliable. Many elderly patients have dementia-related memory loss and baseline confusion. Elderly patients are more vulnerable to delirium caused by their presenting illness, making history taking difficult. Also, hearing loss may be a barrier to an accurate interview. For this reason, obtaining a secondary history from family, a close relative, or caretaker is helpful in this patient population. Important questions to ask the patient and the caretaker include the time of onset of the symptoms, gradual versus sudden onset, and other associated symptoms. Presentations of very serious pathology can sometimes be as subtle as mild nausea or fatigue. It may also be helpful to ask whether these symptoms happened before and what was done for them on prior episodes. Noting whether there was blood in the vomitus or stool is important for deciding on the diagnosis and the disposition for the geriatric patient.

A careful history from either the patient or caretaker is critical in the elderly patient. However, using the patient history in the same manner that you would in a younger patient to guide clinical decisions should be approached with caution, especially when evaluating for a potential GI emergency. These factors may require the emergency physician to begin the evaluation with a very broad work-up in the elderly, including laboratory work, cardiograms, and radiology imaging.

Physical examination

The physical exam in the elderly can be challenging due to altered pain perception and changes in physiology. As in any patient encounter, vital signs are a very important part of the evaluation of an elderly patient although caution should be taken in their interpretation. Elderly patients do not always respond to stress as may a younger patient. This may lead to false assurance in the face of an afebrile patient with vital signs that fall within the normal limits of standards. For example, a normotensive blood pressure in a patient who is hypertensive at baseline may be a sign of early sepsis. If possible, it may be helpful to review a blood pressure recorded from a prior visit for a baseline comparison. Tachypnea is a very important abnormal vital sign to note. Rapid breathing may be a response to pain or underlying metabolic acidosis in the setting of severe illness. Many elderly patients also have underlying lung disease, including chronic obstructive pulmonary disease (COPD) or emphysema. Recognizing tachypnea and signs of respiratory failure is important in this patient population because these patients often do not have the reserve to maintain a rapid rate of breathing and may require early intubation.

The physical exam of the elderly patient should always include the general appearance. It may also be helpful to ask a family member and/or caretaker what their impression is of the patient's general appearance, mental status, or energy level compared to baseline. Systemic infection may present as lethargy and general weakness or as an agitated, confused patient. Despite the chief complaint, a complete physical exam should be performed, including a careful abdominal exam to note any rigidity, change in bowel sounds, rebound, or guarding that may

Geriatric Emergency Medicine, ed. Joseph H. Kahn, Brendan G. Magauran Jr., and Jonathan S. Olshaker. Published by Cambridge University Press.
© Cambridge University Press 2014.

suggest peritonitis. Epigastric pain in the setting of hematemesis should prompt immediate resuscitation and involvement of a gastroenterology specialist to stop the source of the upper GI bleed. A rectal exam is also helpful to assess for GI bleeding, pain, or masses. Repeat physical examinations help the clinician solidify the diagnosis, assist in appropriate disposition, and allow the clinician to monitor progression of the presenting disease. It is prudent to document a repeat abdominal exam in the patient record on every elderly patient who is being discharged from the ED with an abdominal complaint.

Special considerations

In addition to the challenges of an unreliable history and physical exam in the elderly patient, identifying the seriousness and the etiology of abdominal pain can be difficult due to physiologic changes in the elderly. Loss of function of somatic and autonomic nerves can result in changes in pain perception, in addition to misleading vital signs and physical exam findings. There is no single mechanism for altered visceral pain perception in the elderly, but proposed contributors include impaired A Delta fiber function, altered serotonin metabolism, and increased responsiveness of older individuals to non-opioid analgesic pathways at the spinal cord level [3]. In addition to altered pain perception, cognitive impairment and dementia can make history taking challenging and inaccurate. Also, a delay in the patient or caretaker noting signs of a GI emergency leads to a presentation to the ED in the later stages of the disease.

The immune system in the elderly is not as responsive or as effective in responding to pyrogens, leading to a higher susceptibility to infection and decreased reliability of interpretation of white blood cell counts (WBCs). In particular, while evaluating for a surgical abdomen, a third of elderly patients did not display a fever or leukocytosis [4]. Another important consideration is the fact that many patients over the age of 65 have multiple comorbidities and a complicated medication list. Diabetes, hyperlipidemia, and hypertension can lead to more advanced arterial atherosclerosis, which puts these patients at risk for mesenteric ischemia, poor wound healing, poor response to infection, and at a higher risk for metabolic derangement. Diabetes decreases peripheral nerve sensation, making an abdominal exam potentially unreliable. The incidence of bowel pathology such as diverticulitis, colitis, biliary disease, vascular catastrophes, and cancers is also increased in this population, making the ED work-up to rule out these etiologies important.

Medications can contribute to GI pathology in the elderly and mask their presentation. Nonsteroidal anti-inflammatory drugs (NSAIDs) are widely used among the elderly for various forms of osteoarthritic and other chronic pains. This category of medication can lead to peptic ulcer disease, gastric ulcers, and gastritis. Griffin reported that 40% of older adults were prescribed NSAIDs, and their use is an independent risk factor for developing gastroduodenal injury [5]. NSAIDs may also mask an insidious onset of abdominal pain due to dangerous diseases or blunt a fever response. Steroids are often given for COPD and various rheumatologic diseases in the elderly

and may also lead to erosion of gastric mucosa and result in ulcer formation. Steroids can also mask a fever response and cause deranged or elevated leukocyte counts, making laboratory interpretation difficult. Anticholinergics and opiates may lead to gastric dysmotility and physiologic obstruction. Recent antibiotic use may lead to disruption of normal GI flora and risk for *Clostridium difficile* infection, colitis, and toxic megacolon. It is important to review with the patient and family or caretaker the patient's complete medical history, including surgical history, and obtain a complete and accurate medication list while forming a differential diagnosis for an elderly patient with a potential GI emergency.

Diagnostic tests

The evaluation of an elderly patient in the ED for a possible GI emergency may require a complete work-up with laboratory and imaging studies.

Laboratory studies

Laboratory studies are often unreliable in this patient population when used in the evaluation of a potential GI emergency. A work-up may include a complete blood count with differential, complete metabolic panel with liver function tests, and lipase. An amylase is nonspecific for pancreatitis and may be present in simple cases of vomiting. It may be prudent to evaluate for an anginal equivalent with an electrocardiogram (ECG) and perhaps cardiac enzymes in an elderly patient presenting with abdominal pain. Urinalysis with a culture should also be ordered because urinary tract infections are common in the elderly and often present with GI complaints. Plasma biomarkers of inflammation and infection are unreliable and often difficult to interpret. If a fever is present, blood cultures should be sent prior to administering antibiotics. If the patient reports a history of diarrhea for greater than two weeks, recent antibiotic use, hematochezia, or fevers in the presence of diarrhea, a stool sample may be sent for culture, *C. difficile* antigen testing, and ova and parasite analysis. Leukocytosis is commonly absent in the presence of surgical disease in the elderly due to a blunted response to infection or inflammation. Although laboratory tests can be misleading in the elderly, they may be used in conjunction with a prudent physical examination and imaging.

Imaging studies

In an elderly patient with abdominal pain, imaging studies can help distinguish a GI emergency from a benign etiology. This can be very important for treatment decisions and for appropriate disposition for the patient. Imaging studies may include plain radiographs, ultrasound, computed tomography (CT), angiography, and in some cases magnetic resonance imaging (MRI).

Plain radiography may be used as a rapid screening tool for serious etiologies such as peritoneal free air due to perforated viscus, signs of bowel obstruction, and foreign body ingestion or insertion. A minority of patients will show signs of mesenteric ischemia on plain radiography as thumbprinting or thickening of the bowel loops. In general plain radiographs are not a very specific or sensitive test but may aid the evaluating physician in narrowing the differential diagnosis and expedite alerting surgical consultants while the patient waits for more definitive testing.

Ultrasound may be performed at the bedside by the emergency physician, or a complete ultrasound study may be ordered through the radiology department. More emergency physicians are using point-of-care ultrasound to guide their clinical care within the ED. The use of bedside ultrasound has been shown to be safe in the diagnosis of gallbladder disease, and emergency physicians have recorded 94% sensitivity for detecting gallstones [6] (Figure 21.1). Ultrasound is the imaging modality of choice for biliary pathology. Mesenteric and celiac duplex ultrasound can be used for evaluation of chronic mesenteric ischemia, but it is not accurate in evaluating an acute occlusion [7]. Certain vascular catastrophes such as portal vein thrombosis and Budd–Chiari syndrome may be evaluated with Doppler ultrasound.

Computed tomography is the imaging modality of choice for the evaluation of GI emergencies when primary biliary disease is not suspected. The threshold to order a CT to evaluate an elderly patient with an abdominal complaint should be low because history, physical exam findings, and laboratory findings are less reliable in ruling out dangerous pathology in this patient population. With newer machines providing higher image quality, reformatting for angiography, and shorter acquisition times, use of CT scanning allows for definitive diagnosis for many of the GI emergencies that afflict the elderly population. Esses et al. demonstrated how the use of CT scan altered decision making in the care of the elderly patient, including an altered diagnosis in 45% of patients and surgical management in 12% [8]. Most CT scans require intravenous (IV) contrast to adequately evaluate for infectious or ischemic etiologies of abdominal pain. The use of oral contrast as part of the protocol for obtaining an abdominal CT scan leads to delay in obtaining the study because of the long transit time for contrast to move through the bowel. Use of oral contrast has largely fallen off CT abdomen protocols because it rarely increases diagnostic accuracy. CT scans without contrast are reserved for evaluation for renal colic or in cases where the patient cannot receive IV

contrast due to allergy or impaired renal function but emergent imaging is required. However, CT scans are not always available in smaller facilities or in under-resourced areas. Their use is also limited by other contraindications such as their use in patients with poor renal function and with contrast allergy. Patients with healthy renal function usually require careful hydration after a CT scan with IV contrast. Those taking metformin are required to hold their dosing for 24–48 hours after receiving IV contrast, which can be problematic in maintaining adequate glucose control.

Angiography is considered the gold standard for evaluation of mesenteric arterial ischemia. The study requires catheterization of the arterial system and serves as both a diagnostic and potentially therapeutic procedure. Limitations to the study include consideration that it is invasive, it may lead to nephrotoxicity due to IV contrast administration, and it is not always available due to limited resources. CT angiography has been found to have a sensitivity as high as 93% and a specificity as high as 100%. It is often chosen over conventional angiography because it is less invasive and has wider availability [9]. However, in patients for whom the diagnosis of mesenteric ischemia is high on the differential diagnosis, it is reasonable to discuss performing angiography with the interventional radiologist prior to CT scan to prevent two loads of IV contrast. An expedited angiogram may decrease the extent of renal damage and decrease the amount of bowel that is subject to ischemia if the vessel is rapidly reopened.

Magnetic resonance imaging has typically played a limited role in the ED for the evaluation of elderly patients with a potential GI emergency. MRI may be utilized to assess chronic mesenteric ischemia but this is typically performed on a non-emergent basis. Although MR cholangiopancreatography (MRCP) may be utilized to evaluate cholecystitis and choledocholithiasis, typically these tests are ordered after admission to the hospital. However, as access to MRI becomes greater within the ED, there has been advocacy for utilization of MRCP for the evaluation of acute cholecystitis to help facilitate appropriate triage for management. An MRCP may help with the decision for obtaining preoperative biliary drainage, need for endoscopic retrograde cholangiopancreatography, or intraoperative endoscopic rendezvous in the presence of stones [10].

Differential diagnosis

Appendicitis

Acute appendicitis is a common disease that can affect patients of all ages, with a lifetime occurrence of 7%. Although the condition mostly affects young adults, the incidence in the elderly population is rising secondary to prolonged lifespan. The mortality of appendicitis is higher in the older adult population (3%) compared with a younger population (0.2%), and even higher in patients more than 70 years old (32%) [11].

Elderly patients may experience the classic symptoms of appendicitis including fever, nausea, vomiting, migrating pain, right lower quadrant tenderness, rebound pain, and anorexia, but they may also display less impressive symptoms making the diagnosis challenging. The combination of late presentation,

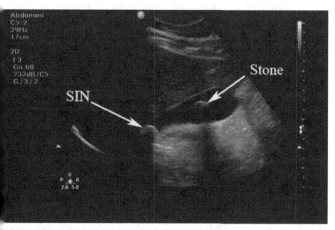

Figure 21.1. Bedside ultrasound demonstrating a stone in the neck (SIN) of the gallbladder and a second stone in the body of the gallbladder.

atypical symptoms, communication difficulty, and delayed diagnosis leads to a disproportionately high perforation rate (up to 35%) [11].

The work-up for appendicitis is similar to the work-up that would be performed for younger patients. Laboratory data, including leukocytosis, presence of a left-shift, and an elevated C-reactive protein (CRP) should be used to supplement the history and physical. However, these tests have been found to be poor predictors of acute appendicitis in the elderly, with sensitivities of 81.4%, 88.3%, and 90%, respectively. If all three values are abnormal, the sensitivity improves (97.4%) but there is a low specificity (12.5%) [12]. Imaging plays a major role in the diagnosis of appendicitis in the elderly patient population. The use of CT with IV contrast is the imaging modality of choice. In regard to the use of oral contrast for visualization of the bowel, CT without oral contrast compared to CT with oral contrast was shown to have equal sensitivity and negative predictive value. A CT without oral contrast was found to be superior in specificity, accuracy, and positive predictive value in one comparative study [13].

Treatment in the acute setting focuses on resuscitation with IV fluids, symptomatic relief, and empiric antibiotics to cover both Gram-negative organisms and anaerobes. Recurrence is common when only medical management is utilized. Therefore, patients may benefit from definitive treatment with the early involvement of a surgeon. While both the laparoscopic and open approaches to an appendectomy have been shown to be safe and effective definitive treatment options in the elderly, multiple studies suggest elderly patients on average have a shorter length of stay with laparoscopic appendectomy [14].

Pancreatitis

In the elderly population, acute pancreatitis is frequently a result of biliary disease and idiopathic etiologies, with alcohol-induced pancreatitis only occurring in a minority of cases. Scoring systems including Ranson's criteria and APACHE II criteria help predict the likelihood for severe disease and complications. In both of these criteria, older age is an independent risk factor for progression to severe disease [15]. Although often used to aid in clinical decision making and disposition of the patient, Ranson's criteria have never been prospectively validated.

Similar to a young population, elderly patients characteristically present with classic symptoms of constant upper abdominal pain, boring in nature, that radiates in a band-like pattern to the back and is associated with nausea and vomiting. The intensity of pain may vary from mild discomfort to severe pain, with peritoneal signs later in the disease. However, some elderly patients present with vague symptoms of nausea and vomiting without pain. Patients may also present in a hypermetabolic state resembling systemic inflammatory response syndrome, with altered mental status or even hypotension. In some elderly patients, however, the diagnosis of acute pancreatitis can be challenging and vague symptoms can cause a delayed diagnosis. Imaging with a CT scan is indicated in patients with moderate to severe pancreatitis to screen for potentially surgical complications such as a pancreatic pseudocyst or necrotizing

pancreatitis. Use of a CT scan is also indicated if there is concern for an alternative diagnosis.

The treatment of acute pancreatitis depends on the severity of the acute disease. Patients with mild pancreatitis experience a prompt uncomplicated course and treatment focuses on symptomatic care for dehydration, vomiting, and pain. In more severe cases, patients suffer from organ failure (pulmonary, renal, or cardiac) and/or local complications such as necrosis, pseudocyst, or abscess. Patients may require more acute critical interventions on initial presentation, including supplemental oxygen or intubation for altered mental status and acute respiratory distress syndrome. In these more severe cases, intensive care unit (ICU) level care is necessary for cardiopulmonary monitoring, aggressive resuscitation, and electrolyte repletion, as well as early surgical consultation [15]. Endoscopic retrograde cholangiopancreatography (ERCP) is recommended therapy for severe gallstone pancreatitis, as it is safe with a high degree of success and low complication rates for elderly patients [16].

Diverticulitis

Diverticular disease commonly affects the adult population in developed countries, with an incidence of 50% in those older than 70 years of age. The exact cause of diverticular disease is unknown, but possible mechanisms include colon wall muscle irregularities, abnormal colon motility, and increased intraluminal pressure. Physical inactivity and a low-fiber diet are two factors thought to contribute to the high prevalence in developed nations [17].

Diverticular disease classically presents as two clinical pictures, specifically diverticulosis (diverticula are not inflamed) or diverticulitis (diverticula are inflamed). In cases of diverticulosis, patients may experience a spectrum of lower GI bleeding, with mild bleeding seen in the majority of cases. Diverticulitis typically manifests with left lower quadrant tenderness, fever, nausea, and change in bowel regimen (constipation, diarrhea, or tenesmus). Some elderly patients with diverticulitis present solely with urinary symptoms as a result of the inflamed colon irritating the bladder. This leads to hematuria and pyuria. Such atypical symptoms can make the diagnosis challenging and lead to misdiagnosis.

A normal WBC does not exclude the diagnosis of diverticulitis. As with most abdominal pathologies in the elderly, physicians should maintain a low threshold to image. A contrast-enhanced CT is the imaging modality of choice when evaluating diverticulitis, and it has the advantage of identifying complications and alternative diagnoses. Elderly patients with uncomplicated diverticulitis associated with mild pain, no systemic symptoms, and strong social support can be managed as outpatients with a low-residue diet and antibiotics against Gram-negative and anaerobic bacteria for 7–10 days. In general, elderly patients with multiple risk factors such as diabetes or coronary artery disease, which would make them more susceptible to complications, should be admitted to the hospital for IV analgesics, antiemetics, fluid resuscitation, and broad-spectrum antibiotics. Surgical consultation is necessary for patients with complicated courses, including perforation, the formation of an abscess or fistula, or obstruction. Direct visualization (colonoscopy and sigmoidoscopy) is avoided in the acute attack, but typically recommended 6 weeks after the symptoms have resolved to rule out cancer and inflammatory bowel disease [18].

Inflammatory and infectious colitis

Colitis is an inflammation of the large bowel and may have an infectious or inflammatory etiology. Colitis may have a similar presentation to diverticulitis, including pain, fevers, and diarrhea. Inflammatory bowel disease includes ulcerative colitis and Crohn's disease. These autoimmune diseases have a bimodal age distribution, and thus a significant portion of new diagnosis is made in the elderly. Older patients make up more than 20% of admissions for Crohn's disease and more than 30% of admissions for ulcerative colitis [19]. Infectious colitis is often caused by *C. difficile* in the elderly and is quoted as the most common cause of infectious diarrhea in nursing homes in the US, with a mortality estimated at more than 17% [20]. Over the last several years, the frequency and severity of the disease has increased at the same time as a high rate of treatment failure. Risk factors for the disease include recent antibiotics, hospitalization, advanced age, and severe underlying illness. Symptoms vary with severity of disease. In mild cases, patients have watery diarrhea with abdominal cramping. In more moderate to severe cases, patients also have signs of systemic infection including fever and dehydration. One complication of *C. difficile* colitis is toxic megacolon, which is characterized by total or segmental nonobstructive colonic dilatation greater than 6.0 cm plus systemic toxicity. If toxic megacolon develops, early surgical intervention is recommended as patients can quickly develop perforation and multiorgan dysfunction.

The gold standard for diagnosis of *C. difficile* infection is the cell cytotoxicity assay. The test is not universally available, and thus most institutions use enzyme immunoassay (EIA) kits. The kits test for toxin A alone or for both toxins, A and B – testing for both toxins is preferred. The sensitivity of EIA can be improved with serial testing. Severe disease is defined as WBC >15,000 and serum creatinine level at least 1.5 times the premorbid level [21].

Treatment is based on the severity of infection and recommendations have recently changed. For the initial episode of mild to moderate infection, therapy is metronidazole (500 mg orally 3 times per day for 10–14 days). For the initial episode of severe infection, vancomycin (125 mg orally 4 times per day for 10–14 days) is recommended. If the patient is being seen for the first recurrence, treatment is the same as the initial episode, as long as the severity has not changed. After the first recurrence, metronidazole should not be used because of the potential for cumulative neurotoxicity [21].

Gallbladder disease

The prevalence and severity of gallstone disease increases with advancing age. Elderly patients present with a spectrum of gallbladder disorders but, when compared with their younger counterparts, the geriatric population more often present with severe disease and more frequently have complicated courses [22].

Gallbladder disorders cause a wide range of symptoms. Classically, intermittent right upper quadrant (RUQ) pain after eating implies biliary colic, while longer-lasting pain with associated nausea, vomiting, belching, or fevers suggests cholecystitis. Elderly patients tend to lack classic symptoms of gallbladder disease and present with a variety of symptoms including mild epigastric pain, dehydration from vomiting, jaundice, pancreatitis, altered mental status, or systemic inflammatory response syndrome (SIRS). In the younger patient population, a positive Murphy's sign has a high sensitivity. In elderly patients, however, this physical exam finding is less reliable.

Diagnosis of acute biliary disease can be challenging when labs and clinical findings are misleading. In one retrospective study done in the ED, 56% of elderly patients were afebrile and 41% had no increase in WBC [23]. Ultrasound is considered the gold standard imaging modality for the diagnosis of cholecystitis. If ultrasound findings are equivocal, CT scans can confirm visualization of stones and are recommended if perforation or emphysematous cholecystitis is suspected [24]. Other studies, including radionuclide cholescintigraphy scans (e.g., hepatobiliary iminodiacetic acid) and abdominal MRI are also useful in the diagnosis of biliary tract disease, but are expensive and have traditionally had limited availability in the ED. As MRI becomes more readily available, its role in coordination of care from the ED may increase [10].

The disposition for elderly patients with symptoms consistent with gallbladder disease can be a challenge in the setting of negative ED imaging. Strong consideration should be given to admitting such patients for observation due to the high morbidity and mortality of gallbladder disease in this population. When a diagnosis of gallbladder disease is secured through imaging, treatment of biliary disease begins with supportive care, but ultimately requires surgical intervention. Antibiotics are indicated for cases of cholecystitis, and should provide coverage against Gram-negative and anaerobic bacteria. Elderly patients who have emergency cholecystectomy tend to do poorly, with a mortality rate of 6–15%. More conservative approaches including ERCP and percutaneous cholecystostomy are preferred, as these minimally invasive interventions are better tolerated, less risky, and have lower mortality rates [13,25].

Peptic ulcer disease

Peptic ulcer disease (PUD) is a common disorder of the GI system that affects patients of all ages. Over recent years, improvements in health care and the implementation of anti-ulcer drugs led to a decreased incidence of PUD in young patients. Conversely, the incidence of PUD and its complications has increased in the elderly population. This trend in the geriatric population is thought to be secondary to a higher prevalence of *Helicobacter pylori* infection and the use of gastroduodenal-damaging drugs (specifically NSAIDs and antiplatelet agents). Moreover, aging causes a loss of mucosal protection and repair mechanisms, thus increasing susceptibility to pathogens [26].

The initial assessment in the ED of the elderly patient with epigastric discomfort focuses on differentiating PUD from other causes of abdominal pain. Elderly patients with PUD most commonly present with epigastric pain, but may also experience nausea, vomiting, GI bleeding, or symptoms of anemia. In cases of perforation, patients endorse sudden severe abdominal pain and physical exam shows a distended rigid abdomen with peritoneal signs. Epigastric discomfort is a common symptom in a number of disease processes, and therefore consideration should be given to non-GI causes such as angina and lower lobe pneumonia when evaluating these patients in the ED.

Diagnosis of PUD occurs through direct visualization or by noninvasive testing. Unless the patient is unstable, upper GI endoscopy is not typically indicated on initial presentation. If *H. pylori* is suspected, the bacteria can be identified through serology, urea breath testing, urine and fecal antigens, or endoscopic biopsy. Of note, the C-urea breath test has higher sensitivity, specificity, and accuracy than measurement of anti-*H. pylori* antibodies [13,26]. If a patient displays clinical signs of perforation, plain radiographs and CT scans can be performed for the detection of free intraperitoneal air.

Treatment centers on healing ulcers with pharmacotherapy agents and preventing recurrence. Proton pump inhibitors (PPIs) are the principal therapy for ulcer healing and prevention of GI bleeding. If *H. pylori* is suspected, the therapy is broadened to include a PPI and two of the following antibacterials: clarithromycin, amoxicillin, and nitroimidazole – metronidazole or tinidazole. Studies suggest elderly patients tolerate the triple therapy regimen well, especially when the therapy is of short duration and uses low doses of both the PPI and clarithromycin [27]. If perforation occurs, emergency physicians should provide aggressive resuscitation, administer broad-spectrum antibiotics to cover Gram-negative and anaerobic bacteria, and obtain emergent surgical consultation.

Esophageal obstruction and perforation

Esophageal obstruction in the elderly typically involves food impaction or accidental ingestion of dentures or other foreign bodies. The majority of these foreign bodies pass spontaneously but occasionally require intervention with endoscopy. Patients present with neck pain and inability to swallow. Complete obstruction is highly suggested in the setting of drooling and inability for the patient to swallow their own saliva. Structural or functional esophageal abnormalities increase the risk for foreign body or food impaction. In one retrospective study in China, the underlying conditions associated with esophageal impactions included esophageal carcinoma (33%), strictures (24%), diverticulum (16%), postgastrectomy (11%), hiatal hernia (10%), and achalasia (6%) [28]. Emergent or urgent endoscopy is the mainstay of treatment in patients with persistent symptoms. A foreign body should not remain in the esophagus more than 24 hours due to the risk of esophageal perforation. Use of glucagon IV to relax the esophageal smooth muscle has been proposed, but there is no evidence to support its efficacy and there is potential to cause harm [29]. Early consultation with a gastroenterologist is important in this age group. Even if spontaneous passage of the foreign body occurs, gastroenterology follow-up for a screening endoscopy is indicated to rule out structural or functional abnormalities.

Mallory–Weiss tears occur after a sharp rise in intra-esophageal/intragastric pressure during episodes of vomiting, retching, or hiccupping. Most cases resolve spontaneously, but a minority of cases will require emergent intervention if a transmural perforation occurs, termed Boerhaave's syndrome. Patients with esophageal perforation often describe a sudden onset of severe chest pain, although this dramatic presentation is frequently absent in the elderly. Other presenting symptoms include vomiting and subcutaneous emphysema. Imaging often begins with a chest radiograph to evaluate for mediastinal or subcutaneous free air. In patients with pneumomediastinum, a frontal view may reveal a V-shaped lucency filled with air in the lower left area of the mediastinum, a finding known as the V-sign of Naclerio. The initial imaging modality of choice for suspected esophageal rupture is contrast-enhanced esophagography, which may depict extravasation of contrast material, submucosal collection of contrast material, and esophagopleural fistula. CT is the modality of choice in patients with equivocal esophagography results. The use of hydrosoluble contrast material is preferred over barium in patients with suspected esophageal rupture because of the risk for mediastinitis, resulting from irritation caused by barium. Common CT findings in esophageal perforation include esophageal wall thickening, periesophageal air collections, pneumomediastinum, mediastinal fluid collections, pleural effusions, extravasation of contrast material, and esophagopleural fistula [30]. A high index of suspicion is crucial for the early diagnosis of esophageal rupture. The mortality rate in one study among patients with a delayed diagnosis of esophageal rupture was 40%, compared with 6.2% among patients who received a diagnosis and treatment within 24 hours. The mortality rate of acute mediastinitis secondary to esophageal rupture may be as high as 90% if repair of the rupture is delayed for longer than 48 hours [31].

Upper gastrointestinal bleed

Hemorrhage from upper GI bleed (UGIB) is common and a life-threatening occurrence in the elderly population, with an incidence of 500 episodes in 100,000 people per year. When compared with a younger patient population, elderly patients have a higher morbidity and mortality due to their comorbid medical conditions and the concomitant use of anticoagulation therapy and NSAIDs [32].

Upper GI bleeds are more common than lower gastrointestinal bleeds (LGIB) in the geriatric population. The most common causes of UGIB are PUD and esophagitis, while Mallory–Weiss tears and gastro-esophageal varices are more commonly found in the younger population [33]. Although patients with UGIB often present with hematemesis and/or melena, it is also common for elderly patients to have vague symptoms of syncope, light-headedness, postural hypotension, and dyspepsia. Diagnosis of GI bleeding is contingent on a careful medical history, identification of pertinent risk factors, and a proper physical examination.

The use of nasogastric aspiration for identification of source is currently a controversial topic. If patients have hematemesis and a clear UGIB, nasogastric intubation and aspiration help quantify the amount of bleeding and determine its rate. When source of bleeding is unclear, nasogatric catheter placement with return of bloody aspirate can confirm presence of UGIB, however a clear lavage does not definitively exclude UGIB [34]. Direct visualization by esophagogastroduodenoscopy (EGD) is the study of choice for UGIB.

Esophagitis is a major cause of UGIB and abdominal pain in the elderly. Although medications (including NSAIDs, potassium, quinine, and tetracyclines) lead to esophagitis, it is thought that esophagitis is more often caused by deterioration in the esophageal clearance mechanisms and weakening of the protective mechanisms in the mucosa [35]. Esophagitis rarely causes overt hemorrhage. Therapy includes suppression of gastric acid secretion with PPIs and avoidance of irritating medications.

Resuscitation and stabilization of elderly patients with UGIB are the mainstays of treatment in the ED. Patients with cardiovascular disease may require early blood transfusion, with careful attention to slow infusion in those with pre-existing congestive heart failure to avoid flash pulmonary edema. Coagulopathic patients may require platelets or fresh frozen plasma. Anemia from GI bleed can lead to generalized weakness, myocardial ischemia, and syncope in the elderly, which makes admission to the hospital for inpatient evaluation the recommended disposition.

Lower gastrointestinal bleed

In the US and Western Europe, the most common causes of lower GI bleed (LGIB) in the elderly are diverticulosis and angiodysplasia. Other etiologies of LGIB include malignancy, inflammatory bowel diseases – ischemic colitis, infectious colitis, idiopathic inflammatory bowel disease, and post-irradiation colitis. Patients with acute LGIB typically present with hematochezia or melena, depending on the source and transit time of the bleed.

Direct visualization by colonoscopy is the investigative study of choice for LGIB. If no definitive source is found for LGIB, repeat colonoscopy or mesenteric angiography is recommended. Video capsule endoscopy (VDE) has emerged as a timely option for diagnosis of small bowel source of bleeding [36].

In general, elderly patients with GI bleeds should be admitted for serial hematocrit testing and urgent inpatient evaluation by a GI specialist. A careful medication review should be performed to identify anticoagulating or antiplatelet medications, which may put these patients at higher risk for significant blood loss. If a clear source of LGIB can be identified by noscope, such as external hemorrhoid, consideration can be made for disposition home with close follow-up with primary care and/or referral to the appropriate specialist. A disposition home in an elderly patient with a lower GI bleed should be considered very carefully and active bleeding, however minor, is best managed as an inpatient in this vulnerable population.

Constipation

Constipation is a disorder that impairs the quality of life in the elderly. It is estimated that approximately 74% of nursing home residents use a daily laxative [37]. As the definition of constipation is inconsistent between patients and practitioners, Rome III Criteria defined constipation for research purposes as having two of the following symptoms over a 3-month period at least 25% of the time: 1) Fewer than three bowel movements per week, 2) straining, 3) lumpy, hard stools, 4) the sensation of anorectal obstruction, 5) the sensation of incomplete defecation, and 6) manual maneuvering to allow defecation.

There are multiple etiologies of constipation in the elderly, making it important for medical providers to obtain a careful medical history. Key historical features to address include onset of symptoms, abdominal pain, fevers, anorexia, weight loss, use of constipating drugs, and laxatives. It is helpful to perform a thorough digital rectal exam to identify structural obstructions, such as a mass, redundant or thrombosed internal hemorrhoids, fissures, rectal stenosis, impacted stool, and neurogenic abnormalities. If clinically indicated, a complete blood count, basic metabolic panel, and thyroid tests can discriminate metabolic disorders and complications from chronic laxative use. Plain abdominal radiographs aid in the detection of other causes of constipation including bowel obstructions, megacolon, volvulus, and mass lesions. Elderly patients who present in pain or who display other physical exam findings concerning for obstruction should be evaluated with abdominal CT. If no obvious etiology for constipation is diagnosed in the ED, the patient needs follow-up with gastroenterology for direct visualization with endoscopy [37].

The treatment for constipation is aimed at correcting the underlying causative abnormality. Manual disimpaction of hard stool, stool softeners, and enemas can be used adjunctively to stimulate defecatory urge. When deciding on a treatment plan, it is important to consider cost, adverse effects, medical history, medication interactions, and baseline cardiac and renal function. If a patient appears to have a perforation from constipation on exam, surgical consultation is indicated.

Small bowel obstruction

Small bowel obstruction (SBO) is a frequent cause of abdominal pain in the geriatric population and is associated with a high rate of mortality (26%) [38]. In the Western world, the majority of obstructions are secondary to prior operative adhesions, with hernias and neoplasms contributing to only a minority of cases. Depending on the type and cause of the obstruction, elderly patients present with variable timing and onset of symptoms. Symptoms originate from the amount of interference of normal transit through the GI system. With proximal blockage, gas and fluid build up and result in nausea and vomiting. Early in the course, peristalsis continues to occur and contributes to vague, colicky abdominal pain and defecation of distal contents. As the course progresses, abdominal volume increases, consequently producing abdominal distention. Eventually arterial compromise and increased intraluminal pressures result in bowel wall necrosis and perforation. Sepsis can occur through bacterial translocation [39].

In the acute setting, laboratory tests do not improve diagnosis or predict need for surgical management. There may be important physical examination findings in patients with acute

SBO. Exam findings of distended, rigid abdomen with absent bowel sounds and presence of rebound and guarding should prompt early surgical consultation. In cases where the physical exam is less diagnostic of bowel obstruction, the use of imaging (abdominal radiographs, CT, ultrasound, contrast studies, and MRI) is the mainstay of prompt diagnosis and early management. Classic findings in abdominal radiographs include distended small bowel (>3 cm in diameter), air–fluid levels, and very little colonic or rectal gas. Multiple other pathologies, including appendicitis, diverticulitis, mesenteric ischemia, and adynamic ileus can have similar radiographic findings, however. Abdominal radiographs are only diagnostic in about 30–70% of cases (specificity of 50%) [39,40]. The American College of Radiology recommends CT scans with IV contrast of the abdomen and pelvis as the modality of choice for SBO (sensitivity 64–94%, specificity 79–95%). Oral contrast is not required because the fluid in the distended bowel loops acts as a natural contrast agent. Oral contrast can be helpful for partial obstructions and should be considered on a case-by-case basis in the ED [40].

In patients who are stable and without signs of strangulation, conservative treatment and non-operative management is successful in 80% of patients within 48 hours. Placement of a nasogastric tube should be considered in the ED to help with decompression of the bowel. If a patient has signs of peritonitis or strangulation or has failed a trial of conservative treatment, early surgical management may reduce complications, morbidity, and mortality.

Large bowel obstruction

Large bowel obstruction (LBO) is less common than SBO. The most common cause of LBO is obstruction from neoplasm, with a much smaller proportion secondary to volvulus and strictures from chronic diverticular disease. Symptoms of LBO are typically insidious in onset when the cause is neoplasm or diverticular disease. Patients experience weight loss, rectal bleeding, diarrhea, abdominal distention, and minimal vomiting for days to weeks prior to presentation. Conversely, when obstruction is secondary to volvulus, symptoms occur more acutely depending on the rapidity of twisting. In the adult population, the most common site in the GI tract for volvulus is the sigmoid colon. Although uncommon, spontaneous volvulus occurs primarily in patients who are male, elderly, have a history of chronic constipation, and are institutionalized on psychoactive medications. These institutionalized patients may present late if caretakers fail to recognize signs of LBO, leading to higher morbidity and mortality [41].

Similar to SBO, the modality of choice for diagnosis of all causes of LBO is CT scan (sensitivity and specificity 90%). Abdominal radiographs may show distinct distention of the colon with a disproportionate dilation of the cecum (>10 cm). Radiographs do not show the cause of obstruction and have poor inter-observer agreement, and thus should be reserved for screening purposes if more definitive imaging is delayed [42].

Management for LBO starts with supportive care and resuscitation. Surgical decompression is dependent on clinical context, degree of distention, and duration of symptoms. Emergent

surgical intervention is indicated in those patients with a perforation or peritonitis, sepsis, or if the patient is unstable. For sigmoid volvulus, non-operative detorsion (barium enema, rigid sigmoidoscopy, or the preferred method of flexible sigmoidoscopy) is treatment of choice in patients who are stable. In unstable patients or in patients who had unsuccessful non-operative detorsion, emergency surgery (resection with a stoma or resection with a primary anastomosis) is the treatment of choice. Prognosis of elderly patients with sigmoid volvulus is overall poor and, despite appropriate treatment, there is a high rate of recurrence (41.7–55.0% in non-operative treatment, 6.7–55.0% in surgical treatment) [41,43].

Acute colonic pseudo-obstruction

Acute colonic pseudo-obstruction (Ogilvie's syndrome) is a rare clinical disorder characterized by impaired bowel motility without evidence of a mechanical obstruction. Massive colonic dilation occurs, which puts the patient at risk for perforation. The syndrome typically occurs in the setting of recent significant medical illness, trauma, burns, spinal injury, or surgery. Patients who present with a colonic pseudo-obstruction have similar symptoms to a patient with a mechanical obstruction. They experience abdominal pain, distention, nausea, vomiting, obstipation, and fevers. Abdominal films show dilation of the cecum and colon with the presence of air in the rectum. CT scans are not essential, but help rule out other causes and complications of obstruction. After confirmation that no other sources of obstruction are present, the initial management addresses correction of underlying medical disorders and discontinuation of medications that potentially exacerbate the problem. Decompression by colonoscopy or rectal tube placement or drug therapy using neostigmine (an acetylcholinesterase inhibitor) can help prevent perforation [44].

Mesenteric ischemia

Mesenteric ischemia is a condition characterized by inadequate blood supply leading to inflammation and injury to the small intestine. Inadequate blood supply occurs through four distinct mechanisms: arterial thrombosis, arterial embolism, venous thrombosis, and nonocclusive mesenteric ischemia (NOMI). Difficulty in diagnosis and delay in treatment, in part, contribute to the high mortality rate (60–100% depending on mechanism of occlusion) [45].

The characteristics of abdominal pain at presentation depend on the source of obstruction. Arterial embolus is typically found in patients with a predisposing cardiac condition (arrhythmias, myocardial infarction, cardiomyopathy, recent angiography, valvular disorders, or ventricular aneurysm). Patients typically present with acute abdominal pain, nausea, vomiting, or diarrhea (bloody or nonbloody) [45]. In cases of arterial thrombosis, patients commonly have underlying atherosclerosis, hypercoagulability, estrogen therapy, or prolonged hypotension. Early in the course, patients have chronic epigastric pain with eating and gradually develop fear of food causing weight loss. These symptoms continue until an acute thrombus occurs and symptoms are more similar to the presentations of those patients with arterial thrombosis. Venous thrombosis is frequently found in elderly patients with malignancy, hypercoagulability, portal hypertension, deep vein thrombosis, clotting disorder, pancreatitis, hepatitis, or sepsis. Patients may present with subacute abdominal pain and diarrhea early in the course of the disease, and peritonitis if the presentation is delayed [46]. NOMI is frequently caused by low-flow cardiac states (including hypotension, hypovolemia, heart failure, or sepsis), medications (digitalis, ergot alkaloids, vasopressors, or beta blockers), or drugs (cocaine). Patients can also experience abdominal distention and nausea and will have pain out of proportion to physical exam findings.

Health care providers should maintain a high index of suspicion, as patients present with vague symptoms and ancillary biochemical tests are not reliable. Elevated lactate levels occur late in the disease process, but waiting for the elevation can lead to delayed diagnosis [45]. Imaging may aid the diagnosis, but determining the ideal mode of imaging is challenging. Pathognomonic findings of thickened bowel loops and

thumbprinting are found on plain radiographs only 40% of the time. More commonly, plain radiographs display nonspecific findings. Doppler ultrasound is of limited use because it is time consuming, operator dependent, and has variable accuracy. Multidetector-row CT with IV contrast is the test of choice for venous thrombus, but is not ideal for other mechanisms of ischemia as findings in both early (dilated bowel loops, air–fluid levels, changes in bowel wall enhancement, vascular opacification) and late disease (air in the bowel wall) are nonspecific [47]. Magnetic resonance oximetry is currently being investigated as a diagnostic modality for chronic mesenteric ischemia [46]. Selective mesenteric angiography is considered the gold standard for the detection of arterial occlusions [45] (Figure 21.2).

Early management of mesenteric ischemia focuses on supportive care, administration of broad-spectrum antibiotics, and emergent surgical consultation. Heparin therapy should be initiated when no contraindications exist. If vasopressors are

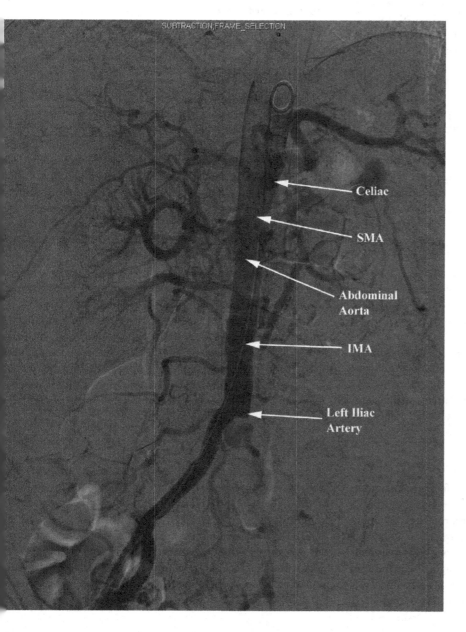

Figure 21.2. Angiograph of the abdominal aorta with complete occlusion of the superior mesenteric artery, inferior mesenteric artery, and left iliac artery.

indicated, vasopressin (pure alpha agonist) should be avoided to minimize vasospasm. Surgical intervention will depend on the clinical scenario.

Ischemic colitis

Ischemic colitis is a medical condition in which inadequate blood supply causes inflammation and injury to the large intestine. Hypoperfusion results from many situations, including systemic hypoperfusion, thromboembolism, small vessel disease, and iatrogenic causes (medications and surgeries). Elderly patients are the most commonly affected by the condition, likely secondary to increased vascular resistance from age-related changes of the colic arteries. The severity of the condition depends on the area of the bowel affected (small portion versus entire bowel), timing of the insult (transient versus permanent), and depth of injury (superficial versus transmural). The majority of cases are mild in nature and resolve without long-term complications.

Symptoms depend on the severity of ischemic colitis. In mild cases, patients present with acute mild left-sided abdominal pain and tenderness. Patients typically experience mild hematochezia within 24 hours of the abdominal pain. When hypoperfusion is more significant and the bowel becomes gangrenous, a patient can present with severe pain, fevers, dehydration, massive hematochezia, and sepsis.

Diagnosis is typically based on clinical presentation in the acute setting. Park et al. showed that a clinical presentation of lower abdominal pain or bleeding, or both, was 100% predictive of ischemic colitis when accompanied by four or more of the following risk factors: hypoalbuminemia, age over 60, hemodialysis, hypertension, diabetes mellitus, and constipation-inducing drugs [48]. Nonspecific tests, including lactate, lactate dehydrogenase, creatine kinase, and amylase, are typically normal in early disease and slightly elevated in later disease suggestive of tissue injury. Stool samples should be sent to exclude infectious sources of colitis. In early presentation, CT findings can be normal. Later in the course, CT scans show nonspecific changes with colonic wall thickening, pericolic streaking, and pneumatosis [49]. Endoscopy is the diagnostic test of choice in establishing the diagnosis of ischemic colitis.

In the acute setting, management focuses on hemodynamic stabilization, bowel rest, empiric broad-spectrum antibiotics, and avoidance of vasoconstrictive agents. Most patients will improve with conservative therapy alone. Patients with peritoneal signs, massive bleeding, or fulminant ischemic colitis may require subtotal or segmental colectomy.

Disposition

The elderly population is at higher risk for infectious, inflammatory, and ischemic GI emergencies that lead to higher morbidity and mortality than their younger counterparts. They also more often present with atypical symptoms, provide an unreliable history, and their physical exam and laboratory tests are unreliable. Therefore, liberal use of testing and imaging is encouraged to screen for dangerous pathology. Serial examinations play a very important role in deciding on the disposition of the elderly

patient in the ED. The physician should have a low threshold for inpatient hospital admission for elderly patients who have persistent symptoms and do not have a clear etiology for their symptoms at the end of the ED work-up. Some disease processes may not fully manifest with diagnosable symptoms until the disease has progressed and the patient has become severely ill. For this reason, a hospital admission for close observation for development of subtle symptoms is recommended, allowing for prompt initiation of treatment once the diagnosis is suspected.

Those patients selected for discharge from the ED should have a clear discharge plan in place. A repeat abdominal exam should be documented, including repeat vital signs. The patient should be able to ambulate safely and tolerate oral nutrition, if this is baseline. Ideally the patient will be able to stay with a family member or in the care of a 24-hour caretaker. Close primary care or visiting nurse follow-up should be arranged in a reasonable time frame. This can often be facilitated by family members, the patient's primary care office, or nursing home, or by an available social worker or case manager. If there is any doubt in regard to safety or lack of appropriate home observation and follow-up, the patient should be admitted to the hospital to ensure these items are in place prior to going home.

Pearls and pitfalls

It is important to maintain a broad differential diagnosis while evaluating an elderly patient for a potentially life-threatening GI emergency. The evaluating physician should not be reassured by normal laboratory tests and imaging studies if the patient continues to feel unwell or displays persistent physical exam findings. It is also important not to ignore abnormal vital signs. In the case of a completely negative work-up with laboratory testing and imaging, an elderly patient with a persistently abnormal vital sign likely will require overnight inpatient hospital observation for a possible occult infection or surgical disease. Elderly patients are more vulnerable to infection and have decreased cardiopulmonary reserve as compared with younger patients, making them much more susceptible to death from infection and surgical pathology.

It is also important to note etiologies that may mimic GI emergencies such as lower lobe pneumonia, acute myocardial infarction, renal colic, and abdominal aortic dissection or aneurysm. An astute physician should keep the differential diagnosis broad and work through these possibilities systematically to ensure that a dangerous disease is not missed and the diagnosis is not delayed.

Summary

There is a rapidly growing geriatric population across the globe due to improved health care and nutrition. The number of elderly patients presenting to the ED is growing and it is important that providers learn the unique physiology and set of diseases that exist in this patient population. Understanding the subtle ways that GI emergencies present in this patient population has the potential to improve patient care and appropriate decision making while caring for the elderly in the ED [50]. Gastrointestinal emergencies are a significant cause of morbidity and mortality among the elderly, and a prudent evaluation of these patients will improve survival and quality of life in this older patient population.

References

1. Marco CA, Schoenfeld CN, et al. Abdominal pain in geriatric emergency patients: Variables associated with adverse outcomes. *Acad Emerg Med.* 1998;5(12):1163–8.

2. McNamara RM, Rousseau E, Sanders AB. Geriatric emergency medicine: a survey of practicing emergency physicians. *Ann Emerg Med.* 1992;21:796–801.

3. Moore AR, Clinch D. Underlying mechanisms of impaired visceral pain perception in older people. *J Am Geriatr Soc.* 2004;52(1):132–6.

4. Potts FE, Vukov LF. Utility of fever and leukocytosis in acute surgical abdomens in octogenarians. *J Gerontol A Biol Sci Med.* 1999;54:M55–8.

5. Griffin MR. Epidemiology of nonsteroidal anti-inflammatory drug-associated gastrointestinal injury. *Am J Med.* 1998;104:23–9S.

6. Miller AH, Pepe PE, Brockman CR, Delaney KA. ED ultrasound in hepatobiliary disease. *J Emerg Med.* 2006;30(1):69–74.

7. AbuRahma AF, Stone PA, Srivastava M, et al. Mesenteric/celiac duplex ultrasound interpretation criteria revisited. *J Vasc Surg.* 2012;55(2):428–36; discussion, 435–6.

8. Esses D, Birnbaum A, Bijur P, et al. Ability of CT to alter decision making in elderly patients with acute abdominal pain. *Am J Emerg Med.* 2004;22(4):270–2.

9. Aschoff AJ, Stuber G, Becker BW, et al. Evaluation of acute mesenteric ischemia: accuracy of biphasic mesenteric multi-detector CT angiography. *Abdom Imaging.* 2009;34(3):345–57.

10. Tonolini M, Ravelli A, Villa C, Bianco R. Urgent MRI with MR cholangiopancreatography (MRCP) of acute cholecystitis and related complications: diagnostic role and spectrum of imaging findings. *Emerg Radiol.* 2012;19(4):341–8.

11. Kraemer M, Franke C, Ohmann C, Yang Q, Acute Abdominal Pain Study Group. Acute appendicitis in late adulthood: Incidence, presentation, and outcome results of a prospective multicenter acute abdominal pain study and a review of the literature. *Langenbecks Arch Surg.* 2000;385(7):470–81.

12. Yang HR, Wang YC, Chung PK, et al. Role of leukocyte count, neutrophil percentage, and C-reactive protein in the diagnosis of acute appendicitis in the elderly. *Am Surg.* 2005;71(4):344–7.

13. Anderson SW, Soto JA, Lucey BC, et al. Abdominal 64-MDCT for suspected appendicitis: The use of oral and IV contrast material versus IV contrast material only. *AJR Am J Roentgenol.* 2009;193(5):1282–8.

14. Yeh CC, Wu SC, Liao CC, et al. Laparoscopic appendectomy for acute appendicitis is more favorable for patients with comorbidities, the elderly, and those with complicated appendicitis: A nationwide population-based study. *Surg Endosc.* 2011;25(9):2932–42.

15. Xin MJ, Chen H, Luo B, Sun JB. Severe acute pancreatitis in the elderly: Etiology and clinical characteristics. *World J Gastroenterol.* 2008;14(16):2517–21.

16. Hu KC, Chang WH, Chu CH, et al. Findings and risk factors of early mortality of endoscopic retrograde cholangiopancreatography in different cohorts of elderly patients. *J Am Geriatr Soc.* 2009;57(10):1839–43.

17. Jacobs DO. Clinical practice. Diverticulitis. *N Engl J Med.* 2007;357(20):2057–66.

18. Hall J, Hammerich K, Roberts P. New paradigms in the management of diverticular disease. *Curr Probl Surg.* 2010;47(9):680–735.

19. Sonnenberg A. Demographic characteristics of hospitalized IBD patients. *Dig Dis Sci.* 2009;54:2449–55.

20. Crogan NL, Evans BC. *Clostridium difficile*: an emerging epidemic in nursing homes. *Geriatr Nurs.* 2007;28:161–4.

21. Cohen SH, Gerding DN, Johnson S, et al. Clinical practice guidelines for *Clostridium difficile* infection in adults: 2010 update by the Society for Health Care Epidemiology of America (SHEA) and the Infectious Diseases Society of America (IDSA). *Infect Control Hosp Epidemiol.* 2010;31(5):431–55.

22. Rahman SH, Larvin M, McMahon MJ, Thompson D. Clinical presentation and delayed treatment of cholangitis in older people. *Dig Dis Sci.* 2005;50(12):2207–10.

23. Parker LJ, Vukov LF, Wollan PC. Emergency department evaluation of geriatric patients with acute cholecystitis. *Acad Emerg Med.* 1997;4(1):51–5.

24. McGillicuddy EA, Schuster KM, Brown E, et al. Acute cholecystitis in the elderly: Use of computed tomography and correlation with ultrasonography. *Am J Surg.* 2011;202(5):524–7.

25. Ali M, Ward G, Staley D, Duerksen DR. A retrospective study of the safety and efficacy of ERCP in octogenarians. *Dig Dis Sci.* 2011;56(2):586–90.

26. Pilotto A. *Helicobacter pylori*-associated peptic ulcer disease in older patients: Current management strategies. *Drugs Aging.* 2001;18(7):487–94.

27. Pilotto A, Salles N. *Helicobacter pylori* infection in geriatrics. *Helicobacter.* 2002;7(Suppl. 1):56–62.

28. Li ZS, Sun ZX, Zou DW, et al. Endoscopic management of foreign bodies in the upper-GI tract: experience with 1088 cases in China. *Gastrointest Endosc.* 2006;64(4):485–92.

29. Weant KA, Weant MP. Safety and efficacy of glucagon for the relief of acute esophageal food impaction. *Am J Health Syst Pharm.* 2012;69(7):573–7.

30. Katabathina VS, Restrepo CS, Martinez-Jimenez S, Riascos RF. Nonvascular, nontraumatic mediastinal emergencies in adults: a comprehensive review of imaging findings. *Radiographics.* 2011;31(4):1141–60.

31. Shaker H, Elsayed H, Whittle I, Hussein S, Shackcloth M. The influence of the 'golden 24-h rule' on the prognosis of oesophageal perforation in the modern era. *Eur J Cardiothorac Surg.* 2010;38(2): 216–22.

32. Lingenfelser T, Ell C. Gastrointestinal bleeding in the elderly. *Best Pract Res Clin Gastroenterol.* 2001;15(6):963–82.

33. Tariq SH, Mekhjian G. Gastrointestinal bleeding in older adults. *Clin Geriatr Med.* 2007;23(4):769–84.

34. Palamidessi N, Sinert R, Falzon L, Zehtabchi S. Nasogastric aspiration and lavage in emergency department patients with hematochezia or melena without hematemesis. *Acad Emerg Med.* 2010;17(2):126–32.

35. Zimmerman J, Shohat V, Tsvang E, et al. Esophagitis is a major cause of upper gastrointestinal hemorrhage in the elderly. *Scand J Gastroenterol.* 1997;32(9):906–9.

36. Chait MM. Lower gastrointestinal bleeding in the elderly. *World J Gastrointest Endosc.* 2010;2(5):147–54.

37. Rao SS, Go JT. Update on the management of constipation in the elderly: New treatment options. *Clin Interv Aging*. 2010;5:163–71.

38. Schwab DP, Blackhurst DW, Sticca RP. Operative acute small bowel obstruction: Admitting service impacts outcome. *Am Surg*. 2001;67(11):1034–8; discussion, 1038–40.

39. Zielinski MD, Bannon MP. Current management of small bowel obstruction. *Adv Surg*. 2011;45:1–29.

40. Maglinte DD, Reyes BL, Harmon BH, et al. Reliability and role of plain film radiography and CT in the diagnosis of small-bowel obstruction. *AJR Am J Roentgenol*. 1996;167(6):1451–5.

41. Osiro SB, Cunningham D, Shoja MM, et al. The twisted colon: A review of sigmoid volvulus. *Am Surg*. 2012;78(3):271–9.

42. Suri S, Gupta S, Sudhakar PJ, et al. Comparative evaluation of plain films, ultrasound and CT in the diagnosis of intestinal obstruction. *Acta Radiol*. 1999;40(4):422–8.

43. Atamanalp SS, Ozturk G. Sigmoid volvulus in the elderly: Outcomes of a 43-year, 453-patient experience. *Surg Today*. 2011;41(4):514–19.

44. Avenel P, Subhas G, Gasquet B, Atwal M, Mittal VK. Acute colonic pseudo-obstruction (Ogilvie's syndrome). *Am Surg*. 2010;76(11):E195–6.

45. Chang RW, Chang JB, Longo WE. Update in management of mesenteric ischemia. *World J Gastroenterol*. 2006;12(20):3243–7.

46. Chang JB, Stein TA. Mesenteric ischemia: Acute and chronic. *Ann Vasc Surg*. 2003;17(3):323–8.

47. Berland T, Oldenburg WA. Acute mesenteric ischemia. *Curr Gastroenterol Rep*. 2008;10(3):341–6.

48. Park CJ, Jang MK, Shin WG, et al. Can we predict the development of ischemic colitis among patients with lower abdominal pain? *Dis Colon Rectum*. 2007;50(2):232–8.

49. Smerud MJ, Johnson CD, Stephens DH. Diagnosis of bowel infarction: A comparison of plain films and CT scans in 23 cases. *AJR Am J Roentgenol*. 1990;154(1):99–103.

50. Biese, KJ, et al. Effect of geriatric curriculum on emergency medicine resident attitudes, knowledge, and decision-making. *Acad Emerg Med*. 2011;18(10)(Suppl. 2):S92–6.

Chapter

22

Genitourinary and gynecologic emergencies in the elderly

Marianne Haughey

Age-related changes in the renal system

When caring for the geriatric population consideration must be given to the physiological, anatomical, and hormonal shifts related to aging in approaching the emergency complications of illness or injury of the genital and urinary systems. Special attention should be paid to the challenges of obtaining a complete and relevant history and physical of the genital and renal systems in the aged. It can be more difficult to achieve these goals in the hustle of the busy emergency department (ED), but with forethought these goals can be met.

The physiologic changes affecting the renal system can be measured as easily as measuring the renal mass of humans as we age. Kidney mass/weight peaks in the 4th decade and then starts to decline (most of the decline is from the cortex). The anatomical changes also include progressive thickening of the basement membrane, focal glomerulosclerosis, and mesangial expansion. Focal sclerosis at first individually and then in aggregate reduces available nephrons [1]. Podocytes, which line the basement membrane and form the filtration barrier of the glomerulus, decrease as a percentage of the cells that make up the glomerular tuft. Connective and fibrous tissue replace parts of the now nonfunctional tubules, and the remaining tubules hypertrophy [2].

While the structure of the nephrons and the kidney undergo these anatomic changes, there are additional changes impacting the function of the renal unit [3]. The rate and amount of blood flow reaching the glomerulus are essential to the filtration potential of the kidney. Renal arteries undergo the same thickening endured by all aging vasculature. The afferent and efferent arterioles of the glomeruli often form an arteriovenous shunt in the sclerosed glomeruli [1]. This, in combination with age-related changes of the vascular system extrinsic to the kidney, results in a significant decrease in the flow of blood to functional glomeruli and renal perfusion drops over time. There is a drop of about 10% on average of renal blood flow per decade after the 4th decade of life [1]. These changes are independent of alterations in renal blood flow and renal damage caused by other comorbid illnesses, which only accelerate the damage.

The elderly also have an age-related drop in muscle mass. Creatinine is a muscle breakdown product that is excreted through the kidney and is a common and easy measurement of renal function. As the creatinine excreted drops in an individual with a lower muscle mass, it often means that the renal flow drop is less obvious as the kidney is asked to filter less creatinine [1]. A normal creatinine does not mean that the frail, 80-year-old woman has kidneys that function normally, but that she can filter the current creatinine that she is being called upon to excrete. If she is given a salt or fluid load beyond her current renal capabilities (but which would be within the capabilities of the normal 30-year-old kidney with the same creatinine value) she may decompensate. Additionally, the damage from a nephrotoxic drug, including commonly used drugs such as nonsteroidal anti-inflammatory drugs (NSAIDs), aminoglycoside antibiotics, or contrast load may be beyond what her kidneys with the apparently "normal" creatinine can handle.

Age-related changes in the genital system

In women, years of gravity and the long-term effect of the trauma of childbirth cause prolapses which can involve the vagina, rectum, uterus, or a combination of organs, and incontinence issues. The hormonal changes in women post-menopause are due to the cessation of secretion of of estradiol and progesterone from the atrophied ovaries. The ovaries secrete androstenedione, which is converted to estrone in adipose tissue [4]. Ovaries in post-menopausal women should be almond sized, and the uterus, lacking the hormonal monthly stimulation, is also much smaller than during the fertile period of a woman's life. The hormonal effects post-menopause are varied, but for the purposes of this chapter the description of its effects will be limited to the pelvic organs. There is atrophy of estrogen-responsive tissues: decreased vaginal rugae, decreased lubrication, decreased detrusor strength, and vaginal tissue becomes thinner and more friable. There is laxity of the pelvic ligaments leading to increased likelihood of prolapse of the various pelvic organs. There can be a decrease in sensation, as well as a decrease in strength of sphincters and detrusor muscles, leading to incontinence of stool and urine and/or retention of urine. The vaginal flora shifts with the pH shift that occurs in the vagina, and the protective barriers against infection are reduced [5].

Geriatric Emergency Medicine, ed. Joseph H. Kahn, Brendan G. Magauran Jr., and Jonathan S. Olshaker. Published by Cambridge University Press.
© Cambridge University Press 2014.

The hormonal changes in men include a slowly and steadily dropping testosterone level. They maintain libido with a minimal amount of testosterone, but other effects include decreased muscle and bone mass, decreased sperm count, and fewer functional sperm [6]. A significant factor in the aging of the male genital system that causes many presentations to the ED is the steady growth of the prostate. Both stromal and epithelial cells give rise to hyperplastic nodules which cause benign prostatic enlargement (BPE) that can proceed to symptomatic hypertrophy (BPH) [7]. BPH arises most commonly in the peri-urethral and transition zones of the gland, and the peri-urethral portion of the gland increases in size especially after age 55, causing higher bladder outlet resistance [7]. This increased resistance results in detrusor muscle hypertrophy and hyperplasia causing decreased bladder compliance which leads to nocturia, urgency, and urinary retention [7]. Patients can then present to the ED in acute retention.

The incidence of BPH, the most common benign tumor in men, is age related. Fifty percent of men have histopathological changes at age 60 consistent with BPH, and by age 85 the rate is about 90% [8]. Symptoms also increase with age [8]. Hormonal factors play a significant role, with prostatic androgen levels (dihydrotestosterone (DHT)) implicated in the development of BPH [7].

History

Elderly patients may be less than ideal historians due to confusion, dementia, or even the sheer difficulty of conveying many complex medical problems that they may only partially understand. The environment of the ED, with the noise and commotion, may worsen the situation. Older immigrants who are less interactive with the community at large may be less likely to have complete fluency in English, so language barriers can pose more of a difficulty than in the non-geriatric age group. Physical problems that make it difficult to relate to one's surroundings, such as hearing or visual difficulties, may make communication more challenging.

Taking the history of patients presenting with genital or urinary issues touches upon the most private aspects of patients' lives. The patient might not be forthcoming about issues of concern unless directly queried by the physician. Any reservations or assumptions regarding practitioner reluctance in discussing sexuality among the elderly must be overcome in order to get a complete history. Sexual activity certainly occurs among the geriatric population, with 71% of men and 51% of women in their 60s reporting that they are sexually active. Among patients in their 80s, about 25% report they are sexually active [9]. One way to approach this question can be: "Are you currently satisfied with your sexual activity?" That can open the conversation and then be followed up by questions regarding number of partners, sexual orientation, and frequency and type of activity. Other pertinent questions can include topics such as penile implants and medications, such as hormone replacement or medications taken for erectile dysfunction.

Physical exam

Physical disabilities and immobility can make performing a physical exam more challenging than in the younger adult population. Specifically, decreased flexibility and reductions in hip range of motion can make the lithotomy position, for men and women, a difficult position to both get into and maintain. The vaginal dryness that can set in after menopause, and the possibility that female patients may have less vaginal elasticity, can contribute to the challenges. Ample lubrication can aid most exams, and 2% lidocaine jelly can be used to ease the discomfort of the exam if needed. The gynecology table with stirrups is not the only place an exam might be done. An aide to help hold a leg in a non-stirrup position may help the less flexible patient. Bedside gynecology exams can be accomplished with the use of an orthopedic bed pan inverted on the stretcher to elevate the hips, or even in the lateral decubitus position on the stretcher. It is also possible to consider evaluating for pelvic pathology via a recto-vaginal exam. For prolapses and hernias, it is also helpful to examine the patient while upright.

The challenges of the male exam include the issue that hernias are best evaluated in the patient who is upright. Prostate exams can be done standing, lying on the side, or in the lithotomy position. Patients with prior care for impotence may have had surgically placed penile implants that are usually either semi-rigid and in the penis or inflatable with the use of a pump normally placed in the adjoining area of the thigh. It is helpful to uncover these facts in the history before encountering a partially erect penis in the patient mid-exam.

Genitourinary and gynecologic issues in the elderly

Acute kidney injury

The age group with the highest rate of initiating treatment for end-stage kidney disease is that 65 or older. Data from the 2006 US renal data system show that 1.5 in 1000 people aged 65 or older initiate treatment for end-stage renal disease [1]. As mentioned above, the geriatric patient generally has less functional kidney than the younger patient and is therefore at increased risk of acute kidney injury (AKI; formerly acute renal failure) when exposed to nephrotoxic drugs, or diminished renal flow due to concurrent illness or sepsis.

The history of patients with AKI can be very vague. Patients can complain of feeling weak, fatigued, being dizzy, or just "feeling sick." They may note changes in their urine: decreased volume, darker color, inability to urinate, or retention. The more concrete symptoms can include those associated with uremia: headache, nausea, vomiting, or fluid overload, either as pulmonary or peripheral edema. The physical exam can range from completely normal to dyspneic with rales, disoriented, or otherwise acutely ill. An enlarged bladder on ultrasound can point toward renal failure secondary to obstructed outflow which can then be relieved. Patients often have other concurrent illnesses such as hypertension or diabetes which have led to the underlying damage causing what is now an AKI.

The kidneys are generally paired organs and either can usually take the load of filtering for the body if needed. When AKI occurs, this is generally something which affects both kidneys either as a systemic illness/injury or as an obstruction from where the system joins either at the bladder or below.

Acute renal failure is essentially a laboratory diagnosis and serum creatinine is the diagnostic test of choice. An electrocardiogram (ECG) may be the first test obtained in the ED to show signs of elevated potassium and should be checked, along with the serum potassium level, if renal failure is suspected. The actual criteria used to define AKI are identified in the Acute Kidney Injury Network (AKIN) paper of 2007 [10], which include: over a 48-hour period either 1) an absolute increase in serum creatinine of greater than or equal to 0.3 mg/dl; 2) a change in serum creatinine of at least 50% (1.5 × baseline); or 3) urine output of less than 0.5 ml/kg/h for more than 6 hours [10]. In the ED we may not have prior data to work with, and essentially we evaluate for signs of uremia or fluid overload in considering whether emergent treatment is acutely necessary, either via medical management or dialysis. Trending the creatinine, if available, can help identify the acuity of the problem. Because one of the few reversible causes of AKI is obstruction, a patient presenting in new acute renal failure should have an evaluation in the ED to determine whether obstruction is the cause of the AKI, because if obstruction can be bypassed or relieved the kidney failure might improve or resolve. This evaluation can be done by either ultrasound (post-void) or a post-void residual (PVR) volume measurement when evaluating whether the problem is a bladder obstruction. If there is concern for bilateral ureteral obstruction, an urgent computed tomography (CT) scan may be required, perhaps identifying pelvic masses causing the obstruction. When a patient presents in shock, a urinary catheter can provide valuable information about renal function. If the patient's level of urinary output becomes inadequate (typically <30 ml/h), this can be an early sign of decreased renal flow and impending AKI. A urine analysis (UA) can provide additional information as intrinsic renal damage can produce casts or other cellular debris. Urine should also be sent for myoglobin in a patient with a high creatinine phosphokinase (CPK) following a fall or injury that did not permit the patient to get up. Rhabdomyolysis can present with cola-colored urine.

Renal failure can be divided into pre-renal, renal, and post-renal causes. Pre-renal causes are united by the fact that they all involve decreased blood flow to the kidney. Typically the blood urea nitrogen (BUN)/creatinine ratio is greater than ten. Decreased blood flow can occur because of systemic hypovolemia (shock), heart failure, severe liver disease, or obstructions in the renal vasculature such as renal artery stenosis. Post-renal causes, which are of especial note in our geriatric population, include either obstruction of outflow of the bladder or bilateral ureteral obstruction. An enlarged prostate can cause bladder outflow obstruction, and pelvic tumors can cause bilateral ureteral obstruction. Renal causes of particular concern in the elderly include nephrotoxic drugs (Table 22.1), rhabdomyolysis can occur secondary to a fall in the elderly, or from anticholesterol drugs), and myeloma. Other causes include glomerulonephritis, interstitial nephritis, and the collagen vascular or immunologic diseases. Patients generally require admission to

Table 22.1. Nephrotoxic drugs. Based on Choudhury and Ahmed [11]

Nephrotoxic drugs (partial list)	Diuretics
	NSAIDs
	ACE inhibitors
	Radiocontrast dyes
	Warfarin
	Heparin
	Streptokinase
	Aminoglycosides
	Amphotericin
	Carbamazepine
	Mithramycin
	Quinolones
	Lovastatin
	Ethanol
	Barbiturates
	Diazepam
	Sulfonamides
	Hydralazine
	Triamterene
	Nitrofurantoin
	Penicillin
	Ampicillin
	Rifampin
	Thiazides
	Cimetidine
	Phenytoin
	Omeprazole
	Lithium

determine the cause and to manage the complications of new-onset renal failure/AKI.

Treatment of the elderly for AKI/renal failure is the same in the geriatric population as it is in the younger population. Urgent hemodialysis should be considered for uremia, fluid overload, hyperkalemia, or toxin ingestion that can be removed by dialysis. Hyperkalemia is always an urgent concern in acute renal failure. An ECG should be done urgently in all patients with suspected AKI/renal failure in order to rapidly diagnose clinically relevant hyperkalemia. Medications can be used to shift potassium and increase its excretion if required, while awaiting hemodialysis. Respiratory status is always a concern in the fluid-overloaded patient, and such patients may require intubation. Age alone is not a consideration in instituting dialysis. However, in addition to being a lifesaving treatment, dialysis is also a burdensome treatment and consideration of the ethics of balancing that burden with a patient's ability to comprehend and participate in that treatment should be taken into account [12].

Geriatric gynecological emergency presentations

Vaginal discharge

The common reasons for vaginal discharge among the younger population do not disappear as people age into the geriatric age group. Sexual activity exists, as do sexually transmitted infections. Patients who have had a lifelong partner may have new sexual partners as marriages break up, or they lose their spouses. As pregnancy is not an issue, condom use might not be the priority it may once have been and patients may be exposed to gonorrhea, chlamydia, trichomonas, herpes, HIV, syphilis, and other sexually transmitted infections (STIs). The history of sexual activity in the cognitively intact geriatric patient is important. In such individuals, it is certainly possible that abdominal pain and tenderness might have an STD as its source and should be investigated with an appropriate gynecological exam. The issue of non-consensual intercourse should also be considered among the cognitively impaired who present to the ED with an STI, whether from an institution or from family care. Sexually transmitted infections such as herpes and HIV are lifelong infections. A herpes outbreak can certainly present as vaginal discharge.

The female geriatric patient can have mucosal changes, as atrophy causes a rise in vaginal pH which can predispose them to bacterial vaginosis [13]. Treatment can be with oral metronidazole, local metronidazole gel 0.75%, or clindamycin cream 2%. Clearly, among the geriatric population, it is often best to treat locally rather than add another oral medication to their regimen. If patients are not symptomatic, they do not require treatment.

Candida is not an uncommon issue for elderly women. If there are issues of incontinence and difficulties with hygiene there can be a constantly moist environment that provides a ripe area for candida to grow. Also of note, patients with glycosuria due to poorly controlled diabetes may complain of vaginal or vulvar irritation and pruritus which may be due to yeast overgrowth. It is prudent to check the serum glucose of elderly patients presenting with yeast infections. Yeast infections are more likely to occur in geriatric patients who are using estrogen therapy.

There are two conditions that are less common in the non-geriatric patient but which are essential to consider in the geriatric female who presents with vaginal discharge. The first condition is a fistula. Fistulas can form for many reasons, including birth trauma, cancers, radiation treatment, and surgical procedures. The cause of fistula in the elderly of industrialized nations is more likely to be increased friability of the involved tissues and increased duration over which the patient has experienced one of the conditions leading towards a fistula, unlike the devastating fistulas often seen from childbirth in a younger population in Third World countries. Patients present with vaginal "discharge" that may be foul smelling if the source of the discharge is an enterovaginal fistula, or liquid if the source is a vesiculovaginal fistula. It is also possible that this foul discharge is the fresh presentation of a new fistula, which can indicate a cancer eroding through gynecological tissue. Endometrial cancers can also present with foul, necrotic-smelling discharge.

There is also a benign vaginal discharge in the elderly, which is the second diagnosis of special consideration in this population. Patients who have an asymptomatic discharge filled with epithelial cells but lacking in white blood cells may

be presenting with "desquamation" [13]. This can present after the replacement of a uterine prolapse or with estrogen therapy [13]. It is self-limiting and does not require treatment.

Vaginal bleeding

Vaginal bleeding in the post-menopausal patient is always abnormal. A physical exam should be done to exclude other bleeding sources. Vulvar abnormalities, such as tumor, can bleed. Rectal bleeds and hemorrhoids can be confused by the elderly or their caregivers with vaginal bleeding. Trauma to the vagina can cause bleeding of relatively friable tissue and may have implications of sexual assault in a cognitively impaired patient.

The geriatric patient with vaginal bleeding should be carefully queried regarding estrogen use, either orally or as a vaginal cream or ointment. Hormone use can promote bleeding in patients who have stopped menstruating.

After checking for hemodynamic stability and repairing any traumatic lacerations, definitive care of the geriatric patient with true vaginal bleeding (including bleeding caused by estrogen use) is done by the gynecologist. Patients require an endometrial biopsy to evaluate for endometrial cancer. Ultrasound is another modality used in diagnosis, but is inadequate on its own. Endometrial cancer is the most commonly diagnosed malignancy of the genital tract [13].

Uterine prolapse

Uterine prolapse is not an uncommon finding in the ED. Fortunately, it is not generally an urgent problem and the patient can usually be reassured and referred for outpatient management. The main complication that needs evaluation in the ED is the possibility of renal failure due to obstruction from the protrusion and/or kinking of the ureters with complete prolapse (procidentia uteri) [14]. Higher parity is associated with increased likelihood of prolapse. As patients age, the laxity of their connective tissue can increase so that the normal position of the uterus is shifted, and in fact can even protrude. Patients with connective tissue disorders, chronic cough, pelvic tumors, chronic constipation, or neurological disorders may have a higher likelihood of uterine prolapse [15].

The history might reveal that the patient has no symptoms, or that they feel a bulge or pressure. They may have urinary complaints, or note they may have to reposition themselves, perhaps including elevating the prolapse, to urinate. There can be vaginal discharge (often a desquamation reaction) or bleeding.

The findings on physical exam depend on the degree of prolapse. The uterus can be prolapsed, yet still be endovaginal. The entire uterus can also be completely protuberant. The prolapse is significant only if it is causing symptoms. There are staging systems for prolapse, but they are not going to change management in the ED. A single-blade speculum may be used to identify a cystocele prolapse (anterior vaginal wall permitting a portion of the bladder to prolapse through to the vagina) or a rectocele (posterior vaginal wall prolapse permitting a portion of the rectum to prolapse through to the vagina) [4]. I may be necessary to examine the patient in the standing position to truly appreciate the prolapse. A cystocele may be large enough to be associated with an elevated PVR [13]. A rectocele is often associated with constipation. Both can be associated with the patient's need to manually reduce the prolapse partially in order to void.

In the ED, issues pertaining to prolapse that are of concern include ensuring that there is no irreducible prolapse, that there is no area of incarceration related to the prolapse, that renal function is intact, and that hydronephrosis is not present and related to the prolapse.

Methods of management of genital prolapse range from medical treatment (with estrogens), mechanical support through a pessary, and surgery, which can be either reconstructive or involve removing the prolapsing organ(s) (usually the uterus). All of these options require close care over time and are best instituted by the gynecologist.

Urinary retention/stricture

Urinary retention can present either as an acute complaint or chronic condition. If acute, it is associated with pain due to a distended bladder from the patient's inability to urinate. When the bladder is drained, pain relief is achieved. Chronic urinary retention causes a distended bladder which may or may not be painful due to the prolonged course of the distention. Symptoms elicited in the history of chronic obstruction can include a progressively weak stream, frequent urination, and incomplete voiding with urination over time.

An essential question on history is whether a patient in retention has had any recent urological interventions. If a patient has had a recent procedure, the urologist should be contacted. Catheter placement is the primary treatment for a patient in retention, but might be contraindicated in the case of a recent procedure. If a patient has undergone recent instrumentation, the path for the catheter might not be as anatomically clear, and attempting to pass a urinary catheter may cause damage. Instrumentation can cause strictures in women as well as men.

Given the polypharmacy common among the elderly, it is important to note that a number of medications can cause retention. This should be considered both in the care of a patient presenting in acute retention and in the discharge of a patient with a non-urological complaint who has some moderate BPH. Medications such as anticholinergics (including the anticholinergic effects of antihistamines), alpha-agonists, antispasmodics, and narcotics are notorious for causing retention, especially if added to the regimen of a patient with partial outlet obstruction who has been able to maintain voiding until the medication was added [16]. Often these medications are added for the patient presenting with exacerbation of chronic obstructive pulmonary disease (COPD), recent anesthesia/surgery, or perhaps an upper respiratory infection, as many of the cold remedies, narcotics, and asthma/COPD medications (atrovent is a prime anticholinergic) contain medications that can potentiate retention in a susceptible patient (Table 22.2).

Table 22.2. A sample of commonly used medications that can cause acute urinary retention [16–20] (especially of note in patients with pre-existing mild BPH symptoms)

Antiarrhythmics	Disopyramide
	Procainamide
	Quinidine
Anxiolytics/hypnotics	Clonazepam
	Diazepam
	Zolpidem
Antidepressants	Amitriptyline
	Citalopram
	Doxepin
	Imipramine
	Venlafaxine
Antiseizure drugs	Carbamazepine
	Gabapentin
	Lamotrigine
	Tiagabine
Antihistamines	Cetirizine
	Chlorpheniramine
	Cyproheptadine
	Diphenhydramine
	Hydroxyzine
Antihypertensives	Clonidine
	Hydralazine
	Nifedipine
Antiparkinsonian drugs	Benztropine mesylate
	Carbidopa/levodopa
	Pramipexole
	Selegiline
Antipsychotics	Aripiprazole
	Clozapine
	Haloperidol
Decongestants	Phenylpropanolamine
	Pseudoephedrine
Dementia agents	Memantine
	Rivastigmine
Gastrointestinal drugs	Atropine/scopolamine/hyoscyamine
	Dicyclomine
	Metoclopramide
Hormones	Estrogens
	Progesterone
	Testosterone
Muscle relaxants	Baclofen
	Cyclobenzaprine
	Diazepam
Pain relievers	Nonsteroidal anti-inflammatory drugs
	Opioids
	Tramadol
Pulmonary drugs	Ipratropium
	Tiotropium
Urologic agents	Darifenacin
	Oxybutynin
	Tolterodine

By asking a few questions before discharging a patient with an unrelated complaint, it can fairly readily be ascertained whether this patient has mild BPH that might be worsened into acute retention by the addition of a concerning medication. It is prudent to inquire about symptoms, such as the sensation of the need to urinate frequently and incomplete emptying, stream strength, nocturia, straining to urinate, and post-void leakage. A scoring system, the American Urological Association symptom index (AUA symptom score), uses these and other symptoms to rate mild, moderate, and severe BPH [8] (see Table 22.3). If the patient has a high score, the practitioner can take that into account before prescribing medications that might tip the patient over to urinary retention, or at least warn the patient of the possibility.

Distention of the bladder can often be diagnosed on physical exam as a tense, tender, full area in the lower abdomen. The distended bladder can easily be identified by post-void ultrasound, or in the absence of ultrasound, PVR volume can be obtained by Foley catheter. Placement of the catheter, in the absence of recent procedures, is therapeutic as well as diagnostic. A UA can be sent, looking for gross hematuria and/or infection.

An exam of the prostate is an important part of the evaluation of urinary retention, but the prostate is a three-dimensional organ and it can feel normal from the rectal angle of the exam but still extend sufficiently into the area of the urethra to cause obstruction. If the prostate is hard and nodular, the patient should be referred for an evaluation for prostate cancer. If the prostate is tender and "boggy," the patient needs treatment for prostatitis. The rectal exam might also reveal fecal impaction, masses, or abnormal sphincter tone and therefore is appropriately completed in women as well as in men presenting in retention. Other elements of the physical include a pelvic examination in order to evaluate for cystocele, uterine prolapse, severe fibroids, and other pelvic or vaginal tumors, any of which can be a cause of retention/obstruction. The male genital exam should evaluate for phimosis, paraphimosis, and meatal stenosis. A neurologic exam is also an important part of the evaluation for urinary retention.

Lab exams that are useful include a urinalysis looking for infection or blood. The presence of blood might indicate infection or stone, but may also be found in cancers of the urinary tract. A urine culture should be done if infection is suspected. A creatinine can determine whether obstruction is causing AKI.

The cause of urinary retention in the elderly is often due to outflow obstruction, either at the level of the bladder or the urethra. This is especially common in the geriatric male population as the prostate is ideally placed to cause obstruction of the urethra. The most common reason for obstruction is BPH, which is normally not a concerning diagnosis in the ED but becomes an emergent cause for concern if it causes urinary retention. When an elderly patient presents with urinary retention, there are a number of other causes in the differential which should be considered. Neurologic causes of retention can occur because of decreased bladder contractility, disturbance in motor or sensory innervations of the bladder, or dissociation between bladder contraction and urethral sphincter relaxation. These diagnoses should be considered: multiple sclerosis, spinal injury/compression causing motor paralysis, spinal shock, tabes dorsalis, and diabetes [21]. Herpes zoster can also lead to retention, either because of the pain of urinating or because of L3 nerve involvement in the infection [13].

Additional anatomic causes of retention include stone, urethral stricture, phimosis, paraphimosis, pelvic tumors, uterine prolapse, cystocele, rectocele, urethral or bladder tumors, meatal stenosis, and prostate cancer. Obstructions may also include urethral foreign bodies, urethral stones, or even constipation or fecal impaction.

After the diagnosis of urinary retention has been made, urinary drainage/bladder decompression should be performed. The insertion of a lubricated 16 or 18 Fr Foley catheter into the urethra is usually the first line of treatment. In men with BPH, a larger catheter or a Coude catheter, which has a firm, curved tip to help navigate the prostatic urethra, may be helpful. If the usual methods of passing a Foley catheter fail, it is possible to consider filiforms and followers. Filiforms are long, thin probes that can pass through strictures and then into the bladder. Followers are tapered catheters that can screw into one end of the filiform and will follow the filiform through the stricture [22]. Since the followers can be of larger diameter when used with the filiforms, followers will progressively dilate the stricture area through which they pass, thus possibly allowing insertion of a standard Foley catheter. Cysto-urethroscopy is the safest and ultimately the most successful way to insert a filiform since it is done using a cystoscope, providing direct vision while passing a filiform through a stricture. If a catheter cannot be passed (due to anatomical obstacles) a percutaneous suprapubic tube may be placed, usually by urology. The Foley catheter will usually remain in place until urology follow-up for a trial of voiding without a catheter. The urologist may eventually choose uroplasty as the definitive method of care [22].

In addition to the mechanical methods of relieving the obstruction, there are medications that can decrease the impedance of urine outflow in patients with BPH. These may be used alone or in combination with a catheter. Alpha blockers such as alfuzosin and tamsulosin lead to relaxation of smooth muscle at the bladder neck/urethral sphincters. Five-alpha reductase inhibitors such as finasteride and dutasteride block conversion of testosterone to dihydrotestosterone leading to reduction in the size of the gland, and are used in men with BPH [8]. Surgery is also an eventual option in patients with BPH, and transurethral resection of the prostate (TURP) significantly reduces the risk of developing urinary retention. Open suprapubic prostatectomy is used for patients with a very large prostate. Laser vaporization is becoming more popular as an eventual treatment choice [8].

Complications can be involved in resolving the obstruction. Post-obstructive diuresis is one such complication, especially for those with prolonged or chronic retention. These patients should have their vital signs and their input and output

Table 22.3. American Urological Association Symptom Index to assess severity of benign prostatic hyperplasia (BPH; score for each item ranges from 0 to 5) [8]

1. Over the past month, how often have you had a sensation of not emptying your bladder completely after you finish urinating? (not at all–almost always)

2. Over the past month, how often have you had to urinate again less than 2.5 hours after you finished urinating? (not at all–almost always)

3. Over the past month, how often have you found you stopped and started again several times when you urinated? (not at all–almost always)

4. Over the past month, how often have you found it difficult to postpone urination? (not at all–almost always)

5. Over the past month, how often have you had a weak urinary stream? (not at all–almost always)

6. Over the past month, how often have you had to push or strain to begin urination? (not at all–almost always)

7. Over the past month, how many times did you most typically get up to urinate from the time you went to bed at night until the time you got up in the morning?

Total score: ≤7 indicates mild BPH; 8–19 indicates moderate BPH; 20–35 indicates severe BPH.

monitored. Some patients may also experience hematuria or hemorrhage due to mucosal disruption from prolonged bladder distention. Hypotension may occur as a result of a vasovagal response due to bladder decompression after significant distention. Renal failure may occur with an elevated creatinine due to the obstruction. Infection is always a risk after instrumentation. When performing bladder decompression, whether urethral or suprapubic, proper sterile technique must be maintained to prevent secondary infection. Strictures can also occur post-instrumentation.

Most patients may be discharged home with the Foley catheter in place and a leg collection bag.

Patients must be instructed in managing the Foley catheter, how to empty the collection bag, and how to monitor urine output. Hospitalization is indicated for patients who have urosepsis from retention or related procedures, or a significant underlying cause of retention such as spinal cord compression from trauma or malignancy. Patients should follow up with urology, obstetrics/gynecology, or their primary care physician depending on the cause of the retention. Those discharged with a Foley catheter in place will need to have the catheter removed at a later time with evaluation of spontaneous micturition ("trial without catheter").

Balanitis

Balanitis is inflammation of the glans of the penis; balanoposthitis is inflammation of the glans and the prepuce (foreskin). The patient often complains of pain, pruritis, burning, or tenderness of the glans. Other complaints can include dysuria, discharge, or swelling of the foreskin. It is usually a localized process and systemic symptoms are not common. Physical exam findings include erythema, swelling, ulcerations, and/or scaling of the glans and prepuce. Subpreputial exudate may be present, and there may be localized lymphadenopathy.

Diagnostic tests done in the ED are limited, as the diagnosis is clinical in most cases. There are tests that can be helpful, but usually not acutely. One acute test that is helpful is a finger stick for blood glucose in suspected cases of *Candida* spp. balanitis. A number of diabetics have balanitis as their presenting symptom. It can be helpful for outpatient care if the following are done in the appropriate setting: a potassium hydroxide slide can help clarify the diagnosis of *Candida* spp., a wet

mount can help visualize *Trichomonas* and/or white cells, and additional testing for gonorrhea, chlamydia, syphilis, herpes, and bacterial culture can aid the consultant in non-urgent follow-up.

Causes of balanitis include hygiene issues (especially in the uncircumcised), drug eruptions, chemical irritants, and infections, with the latter being the most common. The most common of the infections are *Candida* spp. (about 35% of cases), followed by *Streptococcus* and *Staphylococcus* spp. [23]. Other infectious causes include *Chlamydia* and/or *Gonococcus*, *Trichomonas*, *Borrelia*, *Treponema pallidum*, anaerobes, *Gardnerella vaginalis*, herpes, and human papilloma virus [23].

Patients at risk for *Candida* spp. balanitis include diabetics, uncircumcised, and immunocompromised patients. The exam reveals erythema with papules, burning, and pruritus. Infections often present with exudate, erythema, and swelling. There are other non-infectious, and often chronic causes of penile skin discoloration and scarring that may be detected on exam that should be referred to a urologist for further evaluation. Lichen sclerosus (balanitis xerotica obliterans) presents with hypopigmented plaques or papules over the glans/prepuce. Lichen sclerosus may lead to phimosis and scarring of the meatus, with a chronic and relapsing course. Remission may be achieved with treatment, but the risk of malignant transformation is 1% [24]. Circinate balanitis presents with a serpiginous, grayish-white dermatitis with white margins and small, painless ulcers over the glans. It can be associated with reactive arthritis and if identified the patient should be referred to a rheumatologist. Zoon's (plasma cell) balanitis is seen in uncircumcised males of the early and later geriatric population. The exam demonstrates orange–red circumscribed lesion(s) with pinpoint red spots. Any chronic scarring balanitis should be referred to a urologist to evaluate for carcinoma in situ or frank squamous cell cancer. Zoon's balanitis has a chronic course but may resolve with circumcision [25].

Patients may present with a drug eruption on the penis – or anywhere else on the body – after exposure to drugs such as salicylates, sulfonamides, or tetracyclines, among others. Chemical irritation can be caused by soaps, spermicides, and other locally applied lotions. Also, the skin of the penis can exhibit other systemic illnesses that may be confused with balanitis. Among the diagnoses included in the differential are nummular eczema, psoriasis, and scabies.

Treatment is directed at the suspected etiology, infectious being the most common. The patient may be advised to retract the foreskin 1–2 times daily and wash with warm water or saline (soap may be irritating) to clear debris and smegma. Balanitis is treated the same in the geriatric population as it is in the younger patient. The most common cause is *Candida* spp., and this can be treated with antifungal cream. The next most likely cause is bacterial, with the most common organisms being *Staphylococcus* and *Streptococcus* spp., so coverage of those microbes is important [23]. If the balanitis is thought to be caused by a drug allergy or irritant, the offending agent should be discontinued and a mild steroid cream may prove helpful. The diagnosis of lichen sclerosus or Zoon's balanitis is made by biopsy, requiring a referral to urology for follow-up. If circinate balanitis is suspected, look for reactive arthritis as well and treat the associated infection if present, and also refer to urology or dermatology. Particular attention should be paid to the possibility of squamous cell cancer presenting in the elderly population with penile skin changes [15]. Balanitis requires follow-up, as the various etiologies can be confusing in their clinical presentation and there may be a required test of treatment to ensure cure.

Emergent issues in the ED requiring urgent urologic intervention and consultation include paraphimosis, urinary retention, and penile cellulitis. Phimosis might also require urgent intervention, because if the balanitis is severe enough phimosis can cause urinary obstruction.

Male genital infections: prostatitis, epididymitis, orchitis

Pain coming from the prostate, testes, scrotum, and/or urethra is the underlying patient concern for a number of presentations to the ED. In the younger population, most of those complaints are connected to sexually transmitted infections. In the aged, although sexually transmitted infections are always to be considered, they represent a smaller proportion of the etiologies of the complaints. Even if the male genital system is the origin of the problem, the aged population can present with more non-specific symptoms than a younger population. Complaints can range from voiding symptoms of dysuria, frequency, urgency, penile discharge, pain with ejaculation, testicular or epididymal tenderness, perineal pain, back pain, fever, and even sepsis. In patients who have an infection/inflammatory reaction (orchitis, epididymitis, urethritis, prostatitis), this may have seeded to these other areas as all are in continuity.

Urethritis is defined by inflammation of the urethra and can be due to infectious or non-infectious causes. Epididymitis is defined as inflammation or infection of the epididymis with resultant vascular congestion and inflammation of surrounding structures. Orchitis is defined as inflammation or infection of the testicle, most often secondary to epididymitis. Each can be classified based on symptom duration as either acute, subacute (<6 weeks), or chronic (>6 weeks). As the infection ascends through the genitourinary tract, urethritis can progress to epididymitis and, as it travels further, to orchitis and then prostatitis. The complaint of scrotal pain can originate in either the epididymis or testicle, but may be difficult to distinguish on physical exam depending on the chronicity of the infection and the swelling involved. There may be penile tenderness with urethritis, which untreated can develop into epididymal or testicular tenderness, induration, or warmth (from associated epididymitis or orchitis). If an STI is the cause, there may be lesions of other STIs (such as herpes or syphilis). There may also be inguinal lymphadenopathy.

There are infectious and non-infectious etiologies for male genital infections. Generally the causes of infection above age 35 (and certainly in the geriatric age group) are found to be primarily coliforms and other infections commonly found in the urinary tract. Male genital tract infections are divided into gonococcal (*Neisseria gonorrhoeae*) and non-gonococcal causes. The non-gonococcal (in addition to the coliforms) causes of infection include: *Chlamydia trachomatis*, *Mycoplasma genitalium*, *Trichomonas vaginalis*, herpes simplex virus, adenovirus, *Ureaplasma urealyticum*, *Staphylococcus saprophyticus*, and yeasts [26,27]. Unprotected intercourse is a cause of an STI-related urethritis and that consideration should not be omitted in the aged. In STI-related infections, symptoms typically occur 4–14 days after exposure. In the case of chronic infectious epididymitis/orchitis, tuberculosis is also a relatively common etiology and needs to be considered in indolent presentations [28,29]. There are also non-infectious causes of urethritis. Trauma from repetitive catheterizations, foreign body insertion, an indwelling catheter, and urethral procedures can all lead to urethritis.

Orchitis

Orchitis usually presents as the gradual onset of scrotal pain and swelling. The pain is usually unilateral, becoming more generalized as inflammation spreads to the adjacent testicle. Occasionally pain will radiate to the lower abdomen. Symptoms of lower urinary tract infection (UTI) can be present. Symptoms may also include nausea and vomiting. A confounding diagnosis in younger patients with scrotal pain is testicular torsion, which is an extremely rare diagnosis in the geriatric male [30], but is found and treated the same way in the elder population with physical exam, ultrasound, and surgery. The differential can also include areas that provide referred pain to the testicle. These can include ureteral stones, inguinal hernias, appendicitis, cystitis, and pyelonephritis.

On physical exam, patients may find sitting to be uncomfortable. Systemic signs of infection, such as tachycardia and fever, may be present. The epididymis is usually tender and the infection can progress to testicular pain and testicular swelling if untreated. Prehn's sign, which is partial or complete relief of pain with testicular elevation, is suggestive of epididymitis. Urinary retention from bladder outlet obstruction has been seen among the elderly in epididymitis/orchitis. An inguinal exam should be performed looking for lymph nodes which may be associated with epididymo-orchitis, and to exclude hernia. It is important to check for costovertebral angle (CVA) tenderness when looking for co-existing pyelonephritis and to help evaluate for alternative diagnoses.

Epididymitis

Epididymitis most often occurs when pathogens travel retrograde up the genitourinary tract to cause infection. Hematogenous spread is rare. Again, in older populations the etiology is most likely a urinary pathogen. In the population of men who have sex with men, coliform bacteria are common causative agents, and in the HIV population, viral, fungal, and cytomegalovirus have been described [31]. Other possible although less common bacteria include *Klebsiella pneumoniae*, *Pseudomonas aeruginosa* and, in rare cases, *Mycobacterium tuberculosis* [31]. Non-infectious causes include vasculitides and medications such as amiodarone. Dose reduction is generally the method of treatment in amiodarone-induced epididymitis [32].

Physical exam is essential to the diagnosis of these male genital tract infections, but there are some lab tests of value. A urinalysis with urine culture should be done to ensure effective treatment. A urethral swab or urine test for *Chlamydia trachomatis* or *N. gonorrhoeae* should be performed. A blood count might be advisable. In the ill patient, leukocytosis can be suggestive of infectious causes of scrotal pain with systemic effects. Imaging can be used to define the pathology of the testicle. Although in the elderly patient it may not be needed frequently, if there is concern for mass or tumor or abscess, ultrasound can be a useful tool.

Treatment should focus on eradicating infection, relieving symptoms, preventing complications and transmission, and treatment of associated conditions. Most patients with epididymo-orchitis can be treated as outpatients. Supportive care includes: reduced physical activity, scrotal support and elevation, ice packs, NSAIDs, and Sitz baths. A follow-up visit in 72 hours to the urologist to evaluate for improvement is optimal. As always, if an STD is under consideration, then sexual abstinence until the partner receives treatment is mandatory. Rarely, patients require admission; indications for admission include sepsis, large overlying cellulitis, inability to tolerate food or fluids by mouth, and failed outpatient treatment.

Prostatitis

'Prostatitis' is actually a continuum of disease. The range of presentation includes patients with voiding symptoms with genitourinary pain, pain with defecation, back or perineal pain with fever or malaise, sexual dysfunction, and even urinary retention. It is the third most common urological diagnosis among men older than 50 years of age [33]. The prevalence of prostatitis in a North American population ranged from 2 to 16% [34]. Risk factors for prostatitis include: urethritis, UTIs, STIs, urologic instrumentation (including indwelling Foley catheter), and anatomic or neurologic outlet obstruction.

The National Institute of Diabetes and Digestive and Kidney Diseases created a 4-stage classification system for prostatitis in 1995. Of the four classifications, two are generally of concern in the ED and two are useful for general knowledge. Class I is acute bacterial prostatitis (ABP), class II is chronic bacterial prostatitis (CBP), class III is chronic non-bacterial prostatitis/chronic pelvic pain syndrome (CNP/CPPS), and class IV

is asymptomatic inflammatory prostatitis (AIP). Classes III and IV are not particularly relevant to requirement for care in the ED, but classes I and II can present with acute issues that require emergency treatment [35,36].

Acute bacterial prostatitis represents 2–5% of cases of prostatitis [36]. There are local as well as systemic symptoms and it more commonly affects young men. The pathogens are generally uropathogens. Complications can include prostate abscess, acute urinary retention, and sepsis. The infection is responsive to antibiotics. The suggested course of antibiotics required for treatment varies in the literature, but 4–8 weeks' treatment is included in the recommended courses [33,36,37].

Chronic bacterial prostatitis represents 2–10% of prostatitis cases [34]. It occurs more commonly in older men and by definition has symptoms lasting longer than 3 months. The physical exam may be normal and patients do not generally appear ill, but the infection can seed from the prostate. It presents with systemic or local symptoms. Patients are also at risk for complications of prostatic abscess (especially with the additional risk factor of immunocompromise), acute or chronic urinary retention, renal failure from chronic obstruction, and sepsis. The pathogens are typically uropathogens and the infection is responsive to antibiotics, although generally even a longer course than for ABP is required, in the order of 12 weeks [33].

Neither CNP/CPPS nor AIP respond to antibiotics or present with signs of indolent or acute infection. The causes can be as varied as reflux of urine into prostatic ducts (e.g., "chemical prostatitis"), unidentified infectious agents (atypical pathogens), autoimmune disorders, bladder neck/urethral spasms, or pelvic floor muscle tension [33]. There is a scoring system to evaluate symptoms and their impact to be found on the patient National Institutes of Health Chronic Prostatitis Symptom Index questionnaire (NIH-CPSI test). This includes 13 questions that quantify pain symptoms, urinary symptoms, and quality of life (Table 22.4). CNP/CPPS and AIP are best managed by the urologist in an outpatient setting.

Patients with acute prostatitis may present with pain in the lower abdomen, testicles, or perineum and fever, chills, fatigue, and malaise. Chronic prostatitis may present with bladder outlet obstruction or urinary retention. Acute or acute on chronic, prostatitis can be a subtle cause of sepsis in both the obtunded and the alert patient who presents with nonspecific systemic signs of sepsis. The patient in acute retention will usually present with a great deal of pain and discomfort. If chronic, the patient may present with lower urinary tract symptoms such as frequency, urgency, or hesitancy.

Physical exam findings may include an abdomen with suprapubic fullness or tenderness of the CVA coupled with an abnormal genitourinary exam. Prostate tenderness may be the only finding, especially in acute prostatitis. It has been described as a "boggy" to the touch. Prostatic massage in patients with acute infection is contraindicated because of the risk of bacteremia. Likewise, if there is urinary retention and also concern for an acutely infected prostate, a suprapubic tube is an appropriate remedy for retention, due to the concern of bacteremia resulting from the passage of a catheter through the prostate.

Table 22.4. NIH Chronic Prostatitis Symptom Index [38]

A scoring system evaluating the impact of symptoms of Chronic Prostatitis by querying symptoms relating to pain, urinary symptoms and impact on quality of life.	
Query	**Score**
1. Over the last week, have you experienced: Any pain or discomfort in the perineum (area between rectum and testicles), testicles, tip of the penis (not related to urination), below your waist, and/or in your bladder or pubic area?	1 point for each "yes"
2. Over the last week, have you experienced: Pain or burning during urination and/or pain or discomfort during or after ejaculation?	1 point for each "yes"
3. Over the last week, how often have you had pain or discomfort in any of these areas?	From 0 (never) to 5 (always)
4. Over the last week, which number best describes your *average* pain or discomfort on the days that you had it?	From 0 (none) to 10 (severe)
5. Over the last week, how often have you had a sensation of not emptying your bladder completely after you finished urinating?	From 0 (not at all) to 5 (almost always)
6. Over the last week, how often have you had to urinate again less than two hours after you finished urinating?	From 0 (not at all) to 5 (almost always)
7. Over the last week, how much have your symptoms kept you from doing the kinds of things you would usually do?	From 0 (none) to 3 (a lot)
8. Over the last week, how much did you think about your symptoms?	From 0 (none) to 3 (a lot)
9. If you were to spend the rest of your life with your symptoms just the way they have been during the last week, how would you feel about that?	From 0 (delighted) to 6 (terrible)
Total for items 1–4	Mild = 0–9
Urinary symptoms: Total of items 5 and 6	Moderate = 10–18
Quality of life & impact: Total of items 7–9	Severe = 19–31

All portions of the genitourinary tract need examination, as the infection may have arisen from an orchitis or epididymitis. Likewise, when a patient presents with urethritis, orchitis, or epididymitis, it is appropriate to evaluate the prostate, as acute or chronic bacterial prostatitis will require a longer antibiotic treatment course than any of these other diagnoses.

The etiology of ABP/CBP is usually an ascending infection from the urethra or migration from bladder. The most common cause is aerobic Gram-negative uropathogens. The common bacteria identified are *Escherichia coli* (60–80%), other Enterobacteriaceae such as *Klebsiella*, *Proteus*, and *Serratia*, and *Pseudomonas*. Other bacteria include Gram-positive Enterococci, *Staphylococcus epidermis*, and rarely *Streptococcus*. It is also possible to encounter atypical pathogens such as *Chlamydia trachomatis*, *Ureaplasma urealyticum*, *M. tuberculosis*, and viruses [33,36,38,39].

Diagnostic studies to be obtained in the ED include a urinalysis with microscopy – which should demonstrate white blood cells and bacteria, a urine culture, and bladder ultrasound to evaluate for retention. If there is concern for prostatic abscess, a CT or localized ultrasound can define the abnormality [36]. A creatinine can help identify renal insufficiency caused by chronic retention. If the patient is ill enough to consider hospitalization, a complete blood count (CBC) with differential, and blood cultures should be obtained. There are other tests the urologist may choose to perform. A prostate-specific antigen (PSA) can be used as a biomarker to correlate with clinical and microbiological improvement, although it is not of help in the acute, ED presentation and is not used as a screening test. There are various methods of obtaining prostatic secretions that entail collecting urine before and after prostatic massage that the urologist may choose to employ [33].

Management of the infected prostate includes treating discomfort and pain, scrotal elevation, and treating with antibiotics that have appropriate prostate penetration and function against the common urinary pathogens. Stool softeners may be advisable as well. Patients should be alerted to possible complications, including abscess or atypical infections, all of which would require the urologist's intervention. Most patients may be managed as outpatients by the urologist. If a patient presents with signs of sepsis, or has signs of infection with significant comorbidities especially immunocompromise, acute urinary retention, or renal injury, they may be best served by an inpatient hospital stay. The prognosis of acute bacterial prostatitis with aggressive antibiotic therapy and good patient compliance results in 33–60% bacterial cure rates. The more chronic prostate infections are often difficult to treat, and are likely to relapse and require long-term suppressive antibiotics [36].

Antibiotic therapy in male genital system infections in the elderly

Infections of the prostate, testicles, or epididymis in the geriatric population are overwhelmingly due to the usual flora found in urinary infections, which is mainly bowel. The organisms include *E. coli*, *Enterococcus*, Enterobacteriaceae, but can also include Gram-positive organisms and *Pseudomonas*, which may have seeded the prostate from a site other than bowel. Lower UTIs in elderly men should be considered as involving the prostate, as it is likely anatomically that the prostate is seeding the urine, or is being seeded by the urine.

There are particular concerns in considering antibiotic coverage for the infected prostate gland. The healthy prostate has barriers that prevent free dissemination of antibiotics equivalent to the concentrations found in plasma. The prostate tends to be acidic and hence acidic antibiotics have difficulty diffusing into the prostate, while alkaline drugs pass more freely. In the infected and inflamed prostate, however, many of those barriers are less likely to be an impediment [40]. The treatment course of infections of the prostate is generally longer than in other infections – suggested courses can extend to 4–8 weeks for acute prostatitis [33,36,37]. The difficulty of concentrating antibiotic levels in the prostate may be why extended courses help prevent relapse and promote cure.

In the changing milieu of antibiotic resistance, it is important to consider local antibiotic resistance and susceptibility data in selecting the antibiotic for the patient. It is reasonable to begin treatment in the ED with a dose of parenteral antibiotics, if the patient appears ill with systemic signs. Widespectrum oral antibiotics can then follow [41]. Appropriate initial antibiotic regimes can include a combination of penicillin (i.e., ampicillin) and an aminoglycoside (i.e., gentamicin), a second- or third-generation cephalosporin, or one of the fluoroquinolones [37,42]. If outpatient care is the plan, the current optimal choices include fluoroquinolones and trimethoprim-sulfa [37,43]. The rates of resistance to both of these drugs, and extended-spectrum beta-lactamase (EBSL) resistance in the gut flora causing genitourinary infections, are considerations to keep in mind for the patient who is not improving [44,45]. Other issues that complicate antibiotic choice include drug interactions (especially significant in the elderly with polypharmacy) and the side effects of antibiotics. As an example, the fluoroquinolones are associated with tendinopathies and tendon rupture (more common when patients are also on steroids) and QT prolongation – especially of note if patients are on other medications that cause prolongation of the QT interval [46,47]. Also, warfarin is potentiated by a number of antibiotics, including fluoroquinolones, azithromycin, amoxicillin/clavulanate, and isonicotinic acid hydrazide among others [48].

Hematuria

Hematuria is not an uncommon complaint in the aged population. It can be the presenting complaint in problems as diverse as UTI, cancer, and aortic dissection. Although many eventual diagnoses resulting from the complaint of hematuria in the younger population are relatively benign (such as renal stone or infection), many of the diagnostic evaluations of the geriatric patient can reveal cancers, vascular disease, or intrinsic renal disease.

The actual definition of hematuria is the presence of blood in the urine, either macroscopic (visible to naked eye) or microscopic (2–10 red blood cells (RBCs)/high-power field in spun urine sediment) [49]. The first caveat is that a patient who complains of "blood in my urine" must be evaluated to ensure that the source of the blood is actually the urinary system. Complaints of "blood in the urine" may originate from bleeding sources in the vagina or rectum. If clarity of the origin of bleeding is not made with the physical exam, a gentle straight catheterization may be of use and additionally provides a sterile sample for culture. Pseudohematuria can be caused by hemoglobinuria, myoglobinuria, porphyria, or beets, blackberries, rifampin, or phenytoin ingestion [50]. This can be excluded by direct visualization of RBCs under the microscope.

Once the origin of the bleeding is confirmed to be the urinary tract, there are still a number of possible sources for the blood extrinsic to the kidneys, ureters, bladder, and urethra. The bleeding may be due to a hematologic issue, and simply happens to manifest in the urinary tract. Sickle cell or hemophilia is of concern in younger age groups, but in the geriatric age group anticoagulation is more likely. Renal vein thrombosis can cause hematuria. Tumors, especially pelvic tumors, can erode into the urinary tract and cause bleeding. Malignant hypertension or dissection of the aorta into the renal artery are cardiovascular causes of hematuria. Although very rarely patients may receive a first diagnosis of renal stone after the age of 65, this is unusual and should not be accepted as the reason for hematuria at first glance. Other life-threatening causes for hematuria exist in this age group and should be excluded. A classic miss is that of the patient who appears to be presenting with colicky flank pain and hematuria, is given the diagnosis of renal colic/renal stone, but actually has an aortic dissection.

Hematuria can originate from the urinary tract (i.e., the kidneys, ureters, bladder, urethra), and (in the male patient) prostate. Infection is the most common cause for gross hematuria. Other urologic causes include inflammation, malignancy, stones, foreign body, anatomic abnormalities, radiation cystitis resulting from care for other pelvic tumors, and trauma [50]. Renal, ureteral, and bladder tumors may present with hematuria and should be excluded in elderly patients with hematuria.

Important questions on history include the timing of appearance of blood during micturition (initial, throughout, terminal urine, or between voiding) and whether there is dysuria, urinary frequency, or urgency. It is important to ascertain whether there is pain with the bleeding and, if so, when and where – suprapubic pain, unilateral/bilateral flank pain, abdominal pain, back pain – and whether there is radiation of the pain. Other important questions include the following. Is there difficulty in beginning or during micturition? Does this patient have a history of BPH or undergone urologic surgery or instrumentation? Is there a history of hypertension, diabetes, or renal disease? Are there any possibly nephrotoxic drugs taken by the patient? Is there a history of stone disease? Have they had any radiation for a pelvic, prostate, GI, or urologic cancer? Is there a history of coagulopathy? Has there been any recent travel outside the US, such as the Middle East or Africa (which is concerning for schistosomiasis) [49]? Are there associated symptoms of nausea, vomiting, fever, or weight loss?

Pertinent elements of the physical exam include the position of the patient (lying quietly or writhing in pain), vital signs, signs of trauma to urethrogenital area, abdomen, and back, signs of fluid overload such as periorbital edema, pleural effusion or ascites, tenderness in the abdomen or CVA, palpable masses in the abdomen, presence of urethral discharge, or other genital findings.

Lab work should include a urinary analysis. A catheter-collected sample is recommended if there are any perineal lesions, vaginal discharge, bleeding, or doubt as to the origin of the bleeding site. A positive result from the urine dipstick should be confirmed with a formal urinary analysis. The urine should be analyzed for the presence of red blood cells (RBCs) and their morphology, white blood cells, casts, crystals, bacteria, and protein. Abnormal RBC morphology or casts, and proteinuria suggest a glomerular source. Uniform, normal-shaped, or clumped RBCs (microscopic clots) suggest lower urinary tract bleeding [49].

Aged patients, especially those on anticoagulation, merit some blood work in the evaluation of hematuria. Appropriate ED testing includes: 1) checking the renal function with BUN, creatinine, and electrolytes; 2) evaluating for coagulopathy by checking prothrombin time/International Normalized Ratio, partial prothrombin time, and platelets; 3) checking with a CBC for anemia and signs of infection; 4) checking a creatinine phosphokinase (CPK) for muscle breakdown in case the "hematuria" is actually myoglobinuria. Patients can have a multitude of medical reasons for hematuria and nephritis, and may merit other exams in order to begin that evaluation, but these will not determine the cause in the ED.

Useful ED imaging can include an ultrasound evaluating for renal or pelvic masses, hydronephrosis, and abdominal aortic aneurysm [51]. The limits of ultrasound must be considered, especially in the evaluation for arterial dissection. An abdominal or pelvic CT can be used to evaluate for intra-abdominal and retroperitoneal mass, obstruction, stones, aortic aneurysm, and with contrast can evaluate for dissection, tumor, and abscess [49,52]. Some of the pathologies that cause hematuria in the elderly may decrease renal function, so the benefit of contrast in the diagnostic algorithm must be balanced against the risk of nephrotoxicity.

The cause of the bleeding will determine the disposition and care of the patient. The treatment of the illnesses on the differential does not vary according to the age of the patient, but it is of paramount importance to have a higher index of suspicion for the dangerous diagnoses in the geriatric population than in younger age groups.

Eventual referral, either as an inpatient or outpatient, will be to primary care, urology, or nephrology. Nephrolithiasis and urologic tumors require urology consultation or follow-up. Patients with tumors additionally require oncology evaluation. Patients found to have nephritis require nephrology evaluation. Asymptomatic hematuria, if stable, needs primary care physician follow-up for repeat urinalysis within 2 weeks. Gross hematuria with blood clot formation and difficult urination requires urologic consultation if an ED triple-lumen urinary catheter drainage and irrigation is unsuccessful. Most patients can be safely discharged home with necessary follow-up. Some patients require hospital admission, usually due to the etiology of hematuria rather than the hematuria itself.

Phimosis/paraphimosis

Phimosis is the inability to retract the foreskin behind the glans, and can present with dysuria, hematuria, or poor urinary stream. There can be ballooning of the foreskin with urination. Patients, especially diabetics, may present with a concurrent balanitis, presenting challenges in diagnosing the cause of the balanitis (because of access) and treating the glans. The exam of the patient with phimosis may demonstrate a narrowed preputial opening of the foreskin and edema, erythema, and tenderness of the prepuce. There may be cracking of the skin of the prepuce causing the tenderness.

The danger of a phimosis is that the opening permitting urine outflow can sufficiently narrow to cause obstructive uropathy. If there is concern about possible obstruction, it is imperative to check the creatinine for post-renal obstructive failure. A renal ultrasound would show a distended bladder and possibly hydronephrosis in the case of obstructive uropathy. There is merit to checking a glucose level as well, as *Candida* balanitis is often found under the foreskin of diabetics.

Phimosis does not usually require emergent treatment. Recurrent balanitis in the setting of phimosis is an indication for circumcision [53]. Without co-infection or obstruction, appropriate treatment of phimosis alone is a topical steroid to decrease inflammation and increase the pliability of the skin [53]. If there is obstructive uropathy, the obstruction must be relieved with Foley catheter or suprapubic aspiration.

Paraphimosis is congested, edematous foreskin fixed in a retracted position which can cause a tight ring proximal to the glans and then lead to ischemia. The phimotic ring retracts over the glans and is trapped behind the coronal sulcus. It impedes vascular and lymphatic drainage from the glans penis causing edema, and is a surgical emergency. It is very painful for those patients capable of describing their symptoms. Physical exam reveals a retracted foreskin which is unable to be reduced by the patient, with an edematous glans. Risks for paraphimosis include recurrent phimosis, infection, or trauma. Of special note, especially in debilitated patients, another cause of paraphimosis is the failure of health care workers to replace foreskin after catheterization, bathing, or a genital exam.

Paraphimosis is a urologic emergency. The danger of paraphimosis, in addition to obstructive uropathy, is that necrosis of the glans can occur due to constriction of lymphatic and venous drainage and arterial compromise. Reduction must be accomplished urgently, either manually or surgically. It is a painful process, so pain relief should also be in place, either via local blocks (note: no epinephrine in the lidocaine) and/or parenterally, even via conscious sedation.

Reduction success will be improved if the edema can be reduced. Ice may be placed to reduce swelling while preparing for definitive reduction. The penis may be wrapped in elastic bandage or gauze to aid in reduction of the edema. The physician can use a sterile needle to make punctures around the circumference of the swollen foreskin and express edema fluid.

Manual reduction proceeds with steady manual compression applied for a few minutes to reduce the edema. The thumbs compress the glans while fingers pull the foreskin forward over the glans. An alternative method is to grasp the whole penis in the palm of one hand, applying gentle compression then pushing the glans back through the cylinder of fingers with the index finger of the other hand. If manual compression fails, surgical reduction can be accomplished with a dorsal slit through the foreskin, permitting the glans to be reduced. This can be accomplished by the emergency physician, although urologic referral is essential as eventual circumcision may be needed to prevent recurrence of paraphimosis or phimosis due to recurrent balanitis. Patients who have obstructive uropathy, severe infection, ischemia, or necrosis should be considered for hospital admission [54].

Fournier's gangrene

Fournier's gangrene is a life-threatening emergency that can be deceptively subtle, and the geriatric population with their decreased immunity is at higher risk. There is high mortality and morbidity, and a high index of suspicion is needed to detect this illness early for the patient to survive as intact as possible. Fournier's is a progressive infection of the perineum and genitalia that spreads aggressively along fascial planes. The fascia that are typically involved are the superficial perineal fascia (Colles' fascia), then continuing along Buck's and Dartos' fasciae, involving the penis and scrotum, or the anterior abdominal wall via Scarpa's fascia [55]. The treatment is primarily surgical and it is considered a surgical emergency.

Those who are immunocompromised – the elderly, those with diabetes, alcoholism, malignancy, chronic steroid use, HIV, or other issues – are at higher risk. There is rapid progression from cellulitis to blister formation and foul-smelling necrotic lesions. Pain might seem out of proportion to the exam. The patient will frequently have a history of perineal trauma, instrumentation, urethral stricture, or urethral cutaneous fistula.

Fournier's may start as a cellulitis, but early clues that might distinguish it from simple cellulitis include disproportionate fever, systemic toxicity, and exquisite tenderness. The tenderness often extends beyond the borders of erythema. Fournier's commonly starts as cellulitis adjacent to the portal of entry and the skin appearance often underestimates the degree of underlying disease as the infection spreads aggressively along fascial planes [55]. The swelling and crepitus quickly increase and dark purple areas may develop. Progression may involve infection spreading rapidly into the anterior abdominal wall, gluteal muscles, scrotum, and penis. Bullae and skin necrosis are late signs of deep soft tissue destruction.

Fournier's most commonly arises from colorectal, skin, or genitourinary sources. Wound cultures generally yield multiple anaerobic and aerobic organisms which act synergistically to destroy fascial planes. There are on average 4.4 organisms isolated from cultures of necrotizing skin infections such as Fournier's [56]. It is a relatively uncommon illness that occurs most often in middle-aged or older men (85%). Although once thought to involve only men, Fournier's affects women as well, and may be more easily missed as the index of suspicion may be lower [55]. The differential diagnosis includes cellulitis, gas gangrene, pyomyositis, and myositis.

Table 22.5. Calculator tools for Fournier's gangrene: Laboratory Risk Indicator for Necrotizing Fasciitis (LRINEC Score) [57]

Parameter	Points
Serum CRP ≥150 mg/l	4
White blood cell count	
15,000–25,000	1
>25,000	2
Hemoglobin (g/dl)	
11.0–13.5	1
<11.0	2
Serum sodium: <135 mEq/l	2
Serum creatinine: >1.6 mEq/l	2
Serum glucose: >180 mg/dl	1

Total score: ≥6, raise suspicion for necrotizing fasciitis; ≥8, highly predictive for necrotizing fasciitis. CRP, C-reactive protein.

Laboratory findings are generally nonspecific, and blood cultures are of low yield. A set of labs including a CBC, electrolytes, BUN, creatinine, blood glucose, C-reactive protein (CRP), and CPK can be used to create an individual Laboratory Risk Indicator for Necrotizing Fasciitis (LRINEC) score [57] (Table 22.5). Plain films of the abdomen may identify air, and non-contrast CT may show air along fascial planes. Gas is highly specific, but not sensitive (absence of air does not exclude the diagnosis). Imaging should not delay surgical therapy when clinical evidence suggests progressive infection. Surgical exploration is the only way to be certain of the diagnosis and immediate surgical debridement may be indicated. Repeat trips to the operating room for repeated debridement may be necessary [55].

Treatment includes immediate antibiotics with broad coverage against Gram-positive, -negative, and anaerobic organisms. The usual combination includes penicillin (often an extended-spectrum penicillin) for the streptococcal species, third-generation cephalosporin with or without an aminoglycoside for the Gram-negative organisms, plus metronidazole for the anaerobes [58]. There is also benefit to considering adding protein synthesis-inhibiting agents such as clindamycin or linezolid, as these help decrease toxin production [56]. Hydration and tetanus immunization can also be addressed in the ED while rapid surgical and urological consultation is obtained. Hyperbaric oxygen has also been shown to have a useful role as the high oxygen tension it creates has been shown to be toxic to *Clostridium perfringens* [59]. Hyperbaric treatments should be considered after surgical debridement, and may be repeated in conjunction with further debridement. These patients can easily progress to sepsis and septic shock, with multi-organ dysfunction. There is a high mortality rate of 22–40% despite optimal management, and an even higher mortality with colorectal etiology [55].

UTIs

In discussing infections of the urinary tract in the elderly, it is helpful to first clarify some definitions. A UTI can be an infection involving any structure in the urinary system confirmed by a positive culture. This definition can be further subdivided based on the exact location of the infection: urethritis is infection involving the urethra, cystitis is infection involving the bladder, pyelonephritis is infection involving the renal pelvis or parenchyma, and urosepsis is a systemic infection that originates in the urinary system.

"Asymptomatic bacteriuria" is the presence of 100,000 colony-forming units of one uropathogen (growing no more than two species) per milliliter (cfu/ml) in a patient without symptoms in two successive clean-catch midstream samples in women without symptoms, and in men with a single clean-catch midstream sample [60]. Uncomplicated infection is limited to the lower collecting system (bladder and below) in a healthy adult, while a complicated infection is one involving the upper collecting system (kidneys) with systemic symptoms in a patient with comorbidities and/or immunocompromise or structural renal or urinary tract abnormalities. The presence of stone, tumor, bladder neck obstruction, or enlarged prostate can obstruct the urinary tract, leading to a complicated infection, and make the development of pyelonephritis more likely.

Ironically, in the aged population one must be both more and less vigilant in the diagnosis of UTIs than one is in a younger population. In the geriatric population, there is a marked increase in the presence of asymptomatic bacteriuria which does not require treatment [60,61]. This includes positive cultures, but without either signs or symptoms of infection. It also indicates that there is an absence of pyuria or leukoesterase on the urine dipstick, as this is a sign of activated leukocytes. Among the institutionalized elderly, the numbers of cases of incidentally identified asymptomatic bacteriuria are much higher than in the non-institutionalized elderly. In community-dwelling aged, men have a prevalence 6–15% (age >75) of asymptomatic bacteriuria and women older than age 80 have an estimated prevalence of more than 20% [60,62,63]. In long-term care facilities 25–50% of women and 15–40% of men were found to have asymptomatic bacteriuria [62,64]. Yet, there is also an increase in the number of patients that either have decreased sensitivity to symptoms including pyrexia, or among the debilitated aged, a decrease in the ability to convey the specifics of their symptoms [65].

Symptoms in the elderly have a range of presentation. Among community-dwelling functional aged the symptoms can be the same as those found in a younger population: dysuria, frequency, urgency, suprapubic pain, burning on urination, hematuria, foul-smelling urine, or back pain. As the aged can be less specific in their complaints, the signs that the urinary system is infected may not occur until the infection has risen to include the kidneys and the patient presents with fever. The clinical diagnosis of pyelonephritis can be made with evidence of a UTI with fever and flank pain. Among a more debilitated population the symptoms may be more nonspecific and generalized. Patients might present with mental status changes, falls, incontinence, fever, chills, or frank sepsis [65]. They may even present with seemingly unrelated complaints, such as nausea, vomiting, or abdominal pain. Of course, even

in the community-dwelling, otherwise well-compensated elders, infection can alter their system sufficiently that a UTI can present as a mental status change or generalized weakness.

The physical exam findings can be limited and moderately nonspecific. Patients may have mild suprapubic tenderness. Flank pain or CVA tenderness suggests pyelonephritis. Patients presenting to the ED should have a pelvic exam or evaluation of the genitals performed to evaluate for alternative diagnoses. A third of elderly patients with pyelonephritis may not present with fever [66]. Clinical findings often do not distinguish between upper and lower tract infections, and the exam correlates poorly with location of infection [65].

Urinary tract infections are a common problem in the aged population. Infections are most commonly caused by retrograde ascent of fecal bacteria into the urinary system. They may also develop from hematogenous or lymphatic spread into the urinary system. About 80–90% of all UTIs are caused by E. coli, 5–10% by S. saprophyticus [60]. In the elderly (and other immunocompromised patients) there is a greater proportion of infection with otherwise uncommon causes of urinary infections, such as Proteus, Pseudomonas, Klebsiella, Streptococcus, Enterobacter, Clostridium, and Candida [60].

As patients age, the innate defense mechanisms to prevent the colonization of bacteria become less effective. Frequent, complete voiding is the most straightforward of these defenses and it is often impacted in the aged [63]. There are additional risks that increase the likelihood of the geriatric patient having a urine infection. More of the elderly have comorbid conditions that are treated by placement of Foley catheters, or a history of urological surgery. Geriatric patients are more likely to have diabetes, dementia, neurologic disease, or pelvic organ prolapse. Women have decreased estrogen post-menopause, may have cystoceles, may be incontinent, and have sensory changes in the genitals. Additionally genital hygiene may become more difficult for the elderly woman to maintain, creating a more contaminated milieu which may increase the risk of infection by colonic flora.

Testing the urine is the first diagnostic testing step in evaluating the patient with suspected urine infection. The urine sampled can be a clean-catch midstream urine sample. If the patient is catheterized, then ideally the catheter should be replaced and a sample of the fresh urine should be evaluated. If the patient is unable to toilet adequately to get a clean-catch midstream sample, then a straight catheter sample can be taken. The urine dipstick is usually the easiest first test to perform in the ED. The signs of infection are most notably a positive nitrite (which demonstrates that nitrate reductase, a breakdown product of bacterial metabolism, is present) or leukoesterase (which is produced by activated leukocytes) test. The nitrite portion of the test has a specificity of 92–100% and a sensitivity of 25% for infection, and the leukoesterase portion of the test has a specificity ranging from 94 to 98% and sensitivity ranging from 75 to 96% for identifying infection [60,67–69]. It is possible to have a false-positive leukocyte dipstick reaction with imipenem, clavulanic acid, and meropenem, while there can be a false negative with doxycycline, gentamycin, and cephalexin [60]. Be aware that UA may be normal if the urine flow from an infected kidney is obstructed, or if the infection is outside the collecting system. Sterile pyuria can secrete white blood cells in the urine and has multiple causes. On UA, white cell casts are specific for pyelonephritis. A urine culture should be sent from all patients hospitalized and those who return for a failure of cure. Arguably, in the ED it may be prudent to send a culture from patients who lack a primary care provider, but it is imperative to have a system of following those cultures and contacting the patient. For a urine culture the traditional criterion for a positive culture is 100,000 bacterial cfu/ml [60]. Studies such as CT scan or renal urine sampling may be considered if upper tract disease is suspected or if there are alternative diagnoses being considered.

Since there are such high levels of asymptomatic bacteriuria among aged, debilitated institutionalized patients, when these patients are brought to the ED for nonspecific symptoms such as fever, decreased mental status, or other non-direct urologic symptomology, it is imperative to evaluate for other causes of these symptoms rather than being quickly satisfied with the identification of a urine culture positive for bacteria. Also, a urine culture is always of use when urine is suspected as being the cause of infection. It is imperative, however, to understand that a positive culture alone is not an adequate reason to treat the urine as the cause of infection in the elderly [60,65]. It is the recommendation of the Infectious Disease Society of America (IDSA) not to obtain urine cultures in febrile residents of long-term care facilities unless either nitrate or leukocyte esterase is positive on dipstick [70]. This is especially true of patients with indwelling urinary catheters. It is important that catheters be avoided unless absolutely necessary, that strict sterile precautions be used in placing the catheters, and that catheters are removed as soon as no longer needed.

Imaging is not necessary to diagnose pyelonephritis, but is recommended when the diagnosis is not clear or to diagnose complications in patients who do not respond promptly to treatment. In the more debilitated patient, imaging may be needed to identify the location of the infection. Always consider imaging male patients, as obstructive pathology is often present and complicates the treatment [63]. An ultrasound may show an enlarged kidney, hypoechoic parenchyma, and compressed collecting system consistent with hydronephrosis. A CT scan with IV contrast may show enlarged kidney(s), attenuated parenchyma, and/or fat stranding. It is advisable to check renal function through serum levels of BUN and creatinine in the aged. Blood cultures are only recommended with suspected hematogenous etiology or immunocompromised patients, although it must be noted that there are subpopulations of those over 65 who qualify as immunocompromised based on age.

The issues in treatment include decisions about antimicrobial agent, length of treatment course, the need for inpatient or outpatient care, and the need for any other modalities of treatment, especially in complicated infections. As an example, an infected, obstructed kidney may need to be urgently stented or drained by the urological service. Obstruction in the setting of infection should be relieved. Another example is having a Foley passed in obstruction due to BPH. Pyridium, a bladder anesthetic, may be prescribed for patients who are suffering from severe symptoms of dysuria, frequency, and urgency.

The choice of antimicrobial agent must take into account the local resistance patterns of the patient population. Although ciprofloxacin and trimethoprim-sulfamethoxazole have been commonly used agents, there is unfortunately a growing rate of resistance to these agents. If resistance rates locally are more than 20%, another agent should be selected. Macrodantin is commonly used if an outpatient regimen is possible, but it must be recalled that macrodantin is bacteriostatic and not bacteriocidal so that the course of the antibiotic must be extended. In an era of growing resistance patterns, the presence of ESBL-producing uropathogens that may well not be identified without a culture makes it especially important to obtain a culture before instigating antibiotics. These generally require parenteral antibiotics and appropriately can involve a consult for infectious disease. It is also important to consider the patient's current medications when choosing an antibiotic, as many interact with other medications, especially coumadin [60]. If the infection has progressed to sepsis or pyelonephritis with additional symptoms (vomiting, systemic signs of progressive illness, pain) and is now a systemic infection, parenteral antibiotics should be chosen.

The course of antimicrobial treatment for urine infections can range from single-dose treatment to multiple weeks of treatment. There is a balance to be struck between the side effects of extended antibiotic courses and the cure rate of the infection. As per the Cochrane Collaboration, for uncomplicated, symptomatic lower UTIs in elderly women, the recommendations are that a 3–6-day course of antibiotics be prescribed [71]. Of note, nitrofurantoin, which is bacteriostatic and not bactericidal, is at the upper end of this course of treatment [71].

The essence of the management plan of upper tract infections is based on distinguishing between uncomplicated and complicated pyelonephritis. Uncomplicated pyelonephritis is composed of a typical pathogen in an immunocompetent host with normal renal anatomy and function. These patients may be discharged on an oral regimen of antibiotics with appropriate follow-up. Most patients with uncomplicated pyelonephritis are successfully treated on an outpatient, oral regimen.

Complicated pyelonephritis patients will include many of the geriatric age group as this includes the immunosuppressed patient. Also of note, diabetics and those with either structural abnormalities of the genitourinary tract or a prolonged course of illness also qualify. As mortality is higher in men, especially men older than 65 years old, some experts consider all pyelonephritis occurring in men to be complicated [72]. Patients with complicated pyelonephritis are treated as inpatients, begun on parenteral antibiotics, and can be switched to oral therapy if improving in 48–72h [73]. In selecting the antimicrobial agent, it is imperative to always consider local bacterial sensitivities. Urology consultation is indicated for complicated pyelonephritis.

Complications of pyelonephritis include acute bacterial nephritis, which may be focal or multifocal. It is more common in diabetics and can be identified via CT scan with IV contrast demonstrating wedge-shaped areas of decreased enhancement, which likely represents the early stage of abscess formation. Emphysematous pyelonephritis is another complication which is defined as a necrotizing infection by gas-forming organisms. It is almost solely found in diabetics or patients with a mechanical urinary obstruction, and can present with pneumaturia. The mortality is 19–43% and it is considered a surgical emergency [74]. Renal abscess is more likely to occur in those with urinary stasis, kidney stones, neurogenic bladder, or diabetes. Ultrasound may show a low-density lesion with increased transmission, and a CT scan with contrast may show an area or areas of decreased attenuation. Later in the progression of the disease, a higher-attenuation ring around the abscess can be visualized. The treatment may require percutaneous drainage by urology in addition to IV antibiotics [75].

Clear indications for hospital admission include sepsis or any signs of hemodynamic instability, signs of complicated pyelonephritis or complications of pyelonephritis, patients who are unable to tolerate oral feeding and medications, a failure of oral outpatient antibiotics, patients who are immunocompromised, or patients who have worsening renal function. A conservative approach is necessary in patients with one kidney or abnormalities of the collecting system – especially those that cause a urinary tract obstruction. These can be internal to the renal/genitourinary system such as BPH, obstructing calculi, or following hydronephrosis due to external compression (often from tumor, but can also be due to uterine prolapse). It is appropriate to consider admission for patients who are more frail, who have poor social support, history of non-adherence to prescribed treatments, or uncertain access to medications or outpatient care.

Summary

The physiological and anatomical changes related to aging have important implications. To borrow from pediatricians, as children are not always "little adults," geriatric patients are not always just "older adults." Changes in the genital and renal systems may be particularly hidden unless sought out, as there are such societal pressures that mitigate against inquiries into the sexual health and activity of the elderly. The elderly renal system can disguise much renal damage until a stress is put upon the system, such as a drug with renal toxicity or muscle breakdown products, a stress that younger kidneys can handle and maintain normal function. Emergency physicians should be aware of the anatomic and physiologic changes impacting the elderly.

Pearls and pitfalls

Pearls

- A gynecological exam in the elderly patient can be well worth the challenge of doing the exam because of the pathology it can reveal.
- Balanitis can be a sign of high glucose, and can be the presenting sign of a new-onset diabetic.
- The elderly with mental status changes can present with infection. Less obvious sources can include the prostate in men and the genital tract in women.

- Epididymitis and orchitis should lead one to consider that the prostate might also be infected.

Pitfalls

- It cannot be assumed that a normal creatinine means a "normal" kidney in the elderly: a creatinine within the normal range may be so only because of the reduced muscle mass of the elderly patient. This can be especially important when giving a medication that has the potential of renal toxicity.
- The cold and flu season gives the opportunity to cause male patients with controlled BPH to go into retention with various medications ranging from inhalers to diphenhydramine.
- It has been shown that the elderly are overtreated for UTI. There are many cases of asymptomatic bacteriuria in the elderly that do not require treatment. Do not always count on the urine being the answer. If nitrites and leukoesterase are negative, complete the search in order not to miss the real infection.
- Do not mistakenly think all red urine is hematuria. Some food (beets, berries), medications (NSAIDs, phenytoin, rifampin), and diseases (rhabdomyolysis) can turn urine red.

References

1. Wiggins J, Patel SR. Changes in kidney function. In *Hazzard's Geriatric Medicine and Gerontology*, 6th edn, ed. Hazzard WR (McGraw-Hill Medical Publishing Division, 2009).

2. Wharram B, Goyal M, Wiggins J et al. Podocyte depletion causes glomerulosclerosis. Diphtheria toxin induced podocyte depletion in rats expressing the human DTR transgens. *J Am Soc Nephrol.* 2005;16:2941–52.

3. Abdel-Kader, K Palevsky PM. Acute kidney injury in the elderly. *Clin Geriatric Med.* 2009;25:331–58.

4. Lewiss RE, Saul T, Teng J. Gynecological disorders in geriatric emergency medicine. *Am J Hospice Palliative Med.* 2009;26:219–27.

5. Kvale JN, Kvale JK. Common gynecological problems after age 75. *Postgrad Med.* 1993;93:263–8; 271–2.

6. Tenover JL. Sexuality, sexual function, androgen therapy and the aging male. In *Hazzard's Geriatric Medicine and Gerontology*, 6th edn, ed. Hazzard WR (McGraw-Hill Medical Publishing Division, 2009).

7. DuBeau CE. Benign prostate disorders. In *Hazzard's Geriatric Medicine and Gerontology*, 6th edn, ed. Hazzard WR (McGraw-Hill Medical Publishing Division, 2009).

8. AUA Practice Guidelines Committee. AUA guideline on management of benign prostatic hyperplasia (2003). Chapter 1: Diagnosis and treatment recommendations. *J Urol.* 2003;170(2 Pt 1):530–47.

9. Wilson MMG. Sexually transmitted diseases. *Clin Geriatr Med.* 2003;19:637–55.

10. Mehta RL, Kellum JA, Shah SV. Acute Kidney Injury Network: report of an initiative to improve outcomes in acute kidney injury. *Crit Care.* 2007;11(2):R31.

11. Choudhury D, Ahmed Z. Drug-associated renal dysfunction and injury. *Nature Clin Pract Nephrol.* 2006;2;80–91.

12. Del Veccio L, Locatelli F. Ethical issues in the elderly with renal disease. *Clin Geriatr Med.* 2009;543–53.

13. Miller KL, Griebling TL. Gynocological disorders. In *Hazzard's Geriatric Medicine and Gerontology*, 6th edn, ed. Hazzard WR (McGraw-Hill Medical Publishing Division, 2009).

14. Romanzi LJ, Chaikin DC, Blaivas JG. The effect of genital prolapse on voiding. *J Urol.* 1999;161:581–6.

15. Cooper T, Smith OM. Gynecologic disorders in the elderly. In *Brocklehurst's Textbook of Geriatric Medicine and Gerontology*, 7th edn, ed. Fillit HM, Rockwood K, Woodhouse K (Philadelphia, PA: Saunders Elsevier Press, 2010).

16. Thorne MB, Geraci SA. Acute urinary retention in elderly men. *Am J Med.* 2009;122:815–19.

17. Selius BA, Subedi R. Urinary retention in adults: diagnosis and initial management. *Am Fam Physician.* 2008;77:643–50.

18. Edwards JL. Diagnosis and management of benign prostatic hyperplasia. *Am Fam Physician.* 2008;77:1403–10.

19. Micromedex® Evidence/Health Care Series [intranet database] (Greenwood Village, CO: Thomson Health Care, 2009).

20. American Urological Association. *Guideline on the Management of Benign Prostatic Hyperplasia (BPH)* (accessed January 2, 2013 from www.auanet.org/guidelines/bph.cfm).

21. Tseng TY, Stoller ML. Obstructive uropathy. *Clin Geriatr Med.* 2009;25:437–43.

22. Mundy, AR. Management of urethral strictures. *Postgrad Med J.* 2006;82(970):489–93.

23. Lisboa C, Ferreira A, Resende C, Rodrigues AC. Infectious balanoposthitis: management, clinical and laboratory features. *Int J Dermatol.* 2009;48:121–4.

24. Das S, Tunuguntla HSGR. Balanitis xerotica obliterans – a review. *World J Urol.* 2000;18:382–7.

25. Buechner SA. Common skin disorders of the penis. *BJU International.* 2002;90:498–506.

26. US Department of Health and Human Services, Centers for Disease Control and Prevention. *Sexually Transmitted Diseases Treatment Guidelines, 2010: Diseases Characterized by Urethritis and Cervicitis* (accessed September 26, 2012 from www.cdc.gov/std/treatment/2010/urethritis-and-cervicitis.htm#urethritis).

27. US Department of Health and Human Services, Centers for Disease Control and Prevention, Division of STD Prevention. *Sexually Transmitted Disease Surveillance 2009, 2010* (accessed September 26, 2012 from www.cdc.gov/std/stats09/).

28. Lai AY, Lu SH, Yu HJ, Kuo YC, Huang CY. Tuberculous epididymitis presenting as huge scrotal tumor. *Urology.* 2009;73:1163e5–7.

29. Park KW, Park BK, Kim CK. Chronic tuberculous epididymo-orchitis manifesting as a non-tender scrotal swelling: magnetic resonance imaging-histological correlation. *Urology.* 2008;71:755.e5–7.

30. Davol P, Simmons J. Testicular torsion in a 68 year old man. *Urology.* 2005;66:195–7.

31. Centers for Disease Control and Prevention. *Sexually Transmitted Diseases. Treatment Guidelines 2006. Epididymitis* (accessed September 26, 2012 from www.cdc.gov/std/treatment/2010/epididymitis.htm).

32. Gasparich JP, Mason JT, Green HL, et al. Amiodarone-associated epididymitis: drug-related epididymitis in the absence of infection. *J Urol.* 1985;133:971–2.

33. Lummus WE, Thompson I. Prostatitis. *Emerg Med Clin North Am.* 2001;19:691–706.

34. Krieger JN, Riley DE, Cheah PY, et al. Epidemiology of prostatitis, new evidence for a worldwide problem. *World J Urol.* 2003;21:70–4.

35. Kreiger JN, Nyberg L Jr, Nickel JC. NIH consensus definition and classification of prostatitis. *JAMA.* 1999;282:236–7.

36. Tran KB, Wessels H. Genital and infectious emergencies: Prostatitis, urethritis and epididymo-orchitis. In *Urologic Emergencies: A Practical Guide*, ed. Wessels, H, McAninch, JW (Totowa, NJ: Humana Press Inc., 2005).

37. Ludwig M. Diagnosis and therapy of acute prostatitis, epididymitis and orchitis. *Andrologia.* 2008;40:76–80.

38. Litwin MS, McNaughton-Collins M, Fowler FJ, et al. The National Institutes of Health chronic prostatitis symptom index: development and validation of a new outcome measure. *J Urol.* 1999;162:369–75.

39. Kreiger JN. Prostatitis revisited: new definitions, new approaches. *Infect Dis Clin North Am.* 2003;17:395–409.

40. Nickel JC. Prostatitis and related conditions, orchitis, and epididymitis. In *Campbell-Walsh Urology*, 10th edn, ed. Wein AJ, Kavoussi LR, Novick AC, et al. (Mosby, PA: Elsevier Saunders, 2012).

41. Becopoulos T, Georgoulias D, Constantinides C, et al. Acute prostatitis: which antibiotic to use first. *J Chemother.* 1990;2(4):244–6.

42. Benway BM, Moon TD. Bacterial prostatitis. *Urol Clin North Am.* 2008;35:23–32.

43. Wagenlehner FM, Weidner W, Naber KG. Therapy for prostatitis, with emphasis on bacterial prostatitis. *Expert Opin Pharmacother.* 2007;8:1667–74.

44. Ekici S, Cengiz M, Turan G, Alis EE. Fluoroquinolone-resistant acute prostatitis requiring hospitalization after transrectal prostate biopsy: effect of previous fluoroquinolones use as prophylaxis or long-term treatment. *Int Urol Nephrol.* 2012;44:19–27.

45. Ozden E, Bostanci Y, Yakupoglu KY, et al. Incidence of acute prostatitis caused by extended-spectrum B lactamase-producing *Escherichia coli* after transrectal prostate biopsy. *Urology.* 2009:119–23.

46. van der Linden PD, Sturkenboom MC, Herings RM, Leufkens HG, Stricker BH. Fluoroquinolones and risk of Achilles tendon disorders: case-control study. *BMJ.* 2002;324(7349):1306.

47. Briasoulis A, Agarwal V, Pierce WJ. QT prolongation and torsade de pointes induced by fluoroquinolones: infrequent side effects from commonly used medications. *Cardiology.* 2011;120:103–10.

48. Holbrook AM, Pereira JA, Labris R, et al. Systematic overview of warfarin and its drug and food interactions. *Arch Intern Med.* 2005;165:1095–106.

49. Cohen RA, Brown RS. Clinical practice. Microscopic hematuria. *N Engl J Med.* 2003;348(23):2330–8.

50. Margulis V, Sagalowsky AI. Assessment of hematuria. *Med Clin North Am.* 2011;95(2):153–9.

51. O'Connor OJ, McSweeney SE, Maher MM. Imaging of hematuria. *Radiol Clin North Am.* 2008;46(1):113–32.

52. Rucker CM, Menias CO, Bhalla S. Mimics of renal colic: Alternative diagnoses at unenhanced helical CT. *Radiographics.* 2004;24:S11–33.

53. Fakjian N, Hunter S, Cole GW, et al. An argument for circumcision: prevention of balanitis in the adult. *Arch Dermatol*. 1990;126:1046–7.

54. Williams JC, Morrison PM, Richardson JR. Paraphimosis in elderly men. *Am J Emerg Med*. 1995;13:351–3.

55. Black PC, Wessells H. Fournier's gangrene. In *Urologic Emergencies: A Practical Guide*, ed. Wessels H, McAninch JW (Totowa, NJ: Humana Press Inc., 2005).

56. May AK, Stafford RE, Bulger EM, et al. Treatment of complicated skin and soft tissue infections. *Surgical Infections*. 2009;5:467–49.

57. Wong CH, Khin LW, Heng KS et al. The LRINEC (Laboratory Risk Indicator for Necrotizing Fasciitis) score: a tool for distinguishing necrotizing fasciitis from other soft tissue infections. *Crit Care Med*. 2004;32(7):1535.

58. Thwaini A, Khan A, Malik A, et al. Fournier's gangrene and its emergency management. *Postgrad Med J*. 2006;82:516–19.

59. Hollabaugh RS, Dmochowski RR, Hickerson WL, Cox CE. Fournier's gangrene: therapeutic impact of hyperbaric oxygen. *Plast Reconstr Surg*. 1998;1:94–100.

60. Matthews SJ, Lancaster JW. Urinary tract infections in the elderly population. *Am J Geriatr Pharmacother*. 2011;9:286–309.

61. Nicolle LE, Bradley SF, Colgan R, et al. Infectious Diseases Society of America Guidelines for the treatment of asymptomatic bacteriuria in adults. *Clin Infect Dis*. 2005;40:643–5.

62. Van Duin D. Diagnostic challenges and opportunities in older adults with infectious diseases. *Clin Infect Dis*. 2012;54:973–8.

63. Nicolle LE. Urinary tract infections. In *Hazzard's Geriatric Medicine and Gerontology*, 6th edn, ed. Hazzard WR (McGraw-Hill Medical Publishing Division, 2009).

64. Nicolle LE. Urinary infections in the elderly: symptomatic or asymptomatic? *Int J Antimicrobial Agents*. 1999;11:265–8.

65. Beveridge LA, Davey PG, Phillips G, et al. Optimal management of urinary tract infections in older people. *Clin Interventions Aging*. 2011;6:173–80.

66. Walker S, McGeer A, Simor AE, et al. Why are antibiotics prescribed for asymptomatic bacteriuria in institutionalized elderly people? A qualitative study of physicians' and nurses' perceptions. *CMAJ*. 2000;163:273–7.

67. Wilson ML, Gaido L. Laboratory diagnosis of urinary tract infections in adult patients. *Clin Infect Dis*. 2004;38:1150–8.

68. Pappas PG. Laboratory in the diagnosis and management of urinary tract infections. *Med Clin North Am*. 1991;75:313–25.

69. Rahn DD, Boreham MK, Allen KE, et al. Predicting bacteriuria in urogynecology patients. *Am J Obstet Gynecol*. 2005;192:1376–8.

70. High KP, Bradley SF, Gravenstein S, et al. Clinical practice guideline for the evaluation of fever and infection in older adult residents of long term care facilities: 2008 update by the Infectious Diseases Society of America. *Clin Infect Dis*. 2009;48:149–71.

71. Lutters M, Vogt-Ferrier NB. Antibiotic duration for treating uncomplicated, symptomatic lower urinary tract infections in elderly women (review). *Cochrane Database Syst. Rev*. 2008;3:CD001535.

72. Efstathiou SP, Pefanis AV, Tsioulos DI, et al. Acute pyelonephritis in adults: Prediction of mortality and failure of treatment. *Arch Intern Med*. 2003;163(10):1206–12.

73. Ramakrishnan K, Scheid DC. Diagnosis and management of acute pyelonephritis in adults. *Am Fam Physician*. 2005;71:933–42.

74. Pontin A, Barnes RD. Current management of emphysematous pyelonephritis. *Nat Rev Urol*. 2009;6:272–9.

75. Rubenstein JN, Schaeffer AJ. Managing complicated urinary tract infections: The urologic view. *Infect Dis Clin North Am*. 2003: 333–51.

Chapter

23

Rheumatologic and orthopedic emergencies in the elderly

Peter J. Gruber and Chris Chauhan

Rheumatologic emergencies in the elderly

Rheumatologic diseases are common causes of disability in the elderly but may not be diagnosed initially due to the patient's co-existing medical problems [1]. If the problem is recognized, it is often undertreated because of concern for the adverse effects of medications on this population. Therefore, it is important for the emergency physician to be familiar with these problems in the elderly and what options exist for initial treatment.

With 50% of people over 65 years old estimated to have arthritis, musculoskeletal problems are the most frequent complaint and most common cause of chronic disability and loss of independence in the elderly population [1,2].

Certain rheumatologic diseases such as polymyalgia rheumatica, pseudogout, spinal stenosis, and osteoporosis commonly have their onset when the patient is elderly while others such as gout, osteoarthritis, and rheumatoid arthritis generally start when the patient is younger and progress as the patient ages. Septic arthritis can occur at any age but is most common in the very young and the very old.

Septic arthritis

Acute non-gonococcal septic arthritis (SA) is a medical emergency that can rapidly lead to joint destruction as well as sepsis and death if the infectious arthritis is not recognized and properly treated early in its course. Owing to a higher rate of comorbidities and less physiological reserve, morbidity and mortality from joint infections are significantly higher in the elderly compared with the younger patient [3]. Irreversible loss of joint function is common and there is a 10–49% mortality due to sepsis in elderly patients with SA [4]. Gonococcal arthritis is much less aggressive and is rare in patients over 40 years old.

In the elderly, there is often a significant delay in the diagnosis of SA because the majority of these patients have chronic joint disease, and the clinician may attribute the complaints and findings to flare-ups of pre-existing chronic arthritis [4,5]. Therefore, in the patient with underlying joint disease it is important to get a history as to whether their current presentation is out of proportion to their baseline arthritis.

The diagnosis of SA in the elderly is also difficult because they may have an atypical presentation of the disease. Elderly patients with SA frequently are not febrile, do not have a leukocytosis, and have a more indolent course in their initial presentation to the hospital. The difficulty in making the diagnosis results in a mean 24-day delay in the elderly as compared with 3–12 days' delay in unselected patients [4,5].

The presence of prosthetic joints greatly increases the chances of joint infection and is responsible for a large part of infectious arthritis seen in the elderly. Acute prosthetic joint infections usually occur in the first 3 months after implantation of the device and present with severe pain, swelling, erythema, and warmth of the affected joint. Prosthetic infections with less virulent organisms may present months to years after the operation and have a more subtle presentation. These chronic infections are difficult to diagnose as they may only present with localized pain and no significant findings. X-rays in chronic infections generally show loosening of the prosthesis at the bone, but this loosening may occur without infection [6]. Arthrocentesis is often necessary to make the diagnosis, but in the face of a prosthetic device this procedure is usually done by the orthopedist.

Risk factors for SA include advancing age, diabetes mellitus, rheumatoid arthritis (RA), osteoarthritis (OA), oral steroids, recent trauma, skin ulceration, recent joint surgery, joint aspiration or injection, and hip or knee prosthesis [4,5]. Pre-existing joint disease, predominantly RA and OA, was found in approximately two-thirds of elderly patients with SA [4–6].

History

Septic arthritis generally presents with a history of up to 2 weeks of a progressively more painful and swollen joint [3]. The condition commonly involves larger joints such as the knee, hip, ankle, and shoulder, but any joint can be involved. Although SA generally involves only one joint, up to 22% of adult patients with septic joints have polyarticular involvement [7]. When multiple joints are infected, the patient usually has a history of chronic joint involvement and a worse outcome is anticipated [4,8].

Geriatric Emergency Medicine, ed. Joseph H. Kahn, Brendan G. Magauran Jr., and Jonathan S. Olshaker. Published by Cambridge University Press.
© Cambridge University Press 2014.

Physical

The joint is generally very swollen, erythematous, warm, and tender and has very restricted range of motion. Fever and leukocytosis are often not present in the elderly patient, and subtle and nonspecific signs such as confusion or decline in function may be the only indication of sepsis [3].

Diagnostic tests

Patients with SA often will have an elevated erythrocyte sedimentation rate (ESR) or C-reactive protein (CRP). However, these tests are not sufficiently sensitive to reliably rule out the presence of a septic joint, particularly in patients with a low-virulence chronic infection [3,6,9–11].

Given the low sensitivity of the patient's history, physical exam, and lab tests in detecting a septic joint, arthrocentesis with synovial fluid analysis is the best diagnostic tool available [11]. Although it is taught that patients with septic joints will have a synovial fluid white blood cell count (WBC) >50,000 cells/mm³, more than one-third of adult patients with SA have synovial WBC below this value with 10% <10,000 cells/mm³ [10]. Additionally, there is considerable overlap between inflammatory and infectious arthritis, with inflammatory arthritides such as gout and RA often having WBC >50,000 cells/mm [3,4].

Although it is commonly held that patients with SA have synovial polymorphonuclear leukocytes (PMNs) ≥90%, more than one-quarter of patients with SA have synovial PMNs below this number. Lowering the PMN cutoff to 75% avoids missing SA but decreases the specificity of the test [12].

Leukocyte count cutoffs for septic arthritis in prosthetic joint infections are significantly lower than in native joint infections. A synovial fluid count of 17,000 cells/mm³ with neutrophils of more than 65% is considered positive for a prosthetic knee infection [13].

Synovial fluid glucose and protein have not been shown to be sensitive for septic arthritis. Synovial lactate levels have been shown in several studies to have a high sensitivity and/or high specificity and may have value in discriminating SA from other causes of arthritis [9,11,12,14].

Gram stains and cultures should be done on all fluid to help detect whether there is a bacterial infection and what kind of infection it is. However, Gram stains are only positive in 50% of cases of SA while synovial fluid culture is only positive in 82–90% [4,9]. Direct inoculation of synovial fluid into an adult or pediatric blood culture bottle at the bedside improves the likelihood of diagnosing bacterial infection [9,15].

It is generally safe to aspirate or inject a joint if the International Normalized Ratio (INR) is <2.5, though aspirating a deep joint such as the hip with an elevated INR should be avoided as compression of the joint after the injection would be difficult [16]. Given the difficulty in diagnosing SA in the patient with a prosthetic hip or knee, orthopedics should be consulted when these patients present with pain in the joint even years after the surgery.

Differential

The joint fluid should also be examined by polarizing light microscopy for negatively birefringent crystals (gout) or for positively birefringent crystals (pseudogout) to evaluate for crystalline joint disease. However, both crystalline and bacterial infection can occur together – they are not mutually exclusive [17]. Rheumatoid arthritis, endocarditis, and viral arthritis are also in the differential for acute SA while Lyme arthritis and, in the immunocompromised patient, fungal and mycobacterial arthritis are in the differential for chronic SA [4].

Treatment

Although *Staphylococcus* and *Streptococcus* are the most common pathogens in SA in all ages, Gram-negative bacilli are common in the elderly and broad coverage should be provided [3,5,9].

Disposition

As none of the tests on synovial fluid are particularly sensitive for excluding bacterial infection, treatment should be started if clinical suspicion is high. In view of the morbidity and mortality of septic SA in the elderly patient, these patients should be admitted to the hospital at least until synovial fluid cultures return. As cultures can miss at least 10% of patients with SA, patients with negative cultures may continue to be treated if clinical suspicion remains high.

Pearls and pitfalls

In order not to miss this diagnosis in the elderly, it is important to consider SA in any elderly patient presenting with new atraumatic joint inflammation or worsening of their baseline monoarticular or polyarticular joint involvement, and to err on the side of doing arthrocentesis whenever there is any doubt in the diagnosis.

Gout

Gout is the most common inflammatory arthritis in the elderly [18]. It is triggered by uric acid crystals deposited in the synovial fluid. Although it is common in middle-aged men, it increases in frequency in women after menopause, particularly in elderly women taking diuretics [16,17]. Accurate diagnosis and treatment of gout is important, as early intervention can minimize the functional decline that occurs with this disease in the elderly.

Diuretics and aspirin increase the renal absorption of uric acid and the increased use of these medications, along with an increase in longevity and the incidence of hypertension, obesity, metabolic syndrome, and kidney disease, is believed to account for the greatly increased prevalence of gout in both young and old [18,19].

Gout is typically a progressive disease advancing from asymptomatic hyperuricemia to intermittent flares with remission to a more chronic problem. Chronic gout may lead to the development of tophi, most commonly in the upper extremities. Tophi, which over time cause destruction of bone and cartilage, have a much earlier onset and more extensive distribution in the elderly [18,19].

During periods of remission, uric acid crystals may continue to increase and cause periarticular destruction, chronic synovitis, formation of tophi, and urate nephrolithiasis [19]

Therefore, it is important for the patient to be followed by their doctor and take urate-lowering medications during periods when the condition is in remission, in order to prevent the destructive sequelae of the disease.

History

The initial attack is most often monoarticular and it classically involves the first metatarsophalangeal joint. Over time, if untreated, gout may become polyarticular with the ankle, knee, and wrist being most commonly involved. However, the initial attack in the elderly may be less severe and have a polyarticular onset with hand involvement. Elderly women, particularly those with renal disease on diuretics, are most likely to have an initial polyarticular presentation [18].

The acute phase is typically marked by the quick onset of severe swelling and exquisite pain, with maximum severity occurring over several hours. The acute flare may last 1–2 days, with more severe attacks lasting 1–2 weeks [20].

Physical

Patients may present with a hot, swollen, red joint that is exquisitely tender. The inflammation may extend beyond the joint into the soft tissue and appear to be cellulitis or tenosynovitis. The patient may also have fever, chills, malaise, and the presence of tophi [19].

Diagnostic tests

As most patients with hyperuricemia are asymptomatic and patients with gout may have normal to low uric acid at the time of their attack, urate levels are neither sensitive nor specific in the diagnosis of acute gouty arthritis. The typical X-ray findings of well-demarcated erosions are generally not seen until 6–12 years after onset of the disease [21].

Differential

When the elderly patient has a polyarticular or indolent presentation of gout, it may make diagnosis difficult and gout may be mistaken for RA or OA. The tophi of gout may be mistaken for rheumatoid nodules. Tophi can be superimposed on the bony nodes of the hand and be mistaken for OA [18].

The main question when seeing a patient with a swollen and tender joint is whether he/she has a septic joint. If the pain and swelling is over the metatarsophalangeal joint and the patient has had the same pain and swelling in this location before, septic joint is less likely. However, if there is reasonable suspicion for SA, particularly in a first-time presentation, joint aspiration should be performed and synovial fluid cell count with differential, culture, and search for crystals carried out.

Treatment

Non-pharmacologic therapy includes application of ice packs over the joint, as well as elevation and resting of the affected joint. Response to ice packs may be useful to help distinguish gout from other inflammatory arthritides, as in one study only patients with gout reported relief of pain with topical ice [21].

Nonsteroidal anti-inflammatory drugs (NSAIDs), if not contraindicated, should be started as early as possible after the attack has started. If NSAIDs are ineffective or not tolerated, systemic or intra-articular corticosteroids may be used. Caution should be used with chronic steroid use in patients with diabetes or severe osteoporosis. Intra-articular injections of depot corticosteroid can be very effective if one or two joints are involved; this approach avoids the systemic effects of oral medications [19]. Local steroid injection is contraindicated if cloudy fluid is withdrawn or there is any suspicion of SA. In the elderly, colchicine may be used at lower doses to avoid vomiting and diarrhea if NSAIDs and steroids are contraindicated and the patient does not have renal or hepatic impairment [19,20].

Once pain is alleviated, prevention of future attacks may be addressed. Dietary practices may be modified to reduce the meat and fish intake and increase dairy products. As an outpatient, the patient's medications which increase urate may be replaced by those which lower uric acid. In patients with recurrent attacks or signs of chronic gout such as tophi or X-ray findings, medications used specifically to lower urate – such as allopurinol – should be started as an outpatient but not in the ED [19,20]. These chronic agents should neither be stopped nor initiated during an acute attack as this may exacerbate the condition [22].

Disposition

Since there may be overlap between the cell count found in gout and a septic joint, those patients with borderline synovial fluid WBC counts will need to be admitted for intravenous (IV) antibiotics until culture results return. Additionally, the elderly patient should be admitted if the results of the aspiration point to gout but the patient has a high fever, leukocytosis, confusion, or appears ill.

Pearls and pitfalls

A history of intermittent pain and swelling returning to normal in between attacks is typical of gout. Diagnosis of gout is made by the presence of negatively birefringent intracellular crystals, but SA may be present simultaneously with acute gout [17].

Pseudogout

Pseudogout is the most common monoarticular arthritis in the elderly but may present with polyarticular involvement [23,24]. It is an inflammatory arthritis caused by the deposition of calcium pyrophosphate crystals in the synovial fluid.

Chondrocalcinosis is the radiologic presence of calcium pyrophosphate in the hyaline or fibrocartilage of the joint space. Chondrocalcinosis is seen in 60% of the population over age 85 and has a strong association and overlap with osteoarthritis [20]. Although calcium pyrophosphate depositions are generally asymptomatic, pseudogout develops when the crystals create an inflammatory synovitis. It is associated with hypothyroidism and hyperparathyroidism in addition to osteoarthritis [23].

Unlike gout which may occur at a younger age, pseudogout is predominantly a disease of the elderly and is rarely seen in younger patients. It may present as an acute or chronic arthritis [20].

History

Pseudogout presents very similarly to gout but the onset is more gradual, over 6 hours to several days. The patient complains of severe swelling and pain in the shoulder, knee, or wrist and may report morning stiffness.

Physical

The patient has a very swollen, tender, red, and warm joint. Patients with pseudogout often have joint swelling, crepitus, and other signs of osteoarthritis. Most episodes are benign but elderly patients may present with systemic features including a high fever, chills, confusion, leukocytosis, and appear quite ill [20].

Diagnostic tests

Most patients with pseudogout have chondrocalcinosis, but most patients with chondrocalcinosis are asymptomatic [20].

Treatment

Treatment is not different than for gout except that there is no medication to prevent future flares or the development of chronic pseudogout.

Differential

Diagnosis is more difficult when multiple joints are involved. It should be considered in the differential when an elderly patient has findings suggesting RA but who is seronegative for RA. A patient with a very painful, red, and swollen shoulder is more likely to have pseudogout than gout, as gout rarely involves the shoulder.

Disposition

Elderly patients should be admitted until cultures return if there is suspicion of SA. The elderly patient who is presumed to have pseudogout but who has a high fever, significant leukocytosis, confusion, or does not look well should also be admitted for observation and treatment.

Pearls and pitfalls

As with gout, joint aspiration should be performed if there is reasonable suspicion for the diagnosis of SA. The presence of chondrocalcinosis on X-ray in an elderly patient probably will not be helpful as there is a good chance that this is an incidental finding rather than a sign of pseudogout.

Rheumatoid arthritis

Although rheumatoid arthritis can present at any age, it is increasingly becoming a disease of the elderly as patients with RA are living longer, and elderly patients develop new-onset RA [24].

Rheumatoid arthritis is a progressive systemic inflammatory disease causing pain in multiple joints. Joint involvement may be accompanied by systemic features such as malaise, fever, and weight loss. Cardiovascular, pulmonary, neurological, and almost every organ system may be involved.

History

When RA presents for the first time in the elderly, it generally has a more acute onset with frequent involvement of the large joints and more constitutional features compared with younger-onset RA. There is often prolonged and disabling morning joint stiffness that may last for over an hour and generally involves the upper extremities [24].

Physical

The joint swelling is polyarticular and symmetrical and usually involves the proximal interphalangeal (PIP) and metacarpophalangeal joints of the hand as well as the wrist, elbow, feet, ankles, knees, and spine. The joints are swollen and tender.

In patients with longstanding disease such as the elderly with early-onset RA, cartilage loss can lead to subluxation of joints in the hands and feet. This results in ulnar deviation and swan neck and boutonniere deformities of the hand and hammer toes and metatarsal subluxation of the feet. These deformities result in severe disabilities for the patient [24].

Cervical spine instability is a serious complication in patients with advanced RA, with atlanto-occipital subluxation being the most critical complication. The neurological exam of these patients may be very difficult due to limited range of motion and existing neuropathies. Severe neck pain, occipital pain, or tingling or motor or sensory changes in the upper or lower extremities may be the first signs of an unstable spine [1]. RA patients with an unstable spine may also present with urinary retention or incontinence, involuntary muscle spasms in their legs, complaints of their legs feeling heavy like stone, or the sensation of an electric shock running down the spine on flexing their neck [25]. All of the above findings in an RA patient require strict spinal precautions, thorough neurological evaluation, and emergent imaging and treatment.

Diagnostic tests

Rheumatoid factor is elevated in 90% of cases of RA but may also be elevated as a baseline in elderly patients [26]. X-ray findings include soft tissue swelling in the early stages and joint space narrowing and erosions in more advanced disease.

Treatment

As intervention in the first 18 months is critical in slowing or preventing the joint destruction of RA, aggressive treatment early in the disease is important in preventing future pain and dysfunction. Disease-modifying anti-rheumatic drugs (DMARDs) have been shown to minimize joint destruction, decrease joint swelling, and improve physical function. Methotrexate is one of the most effective DMARDs. Biologic therapeutic agents which target specific parts of the immune response to RA have also been shown to be very effective in elderly patients, especially when combined with methotrexate. However, DMARDs and biologic agents have potentially serious side effects and require close outpatient monitoring Sulfasalazine and hydroxychloroquine are alternative medications which are less toxic but less effective than other medications, but may be preferred in elderly patients with significant medical problems and more slowly progressive RA [24].

Low-dose oral glucocorticoids have been shown to reduce pain and stiffness and also may slow the progression of the RA. However, osteoporosis is a major side effect of long-term steroid use. If the patient is likely to need glucocorticoids for an extended time, medication to prevent osteoporosis should be given. NSAIDs, if not contraindicated, relieve pain and inflammation but do not affect progression of the disease. The lowest recommended dose of NSAID should be used for a short duration to prevent potential complications of this medication in the elderly. As DMARDs do not take effect for several weeks, low-dose steroids or NSAIDs may be used to provide symptomatic relief when DMARDs are started [24].

Differential

Acute presentations of RA may present with very tender, swollen, and warm joints and require arthrocentesis to distinguish this condition from SA. Gupta et al. found one-third of adult patients with SA had underlying RA, and these patients were less likely to have fever and leukocytosis [8].

Late-onset RA can mimic polymyalgia rheumatica when it presents with involvement of the shoulders and hips. Polyarticular gout, pseudogout, and OA may present similarly to RA.

Disposition

Patients with RA should be admitted if they have life-threatening complications of the disease or if the diagnosis is unclear and there is suspicion for SA. Admission may also be necessary for RA patients with intractable pain or if they are unable to maintain their daily acts of living and require social intervention.

Pearls and pitfalls

The fact that patients with SA and underlying RA have a mortality of up to 49% and often have atypical presentations underscores how important it is to have a high clinical suspicion for the diagnosis of SA in this group [4,8].

Particular attention should be given to patients with advanced RA who have been involved in trauma where there may have been flexion of the neck. As atlanto-occipital instability may not be apparent on history or exam, flexion or hyperextension of the neck should be avoided in patients with advanced RA [25,27,28]. Spinal precautions should also be taken when intubating a patient with advanced RA. In preparation for intubation, mouth opening should be evaluated as patients with advanced RA may have temporomandibular dysfunction with limited opening of the mouth [25].

Osteoarthritis

Osteoarthritis is a degenerative joint disease which is the leading cause of functional impairment in the elderly and is almost universal by the age of 80 [29,30]. This disease is characterized by erosion of the cartilage and underlying bone of the joint as well as bony overgrowth. Rheumatoid arthritis, gout, trauma, or anything that affects the cartilage and subchondral bone increases the incidence and progression of OA [30].

History

Compared with other arthritides, OA onset is gradual with the patient complaining of deep intermittent pain in one or a few joints. Although the patient may have joint stiffness on awakening, this resolves quickly compared with the course of other arthritides. Morning stiffness typically lasts less than 30 minutes and resolves with activity [29].

Osteoarthritis commonly involves the knee, hip, and spine and the PIP, distal interphalangeal (DIP), and metacarpal (MCP) joints of the hand. Pain in the weight-bearing joints is worsened by standing and walking.

Patients with OA of the knee often complain of pain with activities which involve bending the knee such as climbing or descending stairs or getting out of a chair. They often describe their knees buckling or giving way, and this instability causes significant disability [30].

Physical

On exam there is firm swelling at the joint, decreased range of motion, and crepitus is felt on movement of the joint. Heberden's and Bouchard's nodes are bony swellings of the DIP and PIP joints, respectively, and they cause pain and loss of function of the hand.

Diagnostic tests

In OA, the synovial fluid is clear and the WBC is classically below 2000 cells/mm^3 [3] – mostly monocytes. X-ray findings include the presence of osteophytes, joint space narrowing, and subchondral sclerosis related to loss of cartilage and increased pressure on the bone. However, X-rays may be normal in a patient with OA, correlate poorly with the severity of pain, and many patients with positive X-ray findings may not be symptomatic [29,30].

If ordering a knee X-ray, it is important to get an anteroposterior (AP) view with the patient standing so that a correct interpretation can be made regarding whether there is joint space narrowing. Additionally, it is often prudent to examine the hip and acquire a hip film along with a knee X-ray in the patient with knee pain, as OA of the hip will often present with knee pain [1].

Differential

Unlike the other arthritides, the presentation of OA usually does not overlap with SA. OA has a gradual onset, uncommonly has joint effusions, and the joint is generally not erythematous or warm. Additionally the patient does not have systemic findings such as fever or confusion. Polyarticular indolent presentations of gout may present similarly to OA. OA of the hand should be distinguished from RA involving the hand.

Treatment

Low-impact physical exercise, modest weight loss, and the use of knee braces to correct malalignment have been shown to improve pain and function in patients with OA of the knee. NSAIDs are effective in reducing pain. Intra-articular injection of corticosteroids may be helpful but their benefits only last 1–3 months [29,30].

Disposition

Patients rarely may need to be admitted for social intervention or intractable pain.

241

Pearls and pitfalls

Synovial effusions or redness and warmth are not common with OA, and the presence of any of these findings should make one consider performing arthrocentesis to evaluate for an alternative diagnosis.

Polymyalgia rheumatica and giant cell arteritis

Polymyalgia rheumatica (PMR) and giant cell arteritis (GCA) are systemic inflammatory diseases which occur after 50 years of age and peak between 70 and 80 years of age. The two diseases frequently occur together and are thought to be related. They may have an acute or gradual onset and may present with fever, weight loss, or fatigue in addition to the typical joint pain and headache [31].

History

Polymyalgia rheumatica presents with severe pain and stiffness most commonly in the shoulder, neck, and hip, and may involve the knees and small joints of the hands and feet. The pain may begin on one side but quickly becomes bilateral. The pain in the shoulders and hips usually radiates to the elbows and knees [31]. The patient will often have stiffness lasting more than one hour in the morning or after prolonged rest, and this may severely limit the patient's activity [20].

Giant cell arteritis is also known as temporal arteritis. It generally presents with a severe headache localized to the temporal area and may cause pain in the tongue or jaw with talking or with chewing of even soft foods. The headache is generally gradual in onset but may be sudden. Visual disturbance is an early complaint, and up to 20% of patients develop permanent vision loss in one or both eyes related to ischemia of the ophthalmic artery [31]. Visual disturbances include the presence of zigzag lines, general dimness of vision, and sudden transient loss of vision (amaurosis fugax) [1]. This transient loss of vision is a strong predictor of permanent loss of vision in GCA. If only one eye is affected, the other eye is likely to become affected within 1–2 weeks if treatment is not started [31].

Physical

On examination, PMR and GCA usually have a low-grade temperature but GCA may present with a high fever as its main complaint and finding. PMR presents with diffuse tenderness in the proximal muscles of the shoulder, hip, and other joints. Passive range of motion is better tolerated than active range of motion. Like OA, joint swelling is atypical in PMR and one should think of SA if joint swelling or erythema is present.

Giant cell arteritis presents with discrete or diffuse tenderness in the scalp or temporal area. Decreased vision or vision loss or a field cut may be noted. Neurologic manifestations are common with GCA, with the most common findings being neuropathies of the arms and legs.

Giant cell arteritis can affect the vertebral arteries and cause neurological deficits in the area of vertebrobasilar circulation. This diagnosis will generally not be missed in the elderly person who presents with gait and speech disturbance and dizziness,

and who also presents with the classic symptoms of GCA including severe headache, visual disturbance, and temporal or scalp tenderness. However, if the classic signs and symptoms of GCA are not present in a patient with vertebro basilar findings, the diagnosis of GCA will often be missed or significantly delayed [32].

Thoracic aortic aneurysm was found in one study to be 17 times more likely to develop in patients with GCA as compared with patients without this diagnosis. This complication generally developed 2–6 years after the initial diagnosis of GCA. Half of the patients with GCA who had thoracic aneurysms died suddenly of aortic dissection in this study [33].

Diagnostic findings

An ESR >50 mm/h is used to confirm the disease when a patient presents with the typical findings of GCA/PMR. However, approximately 10% of patients with GCA will have an ESR <50 mm/h, and both PMR and GCA may show a normal ESR at the time of diagnosis [34]. Therefore, a normal ESR should not delay treatment of PMR or GCA if other features are consistent with this diagnosis.

Treatment

Low-dose steroids are almost always effective in treating PMR. In GCA, higher-dose corticosteroids if given within the first 24 hours prevent the further progression of the disease. If visual loss has already occurred, it is irreversible in most cases [32]. As steroids do not interfere with the subsequent biopsy and delay in waiting for the results of the biopsy may result in blindness, steroids should be started immediately in any patient where there is a reasonable suspicion of GCA [1].

Disposition

Admit if there are neurologic findings, vascular complications, or vision loss. If discharged, it is important to arrange for expedited follow-up for biopsy of the temporal artery.

Pearls and pitfalls

An ESR should be performed on patients with a history of GCA presenting with new neurologic symptoms, or if an elderly patient presents with neurological complaints consistent with vertebrobasilar insufficiency, particularly if these symptoms or findings are accompanied by a headache. Do not delay steroid therapy in order to obtain a biopsy.

The clinician should ask about jaw pain with chewing and transient visual loss, as patients often will not offer this information unless specifically asked. It is also recommended to take blood pressures in both arms and obtain a chest X-ray in patients with GCA to check for the development of a thoracic aneurysm.

Back pain and spinal stenosis

The diagnosis of back pain in the elderly is complicated by the number of potential problems that cause back pain in this population, as well as by the number of musculoskeletal problems that most of these patients have as their baseline. These problems include infection, malignancy, vertebral fractures spinal stenosis, and mechanical problems. Narrowing the diagnosis requires a detailed history of the problem, including both a review of constitutional symptoms and a detailed physical examination to help distinguish between systemic, neurologic, and mechanical causes of back pain.

Disk herniation is uncommon in the elderly as the nucleus pulposus loses its gel-like quality and is less likely to herniate. While infection of the disk and vertebrae is a rare cause of back pain in children and adults over 50, the fact that it presents with positional pain makes it difficult to distinguish from mechanical back pain [35]. It should be suspected in patients with a history of artificial heart valves, IV drug abuse, or systemic signs and symptoms of infection.

Lumbar stenosis is a common cause of lower back pain and leg pain in the elderly. Spinal stenosis most commonly occurs in the lumbar spine but may also occur in the cervical and thoracic spine. It is a narrowing of the spinal canal that may result in compression of the spinal nerves. The narrowing may be caused by OA of the spine, spondylolisthesis, disk herniation, or facet hypertrophy.

History

Cervical spine stenosis often presents with parethesias and pain radiating to the shoulder and upper extremity. Patients with severe compression of the cervical nerves present with gradual onset of difficulty walking, dropping objects, or loss of coordination.

Patients with lumbar spinal stenosis report bilateral buttock pain and unilateral or bilateral posterior leg pain. Patients with significant lumbar stenosis may present with radicular pain, weakness, or numbness. Central stenosis of the lumbar spine can compress the cauda equina and patients may present with bladder and bowel dysfunction as well as leg weakness [36].

The pain of spinal stenosis is exacerbated by walking and prolonged standing, and relieved by sitting. This is because extension of the spine in walking or standing reduces the volume of the spinal canal, while flexion of the spine in sitting expands the volume of the canal and relieves pressure on the nerve root. The pain and parathesias of spinal stenosis are known as neurogenic claudication or pseudoclaudication, as the symptoms mimic vascular claudication.

Physical

Patients with spinal stenosis tend to walk bent forward because flexion at the waist improves pain. A wide-based gait and unsteadiness may be noted on Romberg's test, but motor findings are generally minimal [37]. Patients with compression of the cauda equina may present with findings of sensory loss in a saddle distribution, lower extremity weakness, and a postvoid urine residual noted on either ultrasound of the bladder or catheterization of the bladder.

Tenderness of the vertebrae is a sensitive but not specific exam for infection. Patients with mechanical back pain have loss of movement of the spine, but this finding is not strongly associated with any specific diagnosis. The straight leg test is helpful in diagnosing herniated disk but is often negative in patients with spinal stenosis [38].

Diagnostic tests

In patients with lower back pain where systemic disease is suspected, complete blood count, ESR, CRP, and plain lumbar spine X-rays should be obtained as normal findings in these tests makes the diagnosis of systemic disease very unlikely [39]. The role of imaging in other situations is limited because of the poor association between symptoms and anatomical findings.

Differential

Cervical spine stenosis with radiation of pain to the upper extremities must be distinguished from primary causes of upper extremity pain. Lumbar pain with its lower back and leg pain must be distinguished from hip pain, which also presents with buttock and leg pain. Hip pain can be distinguished by its general presentation, with groin pain radiating to the anterolateral thigh whereas lumbar pain is generally in the buttock with posterior radiation to the thigh. Additionally, hip pain is worsened by internal rotation while lumbar pain is worsened by spinal extension [35–37]. The pain in patients with herniated disks is improved by extension of the spine and worsened by flexion. Patients with mechanical lower back pain can be distinguished from spinal stenosis by the former's back pain, with any lumbar movement including changing from lying to sitting or bending forward.

Treatment

Management of mechanical back pain and spinal stenosis is generally conservative, with analgesia and exercise. Spinal stenosis progresses very slowly and emergency intervention is generally not necessary. Surgery is considered if mechanical back pain is intractable, or in spinal stenosis if there are progressive neurological deficits or evidence of cauda equina compression [36,37]. However, the benefits of surgery must be weighed against the risks in the elderly population.

Pearls and pitfalls

Neurogenic claudication of spinal stenosis differs from vascular claudication in that the former is improved by walking uphill or sitting (flexion) and worsened by standing (extension), whereas the latter is worsened by any exertion (e.g., walking uphill) and only relieved by rest (standing or sitting). The pain of vascular claudication is generally in the calf and resolves after a 5-minute rest, whereas the pain of neurogenic claudication is generally located in the hamstrings and resolves after a 10–20-minute rest. Vascular claudication generally has loss of the dorsalis pedis pulse. It is important to distinguish between the two different causes of claudication as their treatment and prognosis are very different.

Orthopedic injuries in the geriatric population

Orthopedic injuries which are well tolerated in younger patients can have devastating consequences in the elderly patient in terms of quality of life and overall health. The pain and the loss of function, mobility, and independence resulting from these injuries often lead to a severe physical and psychological decline that may be life threatening [36]. In order to avoid this downward spiral in the elderly patient, these injuries need to be recognized early and wherever possible fractures need to be rapidly and aggressively treated. Operative intervention is often necessary to quickly restore function and avoid the severe medical problems that accompany prolonged immobilization. It is imperative that the emergency physician performs a complete history and physical exam in the elderly patient even with minor trauma, in order to avoid missing fractures in this population.

The high rate of fractures in the elderly results from the high incidence of falls and the fragile nature of their bones due to osteoporosis. Osteoporosis occurs with aging as the creation of new bone fails to keep up with the adsorption of old bone. Add to this a multitude of other factors compounding the degradation of bones in the elderly including poor diet, lack of exercise, and medications, and the end result is an osteoporotic state leaving many elderly with weak and brittle bones prone to fractures. Seventy-five percent of fractures in the elderly are related to osteoporosis, and one in two women and one in four men over age 50 will have an osteoporosis-related fracture in their lifetime [36].

Falls serve as the most common mechanism for injuries and fractures in the elderly. About one-third of the geriatric population falls each year, and the risk of falls increases proportionately with age. According to the Centers for Disease Control and Prevention, falls are the leading cause of death due to injury in the elderly. Eighty-seven percent of all fractures in the elderly are due to falls. In 2009, 2.2 million fall injuries among older adults were treated in EDs and more than 581,000 of these patients were hospitalized. In 2010, $28.2 billion was spent on treatment of falls in the elderly [40].

In taking the history in an elderly patient with a fall, it is important to try to obtain the reason for the fall. Problems such as syncope, overmedication, intoxication, decreased visual acuity, or loss of balance that may have caused the fall should be identified and addressed. The length of time before the patient got help should also be determined as an indication of possible dehydration, rhabdomyolysis, or electrolyte imbalance.

It is also important to not be distracted by the obvious injury and forget to identify and address other injuries associated with the fall. When examining the elderly trauma patient, it is also important to keep these patients warm because they are more likely to develop hypothermia when their clothes are removed, and hypothermia increases the risk of mortality from trauma.

Even if the injury related to the fall is minor, admission may be required to provide further medical work-up or social services regarding the cause of the fall. If the patient is being discharged, measures to decrease falls including appropriate exercise, proper foot care, and if necessary, home care and the use of devices to assist in ambulation should be discussed with patients and their families.

Hip fractures

The vast majority of hip fractures occur in the elderly, with the mechanism of injury generally being a low-velocity fall from standing. Femoral neck fractures occur predominantly in men in their 70s while intertrochanteric fractures occur predominantly in women in their 80s [41]. Overall, 75% of hip fractures occur in post-menopausal women [42].

With the aging of the population, not only is the number of hip fractures increasing but also the average age of the patient with hip fracture. The average age of patients with hip fractures treated at one orthopedic hospital increased from 78 to 88 years between 1991 and 2001 [36].

The effect of hip fractures is devastating from the physical, psychological, and financial points of view. One out of five hip fracture patients dies within a year of their injury and less than one-third recover their pre-fracture level of function [43]. Considerable Medicare costs are spent on hospital admissions for such fractures, as well as nursing home costs and extensive rehabilitation.

The ball-and-socket hip joint is formed by the cup-like acetabulum and the head of the femur. A large number of ligaments and powerful muscles encapsulate the hip joint, allowing humans to be bipedal. The hip is comprised of the femoral head, femoral neck, and the intertrochanteric and subtrochanteric regions.

Potential complications of hip fractures are often related to the vasculature of the hip. In most cases only a small vessel supplies the proximal femoral head, while very large branches of the external iliacs course through the thigh forming a rich blood supply to the intertrochanteric area and distal femur. Thus, disruption of the vasculature via a femoral neck fracture can cause avascular necrosis, while extensive bleeding and shock may result from disruption of the large vessels from a more distal hip or femoral fracture.

Hip fractures in the elderly primarily involve the femoral neck or the intertrochanteric area. Femoral head fractures are less common and are often associated with hip dislocations.

The main concern with femoral neck fractures is that the blood supply to the proximal femur may be disrupted by a displaced fracture of the femoral neck. Minimally displaced or impacted fractures of the femoral neck are unlikely to disrupt the circulation, whereas displaced fractures have a high likelihood of disrupting the blood supply and causing non-union and avascular necrosis of the femoral head. Early detection and treatment of a nondisplaced fracture is important to prevent this from turning into a more serious displaced fracture.

Compared with the femoral neck, the intertrochanteric region has a rich supply of blood. Although this results in much better potential for healing, intertrochanteric fractures can have significantly more bleeding than is seen with femoral neck fractures.

History

Whenever an older adult is unable to get up or bear weight after a fall, a hip fracture should be suspected. The patient will often complain of groin or hip pain but may have thigh or referred knee pain. Occasionally, patients will be able to bear weight with a hip fracture but will report pain with standing or ambulation.

Physical

Displaced fractures are obvious when presenting with a shortened and externally or internally rotated leg. This presentation is due to the quadriceps and hamstrings pulling on the bone fragments causing overlap and misalignment. It is important to diagnose subtle, nondisplaced fractures early to prevent subsequent displacement of the fracture. These fractures may only present with groin pain worsened by any range of motion or by axial loading on the heel. A detailed neurovascular exam should be performed.

Diagnostic findings

The majority of hip fractures are diagnosed via plain radiography. Pelvis and AP and lateral views of the hip are usually sufficient [44]. A pelvis X-ray should be included as this gives a comparative view of the unaffected hip and may reveal a pelvic fracture in the patient with hip pain.

Subtle findings of hip fractures include breaks in the continuity of the cortex of the proximal femur or disruption of the trabecular lines from the femoral shaft to the femoral head. If a fracture is not seen on plain view but is suggested clinically because of tenderness, pain, prior hardware, or inability to ambulate, higher-resolution imaging is needed. Magnetic resonance imaging (MRI) is preferable, but computed tomography (CT) is generally done if MRI is not readily available or is at a distance from the ED and the patient requires close monitoring [44].

Treatment

Traction splints placed pre-hospital can cause or worsen neurologic injury of the leg and the development of pressure ulcers if left on for a prolonged period of time. These splints are intended to be used for isolated mid-shaft femur fractures, but it is often difficult to know what kind of injury the patient has when the splint is applied in the field. Injuries considered contraindications to traction splints such as pelvic, proximal hip, knee, or lower leg fractures are often ignored [45]. As there is no demonstrated benefit to pre-hospital traction splints for hip fractures in adults in terms of reduced bleeding, pain control, or fracture reduction, traction splints should be replaced in the ED with immobilization without traction in adult patients with hip fractures [46].

Patients with suspected hip fractures are generally transported to the ED on backboards. These devices should be removed in the ED as quickly as possible as they are hard and uncomfortable. Pain control should be started early in the ED management of the patient with a hip fracture and is best accomplished with small doses of narcotic medication that can be titrated to pain relief.

The main goals of repair are to stabilize and align the joint to allow patients to regain function and mobility early on, and prevent the downward spiral that often occurs with these injuries. Conservative treatment with traction and bed rest has fallen by the wayside given the large amount of complications associated with such treatment.

Nondisplaced femoral neck fractures are generally fixed by the minimally invasive placement of percutaneous cannulated screws. In contrast, displaced femoral neck fractures in all but the frailest nonfunctional elderly patients are treated with prosthetic replacement of the femoral head or total replacement of the hip, because of the high rate of non-union and avascular necrosis (AVN) that occurs with disruption of the vascular supply in these injuries. With the generous supply of blood to the intertrochanteric area, intertrochanteric fractures generally heal well with closed or open reduction using intramedullary nails and sliding screws, and do not require replacement of the femoral head or hip.

Differential

Hip dislocation, acetabular or pubic ramus fracture, hip or pelvic contusion, septic joint, referred pain from knee injury, trochanteric bursitis, and lumbar spine injury presenting with leg pain are in the differential for hip fracture.

Disposition

Patients should be prepared for surgery by observing nil per os, placing a Foley catheter, and in most cases gentle IV hydration as dehydration is common. Underlying problems should be corrected as expeditiously as possible as patients are generally at their healthiest when they initially come to the hospital, and delaying surgery by more than 24–48 hours increases morbidity and mortality [47]. However, any decompensation must be stabilized prior to surgery.

Pearls and pitfalls

Consider obtaining a CT or MRI in an elderly patient who complains of groin or hip pain or has difficulty bearing weight after trauma if X-rays are negative. Do not be dissuaded from the diagnosis of hip fracture if a patient has hip pain but is able to stand or ambulate, or if the patient has no recollection of trauma. Be attentive to subtle X-ray findings of fractures of the hip such as those described above under "Diagnostic findings." Early detection of nondisplaced fractures is important, as these fractures may become displaced and thus have worse outcomes. Be attentive to hip dislocation as this is an orthopedic emergency and needs to be reduced quickly to avoid AVN. Traction splints placed pre-hospital should be discontinued in the ED in patients who are found to have hip fractures.

Hip dislocations

Dislocations of native hips are true emergencies, as hip dislocations left out longer than 6–12 hours have a high rate of AVN [48]. Prompt reduction restores blood flow to the femoral head and avoids the severely debilitating and painful arthritis associated with AVN. Reduction of a prosthetic hip is important but may not be as emergent as there is no danger of developing AVN. However, any signs of neurovascular injury in a native or prosthetic hip necessitate immediate reduction. Reduction of a dislocated hip can be difficult in the setting of a patient with multiple trauma where spinal immobilization prevents movement of the patient, and other injuries to the patient may take precedence over reduction of the hip.

As a large force is needed for a dislocation of a native hip, a thorough exam should be done looking for associated injuries.

The elderly patient is much more likely than a younger patient to have a concomitant femoral head fracture with their hip dislocation. These fractures are much more common with anterior hip dislocations and indicate a significant force was involved in the injury [49].

History

In elderly patients the majority of hip dislocations arise from falls. In elderly individuals who have had a hip replacement, often only minimal trauma is needed to dislocate a prosthetic hip. As with native hips, the majority of dislocations of prosthetic hips are posterior.

Physical

The patient with a posterior dislocation typically presents with the hip flexed, adducted, and internally rotated, and the leg is generally shortened. A patient with an anterior dislocation holds the hip flexed, abducted, and externally rotated. The typical presentation of a hip dislocation may be absent when there is an associated femoral fracture [50].

As with all dislocations and fractures it is important to assess for neurovascular injuries before and after reduction. In posterior hip dislocations the peroneal nerve branch of the sciatic nerve is most often injured. One should look for weakness in extension of the big toe and dorsiflexion of the foot, as these are sensitive signs of peroneal nerve injury. In anterior hip dislocations the femoral nerve and/or artery are often injured [51].

Diagnostic findings

Diagnosis is almost always made by an AP pelvis X-ray. If a dislocation is found or suspected, a lateral view may be obtained to provide more information on the presence and nature of the dislocation. Although hip dislocations are generally obvious on the pelvis X-ray, a subtle sign of hip dislocation or fracture is a disruption of the smooth line drawn from the superior border of the obturator foramen along the medial aspect of the distal femur (Shenton's line).

Another sign of a hip dislocation is that the femoral head appears smaller in a posterior dislocation as the hip is closer to the X-ray cassette than the unaffected side, and appears larger in an anterior dislocation as the hip is further away from the X-ray cassette. In the posterior dislocation, the femoral head is generally superior to the acetabulum while in the anterior dislocation, the femoral head is inferior to the acetabulum. Femoral head fractures may be subtle but can be detected by looking closely at the border of the dislocated femoral head and the cup of the acetabulum for a small fracture fragment, which is usually seen as a retained fragment in the joint [50].

Treatment

The same techniques are used to reduce prosthetic and native hip dislocations. Three of the most commonly used methods for reduction of a posterior hip dislocation are the Allis, Whistler, and Morgan maneuvers. All three keep the hip stable with the knee and hip flexed while the femoral head is distracted inferiorly to disengage the head from the acetabulum. Longitudinal

traction is then applied under different fulcrums to reengage the femoral head. After reduction, the hip is extended, externally rotated, and a knee immobilizer and abduction pillow are placed to prevent repeat dislocation. All techniques require procedural sedation, and repeat X-rays should be obtained after the procedure to confirm proper reduction.

As with all dislocations, reduction should use gentle, slow, and sustained manipulation to avoid injury to the hip. In general, no more than two reduction attempts should be made in the ED before taking the patient to the OR, to avoid damage to the femoral head. Special care is required with prosthetic hip dislocations as there is a risk of loosening or moving the prosthesis or fracturing surrounding bone with reduction of the hip [50].

Disposition

Most hip dislocations require urgent orthopedic consultation and admission. Unlike other hip dislocations, patients with prosthetic hip dislocations often may be discharged home after reduction and consultation with orthopedics. Where there is an associated femoral neck or more distal fracture of the leg that precludes using the leg to manipulate the hip, reduction is done by orthopedics most commonly by open reduction in the operating room. Hip dislocations with femoral head fractures are generally done with closed reduction.

Differential

Hip or pelvic fracture, hip or pelvic contusion, referred pain from knee injury, and septic joint are in the differential for hip dislocation.

Pearls and pitfalls

Native hip dislocations are true orthopedic emergencies and require prompt reduction to avoid avascular necrosis of the hip. However, airway, breathing, circulation, and neurologic deficits must be evaluated and addressed prior to the patient being sedated for hip reduction. It is important to search the X-ray of a hip dislocation for an associated fracture, as this finding changes the management of the patient.

Pelvic fractures

The pelvis is comprised of the ilium, ischium, and pubis. Together these bones form an anatomical ring with the sacrum. Considerable force is usually required to disrupt the pelvis given its interwoven ligamental structure and the multitude of muscles that course throughout it. Thus, approximately 85% of pelvic fractures seen in adolescence through middle age are via significant trauma, mainly motor vehicle accidents or pedestrians who are struck by vehicles [51].

In contrast, pelvic fractures in the elderly are usually due to minor forms of trauma such as a fall from a standing position but can also result from normal stress in patients with severe osteoporosis. These fractures are known as insufficiency fractures or fragility fractures and are contrasted with the fatigue stress fractures that occur in younger patients with normal bone exposed to repeated abnormal stresses. Pelvic insufficiency fractures most commonly involve the pubic rami and the sacrum and often are misdiagnosed initially as degenerative back problems [52]. Although these fractures are rarely life threatening, they can cause significant disability and loss of independence.

As the pelvis is a rigid ring, there are generally two fractures of the pelvis when it is broken. A fracture in the anterior pelvis such as a pubic ramus fracture is almost always accompanied by another pubic ramus fracture or posteriorly by a sacral fracture. It is important to identify patients with sacral fractures as these patients are at risk of cauda equina injury. Unlike other pelvic fractures which generally occur with more than one fracture, insufficiency fractures and fractures from minor falls in the elderly often occur as an isolated fracture.

Although most pelvic fractures in the elderly are isolated fractures from falls from standing, life-threatening pelvic fractures in the elderly may result from a larger amount of force such as in a motor vehicle accident or a pedestrian–motor vehicle collision. Pelvic fractures are considered unstable if they involve all four pubic rami, or widening of the symphysis pubis or sacroiliac joint or involve the anterior and posterior arches of the pelvic ring. These major pelvic fractures are associated with bladder and urethral injuries and significant retroperitoneal bleeding.

Overall mortality in the elderly with pelvic fractures is 30% and if hypotension is noted on arrival this climbs to 40–50% [53,54]. Elderly patients with open book pelvic fractures have a mortality of up to 81% [53]. Although complex pelvic fractures are more likely to require transfusion, it is important to remember that even minor pelvic fractures resulting from trauma can be a source of significant bleeding in the elderly [53,55].

History

A pelvic fracture should be considered in any elderly patient complaining of groin, hip, or back pain. The patient with a pelvic fracture will usually complain of groin pain worsened with sitting, standing, movement of the hip, or defecation. Lower back pain, as well as groin pain, should raise the suspicion of an associated sacral fracture. It may be difficult to distinguish between a pelvic and a hip fracture based solely on the history and physical exam.

Whereas hip fractures are often caused by a fall laterally, pelvic fractures are most commonly caused by a fall backwards or forwards. A fall backwards onto the buttocks is the most common mechanism of injury [36]. Patients with insufficiency pelvic fractures may describe persistent groin or back pain, or difficulty ambulating for weeks or months.

Physical

A pelvic fracture is suggested by tenderness or laxity on palpation of the bony pelvis. Extensive manipulation of a fractured pelvis should be avoided during physical exam as this increases pain and may disrupt vasculature and increase bleeding.

A discrepancy in leg length or pain with range of motion of the hip suggests a hip or pelvic fracture. Tenderness over the spine or sacrum suggests an associated spinal or sacral fracture. A full neurological exam of the lower extremities and evaluation of perianal sensation and rectal tone is necessary to exclude a cauda equina injury associated with a pelvic fracture.

Other signs indicating a pelvic fracture include gross hematuria or a superficial hematoma above the inguinal ligament or over the scrotum, perineum, or proximal thigh (Destot's sign). The presence of these signs or the inability to urinate should direct attention to evaluate for urethral or bladder injuries.

Diagnostic findings

Compared with CT and MRI, pelvic X-ray has a sensitivity of only 64–86% in the diagnosis of all pelvic fractures and 53–66% in the diagnosis of sacral fractures in blunt trauma patients [56–59]. Given its speed and accuracy in identifying complex and unstable pelvic trauma, CT is the imaging test of choice in evaluating significant pelvic trauma in all but the most hemodynamically unstable patients [58].

The sensitivity of CT for detecting occult minor pelvic fractures is limited when compared with MRI. Henes et al. found CT had a sensitivity of 77% for occult pelvic fractures and a sensitivity of 66% for occult sacral fractures, whereas the corresponding findings for MRI were 96 and 98%, respectively [59]. MRI also determined a cause for pain in 73% of patients where a fracture was not found [57].

As with hip injuries, elderly patients with minor pelvic injury who are unable to ambulate should have a MRI or CT of the pelvis if their pelvis X-ray is normal. If CT is negative but suspicion for pelvic fracture remains, MRI should be the next step in the work-up [59].

In cases where pelvic injury is suspected and more than a low-velocity mechanism is involved, CT with IV contrast helps delineate pelvic fractures and whether there is internal injury including hematoma and active bleeding. In cases where the patient is too unstable to undergo CT, pelvic X-ray is very useful for identifying complex pelvic fractures which may require monitoring or management of pelvic hemorrhage [58].

Elderly patients with suspected or documented pelvic fractures from more than low-velocity trauma should be typed and crossed, have serial hematocrits, and have their vital signs monitored closely. As elderly patients may not initially manifest the fact that they are in compensated shock, an abnormal base deficit or lactate can give an early indication of how sick the apparently stable normotensive or hypertensive elderly trauma patient is before he/she mounts a tachycardia or drops their blood pressure. Serial lactates or base deficits can help evaluate and guide the resuscitation. However, approximately 15% of elderly patients may have significant injuries from trauma and have a normal lactate or base deficit [60,61].

Treatment

Most pelvic fractures are stable and are treated with pain control, thromboprophylaxis, physical therapy, and weight bearing as tolerated.

Where a grossly unstable pelvis is found, external pelvic compression using a sheet or a commercially available pelvic binder may be used to stabilize and close an open pelvis and control bleeding from the fracture site.

Depending on the stability of the patient and their associated injuries, patients with significant pelvic fractures may require the use of a massive transfusion protocol for blood loss and the use of external fixators in addition to external compression devices. Decisions need to be made regarding whether the patient is stable to undergo CT or should go directly to the operating room, intensive care unit, or interventional radiology.

Differential

Hip or lumbar spine fracture or contusion, spinal stenosis, referred pain from the knee, OA of the hip, and inguinal hernia are in the differential for a pelvic fracture.

Disposition

Even though many pelvic fractures in the elderly involve only one part of the ring and are thus deemed stable fractures, most of these patients require admission for pain control and to be set up for home care and physical therapy. Many of these fractures can take up to 8–12 weeks to heal.

Pearls and pitfalls

Pelvis X-rays can miss fractures of the pelvis. Therefore, CT or MRI should be done if suspicion for this injury is high despite negative X-rays. Even minor pelvic fractures in the elderly can have significant bleeding and these patients need to be closely monitored and aggressively managed. In view of the potential danger of unstable pelvic fractures and the complicated work-up and treatment for such patients, it is vital that senior emergency medicine, trauma, and orthopedic physicians be involved in the ED management of the patient and discuss the sequencing of the steps to be done.

Vertebral fractures

Vertebral compression fractures affect approximately 25% of all post-menopausal women and 40% of women over 80 years old in the US [62]. These fractures are the most common consequence of osteoporosis. Although most osteoporotic vertebral compression fractures are asymptomatic, they can cause significant pain, disability, and increased hospitalization and death [63]. Having radiologic evidence of a vertebral compression fracture increases by fivefold the risk that a woman will have another compression fracture [64].

Multiple vertebral compression fractures may lead to loss of height, and wedge-shaped fractures can cause significant kyphosis. Gastrointestinal and pulmonary problems may result from the shorter spine compressing the bowel and impeding expiratory expansion of the rib cage [63].

History

Vertebral compression fractures may present with an acute onset of back pain or may have an insidious presentation. Standing or walking aggravates the pain, while lying supine alleviates the pain. Often the patient may present with atraumatic mild, nonspecific back pain and have difficulty localizing the pain. As with other such fractures in the elderly, no large amount of trauma needs to take place. Simply misstepping, bending, coughing, or sneezing can cause such a fracture. In fact up to 30% of such fractures occur while the patient is in bed [65].

Physical

Most vertebral compression fractures related to osteoporosis occur at the thoracolumbar junction. Percussion of the vertebrae will indicate the level of injury. Patients may present with weakness or pain radiating down the leg or across the chest wall, but neurologic findings are uncommon with compression fractures [36].

Diagnostic findings

Diagnosis is generally made via spinal X-rays, with the fracture most readily seen on the lateral view. Most vertebral compression fractures occur in the lower thoracic or lumbar vertebra, but often multiple compression fractures occur simultaneously and physicians should evaluate the entire spine during the work-up. A decrease in vertebral height of 20% or more, or a decrease of at least 4 mm compared with baseline height of the vertebra, is considered a vertebral compression fracture [1].

Computed tomography is useful to assess the stability of a compression fracture and whether there is retropulsion of fracture fragments and potential involvement of the spinal canal. MRI is indicated where there is a neurologic deficit or there is a question about an underlying malignancy. Either imaging test will help determine whether the fracture is acute or old. ESR, CRP, CBC, and alkaline phosphatase are indicated when a prolonged course puts infection or malignancy in the differential.

Treatment

Most compression fractures of the spine are stable fractures and management is supportive, including pain control and physical therapy. Medications to treat osteoporosis are not only important to prevent future fractures but may also be helpful in treating the acute and chronic pain of vertebral compression fractures [36]. Vertebroplasty and kyphoplasty may be considered when conservative therapy fails, but the long-term benefits of these procedures have not been evaluated [66].

Differential

Osteoarthritis of the spine, osteomyelitis or epidural abscess, malignancy, and musculoskeletal back pain are differentials for compression fracture.

Disposition

Most vertebral compression fracture cases can be discharged home with pain medication and orthopedic follow-up but those patients with refractory pain or neurologic deficits will require admission, with the latter requiring urgent neurosurgical or orthopedic consultation.

Pearls and pitfalls

Have a low threshold for imaging and blood tests in the elderly with back pain. These patients may sustain fractures with minimal or no recalled trauma. As most vertebral compression fractures related to osteoporosis occur in the lower thoracic or upper lumbar spine, a solitary vertebral compression fracture higher than the 4th thoracic vertebra suggests a cause other than osteoporosis.

Proximal humeral fractures

The shoulder is comprised of the clavicle, scapula, and humerus. Together with tendons, muscles and ligaments, three distinct joints are formed: the glenohumeral, sternoclavicular, and acromioclavicular. With a rich vasculature and a multitude of nerves coursing out of the brachial plexus, the arm can produce both powerful and fine dexterous movements that are unique to humans. Fractures of the proximal humerus can thus be devastating to one's way of life if not recognized or properly treated. These fractures occur most commonly in elderly osteoporotic patients.

History

The most common mechanism for proximal humeral fractures is a fall on an outstretched hand (FOOSH). Patients will usually present with pain, swelling, and inability to move the arm.

Physical

There is marked swelling, tenderness, ecchymosis, and oftentimes a palpable deformity of the proximal humerus, and 36% of these fractures are associated with neurovascular injuries [67]. The most common complications arise from injury to the brachial plexus and the radial and axillary nerves, resulting in wrist drop and sensory deficits. Neurologic symptoms typically resolve within several months.

Diagnostic tests

X-rays consisting of the AP, lateral, and axillary views should be obtained to fully assess the nature of the fracture, as well as to outline an effective treatment plan. The Velpeau view allows the patient to keep their arm in a sling and may be used as a modified axillary view if the patient is in too much pain to obtain a standard axillary view.

Treatment

Proximal humerus fractures which are minimally displaced, angulated, or are impacted may be treated with an arm sling or shoulder immobilizer with orthopedic referral and early mobilization. Patients with severe pain are treated with a coaptation splint. Significantly displaced or angulated fractures involving multiple fragments of bone require surgery, including closed or open reduction or arthroplasty.

Differential

Differential diagnosis includes shoulder dislocation, rotator cuff tear, calcific tendinitis, acute hemorrhagic bursitis, pathologic fracture, biceps tendon rupture, and acromioclavicular separation.

Disposition

Most cases of proximal humerus fracture can be discharged with orthopedic referral within 2 weeks. Any complicated proximal humeral fracture including fracture dislocation, grossly comminuted and displaced fractures, open fractures, or fractures with neurovascular compromise require an orthopedic consult in the ED as these patients are at increased risk for neurovascular complication and infection. Many of these fractures will likely require surgical correction. If transferring a patient with a proximal humeral fracture, a U-slab splint should be used with free access to evaluate distal pulses.

Pearls and pitfalls

It is important to do a complete neurovascular exam in proximal humeral fractures as neurovascular complications are common with these injuries. On reviewing the X-rays, special attention should be given to the relationship of the humeral head to the glenoid fossa to avoid missing a dislocation associated with a proximal humeral fracture.

Shoulder dislocations

As the shoulder is the most mobile and unstable joint in the body, it accounts for the majority of all joint dislocations. Approximately 25% of all dislocations occur in the elderly and, as in younger patients, most shoulder dislocations are anterior. While men account for most shoulder dislocations in young adults, in the elderly population, women account for the majority [68].

Neurovascular complications with shoulder dislocations or with their reduction are more frequent in the elderly. Axillary nerve dysfunction is common with anterior shoulder dislocations but generally resolves with reduction within 4–6 months without further intervention. Axillary nerve injury occurring with reduction of the shoulder is rare and is managed conservatively [68].

Although shoulder dislocations are rarely complicated by vascular injuries, more than 90% of these injuries occur in elderly patients at the time of the dislocation or during the attempt at reduction. The increased incidence of axillary artery injury in the elderly is thought to be due to the loss of arterial elasticity secondary to atherosclerosis. Vascular injuries related to shoulder dislocations can occur as either an acute transection or a delayed pseudoaneurysm [69].

Stayner et al. reported that damage to the axillary artery is most commonly seen when shoulder reduction is attempted in elderly patients who dislocated their shoulders weeks to months prior to the procedure. These patients, whose chronic shoulder dislocation may have been mistaken for an acute injury, had a high rate of loss of limb and life when the axillary artery was damaged during the attempted shoulder reduction [68]. Vascular injury should be suspected when pulses are diminished on the side of the dislocation, there is an expanding axillary or deltopectoral mass, or when pain increases after shoulder reduction.

More than half of elderly patients with first-time anterior shoulder dislocations have an associated rotator cuff injury, but this injury is often missed on initial presentation [66]. Many of these patients will require tendon and capsular repair to restore shoulder stability and function. Early diagnosis of rotator cuff injury is important, as operative repair within 3 weeks has been shown to improve functional outcome compared with later surgery [68].

History

Whereas most dislocations in younger patients are secondary to a blow to an externally rotated arm, most dislocations in the elderly are secondary to a fall. The patient classically presents with pain and inability to move the arm. Rotator cuff injury should be suspected in the patient who returns with persistent pain or weakness of the shoulder weeks after it has been reduced [68].

Physical

The arm is typically held slightly abducted and externally rotated in an anterior dislocation of the shoulder. The normal rounded appearance of the shoulder is replaced with a squared-off appearance.

The function of the axillary nerve can be assessed by testing for sensation over the lateral aspect of the shoulder and by feeling for strength and muscle contraction when the patient attempts to abduct the shoulder. The motor test is more accurate than the sensory test, as there are several nerves which overlap in providing sensation to the shoulder.

Rotator cuff tears often present with tenderness over the lateral deltoid and difficulty initiating and maintaining abduction of the shoulder. Limitation in active range of motion but preserved passive movement is characteristic of rotator cuff injuries [68,70]. In the setting of a rotator cuff tear, inability to abduct the shoulder may be misinterpreted as an axillary nerve injury [71]. Diagnosis of this injury may be difficult immediately after injury and is often made at follow-up when the patient has difficulty with arm abduction.

Diagnostic findings

Shoulder dislocations can often be diagnosed clinically. However, pre- and post-reduction X-rays of the shoulder are particularly important in the elderly as fractures are common even with non-traumatic events such as throwing a ball or stretching, and can occur with shoulder reduction. X-rays including AP, scapular Y, and axillary views are almost always sufficient to diagnose shoulder dislocations.

In the elderly, more so than in any other population, fractures often accompany dislocation. Avulsion fractures of the greater tuberosity of the humerus occur in 10–15% of anterior dislocations and are more common in elderly females [72]. Although standard X-rays are usually normal in acute rotator cuff tears, superior displacement of the humeral head such that the acromio-humeral distance is decreased (<7 mm) may be noted on plain films in non-acute complete rotator cuff tears [67].

Treatment

There are many techniques used to relocate an anterior shoulder dislocation, most using traction or leverage of the arm or scapula manipulation to engage the humeral head back into the glenohumeral fossa. All techniques should use gentle, slow, and sustained manipulation. Sudden and forceful maneuvers may cause injuries to the shoulder.

Certain methods such as the Stimson method, in which the patient is placed prone and a weight is attached to the affected arm, may pose risk to the elderly patient especially when sedation is used, as the respiratory status may be compromised in the prone position. Other methods of reduction, such as scapular manipulation with the patient in the sitting position or the external rotation technique, may be better tolerated by the elderly patient and do not require sedation. Gentle traction/counter-traction is effective but generally requires conscious sedation and close monitoring. Intra-articular injection of lidocaine may be tried as an alternative to conscious sedation but is less effective in the patient who presents more than 6 hours after injury [73].

After reduction of an uncomplicated shoulder dislocation (i.e., without associated fracture), the shoulder is immobilized for only 1–2 weeks in patients older than 40 years of age as compared with 3–6 weeks in younger patients. A longer period of immobilization is not required in the older patient, as the risk of recurrent dislocation of the shoulder is very small in this population. More importantly, the shorter period of immobilization and earlier initiation of shoulder exercises helps reduce the risk of developing shoulder stiffness and adhesive capsulitis (frozen shoulder) [74].

Disposition

Most shoulder reductions are reduced by the emergency physician (EP). However, orthopedics should be consulted in the reduction of dislocations and associated fractures as there is an increased risk of additional fractures and worsening of the existing fracture during reduction in these patients [75]. Orthopedics should be consulted in the very frail patient where there is a high risk of a fracture occurring with reduction of the shoulder. The EP should not reduce a shoulder in an elderly patient who presents more than 1–3 days after shoulder dislocation as there is an increased risk of vascular injury associated with reduction of the chronically dislocated shoulder, and open reduction in the operating room is often required even in patients who are less than a week out from their dislocation [76].

Patients can be discharged home with orthopedic follow-up after reduction of an uncomplicated shoulder dislocation. As the diagnosis of rotator cuff injury may not be apparent on the initial visit and early repair of this injury improves outcome, orthopedic follow-up should be arranged as soon as possible in all elderly patients with a shoulder dislocation.

If conscious sedation is used, the patient should be observed to be back to baseline mental status and able to walk. Admission may be required for neurologic deficit or if shoulder reduction is unsuccessful.

Pearls and pitfalls

It is important to do a thorough neurovascular exam in elderly patients with shoulder dislocation before and after reduction. Do not forget to evaluate the elderly patient for rotator cuff injury and arrange for early orthopedic follow-up. Search the X-ray for an associated humeral fracture, as this finding will change the management of the patient. It is also important to ask specifically whether the dislocation is acute or chronic, as the patient may not be forthcoming with this information and the management plan is very different depending on the length of time from the injury.

Distal radius fractures

The distal radius and ulna form the radioulnar joint which abuts the proximal row of carpal bones. The wrist, held together by a group of ligaments interwoven with a delicate network of nerves and vasculature, gives humans the unique dexterity seen only in our species. The loss of function resulting from a distal radius fracture can lead to significant loss of function in an elderly patient.

Given the high rate of falls in the elderly and the fragile nature of their bones, distal radius fractures are common among the elderly. A Colles' fracture, which is a transverse fracture of the distal radius with dorsal displacement and angulation, is the most common wrist fracture seen in adults and the elderly.

Median nerve injury is the most common neurologic complication of wrist fractures. Like carpal tunnel syndrome, median nerve injury in wrist fractures results from increased pressure in the carpal tunnel and presents with parasthesias, loss of sensation, or decreased strength in the median distribution of the hand. Although both are treated with carpal tunnel release, this procedure must be done emergently with median nerve compression from trauma [77].

Compression of the median nerve from trauma is distinguished from contusion or neuropraxia of the median nerve by the fact that sensation is normal initially in the former and subsequently develops sensory loss over hours to days. This is in contrast to a median nerve contusion, which presents with immediate sensory loss that is not progressive. It is important to distinguish the two as a median nerve compression requires emergent surgery and a median nerve contusion only requires observation [77].

History

The mechanism for most wrist fractures in the elderly involves FOOSH.

Physical

The patient with a distal radius fracture holds the wrist close to the body supported by the opposite hand. The classic finding with a Colles' fracture is a dorsally displaced distal radial segment known as a "dinner fork" deformity, but this finding may not be apparent on physical exam.

Diagnostic findings

X-rays are the cornerstone for diagnosing wrist fractures. The X-ray is used to confirm the diagnosis of the fracture and also to determine whether the fracture is comminuted or displaced and whether it is intra- or extra-articular. The posterior-anterior (PA) view shows the amount of radial shortening present and whether the fracture extends into the radiocarpal or radioulnar joints. The lateral view best shows the degree of angulation and displacement.

Differential

Differential diagnosis includes wrist sprain, scaphoid fracture, hand fracture, and septic arthritis of the wrist.

Treatment

The goal in treating Colles' fractures is to restore the radial length and correct dorsal angulation. Management of most Colles' fractures involves early reduction followed by splinting with a well-padded sugar tong splint or cast. The splint must be placed such that the patient has unrestricted movement of the metocarpophangeal joints and thumb. The patient and caregiver should be instructed to use the sling to keep the hand elevated but to remove the arm from the sling frequently to allow movement of the elbow and shoulder. These measures help prevent the development of stiffness in the hand, elbow, and shoulder.

Open fractures and or fractures where there is neurovascular compromise require immediate orthopedic consult in the ED and operative repair. However, the management of Colles' fractures with significant deformity which are not open and do not have neurovascular compromise depends on the level of functioning of the elderly patient.

Operative repair is generally recommended for fractures which are significantly displaced, angulated, comminuted, or with intra-articular extension, as reduction in the ED is frequently unsuccessful with these injuries. High-functioning elderly patients with these complicated wrist fractures will likely benefit from surgical intervention. However, other elderly patients with these injuries have been shown to have good functional outcome with conservative fracture management and rehabilitation even if their wrist has significant deformity. Up to 30° angulation and 5 mm shortening of the distal radius may be acceptable in the elderly patient who is not high functioning [78].

Disposition

Most elderly patients with distal radius fractures can be discharged home with orthopedic follow-up unless there is a problem with pain management or home care. Fractures which are open or have neurovascular compromise require immediate orthopedic attention and admission. Colles' fractures which are not open and do not have neurovascular compromise need a splint and to be seen by orthopedics either in the ED or the next day, depending on the deformity of the wrist and level of functioning of the patient.

Pearls and pitfalls

As median nerve injury may occur with wrist fracture, fracture reduction, splinting, or at some time thereafter, sensation along the median nerve distribution in distal radius fractures must be checked before and after reduction, splinting, and during subsequent visits. The patient should also be given discharge instructions which include returning to the ED immediately if they develop increasing pain or any symptoms of median nerve compression.

References

1. Gonzalez EB, Goodwin JS. Musculoskeletal disorders. In *Practice of Geriatrics*, 4th edn, ed. Duthie EH Jr, Katz PR, Malone ML (Philadelphia, PA: Saunders Elsevier, 2007).

2. Centers for Disease Control and Prevention (CDC). Prevalence of doctor-diagnosed arthritis and arthritis-attributable activity limitation – United States, 2007–2009. *MMWR.* 2010;59(39);1261–65.

3. Mathews CJ. Septic arthritis in the elderly. *Aging Health.* 2010;6(4):495–500.

4. Shirtliff ME, Mader JT. Acute septic arthritis. *Clin Microbiol Rev.* 2002;15(4):527–44.

5. Gavet F, Tornadre A, Soubrier M, Risti JM, Dubost JJ. Septic arthritis in patients aged 80 and older: a comparison with younger adults. *Am Geriatr.* 2005;7:1210–13.

6. Del Pozo JL, Patel R. Infection associated with prosthetic joints. *N Engl J Med.* 2009;361;(8):787–94.

7. Dubost JJ, Fis I, Denis P, et al. Polyarticular septic arthritis. *Medicine.* 1993;72(5):296–310.

8. Gupta MN, Sturrock RD, Field M. A prospective 2-year study of 75 patients with adult-onset septic arthritis. *Rheumatology (Oxford).* 2001;40:24–30.

9. Mathews DJ, Kingsley G, Field M, Jones A et al. Management of septic arthritis: a sytematic review. *Ann Rhem Dis.* 2007;66:440–5.

10. Li SF, Henderson J, Dickman E, Darzynkiewicz R. Laboratory tests in adults with monoarticular arthritis: can they rule out a septic joint. *Acad Emerg Med.* 2004;11(3):276–80.

11. Margaretten ME, Kohlwes J, Moore D, Bent SD. Does this adult patient have septic arthritis? *JAMA.* 2007;297(13):1478–88.

12. Shmerling RH, Delbanco TL, Tosteson AN, Trentham DE. Synovial fluid: what tests should be ordered? *JAMA.* 1990;264:1009–14.

13. Trumpuz A, Hanssen AD, Osmon DR, et al. Synovial fluid leukocyte count and differential for diagnosis of prosthetic knee infection. *Am J Med.* 2004;117:556–62.

14. Carpenter CR, Schuur JD, Everett WW, Pines JM. Evidence-based diagnostics: adult septic arthritis. *Acad Emerg Med.* 2011;18:782–96.

15. Garcia-DeLaTorre I. Advances in the management of septic arthritis. *Infect Dis Clin North Am.* 2006;20:773–88.

16. Thumboo J, O'Duffy JD. A prospective study of the safety of joint and soft tissue aspirations and injections in patients taking warfarin sodium. *Arthritis Rheum.* 1998;41(4):736–9.

17. Yu KH, Luo SF, Liou LB, et al. Concomitant septic and gouty arthritis – An analysis of 30 cases. *Rheumatology (Oxford).* 2003;42(9):1062–6.

18. Ene-Stroescu D, Gorbien MJ. Gouty arthritis: a primer on late-onset gout. *Geriatrics Suppl.* 2005;60:24–31.

19. Ning TC, Keenan RT. Gout in the elderly. *Clin Geriatr.* 2010:19(1):20–5.

20. Scott DL. Arthritis in the elderly. In *Brocklehurst's Textbook of Geriatric Medicine and Gerontology*, 7th edn, ed. Fillit HM, Rockwood K, Woodhourse K (Philadelphia, PA: Saunders Elsevier, 2010).

21. Schlesinger N. Management of gout in seniors: addressing barriers and setting goals for optimal control. In: Management of gout in the elderly: new solutions to an age-old disease. *Clin Geriatr.* 2009;(Suppl.):1–15.

22. Keith MP, Gilliland WR. Updates in the management of gout. *Am J Med.* 2007;120:221–4.

23. Wise CM. Crystal-associated arthritis in the elderly. *Rheum Dis Clin North Am.* 2007; 33:33–54.

24. Cherukumilli VS, Kavanaugh A. Elderly onset rheumatoid arthritis. In *Geriatric Rheumatology: A Comprehensive Approach*, ed. Nakasato Y, Young D (New York: Springer, 2011).

25. Meijers KSE, Cats A, Kremer HP. Cervical myelopathy in rheumatoid arthritis. *Clin Exp Rheumatol.* 1984;2:239–45.

26. Silvestris F, Anderson W, Goodwin JS, Williams RC Jr. Discrepancy in the expression of autoantibodies in healthy aged individuals. *Clin Immunol Immunopathol.* 1985;35:234–44.

27. Slobodin G, Hussein A, Rosenbaum M, Rosner I. The emergency room in rheumatic diseases. *Emerg Med J.* 2006;23:667–71.

28. Bandi V, Munnur U, Braman SS. Airway problems in patients with rheumatologic disorders. *Crit Care Clin.* 2002;18:749.

29. Altman RD. Osteoarthritis in the elderly population. In *Geriatric Rheumatology: A Comprehensive Approach*, ed. Nakasato Y, Young D (New York: Springer, 2011).

30. Felson DT. Osteoarthitis of the knee. *N Eng J Med.* 2006;354:841–8.

31. Salvarani C, Cantini F, Boiardi L, Hunder GG. Polymyalgia rheumatica and giant-cell arteritis. *N Engl J Med.* 2002; 347:261–71.

32. Slobodin G, Hussein A, Rosenbaum M, Rosner I. The emergency room in rheumatic diseases. *Emerg Med J.* 2006;23:667–71.

33. Evans J, O'Fallon W, Hunder G. Increased incidence of aortic aneurysm and dissection in giant cell (temporal) arteritis. *Ann Intern Med.* 1995;122:502–7.

34. Salvarani C, Hunder GG. Giant cell arteritis with a low erythrocyte sedimentation rate: Frequency of occurence in a population-based study. *Arthritis Rheum.* 2001;45:140–5.

35. Cooney LM Jr. Back pain and spinal stenosis. In *Hazzard's Geriatric Medicine and Gerontology*, 6th edn, ed. Halter JB, Ouslander JG, Tinetti ME, Studenski S, High KP, Asthana S (New York: McGraw-Hill, 2009).

36. Cornell, CN, Sculco TP. Orthopedic disorders. In *Practice of Geriatrics*, 4th edn, ed. Duthie EH, Katz PR, Malone ML (Philadelphia, PA: Saunders Elsevier, 2007).

37. Katz JN, Harris MB. Lumbar spinal stenosis. *N Engl J Med.* 2008:358:818–23.

38. Deyo RA, Weinstein JN. Low back pain. *N Engl J Med.* 2001:344:363–70.

39. Jarvik JG, Deyo RA. Diagnostic evaluation of low back pain with emphasis on imaging. *Ann Intern Med.* 2002;137:586–97.

40. Bills EA. *Public Health: Fall Prevention for Older Adults* (Explorebigsky.com Contributor, November 29, 2011, posted by EMILY in HEALTH).

41. Sernbo I, Johnell O. Changes in bone mass and fracture type in patients with hip fractures. *Clin Orthop.* 1989;238:139.

42. Gourlay M, Richy F, Reginster JV. Strategies for the prevention of hip fracture. *Am J Med.* 2003;115:309–17.

43. Lane NE. Epidemiology, etiology, and diagnosis of osteoporosis. *Am J Obstet Gynecol.* 2006;194:S3.

44. Lubovsky O, et al. Early diagnosis of occult hip fractures MRI versus CT scan. *Injury.* 2005;36:788–92.

45. Wood SP, Vrahas M, Wedel SK. Femur fracture immobilization with traction splints in multisystem trauma patients. *Prehosp Emerg Care.* 2003;7:241.

46. Handoll HH, Queally JM, Parker MJ. Pre-operative traction for hip fractures of the femur in adults. *Cochrane Database Syst Rev.* 2011;12.Art. No. CD000168.

47. Aharonoff GB, Koval KJ, Skovron MD, Zuckerman JD. Hip fractures in older adults: Predictors of one-year mortality. *J Orthop Trauma.* 1997;11:162–5.

48. Sahin V, et al. Traumatic dislocation and fracture dislocation of the hip: A long-term follow-up study. *J Trauma.* 2003;54:520.

49. Potter HG, et al. MR imaging of acetabular fractures: Value of detecting femoral head injury, intraarticular fragments, and sciatic nerve injury. *AJR.* 1994;163:881.

50. Fiechtl JF, Fitch RW. Femur and hip. In *Marx: Rosen's Emergency Medicine*, 7th edn, ed. Marx JA, Hockberger RS, Walls RM, Adams JG, et al. (Philadephia, PA: Moseby/Elsevier, 2010).

51. Cornwall R, Radonmisli H. Nerve injury in traumatic dislocation of the hip. *Clin Orthop Res.* 2000;377:84.

52. Sindler OS, Watura R, Cobby M. Sacral insufficiency fractures. *J Orthop Surg.* 2007:15:339.

53. Martin RE, Teberian G. Multiple trauma and the elderly patient. *Emerg Med Clin North Am.* 1990;8:411.

54. Carrafiello G, Mangini M, Ierardi AM, et al. Vascular emergencies of the retroperitoneum: Emergency radiology of the abdomen. *Med Radiol.* 2012;189–205.

55. Sarin EL, Moore EE, et al. Pelvic fracture pattern does not always predict the need for embolization. *J Trauma.* 2005;58:973.

56. Berg EE, Chebuhar C, Bell RM. Pelvic trauma imaging: a blinded comparison of computed tomography and roentgenogram. *J Trauma.* 1996;41:994.

57. Kirby MW, Spritzer C. Radiographic detection of hip and pelvic fractures in the emergency department. *AJR.* 2010;194:1054.

58. Kessel B, Sevi R, Jeroukhimov I, et al. Is routine portable pelvic X-ray in stable multiple trauma patients always justified in a high technology era? *Injury.* 2007;38:559.

59. Henes FO, Nuchtern JV, Groth M, et al. Comparison of diagnostic accuracy of magnetic resonance imaging and multidector computed tomography in the detection of pelvic fractures. *Eur J Radiol.* 2012;81:2337–42.

60. Davis JW, Kaups KL. Base deficit in the elderly: a marker of severe injury and death. *J Trauma.* 1998;45:873.

61. Callaway DW, Shapiro NI, Donnino MW, Baker C, Rosen CL. Serum lactate and base deficit as predictors of mortality in normotensive elderly blunt trauma patients. *J Trauma.* 2009;66(4):1040–4.

62. Mazanec DJ, Mompoint A, Podichetty V, Potnis A. Vertebral compression fractures; manage aggressively to prevent sequelae. *Cleveland Clinic J Med.* 2003;70:147–56.

63. Truumees E. Medical consequences of osteoporotic vertebral compression fractures. *Instr Course Lect.* 2003; 52:551–8.

64. Ross PD, Davis JW, Epstein RS, Wasnigh RD. Pre-existing fracture and bone mass may predict vertebral fracture risk in women. *Ann Intern Med.* 1991;114:919–23.

65. Calvert M, Old J. Vertebral compression fractures in the elderly. *Am Fam Physician.* 2004;69(1):111–16.

66. Kim JH, Yoo SH, Kim JH. Long-term follow-up of percutaneous vertebroplasty in osteoporotic compression fracture: Minimum of 5 years follow-up. *Asian Spine J.* 2012;6(1):6–14.

67. Mali S, Chiampas G, Leonard H. Emergent evaluation of injuries to the shoulder, clavicle, and humerus. *Emerg Med Clin North Am.* 2010;28:739–63.

68. Stayner LR, Cummings J, Anderson J, Jobe CM. Shoulder dislocations in patients older than 40 years of age. *Orthop Clin North Am.* 2000;31:231.

69. Palcau L, Gouicem D, Dufranc J, Mackowiak E, Berger L. Delayed axillary artery pseudoaneurysm as an isolated consequence to anterior dislocation of the shoulder. *Ann Vasc Surg.* 2012;26:279.

70. Brunelli MP, Gill TJ. Fractures and tendon injuries of the athletic shoulder. *Orthop Clin North Am.* 2002;33:497.

71. Simank HG, et al. Incidence of rotator cuff tears in shoulder dislocations and results of prospective randomized trial. *Injury.* 1997;28:283.

72. Neil J. Techniques for reduction of anteroinferior shoulder dislocation. *Emerg Med Australas.* 2005;17:463–71.

73. Riebel GD, McCabe JB. Anterior shoulder dislocations: A review of reduction techniques. *Am J Emerg Med.* 1991; 9:180.

74. Kwon YW, Kulwicki KJ, Zuckerman JD. Glenohumeral joint subluxations, dislocations and instability. In *Rockwood and Green's Fractures in Adults*, 7th edn, ed. Bucholz RW, Heckman JD, Court-Brown CM, Tornetta P (Philadelphia, PA: Wolters Kluwer Health/Lippincott Williams & Wilkins, 2010).

75. Atoun E, Narvani A, Even D. Management of 1st time dislocation of the shoulder in patients over 40 years of age: the prevalence of iatrogenic fractures. *J Orthop Trauma.* 2013;27:190–3.

76. Goga, IE. Chronic shoulder dislocations. *J Shoulder Elbow Surg.* 2003;12(5):446–50.

77. Mack GR, McPherson SA, Lutz RB. Acute median neuropathy after wrist trauma. The role of emergent carpal tunnel release. *Clin Orthop Relat Res.* 1994;300:141–6.

78. Kelly, AJ, Warwick D, Crichlow TP, Bannister GC. Is manipulation of moderately displaced Colles' fracture worthwhile in patients older than 60 years. *Am J Sports Med.* 2012;40(4):822–7.

Chapter

24

Infectious diseases in the elderly

Robert S. Anderson Jr. and Stephen Y. Liang

Introduction

It is hard to conceive of a scenario more conducive to infection than that which exists for our older patients. Natural host defenses are compromised, risk factors are plentiful, and clinical markers of disease are altered. To make matters more challenging, those over 85 years of age represent the fastest growing demographic and are at the greatest risk for health-related complications and death [1]. Relative mortality rates for sepsis and pneumonia are three times that of young people, while mortality rates for appendicitis may be as high as 20 times that of younger adults [2].

Age-related impairment of defenses

It has been argued that geriatric patients represent the largest group of immunocompromised patients treated by emergency physicians (EPs) [3]. Immunosenescence reflects the reality of worn-out adaptive immunity, where T cells are exhausted from a lifetime of antigenic exposure [4]. B cells also suffer from a lack of T-cell regulation leading to attenuated antibody responses [5]. Functional and anatomic changes likewise render older patients more vulnerable to infection. Urinary stasis from either neuromuscular dysfunction or obstruction promotes bacterial growth. The epithelial shield is less apt to present a robust mechanical barrier to skin and other outside flora. A previously stalwart pulmonary system can fall apart on many levels. Delayed cough reflex, poor mucociliary clearance, floppy airways, a stiff thoracic cage, and impaired thoracic muscle endurance can predispose a senior to infection. Chronic malnourishment further depletes existing reserves. Finally, thermoregulatory failure blunts the traditional febrile response, impeding host response to and clinician recognition of ongoing infection.

An onslaught of risks

With advancing age often comes the triple threat of disease burden, polypharmacy, and frequent interactions with health care systems. Chronic illnesses such as diabetes mellitus, rheumatoid arthritis, systemic lupus erythematosus, chronic obstructive pulmonary disease (COPD), malignancy, and stroke carry a predilection for infection. Medications including beta blockers, nonsteroidal anti-inflammatory drugs, immunosuppressants, anticholinergic agents, and gastric acid suppressants can blunt physiologic responses and hamper defenses [6]. Elders who come into contact with health care on a regular basis (e.g., hemodialysis, residence in a long-term care facility) or who require frequent hospital admissions are at heightened risk for health care-associated infections, often with drug-resistant organisms.

Altered clinical markers

Vital signs have been the traditional bellwether of patient stability, or lack thereof. They are a set of values that clinicians can interpret instinctively and rapidly. Unfortunately, as in pediatrics, interpretation of geriatric vital signs requires caution. Unlike in children, age and weight for geriatric patients do no beget a set of expected values. The heterogeneous geriatric population is bombarded by an array of physiologic and pathologic insults. Vital signs in older patients may not only diverge from what we consider normal but settle into a confined range that is unique to each individual patient [4]. For this reason, trends in vital signs for an older adult are particularly important and high-yield for the busy EP.

Fever remains a common reason for transfer from a long-term care facility (LTCF) to the emergency department (ED). It remains highly suggestive of infection and carries mortality as high as 10% [1,7]. Yet, impaired thermoregulation in the elderly has been recognized since Sir William Osler's time. Hypothermia is thus an important and often underappreciated sign of infection. The mechanisms of impaired febrile response are well described [8,9]. Fever, traditionally defined as a temperature ≥38°C, can be absent or blunted in up to 30% of elders presenting with severe infection [10]. Fever in older adults has now been redefined as a consistent oral temperature of ≥37.2°C, a rectal temperature of ≥37.5°C, or a 1.1°C increase in temperature from baseline [9]. In patients presenting from LTCFs, a single oral temperature of ≥37.8°C constitutes a fever.

Geriatric Emergency Medicine, ed. Joseph H. Kahn, Brendan G. Magauran Jr., and Jonathan S. Olshaker. Published by Cambridge University Press.
© Cambridge University Press 2014.

Approach to the elderly ED patient with suspected infection

History

Older patients do not present to the ED in a vacuum, but in the context of chronic diseases, multiple medications prescribed by multiple providers, varying exposure to health care systems, likely cognitive deficits, and fluid living situations. Sorting out the details of these complex patients can be challenging and time consuming. A structured approach to the elderly patient with suspected infection can help streamline the assessment.

First, close attention to and documentation of the patient's mental status is critical. Any acute change from baseline should be taken seriously. Mental status changes can be a presentation of almost any illness, but have a high correlation with infectious diseases. This critical aspect of the history is helpful if detected, but is often missed. Two-thirds of delirious patients have underlying dementia, underscoring the importance of obtaining collateral history from family members, facilities, and other health care providers [11]. The simple phrase "attentive without an acute change in cognition" elegantly reflects a chart that has taken into account an elderly patient's mental status.

Second, it is important to be selective and consistent in obtaining ancillary history. High-yield items include the ability to detect illness through subtle changes in vital signs collected prior to and during the current illness, as well as an appreciation of the patient's baseline mental and functional status. Knowledge of prior contact with health care in the preceding 3 months, antibiotic use within the previous 90 days, and the presence of immunosuppressing drugs or conditions can greatly influence an EP's choice of empiric antibiotic therapy.

Physical examination

The importance of identifying trends in a patient's vital signs in relation to their baseline cannot be overemphasized. A patient presenting with a blood pressure of 110/70 in the ED may be quite ill if the blood pressure earlier in the day was 180/90. Respiratory rates hold special importance in the elderly. A respiratory rate of ≥27 breaths per minute has been correlated with poor outcomes and can be a better marker of severe illness than blood pressure [12]. As mentioned before, hypothermia in an elderly patient should always be considered a significant finding.

Neurologic examination should focus on ascertaining the patient's mental status, though validation of a rapid delirium evaluation tool in the emergency setting is lacking. We suggest that any acute change from baseline be considered delirium. Patient caregivers can accurately report a change in mental status, even in patients with advanced dementia.

Dermatologic evaluation can be extremely revealing but often requires coordination with staff to roll the patient and examine the back and other hidden surfaces. The perineum should be examined, particularly in ill diabetics. Similar to a child presenting with fever, an otoscopic examination should be performed and the mastoid sinuses percussed. The oral cavity should always be inspected to exclude dental infection.

Detecting pathology in the elderly abdomen can be difficult. The leading surgical cause of abdominal pathology is acute cholecystitis [13]. With up to one-third of patients lacking serious pain, careful attention to the abdominal examination is important. Any pain, regardless of peritoneal signs, should raise concern. The cardiopulmonary exam is not geriatric-specific except to point out that murmurs and other findings may be chronic and require review of the medical record.

Differential diagnosis of fever in the elderly

While suspicious for infection, fever may also be the presenting sign of a number of other conditions, including collagen vascular disease (temporal arteritis, rheumatoid arthritis, polymyalgia rheumatica), malignancy, and adverse drug reactions. Temporal arteritis can present with headache, a palpable temporal artery, and elevated erythrocyte sedimentation rate (ESR). Malignancy is often accompanied by constitutional symptoms and may be uncovered during a thorough lymph node exam.

Laboratory evaluation and imaging in the ED should be guided by the history and physical examination. With atypical presentations being the norm in geriatrics, clinicians often order studies to look for rather than to confirm diagnoses. While often unavoidable, extra care should be exercised in interpreting diagnostic results without first establishing the pretest probability of disease.

Several tests, when negative, can greatly reduce the likelihood of certain infections. A normal C-reactive protein strongly argues against a serious bacterial infection [10]. A good-quality chest radiograph with posteroanterior (PA) and lateral views in an immunocompetent elder lowers the likelihood of bacterial pneumonia, regardless of intravascular volume status [7]. A urine sample, clean-catch or catheterized, without white blood cells, bacteria, or their surrogate markers (leukocyte esterase, nitrite) can almost eliminate the possibility of a bacterial urinary tract infection.

Unfortunately, most tests have pitfalls. An elevated white blood cell (WBC) count is absent in up to one-third of cases of acute cholecystitis in the elderly [13]. Clinical guidelines exist regarding the interpretation of the WBC count in residents of LTCFs [3]. Bacterial infection should be suspected in the presence of a WBC count ≥14,000 cells/mm^3, a left shift (defined as band neutrophils >6%), or a total band count >1500 cells/mm^3.

Pneumonia

Community-acquired pneumonia (CAP) remains one of the most common infectious processes encountered in elderly patients. Hospitalization rates for pneumonia in US adults aged 64–74 have increased significantly over time [14]. At least 1 in 20 seniors over the age of 85 years is hospitalized for pneumonia each year [14]. In parallel, mortality from CAP has improved dramatically, due in part to increasingly widespread vaccination of elders against pneumococcus and influenza [15]. Elderly patients with a history of COPD, asthma, congestive heart failure (CHF), diabetes mellitus, lung cancer, immunosuppression, malignancy, malnutrition, tobacco use, or a past history of pneumonia are especially prone to developing CAP [16]. Those residing in LTCFs are likely to have many of these comorbidities in addition to predisposing factors (e.g., difficulty swallowing, poor oral hygiene), placing them at even greater risk for pneumonia.

Streptococcus pneumoniae is the most common microorganism implicated in CAP affecting the elderly. Other organisms include *Haemophilus influenzae*, *Legionella pneumophila*, *Chlamydia pneumoniae*, *Mycoplasma pneumoniae*, as well as respiratory viruses (e.g., influenza, respiratory syncytial virus, human metapneumovirus). *Staphylococcus aureus* and Gramnegative bacilli such as *Klebsiella pneumoniae* and *Pseudomonas aeruginosa* are more likely to be found in older adults with chronic lung disease or who have had frequent exposure to health care or nursing homes. These same patients carry a greater risk of infection with antibiotic-resistant organisms. Methicillin-resistant *S. aureus* (MRSA) is an important cause of severe, necrotizing pneumonia. Pulmonary tuberculosis, often secondary to reactivation of latent disease, should also be considered in the differential diagnosis of an elderly patient with pneumonia, particularly if they are presenting from a nursing home. Influenza can also lead to pneumonia, with the potential for superimposed bacterial infection with *S. aureus*.

Classic signs and symptoms associated with pneumonia including cough (with or without sputum production), dyspnea, pleuritic chest pain, and fever are frequently muted or even absent in elderly patients. In one study, a constellation of cough, dyspnea, and fever was present in only one-third of elders diagnosed with pneumonia, while delirium was a key finding in more than half [17]. More than one-third failed to mount a fever altogether. Sometimes, tachypnea and tachycardia may be the only tip-offs to an active pneumonia. Nonspecific complaints including weakness, myalgias, poor appetite, abdominal pain, and functional decline are commonplace. Given the wide range of atypical presentations possible, the physical examination can be misleading. A normal lung examination devoid of rales or bronchial sounds does not rule out pneumonia.

Diagnostic evaluation should always start with a high-quality chest radiograph with PA and lateral views to assess for lobar consolidation, interstitial infiltrates, or cavitary lesions. In immunosuppressed patients (e.g., neutropenic fever, human immunodeficiency virus infection), plain chest radiography can be deceivingly normal and computed tomography (CT) of the chest should be considered. Patients with severe CAP, particularly with a history of immunosuppression, should have two blood cultures drawn prior to antibiotic administration as they are more apt to develop bacteremia with pneumonia, often with organisms not covered by standard empiric therapy [18]. Likewise, Gram stain and culture of the sputum should be sent to help guide antibiotic therapy in severely ill patients. When available, urinary antigen testing for *L. pneumophila* (serogroup 1) and *S. pneumoniae* can facilitate rapid diagnosis. In the case of *Legionella*, hyponatremia (<130 meq/l) may also be a useful clue to diagnosis, though many elderly patients may be hyponatremic for unrelated reasons. Depending on

Table 24.1. CURB-65 criteria

- Confusion
- Uremia (blood urea nitrogen level >7 mmol/l or 20 mg/dl)
- Respiratory rate ≥30 breaths/min
- Low blood pressure (systolic blood pressure <90 mmHg or diastolic blood pressure ≤60 mmHg)
- Age ≥65 years

the season, nasopharyngeal samples should be sent to evaluate for respiratory viruses including influenza A and B. Current rapid influenza antigen tests lack sensitivity and should be confirmed with reverse transcriptase polymerase chain reaction (RT-PCR)-based assays or other available methods. If influenza is strongly suspected, empiric antiviral therapy is warranted, even in the presence of a negative rapid antigen test, pending additional work-up.

Severity-of-illness and prognostic scoring systems can inform ED decision making about an elderly patient's need for hospital admission and intensive care. The CURB-65 criteria, based on the modified British Thoracic Society assessment tool, provide a simple means of estimating pneumonia severity and 30-day mortality [19]. A single point is awarded for each of the following elements: **C**onfusion, **u**remia, **r**espiratory rate, low **b**lood pressure, and age ≥**65** years (Table 24.1). Patients with a score of 0 or 1 are considered at low risk of mortality (<2%) and may be treated on an outpatient basis. Those with a score of 2 bear an intermediate risk (9%) and are likely to benefit from hospital admission. A score of ≥3 denotes a high risk of mortality that requires admission, potentially to an intensive care unit (ICU). Based on a US pneumonia cohort, the Pneumonia Severity Index (PSI) also provides an estimation of 30-day mortality to aid clinicians in identifying patients at low risk for death and other complications of CAP [20]. More complicated than the CURB-65 criteria, the PSI stratifies patients into five mortality risk classes based on demographic factors, comorbid conditions, physical examination findings, and laboratory and radiographic abnormalities. Both the CURB-65 criteria and PSI have been evaluated in the ED population and are best suited to identifying elderly patients at low risk of death from pneumonia [21–23].

Practice guidelines available from the Infectious Diseases Society of America (IDSA) provide a rational framework for managing elderly patients with CAP in the ED [18]. For previously healthy individuals deemed appropriate to receive outpatient treatment, empiric therapy should consist of either a macrolide (azithromycin, clarithromycin, or erythromycin) or doxycycline. Patients with underlying chronic conditions (e.g. CHF, COPD, diabetes mellitus, renal disease) should receive a respiratory fluoroquinolone (moxifloxacin, levofloxacin) or a combination of a β-lactam (high-dose amoxicillin, amoxicillin-clavulanate) with a macrolide. If the patient is to be admitted to a hospital ward, either a respiratory fluoroquinolone or a combination of a β-lactam (ceftriaxone, cefotaxime) with a macrolide is likewise recommended. If the patient is critically ill and *Pseudomonas* is a concern, the combination of an anti-pseudomonal β-lactam (piperacillin-tazobactam, cefepime meropenem) with either ciprofloxacin or levofloxacin is advisable. If MRSA pneumonia is suspected, vancomycin or linezolid should be added. While a definitive time frame for administering empiric antibiotics against pneumonia is debatable, most experts agree that the first dose should be administered as soon as the diagnosis has been made in the ED, and preferably after cultures have been obtained.

Urinary tract infection

Urinary tract infections (UTIs) account for almost one-quarter of all infections identified in non-institutionalized elders [24]. The yearly incidence of UTI in women over the age of 60 years approaches 10%, while that of men nearing the age of 80 is 5.3% [25]. Urinary catheters are frequently found in elders and pose an added risk of iatrogenic infection.

Coliform bacteria, particularly *Escherichia coli*, are the primary drivers of UTI in the elderly [26]. *Proteus mirabilis*, *K. pneumoniae*, and group B streptococcus (*Streptococcus agalactiae*) are also common offenders. In elderly men, infections involving *Enterococcus* spp., and coagulase-negative staphylococci may be encountered. In addition to these, elders with chronic indwelling urinary catheters are at risk for UTI with *P. aeruginosa*, *Candida* spp., and other organisms associated with health care. It is important to emphasize that anytime *S. aureus* is isolated from the urine, it is likely a manifestation of bacteremia, often related to an endovascular infection, rather than primary UTI, and should be evaluated and treated as such.

The underlying problem with diagnosing UTI in the elderly is the unreliability of its traditional clinical signs and symptoms. Irritative voiding symptoms are often absent and fever nonspecific. This is compounded further by the limited diagnostic value of the urinalysis in the elderly and poorly defined parameters for how to interpret and act upon them. Unfortunately, these facts are of little consolation to the EP tasked with making treatment decisions based on limited data.

Bacteriuria refers to the presence of bacteria in the urine. It may or may not be associated with the classic symptoms of dysuria, frequency, urgency, suprapubic pain, or hematuria, which define and usually prompt the diagnosis of a UTI. When bacteriuria is uncovered in a patient without signs or symptoms of a UTI, it is termed asymptomatic bacteriuria. Up to 50% of women and 30% of men over age 65 have asymptomatic bacteriuria [27]. Different colony-forming unit (CFU) thresholds exist for each clinical scenario and are not particularly useful to EPs. Pyuria refers to the presence of WBC in the urine. Traditionally considered strong evidence for infection when more than 10 WBC per high-powered field, recent guidelines offer strong evidence to the contrary [28]. In fact, pyuria in the presence of asymptomatic bacteriuria (ASB) does not warrant antimicrobial treatment regardless of the degree. Furthermore, in catheterized samples, pyuria is diagnostic of neither bacteriuria nor UTI [28].

The distinction between asymptomatic and symptomatic bacteriuria is of critical importance because it dictates the diagnosis and treatment. In those elders that present with vague, nonspecific complaints, there is no simple algorithm or answer. The impulse to ascribe nonspecific symptoms to UTI should

be tempered and other infectious and non-infectious etiologies considered within the clinical context. In the elderly patient with altered mental status, UTI should ideally be a diagnosis of exclusion rather than of convenience. We recommend that an approach to UTI in the elderly focuses on the presenting characteristics of the patient rather than the discharge destination. This is not to suggest, however, that an abnormal urinalysis should be ignored. In an ill patient with a urinalysis consistent with infection, treatment for urinary tract infection should always be pursued.

Community-dwelling elders

Elders coming from home are less likely to suffer from functional decline, cognitive impairment, or frailty compared to those residing in LTCFs. They are also less likely to have asymptomatic bacteriuria, simplifying the diagnosis of UTI.

Selection of antibiotic therapy should be based upon the clinical status of the patient, local antibiotic resistance patterns, renal function, and consideration of adverse drug–drug or drug–disease interactions. Growing resistance of *E. coli* to trimethoprim/sulfamethoxazole (TMP/SMX) has shifted recommendations for first-line empiric coverage towards the use of fluoroquinolones (e.g., ciprofloxacin). While there is no strong evidence to support the routine practice of obtaining a urine culture prior to treatment, it is encouraged, particularly in patients with a history of recurrent or refractory UTI.

Duration of therapy is dictated by the complexity of the infection. Some authors argue that the distinction between uncomplicated and complicated UTI becomes less meaningful with age and that most UTIs in the elderly should be considered complicated infections. While a 3-day course may suffice for some, a 7-day course is generally recommended. Certain types of patients have been defined as complicated and may benefit from up to 2 weeks of therapy [29]. These patient subgroups include those with diabetes mellitus, genitourinary abnormalities (e.g., benign prostatic hypertrophy, cystocele), nephrolithiasis, immunosuppression, renal failure or transplantation, as well as men [30].

Elders presenting to the ED from LTCF

This group of seniors will, by definition, have complicated UTIs that require a minimum of 7–14 days of treatment. In addition, these patients are more likely to present with sepsis and may require ICU admission. They are also more likely to become infected with atypical as well as multidrug-resistant organisms, particularly extended-spectrum beta-lactamase producing (ESBL) organisms, which can present significant challenges to antibiotic selection. The stakes are higher and the choice of antibiotics harder. Consultation with clinical pharmacists or infectious disease specialists can be especially helpful and should be sought in the ED if available.

Elders presenting to the ED with indwelling catheters

Catheter-associated UTIs (CAUTIs) are the most common cause of health care-associated infection worldwide and account for up to 40% of infections in US hospitals related to urinary catheter use. Yet, multiple guidelines clearly discourage routine screening for bacteriuria in these patients in the absence of symptoms. Urine, collected from the catheter port using sterile technique, should only be examined when the provider has no other alternative diagnosis to explain an elderly patient's symptoms or signs.

Accurate interpretation of the urinalysis obtained from a catheterized patient can be challenging. Making a diagnosis of CAUTI in the ED is likewise cumbersome, unless the patient presents with a pre-existing culture identifying a causative organism. IDSA guidelines state that neither the presence nor degree of pyuria is helpful in distinguishing UTI from asymptomatic bacteriuria. Therefore, pyuria with ASB is not an indication for antibiotics. Conversely though, the absence of pyuria is diagnostic and strongly argues against UTI (Table 24.2 and Table 24.3).

Once a UTI has been diagnosed, it is advisable to replace the catheter and obtain a urine culture from the *new* catheter prior to initiation of antibiotic therapy. Broad-spectrum antibiotics are indicated but can be de-escalated as culture data become available. Treatment should last a minimum of 7 days and be based on patient response. If timely outpatient follow-up cannot be arranged to re-evaluate the patient, it is reasonable to prescribe a 10–14-day course of therapy. IDSA guidelines state that for those "not severely ill," a 5-day course of a fluoroquinolone such as levofloxacin is acceptable. Moxifloxacin, however, should be avoided because of its lack of effective concentration in the urine (Table 24.4).

Abdominal infections

Abdominal infections can be particularly devastating for older patients. The relative mortality rate for cholecystitis is almost 8 times that of younger adults, with appendicitis approaching nearly 20-fold [31]. Furthermore, the causes of

Table 24.2. IDSA definition of CAUTI

- Signs and symptoms compatible with UTI
- No other competing source of infection
- Greater than 10^3 CFU/ml of ≥1 bacterial species

Table 24.3. IDSA signs and symptoms compatible with CAUTI

- Fever with no other identifiable cause
- Rigors with no other identifiable cause
- Altered mental status with no other identifiable cause
- Malaise or lethargy with no other identifiable cause

Table 24.4. Antibiotic choices for treatment of UTI in elders presenting from long-term care facilities or with CAUTI

- Carbapenems
- Third- or fourth-generation cephalosporins
- Fluoroquinolones
- Piperacillin
- Aztreonam
- Aminoglycosides

Table 24.5. Antimicrobial choices for treatment of intra-abdominal sepsis

- Third- or fourth-generation cephalosporin + metronidazole
- Piperacillin-tazobactam
- Ertapenem
- Meropenem
- Aztreonam + metronidazole
- Ciprofloxacin + metronidazole

intra-abdominal sepsis are more varied in those over 65 years compared with younger adults, with more than half attributable to either appendicitis or diverticulitis and one-quarter attributable to either cholecystitis or cholangitis [32]. Finally, with higher rates of admission for any number of reasons, the elderly are at particular risk for iatrogenic infections such as *Clostridium difficile*-related diarrhea. Antibiotic therapy for suspected abdominal sepsis should be administered with the same considerations for renal toxicity, drug–drug interaction, and drug–disease interaction applied to any drug prescribed for an elderly patient (Table 24.5).

Appendicitis

Once considered a disease of the young, experience has borne out the bimodal age incidence of this surgical emergency. With a longer duration of symptoms before presentation, compromised reserves, and comorbid conditions, it is not surprising that older patients fare so poorly with appendicitis. They are more likely to present after perforation with an associated intra-abdominal abscess. The key to successful treatment is to maintain a low threshold for investigation and not to be dissuaded by a lack of fever or leukocytosis. The diagnosis of appendicitis can be clinical, but is just as likely to be radiographic. In fact, given the reality of atypical presentation, it is very reasonable to lower one's threshold for imaging as discussed elsewhere in this text.

Diverticulitis

Diverticula are ubiquitous with aging, the majority being asymptomatic. However, when the diagnosis is considered early CT scanning is recommended as the severity of the disease may not correlate with the symptoms. Indications for surgical consultation include recurrent diverticulitis, complicated diverticulitis (perforation, abscess, obstruction), and bleeding. For nonsurgical cases, the decision for inpatient versus outpatient antibiotics is often difficult (Table 24.6).

Acute cholecystitis

In much the same way that benign diverticula are common with aging, so is the prevalence of asymptomatic gallstones. However, when biliary disease is present in older adults, it occurs with a higher complication rate compared with younger patients [32]. The most commonly performed abdominal surgery for the elderly is biliary surgery. Of particular concern are elderly men who are twice as likely as elderly women to require emergency surgery and have a fivefold increased risk

Table 24.6. Indications for medical admission for elderly diverticulitis. Information obtained from reference [33]

- High fevers and/or leukocytosis
- Nausea and vomiting
- Significant comorbidities
- Older than 85 years of age
- Inadequate home support

of suppurative, necrotizing, or hemorrhagic cholecystitis. They are also at increased risk for emphysematous cholecystitis, which can increase mortality fivefold [13]. As discussed elsewhere in this text, biliary disease may present without pain or with pain that localizes elsewhere in the abdomen, chest, or back. Successful diagnosis and treatment may lie in having a lower threshold for imaging and surgical consultation.

Clostridium difficile-related diarrhea

Older patients presenting from LTCFs are at particular risk for both morbidity and mortality from this disease. With a high rate of colonization in the setting of precarious baseline health status, proliferation of *C. difficile* can be devastating. In addition to the inherent risks of starting antibiotic treatment, volume loss can initiate a cascade of organ dysfunction. *C. difficile* can also precipitate toxic megacolon, presenting as an acute abdomen without diarrhea.

Clostridium difficile infection is diagnosed most commonly by enzyme immunoassay of the stool for toxin. While very specific, the toxin assay is less sensitive. Therefore, repeat testing of the stool may be necessary to establish the diagnosis. While resistant strains of *C. difficile* exist, oral metronidazole remains a reasonable first choice for antibiotic therapy. Oral vancomycin may be used for recurrent and severe infections. Stool transplant has been used in particularly difficult cases.

Central nervous system infections

The epidemiology of bacterial meningitis has changed dramatically over the past 15 years since the advent of effective pneumococcal and *H. influenzae* type B conjugate vaccines. While pediatric cases have dropped considerably, adults ≥65 years of age contribute a significant proportion of cases today, with case fatality rates approaching 23% compared with 3.9% among patients 18–34 years [34]. Death in the elderly is attributable to sepsis or cardiorespiratory failure, due in part to comorbid diseases, rather than brain herniation [35]. Elders are also more likely to incur serious complications from bacterial meningitis including cerebral infarction, hydrocephalus, subdural empyema, seizure disorders, and coma. Therefore, prompt recognition and treatment of elderly patients with bacterial meningitis presenting to the ED is imperative.

As with pneumonia, invasive infection with *S. pneumoniae* is the most common cause of bacterial meningitis in the elderly, accounting for up to two-thirds of identified cases [35,36]. *Neisseria meningitidis*, *H. influenzae*, and group B streptococcus comprise a smaller share. *Listeria monocytogenes* remains a noteworthy pathogen in the elderly, particularly in the setting of immunosuppression or malignancy. *Klebsiella pneumoniae*,

E. coli, *P. aeruginosa*, and MRSA are also important organisms which may cause meningitis in the elderly, typically associated with hematogenous dissemination from other sites of infection (e.g., pneumonia, UTI, endocarditis, intra-abdominal infection), surgery, or trauma.

Fever, neck stiffness, and altered mental status may manifest together in up to 58% of elderly patients presenting with bacterial meningitis, with the latter being the predominant symptom [35]. However, in 30% of elderly patients presenting to the ED in one study, fever was absent [36]. Nuchal rigidity and other classic meningeal signs may be difficult to assess in the setting of pre-existing osteoarthritis and other conditions that may limit flexion of the neck, back, or knees. As many as one-third of elderly patients with bacterial meningitis may present with focal neurological deficits (e.g., aphasia, paresis, cranial nerve palsies). As with other infections in the elderly, atypical presentations and muted physical findings underscore the importance of having a low threshold for proceeding with diagnostic evaluation when bacterial meningitis is suspected.

Lumbar puncture to obtain cerebrospinal fluid (CSF) for cell count, protein, glucose, Gram stain, and aerobic bacterial culture is necessary to establish a diagnosis of bacterial meningitis. Low CSF glucose (<40 mg/dl), low CSF to serum glucose ratio (<0.4), high CSF protein (>150 mg/dl), and a neutrophilic CSF pleocytosis (CSF WBC >500 cells/mm³) are particularly concerning for bacterial infection. Gram staining of the CSF is positive in more than half of all cases, excluding *L. monocytogenes* infection [35,36]. If the patient is immunocompromised or considered high risk for tuberculosis, additional CSF should be submitted for fungal and acid-fast bacilli cultures. It is good practice to save CSF for additional testing if needed at a later time. An opening pressure should be documented at the beginning of the lumbar puncture and blood cultures sent. Computed tomography of the head prior to lumbar puncture is generally warranted in elderly patients to exclude a mass lesion and evaluate for other potential causes of altered mental status.

Empiric therapy for bacterial meningitis in the ED should be initiated as soon as the diagnosis is considered, and prior to lumbar puncture if the suspicion is high. IDSA guidelines recommend that elderly patients with suspected bacterial meningitis receive an empiric antibiotic regimen consisting of intravenous (IV) vancomycin, a third-generation cephalosporin (e.g., ceftriaxone), and ampicillin to provide expanded coverage for penicillin-resistant *S. pneumoniae* and *L. monocytogenes* [37]. Adjunctive corticosteroids (dexamethasone) have been shown to improve outcomes in patients with pneumococcal meningitis and are warranted as part of the empiric therapy for bacterial meningitis in elderly patients presenting to the ED [37,38].

Herpes simplex meningoencephalitis (HSME) is an important part of the differential for any elderly patient presenting with fever, behavioral changes, memory deficits, disorientation, or decreased level of consciousness, with or without aphasia or seizure [39]. Usually caused by reactivation of latent herpes simplex virus type 1 (HSV-1), HSME carries a high mortality and morbidity even when treated appropriately. If

HSME is suspected, empiric therapy with IV acyclovir should be initiated immediately. The CSF profile can be deceivingly unremarkable with little or no pleocytosis; polymerase chain reaction (PCR) testing for HSV-1 is necessary to confirm the diagnosis. Likewise, CT of the head can be normal. Magnetic resonance imaging is more sensitive for identifying classic temporal and frontal lobe disease associated with HSME.

Brain abscesses can arise from contiguous spread of infection (e.g., sinusitis, otogenic or odontogenic infection) or hematogenous seeding associated with an endovascular or pulmonary infection. Symptoms may include fever, headache, and focal neurologic deficits, though it is uncommon to see all three together in the elderly patient. Imaging of the brain (e.g., CT, MRI) is needed to establish the diagnosis. Empiric antibiotic therapy should consist of IV vancomycin, cefepime, and metronidazole. In some instances, surgical aspiration may be necessary.

Skin and soft tissue infections

Aging skin is prone to tearing and ulcer formation, creating avenues for bacterial invasion of soft tissues. Diabetes mellitus, peripheral vascular disease, malignancy, and impaired physical mobility not only impede wound healing but further predispose an elder to infection. Cellulitis, an infection of the subcutaneous tissues, is particularly common in elders with lower extremity ulcers, dermatophytic foot infections, lymphedema, and venous insufficiency. Elders who have undergone saphenous venectomy during coronary artery bypass surgery or lymph node dissection as part of breast cancer surgery are also prone to developing cellulitis. Cellulitis is marked by diffuse erythema, edema, induration, and pain. In contrast, erysipelas, an infection of the upper dermis and superficial lymphatics, is characterized by well-demarcated areas of erythema, edema (*peau d'orange*), and induration, sometimes accompanied by vesicles, bullae, skin streaking, and regional lymphadenopathy.

The most common organisms responsible for cellulitis and erysipelas are *Streptococcus pyogenes* and *S. aureus*. IDSA guidelines recommend the use of an oral penicillinase-resistant penicillin such as dicloxacillin or a first-generation cephalosporin such as cephalexin for mild cases of cellulitis [40]. Moderate to severe cases warranting hospital admission may be treated with IV nafcillin or cefazolin. In the modern era of community-acquired MRSA, TMP-SMX, clindamycin, and doxycycline have emerged as acceptable empiric oral agents for treating mild cellulitis while IV vancomycin, daptomycin, and linezolid are reserved for severe infections [41]. It should be noted that TMP-SMX and doxycycline lack coverage for *Streptococcus* and should not be used if that species is high on the differential for offending organisms. Erysipelas is best treated with a penicillin or a first-generation cephalosporin. Most cases of cellulitis and erysipelas are treated for 7–10 days, though deep-seated infections may require longer courses of therapy.

Necrotizing skin and soft tissue infections (NSTI) target fascia and muscle. Commonly associated with trauma, surgery, peripheral vascular disease, diabetes mellitus, and skin ulcers, NSTIs may be easily mistaken for cellulitis or abscess in the earliest stages. In fact, more than two-thirds of NSTIs are initially identified as cellulitis or abscess [42]. Mortality in elderly patients with NSTIs is historically high, particularly in the setting of delayed diagnosis [43]. Skin changes including ecchymosis, hemorrhagic bullae, cyanosis, and skin necrosis may be encountered as the infection progresses. Crepitus, pain out of proportion to physical findings, and skin anesthesia further increase the likelihood of NSTI. Fever, hemodynamic instability, and altered mental status are the heralds of systemic illness.

Necrotizing fasciitis can be polymicrobial (type I) with Gram-positive bacteria (e.g., streptococci, staphylococci, enterococci), enteric Gram-negative bacteria, and anaerobes, or monomicrobial (type II), most commonly with group A streptococci or *S. aureus*. While visualization of gas along fascial planes on plain radiography or CT is indicative of NSTI, the diagnosis remains a clinical one. Timely surgical consultation for debridement is necessary to remove infected tissue and halt the progression of the disease. Empiric therapy for polymicrobial infections should consist of a combination of ampicillin-sulbactam, clindamycin, and ciprofloxacin [40]. In monomicrobial infection, penicillin with clindamycin is recommended. If MRSA is of concern, vancomycin should be added.

Herpes zoster, or shingles, is a disease of advancing age and waning host cellular immunity. Caused by the reactivation of latent varicella zoster virus (VZV), the rash of herpes zoster is typically preceded by pain along a unilateral dermatomal distribution secondary to acute neuritis. A maculopapular eruption gives way to clusters of vesicles that progress to pustules within days. Healing may require several weeks and elderly patients are at significant risk for developing postherpetic neuralgia (PHN). Prompt ED recognition and initiation of acyclovir or valacyclovir within 72 hours of clinical symptom onset not only accelerates healing but reduces the likelihood and duration of PHN [44].

Human immunodeficiency virus

The elderly represent one of the fastest growing populations at risk for infection with human immunodeficiency virus (HIV). In 2005, persons aged 50 and over accounted for 15% of all new HIV/AIDS diagnoses and 24% of persons living with HIV/AIDS [45]. While universal HIV screening has been encouraged for patients between the ages of 13 and 64 residing in areas where the prevalence of disease is >0.1%, elderly patients are less likely to be screened routinely [46]. It is important to consider primary HIV infection, or acute retroviral syndrome, in any patient presenting to the ED with a constellation of fever, lymphadenopathy, rash, myalgias, arthralgias, sore throat, or headache. Commonly held misconceptions that elders are unlikely to engage in risky behavior or use illicit drugs have greatly hindered early diagnosis of HIV and linkage to care in this highly vulnerable population.

Infectious diseases in special geriatric populations

Traditional geriatric literature has thought of the geriatric population in three subsets: the young-old (age 65–75 years), th middle old (age 76–85 years), and the old-old (age ≥85 years). Clinical practice teaches us that in some regards, age is relative. For example, a fit 75-year-old will cope with the stress of an infection much better than a diabetic 60-year-old with poorly controlled hypertension, hyperlipidemia, and renal insufficiency. Regardless of baseline health status or the type of illness, the old-old are at substantial risk for acute decompensation. In approaching the management of infections, these patients must be treated differently. Frequent vital signs with special attention to trends are requisite. Early, broad-spectrum antibiotics can be lifesaving. Efforts to reduce iatrogenic insults, avoid overaggressive hydration, limit invasive or restrictive monitors and catheters, treat pain, and provide comfort and orientation are just as important.

A busy shift in the ED hardly seems the place or time to have an in-depth and often painful conversation with patients and their families about end-of-life care. Unfortunately, these discussions are becoming increasingly commonplace and often occur in the context of an acute infectious illness. The treating physician may feel conflicted in offering perceived life-sustaining antibiotics in these cases. It is crucial that EPs understand that hospice patients routinely receive antibiotic therapy for pneumonia and UTI in an effort to improve quality of life rather than to extend it [47]. Even IV antibiotics may be considered an option with home hospice. Each case is unique and not always certain. In some cases, the infectious disease process may be the terminal event in which case the treating provider must revisit goals of care.

Antibiotics and the elderly patient

While pharmacological considerations in the elderly have been discussed elsewhere, it is important to highlight that most antibiotics carry a significantly increased risk for bleeding when taken in combination with warfarin, ranging anywhere from two- to fivefold [48]. Although azoles are associated with the highest risk of bleeding, more commonly used antibiotics including fluoroquinolones and TMP-SMX, particularly in the management of UTI, also carry an appreciable risk. Regardless of which antibiotic is selected, it is advisable that all elderly patients receiving warfarin undergo more frequent prothrombin time (PT) and international normalized ratio (INR) testing upon discharge from the ED to ensure that supratherapeutic values are promptly addressed and warfarin dosage appropriately titrated while receiving antibiotic therapy.

Conclusion

Infectious diseases remain a significant cause of morbidity and mortality in elders presenting to the ED. Atypical presentations abound and diagnoses are seldom straightforward. Through early recognition of common infectious processes in aging patients and appropriate selection of empiric antibiotic therapy, EPs can make a tremendous impact on infectious disease outcomes.

Pearls and pitfalls

Vital signs can by influenced by age, disease, and medication, but tend to remain in a range that is specific to each elderly patient. Appreciate that textbook "normal"

vital signs may actually represent a significant change from an individual's usual baseline.

- Altered mental status is a common presentation of infection in the elderly.
- Cough, dyspnea, and fever are present in only one-third of elderly patients with pneumonia. Tachycardia and tachypnea can be subtle clues and should prompt evaluation with chest radiography.
- Up to 50% of women and 30% of men over 65 years of age have asymptomatic bacteriuria. A diagnosis of UTI in this age group should be one of exclusion.
- The most commonly performed abdominal surgery in the elderly is biliary surgery. Elderly men are at increased risk for suppurative, necrotizing, hemorrhagic, and emphysematous cholecystitis.

References

1. Yoshikawa TT. Epidemiology and unique aspects of aging and infectious diseases. *Clin Infect Dis.* 2000;30(6):931–3.
2. High KP. Infections in the elderly. In *Principles of Geriatric Medicine and Gerontology*, ed. Hazzard WR (New York: McGraw-Hill, 2003).
3. High KP. Why should the infectious diseases community focus on aging and care of the older adult? *Clin Infect Dis.* 2003;37(2):196–200.
4. Chester JG, Rudolph JL. Vital signs in older patients: age-related changes. *J Am Med Dir Assoc.* 2011;12(5):337–43.
5. Liang SY, Mackowiak PA. Infections in the elderly. *Clin Geriatr Med.* 2007;23(2):441–56.
6. Strausbaugh LJ. Emerging health care-associated infections in the geriatric population. *Emerg Infect Dis.* 2001;7(2):268–71.
7. Katz ED. Fever and immune function in the elderly. In *Geriatric Emergency Medicine*, ed. Meldon SW (New York: McGraw-Hill, 2004), pp. 55–70.
8. Kenney WL, Munce TA. Invited review: aging and human temperature regulation. *J Appl Physiol.* 2003;95(6):2598–603.
9. Norman DC. Fever in the elderly. *Clin Infect Dis.* 2000;31(1):148–51.
10. Gavazzi G, Krause KH. Aging and infection. *Lancet Infect Dis.* 2002;2(11):659–66.
11. Han JH, Wilson A, Ely EW. Delirium in the older emergency department patient: a quiet epidemic. *Emerg Med Clin North Am.* 2010;28(3):611–31.
12. Fieselmann JF, et al. Respiratory rate predicts cardiopulmonary arrest for internal medicine inpatients. *J Gen Intern Med.* 1993;8(7):354–60.
13. Ragsdale L, Southerland L. Acute abdominal pain in the older adult. *Emerg Med Clin North Am.* 2011;29(2):429–48.
14. Fry, AM, et al. Trends in hospitalizations for pneumonia among persons aged 65 years or older in the United States, 1988–2002. *JAMA.* 2005;294(21):2712–19.
15. Ruhnke GW, et al. Marked reduction in 30-day mortality among elderly patients with community-acquired pneumonia. *Am J Med.* 2011;124(2):171–8.
16. Jackson ML, et al. The burden of community-acquired pneumonia in seniors: results of a population-based study. *Clin Infect Dis.* 2004;39(11):1642–50.

17. Riquelme R, et al. Community-acquired pneumonia in the elderly. Clinical and nutritional aspects. *Am J Respir Crit Care Med.* 1997;156(6):1908–14.

18. Mandell LA, et al. Infectious Diseases Society of America/American Thoracic Society consensus guidelines on the management of community-acquired pneumonia in adults. *Clin Infect Dis.* 2007;44(Suppl. 2):S27–72.

19. Lim WS, et al. Defining community acquired pneumonia severity on presentation to hospital: an international derivation and validation study. *Thorax.* 2003;58(5):377–82.

20. Fine MJ, et al. A prediction rule to identify low-risk patients with community-acquired pneumonia. *N Engl J Med.* 1997;336(4):243–50.

21. Chen JH, et al. Comparison of clinical characteristics and performance of pneumonia severity score and CURB-65 among younger adults, elderly and very old subjects. *Thorax.* 2010;65(11):971–7.

22. Howell MD, et al. Performance of severity of illness scoring systems in emergency department patients with infection. *Acad Emerg Med.* 2007;14(8):709–14.

23. Ochoa-Gondar O, et al. Comparison of three predictive rules for assessing severity in elderly patients with CAP. *Int J Clin Pract.* 2011;65(11):1165–72.

24. Ruben FL, et al. Clinical infections in the noninstitutionalized geriatric age group: methods utilized and incidence of infections. The Pittsburgh Good Health Study. *Am J Epidemiol.* 1995;141(2):145–57.

25. Foxman B, Brown P. Epidemiology of urinary tract infections: transmission and risk factors, incidence, and costs. *Infect Dis Clin North Am.* 2003;17(2):227–41.

26. Nicolle LE. Urinary tract pathogens in complicated infection and in elderly individuals. *J Infect Dis.* 2001;183(Suppl. 1):S5–8.

27. Fircanis S., McKay M. Recognition and management of extended spectrum beta-lactamase producing organisms (ESBL). *Med Health R I.* 2010;93(5):161–2.

28. Hooton TM, et al. Diagnosis, prevention, and treatment of catheter-associated urinary tract infection in adults: 2009 International Clinical Practice Guidelines from the Infectious Diseases Society of America. *Clin Infect Dis.* 2010;50(5):625–63.

29. Nicolle LE. A practical guide to antimicrobial management of complicated urinary tract infection. *Drugs Aging.* 2001;18(4):243–54.

30. Caterino JM. Evaluation and management of geriatric infections in the emergency department. *Emerg Med Clin North Am.* 2008;26(2):319–43.

31. Mezey E. Hepatic, biliary and pancreatic disease. In *Principles of Geriatric Medicine and Gerontology*, ed. Hazzard WR (New York: McGraw-Hill, 2003), pp. 601–13.

32. Podnos YD, Jimenez JC, Wilson SE. Intra-abdominal sepsis in elderly persons. *Clin Infect Dis.* 2002;35(1):62–8.

33. Sinanan M, Kao L, Vedovatti PA. Surgery in the elderly population. In *Principles of Geriatric Medicine and Gerontology*, ed. Hazzard WR (New York: McGraw-Hill, 2003), pp. 385–99.

34. Thigpen MC, et al. Bacterial meningitis in the United States, 1998–2007. *N Engl J Med.* 2011;364(21):2016–25.

35. Weisfelt M, et al. Community-acquired bacterial meningitis in older people. *J Am Geriatr Soc.* 2006;54(10):1500–7.

36. Cabellos C, et al. Community-acquired bacterial meningitis in elderly patients: experience over 30 years. *Medicine (Baltimore).* 2009;88(2):115–19.

37. Tunkel AR, et al. Practice guidelines for the management of bacterial meningitis. *Clin Infect Dis.* 2004;39(9):1267–84.

38. de Gans J, van de Beek D, and European Dexamethasone in Adulthood Bacterial Meningitis Study Investigators. Dexamethasone in adults with bacterial meningitis. *N Engl J Med.* 2002;347(20):1549–56.

39. Riera-Mestre A, et al. Herpes simplex encephalitis in older adults. *J Am Geriatr Soc.* 2010;58(1):201–2.

40. Stevens DL, et al. Practice guidelines for the diagnosis and management of skin and soft-tissue infections. *Clin Infect Dis.* 2005;41(10):1373–406.

41. Liu C, et al. Clinical practice guidelines by the Infectious Diseases Society of America for the treatment of methicillin-resistant *Staphylococcus aureus* infections in adults and children. *Clin Infect Dis.* 2011;52(3):e18–55.

42. Wong CH, et al. Necrotizing fasciitis: clinical presentation, microbiology, and determinants of mortality. *J Bone Joint Surg Am.* 2003;85-A(8):1454–60.

43. Brandt MM, Corpron CA, Wahl WL. Necrotizing soft tissue infections: a surgical disease. *Am Surg.* 2000;66(10):967–70; discussion 970–1.

44. Beutner KR, et al. Valaciclovir compared with acyclovir for improved therapy for herpes zoster in immunocompetent adults. *Antimicrob Agents Chemother.* 1995;39(7):1546–53.

45. Centers for Disease Control and Prevention. *HIV/AIDS Surveillance Report, 2005*, Vol. 17, Rev. edn (Atlanta, GA: US Department of Health and Human Services, Centers for Disease Control and Prevention), pp. 1–54 (also available at www.cdc.gov/hiv/topics/surveillance/resources/reports/).

46. Branson BM, et al. Revised recommendations for HIV testing of adults, adolescents, and pregnant women in health-care settings. *MMWR Recomm Rep.* 2006;55(RR-14):1–17.

47. Lamba S, Quest TE. Hospice care and the emergency department: rules, regulations, and referrals. *Ann Emerg Med.* 2011;57(3):282–90.

48. Baillargeon J, et al. Concurrent use of warfarin and antibiotics and the risk of bleeding in older adults. *Am J Med.* 2012;125(2):183–9.

Chapter 25

Hematologic and oncologic emergencies in the elderly

Michael P. Jones

Introduction

As the nation's population continues to age, emergency physicians will encounter an increasing number of elderly patients suffering from complications of their hematologic and oncologic diseases and the treatments of those diseases. This chapter on geriatric hematologic and oncologic emergencies will discuss fever and leukopenia, tumor lysis syndrome, hypercalcemia, SVC syndrome, hyperviscosity syndrome, coagulopathy, anemia, thrombocytopenia, transfusion of blood components, administration of vitamin K, and other hematologic/oncologic emergencies.

Overview of hematologic diseases

Hematologic diseases are vast and are related to derangements of the hematopoietic system. Curiously, this system when unperturbed maintains a fairly constant level of circulating cells. Emerging research suggests that age has no influence on homeostasis of the hematopoietic system. What is often different, however, is the ability of this system to respond to stress, frequently in relation to other diseases [1]. There are relatively few deficiencies in blood cell function in the elderly, but rather cumulative functional deficiencies when acute or chronic disease stress produces a demand that overwhelms production capacity [2].

Overview of oncologic diseases

Cancer is a rampant public health problem for all patients, young and old – it is the second leading cause of death after heart disease in the US. Cancer accounted for 22% of deaths in the over-65s in 2009. In fact, the age-adjusted US mortality from neoplastic disease in 2009 was 55 per 100,000 in those under 65, 693 per 100,000 in those 65–74, and 1300 per 100,000 in those over 75 [3]. Over 50% of all cancer diagnoses in the US between 2005 and 2009 were made in those over 65 (some studies in other populations put that figure at 60%) [2]. The risk of oncologic diseases is clearly more likely as an individual ages. Certain cancers, including breast, colorectal, prostate, pancreatic, lung, bladder, and stomach cancers, are related to aging and the physiologic changes that occur with the aging process.

The relationship between aging and neoplastic transformation is poorly understood and complex. Data certainly support that aging and cancer incidence are inextricably linked. Current theories include changes in host tumor defenses (e.g. decreased DNA repair ability, tumor suppressor gene loss, decreased immune surveillance, or oncogene activation) that occur with aging, as well as increased exposure (and perhaps susceptibility) to carcinogens over a vastly longer lifetime as contributors to this increase in incidence [4].

Management of the elderly individual with cancer is complicated. Early diagnosis and prevention is widely regarded to be the key in successful management of neoplastic diseases at all age levels. Physicians have been noted to be less aggressive in screening and treatment decisions in the elderly, and older patients have been noted to view cancer as a hopeless, untreatable diagnosis and ultimately fatal [2]. Both physician and patient bias is a significant factor in creating an appropriate patient-specific decision process related to: whether to screen for cancer, whether to pursue diagnostic testing, and whether and how intensely to treat [2]. Even though therapy should be comparable in elderly versus young patients, this is often not the case [5–7].

Treatment options need to incorporate an evaluation of a wide breadth of considerations specific to the elderly. Surgical removal is often the treatment of choice along with adjuvant chemotherapeutics and/or radiation. The perception has always been that the myriad comorbid conditions and physiologic changes, such as diminished cardiopulmonary function, decreased immune response, changes in excretion and metabolism mechanisms, diminished mental acuity, and diminished hematopoiesis, make the elderly poor candidates for treatment [6,7]. However, many studies demonstrate that this is not the case and, in fact, improvements in functionality and quality of life measures are noted in those elderly patients who receive a more aggressive treatment course [8–12].

Specific disease conditions

Fever and leukopenia

Fever (a single temperature of >38.3°C or recurrent temperatures >38°C, preferably measured rectally) combined with

Geriatric Emergency Medicine, ed. Joseph H. Kahn, Brendan G. Magauran Jr., and Jonathan S. Olshaker. Published by Cambridge University Press.
© Cambridge University Press 2014.

leukopenia (particularly neutropenia, an absolute neutrophil count <500 cells/ml) is a medical emergency. In the elderly cancer patient, the body's host defenses are often diminished, either in relation to underlying pathologic condition or due to recent or ongoing chemotherapeutic and radiotherapeutic treatments. Rapidly progressive infection can be life threatening in these immunocompromised patients and warrants aggressive management.

History and physical exam is usually of little import in the immunocompromised patient who presents with fever. Symptoms and findings on examination can often be lacking, despite the rapidity with which an overwhelming infection can present. Patients who have underlying comorbid diseases (particularly common in the elderly), altered mucosal immunity, neutropenia (even greater when >10 days in duration), defects in humoral or cellular immunity, or indwelling catheters are at increased risk of developing life-threatening infections and inquiry directed towards these factors can be helpful. Diagnostic testing should include a complete blood count with manual differential analysis, blood and urine cultures, and chest radiograph (although this may be normal due to the lack of neutrophilic response causing opacification). Indwelling catheters and skin sites should be cultured, if practical. Further diagnostic testing, such as viral testing, cerebrospinal fluid (CSF) studies, computed tomography (CT), or magnetic resonance imaging (MRI) is not routinely warranted unless there are specific focal symptoms to suggest those studies might have diagnostic benefit, initial evaluation is negative, or the patient's clinical condition is deteriorating or just not improving.

Resuscitative measures should be instituted immediately for any patient that is unstable hemodynamically. Because the initial evaluation of the febrile, neutropenic patient does not typically identify a focus of infection, broad-spectrum antibiotics should be given empirically, even if this may potentially mask identification of a cause. Patients can be stratified into high- and low-risk, the latter being potentially treated as outpatients. Those at highest risk of complications, and thus should be treated as inpatients, include those with neutropenia expected to last >7 days or profound absolute neutrophil count ≤100 cells/ml, or the presence of comorbid conditions such as hypotension, pneumonia, new-onset abdominal pain, or neurologic changes. Alternatively, the Multinational Association for Supportive Care in Cancer (MASCC) score can be used to classify patients, with those scoring <21 falling into the high-risk category. In these patients, strong Gram-negative and -positive bacterial coverage should be considered as well as an anti-pseudomonal agent and coverage for methicillin-resistant *Staphylococcus aureus* and penicillin-resistant *Streptococcus pneumoniae*. Suggested initial regimens include cefepime, a carbapenem, or piperacillin-tazobactam plus vancomycin or linezolid if suspecting a catheter infection, skin or soft tissue infection, pneumonia, or if there is hemodynamic instability. Penicillin-resistant patients can receive cephalosporins, but ciprofloxacin plus clindamycin or aztreonam plus vancomycin have been suggested as alternatives [13]. Also, consider the use of antimicrobial agents targeting viral or fungal etiologies.

The decision on antibiotic therapies and inpatient versus outpatient treatment for the leukopenic febrile patient should involve the patient's geriatrician and/or oncologist. In addition, the emergency physician should make all efforts to provide for a sterile, isolated environment for the patient. In the elderly, consideration should be given to the psychosocial ramifications of such therapy [14].

Tumor lysis syndrome

Tumor lysis syndrome is a condition associated with death of neoplastic cells that involves multiple metabolic derangements caused by the sudden release of intracellular contents and electrolytes into the bloodstream. It typically occurs 1–3 days after chemotherapy or radiotherapy and is considered the most common disease-related emergency in all patients with hematologic cancers. It typically includes hyperuricemia, hyperphosphatemia, hyperkalemia, hypocalcemia (secondary to hyperphosphatemia and the subsequent sequestration of calcium in tissues), and acute kidney injury.

Patients with tumor lysis syndrome may present to the emergency department (ED) with a multitude of vague symptoms due to the metabolic derangements that are occurring. Patients can present with lethargy, nausea, and/or vomiting. The may also have clinical manifestations of hypocalcemia, such as muscle spasm, neuromuscular irritability, or seizures. The other electrolyte disturbances, particularly hyperkalemia, can independently, or in conjunction with the compounding effects from acute renal injury, lead to fatal cardiac arrhythmias.

There are two classification systems for tumor lysis syndrome. The clinical classification system identifies some of the more serious historical and examination findings in patients with tumor lysis syndrome and requires the presence of increased creatinine level, seizures, cardiac dysrhythmia, or death in conjunction with the laboratory classification system. The laboratory classification system requires two or more of the following occurring concurrently within 3 days before or 7 days after the start of therapy: hyperuricemia (uric acid >8.0 mg/dl), hyperkalemia (potassium >6.0 mmol/l), hyperphosphatemia (phosphorus >4.5 mg/dl), and hypocalcemia (corrected calcium <7.0 mg/dl or ionized calcium <1.12 mg/dl).

Evaluation by the emergency physician of the elderly patient with nonspecific symptoms after chemotherapy or radiotherapy should focus on initial resuscitative measures and consideration of a broad differential diagnosis. Specific evaluation that should be performed are an ECG for evidence of hyperkalemia, the most deadly complication of this disease, as well as an electrolyte panel looking for the specific abnormalities noted (hyperkalemia, hyperphosphatemia, hyperuricemia, and hypocalcemia). In addition, measurement of urinary output may be useful in identifying acute kidney injury and in management of fluid resuscitation, particularly in the elderly patient with comorbid conditions. Treatments should be directed towards the specific electrolyte disturbances encountered.

In the elderly patient, avoidance of tumor lysis syndrome is paramount as their comorbid medical conditions will often place them at higher risk of sudden cardiac arrhythmias and acute kidney injury, even with just a minimal release of toxi mor metabolites. A low-intensity initial therapy has been suggested to slow the lysis of cancer cells and allow the renal homeostatic mechanisms sufficient time to compensate for the rapid changes in electrolytes. Low-dose treatments prior to the start of intensive chemotherapy have been effective with several diseases and are recommended [4,15].

Hypercalcemia

Hypercalcemia is defined as total measured serum calcium greater than 10.5 mg/dl or an ionized calcium level exceeding 7 mEq/l. Calcium homeostasis is tightly controlled through parathyroid hormone (PTH), calcitonin, and vitamin D. Often, hypercalcemia is due to hyperparathyroidism or malignancy. In addition to malignancy, other common causes of hypercalcemia that may be encountered in the ED, particularly in the elderly, are lithium toxicity and granulomatous disease, such as sarcoidosis and tuberculosis.

Patients with hypercalcemia often have diverse and vague symptoms, but can be generalized by the mnemonic "stones, bones, moans, and groans," or similar varieties of this phrase, representing the more common symptoms of renal or biliary calculi, bone or joint pain, neuropsychiatric disorders such as depression, confusion, memory loss, and abdominal pain with GI irritability, ulcerative disease, or pancreatitis.

Typical findings on examination are subtle or non-existent but generally include decreased neuromuscular activity (diminished sensation, strength, and reflexes) and mental status changes. Diagnostic testing of utility in the ED includes a serum and ionized calcium level as well as an electrocardiogram (ECG), which can show ST segment depressions, wide T waves, QT interval narrowing, and heart blocks. Further evaluation is aimed at identifying and treating the underlying causes.

Dehydration is quite common in hypercalcemia secondary to polyuria from the diminished ability of the kidneys to concentrate urine. Subsequently, most treatment is aimed at correcting dehydration and then increasing both renal excretion and decreasing bone mobilization of calcium. Furosemide or other loop diuretics affect the former, while calcitonin, glucocorticoids, and – less frequently in the ED – bisphosphonates affect the latter.

Specific considerations for the elderly in hypercalcemia revolve mostly around the underlying etiologies and the need for gingerly treating hypercalcemia. The elderly typically have less capacity at managing a homeostatic balance in various organ systems, and as such, the ability to respond effectively to rising levels of calcium may be blunted. Additionally, many of the most common diseases that cause hypercalcemia increase in prevalence as individuals age. Furthermore, the evaluation of vague gastrointestinal or psychiatric complaints should prompt the clinician to consider hypercalcemia in the elderly. But, perhaps of greatest concern in the elderly are the difficulties associated with the most effective treatment for hypercalcemia – large-volume hydration with intravenous (IV) normal saline, which may exacerbate heart failure that is prevalent in the elderly, causing pulmonary congestion and respiratory distress (Table 25.1).

Table 25.1. Treatment of hypercalcemia [26]

Serum calcium level (mg/dl)	Clinical manifestations	Therapy
10.5–12.0	Asymptomatic	Oral hydration, discontinuation of inciting agent (e.g., lithium, thiazide)
12.0–14.0	Mild GI upset, malaise	Oral or IV hydration
>14.0	ECG changes, altered mental status	Aggressive IV hydration (consider loop diuretics in patients with renal or heart failure), calcitonin, bisphosphonates, glucocorticoids. Consider hemodialysis for patients with levels >18.0 and with neurologic symptoms for guiding therapy as this more effectively distinguishes between acute and chronic.

Note: Symptomatology is a more important marker for guiding therapy as it more effectively distinguishes between acute and chronic cases and the body's compensatory mechanisms.

Superior vena cava syndrome

Superior vena cava (SVC) syndrome is typically a slowly progressive condition that involves the compression of the superior vena cava. The most common cause is bronchogenic carcinoma (accounting for nearly 80% of cases), but can also be caused by other malignancies of the chest and neck. Syphilis and tuberculosis have also been documented to have caused SVC syndrome. Mass effect to the SVC causes reduced venous return.

Patients with SVC syndrome often present with dyspnea. Other symptoms may include upper extremity or trunk swelling. Chest pain, cough, and vocal complaints are less common presenting symptoms. Typically, physical exam findings are not present until the malignancy increases in size and/or invasiveness, but can include upper body edema, jugular venous distention, and cyanosis. Rarely, a Horner's syndrome, vocal cord paralysis, phrenic nerve involvement, or acute airway difficulty can occur.

Elderly patients might present to the ED with shortness of breath, chest pain, or upper body swelling. More life-threatening conditions such as acute coronary syndrome, aortic dissection, or aneurysm should be considered first in these patients. An ECG should always be performed with these symptoms, and a chest radiograph may show a widened mediastinum or other evidence of malignancy. CT scan with contrast is diagnostic and should be the first step in patients with clinical symptoms or chest radiograph suggestive of SVC syndrome. Interestingly, a simple examination technique, the Pemberton's maneuver, may also be diagnostic (elevation of both patient's arms above his/her head simultaneously causing facial flushing, distended head or neck veins, inspiratory stridor, and elevated jugular venous pressure) [16,17].

Hyperviscosity syndrome

Viscosity is a measure of the resistance of a fluid which is being stressed by outside forces – less viscous fluid flows with greater ease. This is of importance in regard to blood delivering nutrients throughout the body. The viscosity of blood is directly related to its predominant components: water, cells, and circulating proteins. Hyperviscosity syndrome is a pathologic condition characterized by increased blood viscosity, causing diminished blood flow. This is primarily caused by increased number of cells that occurs in leukemia, polycythemia, or myeloproliferative diseases, or by an increase in proteins, specifically immunoglobulins, as seen in Waldenstrom's macroglobulinemia or multiple myeloma.

Clinical symptoms generally include mucosal bleeding, visual changes, and neurologic symptoms. These symptoms are related to the diminished blood flow seen in hyperviscosity syndrome, as well as to platelet inability to form clots appropriately. Additionally, cardiopulmonary collapse can occur due to reduced or stagnant coronary and pulmonary circulation. Physical findings seen commonly in the ED are evidence of mucosal bleeding, neurologic deficits, and ophthalmologic findings, such as diminished acuity, retinal vein dilatation, or retinal hemorrhage.

The most useful ED test in diagnosing hyperviscosity syndrome is a complete blood count, which may show elevated cell lines or a Rouleaux formation. In addition, an elevated globulin gap (total protein minus albumin >4) may be present, suggesting elevated levels of immunoglobulins. Other testing may identify concomitant metabolic derangements, such as electrolyte disorders, or the underlying etiology.

As the most common causes of hyperviscosity syndrome are blood dyscrasias, and these are most frequently found in the elderly, this syndrome is almost exclusively diagnosed in the geriatric population [18]. Management is largely supportive, although plasma/cellular pheresis may be indicated in consultation with a hematologist/oncologist. Large-volume phlebotomy and repletion with saline has been suggested as an emergent temporizing measure, but should be used cautiously in the elderly population where large volume shifts may not be well tolerated. Definitive treatment requires identification of the underlying, inciting cause.

Coagulopathy

Coagulopathy is a bleeding disorder leading to prolonged or excessive bleeding. This can occur spontaneously or during medical or dental procedures. Coagulation of blood is dependent on the complex intrinsic and extrinsic clotting cascade as well as platelets. Dysfunction or reduced production of the clotting factors, co-factors or platelets can lead to a coagulopathy.

A primary coagulopathy, such as hemophilia or von Willebrand's disease, is an uncommon diagnosis in the elderly. Many of the genetic coagulopathies are diagnosed through pre- or perinatal screening or during early life when symptoms such as heavy menstruation, easy bruisability, and gingival bleeding are investigated further. The more common coagulopathies found in the elderly are often related to medication side effects or underlying disease pathology resulting in platelet suppression or liver dysfunction, sepsis, or vitamin K deficiency leading to insufficient coagulation factors. In particular, treatment with vitamin K antagonists such as warfarin is commonplace in the elderly, and numerous interactions through potentiation or inhibition of the cytochrome P450 system by other medications, such as antibiotics or proton pump inhibitors (PPIs), can lead to devastating coagulopathies.

Historical information of import includes easy bruisability, gingival or mucosal bleeding, melena, frank hematochezia, or hematuria. Other aspects to investigate are neurologic symptoms suggesting intracranial bleeding or generalized fatigue, weakness, or any other complaints consistent with anemia. Examination should look for particular aspects of bleeding diatheses such as petechiae and purpura on the skin, blood in the stool, or even swollen joints in the case of a hemarthrosis. Basic diagnostic testing for suspected coagulopathy should include a complete blood count (and perhaps a specific platelet count), prothrombin time/international normalized ratio, partial thromboplastin time, and less important in the ED, a bleeding time.

Any elderly patient with a coagulopathy should be thoroughly evaluated for the underlying cause. In the ED, this evaluation should focus on medication effects, the possibility of oncologic disease or sepsis, as well as the safety of disposition to home of a patient with a potential increased risk of bleeding. As the elderly are more prone to falls and other traumatic injuries, a low threshold for admission to the hospital should be used with the coagulopathic elderly patient [19].

Anemia

Anemia is the most common disorder of the blood and is characterized by a reduced number of red blood cells or hemoglobin in the blood. The World Health Organization in 1968 defined anemia as <11–13 g/dl in adults, and little change has been brought to that definition. Numerous studies have attempted to identify the average hemoglobin based on a variety of factors, and age seems to have no specific variability on hemoglobin concentration because some studies show a rise and others show a fall in hemoglobin concentrations as patients age [20]. The currently accepted value for anemia in the elderly is consistent with this early definition.

Anemia generally is the result of impaired red blood cell production, increased red blood cell destruction, or blood loss but can also be due to fluid overload, causing a dilutional-type anemia. Historical data helpful in the anemic patient include information about previous anemia and illness. Additionally vague symptoms such as fatigue and malaise may be present. In more severe cases, symptoms such as chest pain and fainting may be recorded due to substantially diminished oxygen carrying capacity.

Physical examination may find patients to be pale, although this is not considered to be reliable. Tachycardia, hypotension, and orthostatic hypotension are far more important as these represent hard findings of true symptomatic anemia and should potentially trigger transfusion in the right clinical scenario. Further examination should be targeted at the etiology of anemia, such as koilonychias in iron deficiency, jaundice in hemolytic anemia, and guiaic-positive stool or hematochezia in frank gastrointestinal bleeding. Laboratory examination and work-up should be directed at identifying the underlying cause – a complete blood count, coagulation studies, and a type and screen/cross-match should be ordered for suspected anemic patients. Prior to possible resuscitative measures, including transfusion, other more specific blood tests might be ordered to help identify the underlying cause after analyzing the initial blood count and mean corpuscle volume. These tests may include hemoglobin electrophoresis (although, not as typically useful in the elderly), lactate dehydrogenase, reticulocyte counts, iron studies, B$_{12}$ and folate levels, and perhaps most importantly, a manual peripheral smear to evaluate red blood cell morphology.

As mentioned, the elderly don't necessarily suffer from increased hematologic problems as they age, but rather are more prone to aberrations in their homeostatic mechanisms that cause conditions such as anemia to have more deleterious effects. As such, identifying the underlying cause is most important and treatment should be directed towards that cause.

Thrombocytopenia

Thrombocytopenia is a condition where the number of circulating platelets is <150,000/μl. Platelets are necessary for the initiation of the clotting cascade when there is endothelial blood vessel damage. The clinical significance of thrombocytopenia can be vast, from simply an incidental findings on routine blood tests to life-threatening hemorrhage requiring transfusion of platelets. The causes of thrombocytopenia can be grouped into decreased production (vitamin deficiency, neoplastic diseases, and sepsis), increased destruction (immune thrombocytopenic purpura, thrombotic thrombocytopenic purpura [TTP], and disseminated intravascular coagulation [DIC]), and medication-induced (heparin-induced thrombocytopenia [HIT], PPIs, and methotrexate). Idiopathic (or immune) thrombocytopenic purpura is a condition in which thrombocytopenia has no readily apparent clinical cause and is thought to result from an alteration in immune response. Thrombotic thrombocytopenia purpura can be described easily by the pentad of thrombocytopenia, microangiopathic hemolytic anemia, neurologic symptoms, renal failure, and fever. Disseminated intravascular coagulation is an aberration in the delicate balance between coagulation and fibrinolysis and can occur in a myriad of disease states, most prominently sepsis. It leads to clotting of blood and consumption and subsequent decline of clotting factors in the bloodstream leading to bleeding. Medications can cause thrombocytopenia as well, as in the use of heparin, which can precipitate HIT, an autoimmune response to heparin that targets platelets. Additionally, the clinician should be alert to commonly used medications that cause reduced platelet function that could be qualified as a "relative" thrombocytopenia, such as aspirin, clopidogrel, and NSAIDs [21].

Historical and physical examination information is largely similar to basic coagulopathies, as this is a subset of such. This includes easy bruisability, petechiae and purpura on the skin, as well as mucosal bleeding. Basic diagnostic testing should include a complete blood count, as well as a prothrombin time/international normalized ratio and partial thromboplastin time, to exclude other potential causes of bleeding. In addition, the clinician should attempt to exclude pseudothrombocytopenia caused by platelet clumping when using EDTA as a test medium. Sending a specimen diluted with heparin is a more accurate evaluation of platelet count [22]. Along with decreased platelet count, bleeding time will be prolonged and will be the only aberrant coagulation parameter.

Thrombocytopenia is more common in the elderly due to increased medication use and greater likelihood of malnutrition. The emergency physician who is presented with the thrombocytopenic elderly patient should make extensive efforts to identify the underlying causes, as this may be a harbinger of more insidious disease processes. Additionally, the elderly thrombocytopenic patient at high risk for falls or with active bleeding should be admitted to the hospital, as the potential for complications is far greater in this population.

Transfusion of blood components

Transfusion of blood components is warranted in certain clinical conditions. However, the emergency physician must carefully think out the benefits of transfusion versus the risks of infection, transfusion, and volume overload in caring for the elderly patient. Profound symptomatic anemia and life-threatening coagulopathy are the primary indications for blood transfusion in the elderly. As such, the primary transfusion components are packed red blood cells, platelets, and fresh frozen plasma. Prothrombin complex concentrate is a newer synthetic blood component that can be used in the case of life-threatening coagulopathy, however, it is currently cost-prohibitive and there are questions regarding its safety with regard to increased thrombogenesis.

There are many clinical guidelines related to the use of red blood cell transfusion. In general, most of these guidelines recommend red blood cell transfusion at levels of hemoglobin between 6.0 and 8.0 g/dl [23]. However, in the elderly, who often represent a cohort of sicker patients, despite the diminished response to anemia due to lower cardiac output, increased coronary artery atherosclerosis, and increased myocardial oxygen demands, evidence suggests a more aggressive approach might decrease mortality rates [24].

The use of platelets is generally reserved for the thrombocytopenic patient with trauma or life-threatening hemorrhage. In surgery or trauma, platelet levels <50,000/μl represent the generally accepted threshold for transfusion, with <10,000/μl the threshold for transfusion for spontaneous bleeding. However, other conditions with life-threatening hemorrhage, such as concomitant use of aspirin or clopidogrel or profound uremia, which inhibits platelet function, may lead to platelet transfusion. Additionally, studies have shown poor outcomes in transfusing platelets in those with TTP or HIT type II, as the platelets are thought to be catalysts for further thrombosis [25].

The use of fresh frozen plasma, and more recently prothrombin complex concentrate (a synthetic or pooled superconcentrate usually containing factors II, VII, IX, X and proteins C and S), holds similar indications in that it is reserved for patients with trauma or life-threatening hemorrhage in the coagulopathic patient. This can be most commonly found in patients with hepatic failure, DIC, or warfarin anticoagulation.

Data are slowly emerging about the utility of transfusions of blood products for patients on new designer anticoagulants that fall into the direct thrombin and factor Xa inhibitor classes, such as Xarelto (rivaroxaban) and Pradaxa (dabigatran). Considerable caution should be exercised in placing elderly patients on these medications (and all anticoagulants) due to the inability to effectively reverse their effects with blood components or other methods [25]. Additionally, caution over transfusions in the elderly should focus mainly on the volume status of the patient, as transfusion could trigger potential cardiopulmonary collapse due to rapid volume expansion. Co-administration with furosemide or other diuretics has generally been practiced to eliminate the unnecessary water volume of transfusion but maintain the components' function [26].

Administration of vitamin K

Vitamin K is commonly known as a factor necessary for the coagulation of blood. It is also involved in other processes within the body, including bone metabolism. It is found as a natural component of leafy green vegetables that is necessary for photosynthesis as well as a product of natural bacterial gut flora. In the elderly, this natural production of variants of vitamin K is reduced [27]. Additionally, the elderly are often prescribed medications that may reduce the function, absorption, or production of vitamin K (medications such as Coumadin or antibiotics are implicated in this). As such, supplementation of vitamin K or use as an antidote for vitamin K-dependent coagulopathy (factors II, VII, IX, X and proteins C, S, and Z are dependent on vitamin K) may become necessary in the elderly population [28].

Vitamin K can be administered orally, subcutaneously, or IV. Intravenous administration is only recommended in the setting of life-threatening or serious bleeding. Otherwise, the preferred method is oral administration. However, in either case, the effective onset of therapeutic action will be delayed (up to 24 hours) and as such, administration of fresh frozen plasma (FFP), prothrombin complex concentrate (PCC), or other blood products may be advised in life-threatening emergencies. The appropriate dosing of vitamin K is dependent on the clinical scenario as well as the various coagulation parameters [28,29]. In situations of life-threatening bleeding, vitamin K should be given at its maximum dose of 10 mg by slow IV infusion, with simultaneous administration of FFP (or PCC or recombinant factor VIIa) to rapidly reverse the anticoagulation effects [30].

Summary

The vast majority of hematologic and oncologic diseases that the emergency physician encounters are in elderly patients. By fully understanding the complexities of these diseases and how specifically they affect elderly patients, the emergency physician

will be best equipped to appropriately and compassionately treat the geriatric population with hematologic or oncologic diseases, and most importantly for the elderly, be well equipped to have a meaningful discussion about diagnosing and treating these conditions.

Pearls and pitfalls

- With a growing elderly population, the emergency physician will be more frequently exposed to and manage patients with hematologic and oncologic emergencies.
- The pathophysiologic changes on the hematopoietic system are primarily a diminished capability of responding to stressors as opposed to a blatant decline in function.
- Oncologic diseases are common in the elderly and require a degree of sensitivity and vigilance in their management and the frequent effects they can have on the cardiopulmonary, renal, and gastrointestinal systems.
- Despite trends to the contrary, it is appropriate to offer the geriatric population similar screening and treatment options as younger patients, and in fact, despite common misconceptions, geriatric patients benefit enormously from receiving the same options as the young.
- Elderly patients who present to the ED should be screened for potential hematologic conditions by performing a complete blood count. This can be helpful in uncovering the cause of the visit or asymptomatic hematologic disturbances that in the elderly can rapidly progress to fatal conditions with a minor physiologic stressor.
- The complications of oncologic disease and their treatments can often be more devastating than the disease itself; particular attention should be paid to electrolyte disturbances and cardiopulmonary status in managing these patients.

References

1. Chambers SM, et al. Aging hematopoietic stem cells decline in function and exhibit epigenetic growth dysregulation. *PLoS Biol* 2007;5(8):e201.
2. Hazzard WR, Halter JB. *Hazzard's Geriatric Medicine and Gerontology*, 6th edn (New York: McGraw-Hill Medical, 2009).
3. Howlader N, Noone AM, Krapcho M, et al. (ed.) *SEER Cancer Statistics Review, 1975–2009 (Vintage 2009 Populations)* (Bethesda, MD: National Cancer Institute, http://seer.cancer.gov/csr/1975_2009_pops09/, based on November 2011 SEER data submission, posted to the SEER website, 2012).
4. Fillit H, Rockwood K, Woodhouse KW, Brocklehurst JC. *Brocklehurst's Textbook of Geriatric Medicine and Gerontology*, 7th edn (Philadelphia, PA: Saunders/Elsevier, 2010).
5. Edwards BK, Brown ML, Wingo PA. Annual report to the nation on the status of cancer, 1975–2002, featuring population-based trends in cancer treatment. *J Natl Cancer Inst.* 2005;97:1407–27.
6. Murthy VH, Krumholz HM, Gross CP. Participation in cancer clinical trials: race, sex-, and age-based disparities. *JAMA.* 2004;291:2720–6.
7. Samet J, Hunt WC, Key C, et al. Choice of cancer therapy varies with age of patient. *JAMA.* 1986;255:3385–90.

8. Walsh TH. Audit of outcome of major surgery in the elderly. *Br J Surg.* 1996;83:92–7.

9. Gosney M. Cancer. In *Drugs and the Older Population*, ed. Crome P, Ford G (London: Imperial College Press, 2000), pp. 601–51.

10. Tam-McDevitt J. Polypharmacy, aging, and cancer. *Oncology.* 2008;22:1052–5.

11. Balducci L, Beghe C. Pharmacology of chemotherapy in the older cancer patient. *Cancer Control.* 1999;6:466–70.

12. Chen H, Cantor A, Meyer J. Can older cancer patients tolerate chemotherapy? A prospective pilot study. *Cancer.* 2003;97:1107–14.

13. Freifeld AG, Bow EJ, Sepkowitz KA, et al. Clinical practice guidelines for the use of antimicrobial agents in neutropenic patients with cancer: 2010 update by the Infectious Diseases Society of America. *Clin Infect Dis.* 2011;52:e56.

14. Pizzo PA. Fever in immunocompromised patients. *N Eng J Med.* 1999;341:893–900.

15. Howard SC, Jones DP, Pui CH. The tumor lysis syndrome. *N Eng J Med.* 2011;364:1844–54.

16. Pemberton HS. Sign of submerged goitre. *Lancet.* 1946;251:509.

17. Wilson LD, Detterbeck FC, Yahalom J. Superior vena cava syndrome with malignant causes. *N Engl J Med.* 2007;356(18):1862–9.

18. Adams BD, Baker R, Lopez JA, Spencer S. Myeloproliferative disorders and the hyperviscosity syndrome. *Emerg Med Clin North Am.* 2009;27(3):459–76.

19. Drews RE. Critical issues in hematology: anemia, thrombocytopenia, coagulopathy, and blood product transfusions in critically ill patients. *Clin Chest Med.* 2003;24(4):607–22.

20. Beutler E, Waalen J. The definition of anemia: what is the lower limit of normal of the blood hemoglobin concentration? *Blood.* 2006;107(5):1747–50.

21. Konkle BA. Acquired disorders of platelet function. *The Education Program of the American Society of Hematology.* 2011;2011:391–6.

22. Sekhon SS, Roy V. Thrombocytopenia in adults: A practical approach to evaluation and management. *South Med J.* 2006;99(5):491–8; quiz, 499–500, 533.

23. Goodnough LT, Bach RG. Anemia, transfusion, and mortality. *N Engl J Med.* 2001;345(17):1272–4.

24. Vincent JL, Baron JF, Reinhart K, et al. Anemia and blood transfusion in critically ill patients. *JAMA.* 2002;288(12):1499–507.

25. Hoffman R. "Anticoagulants: Beyond Coumadin." Lecture at Third All NYC EM Conference, August 29, 2012.

26. Popovsky MA. Transfusion and the lung: circulatory overload and acute lung injury. *Vox Sang.* 2004;87(Suppl. 2):62–5.

27. Hodges SJ, Pilkington MJ, Shearer MJ, Bitensky L, Chayen J. Age-related changes in the circulating levels of congeners of vitamin K2, menaquinone-7 and menaquinone-8. *Clinical Science.* 1990;78(1):63–6.

28. Crowther MA, Julian J, McCarty D, et al. Treatment of warfarin-associated coagulopathy with oral vitamin K: a randomized controlled trial. *Lancet.* 2000;356(9241):1551–3.

29. Guyatt GH et al. Executive Summary: Antithrombotic Therapy and Prevention of Thrombosis, 9th edn: American College of Chest Physicians Evidence-Based Clinical Practice Guidelines. *Chest.* 2012;141(Suppl. 2):7–47S.

30. Ansell J, Hirsh J, Hylek E, et al. Pharmacology and management of the vitamin K antagonists: American College of Chest Physicians Evidence-Based Clinical Practice Guidelines (8th edn). *Chest.* 2008;133(6 Suppl.):160–98S.

Chapter

26

Psychiatric emergencies in the elderly

Joanna Piechniczek-Buczek

Introduction

The vast majority of elderly patients visit the emergency department (ED) for medical rather than behavioral problems. Geriatric patients account for about 5–6% of all psychiatric emergency services encounters, yet they constitute 12% of the general population. This relatively small subset of emergency presentations can, however, be among the most difficult to accurately diagnose and treat.

The goals of psychiatric assessment in the ED are to conduct adequate evaluation, assure safety, ascertain tentative diagnosis, provide appropriate acute treatment, and establish adequate disposition.

This chapter will review key psychiatric problems among the elderly presenting to the ED and provide guidelines for the diagnosis, assessment, and management of these common geriatric emergencies.

Specifically, elderly suicide, depression, substance abuse, and agitation linked to psychosis or dementia are discussed in detail.

Suicide

Background and epidemiology

Suicide is a tragic event affecting the individual, families and friends, communities, and the population at large. Almost one million lives are lost annually worldwide through suicide, accounting for 1.5% of global burden of disease or more than 20 million disability-adjusted life-years. Suicide rates vary greatly among countries and regions, with the greatest burden reported in Eastern Europe and lowest in Latin America and the Muslim world [1].

The estimated national burden of suicide is over 36,000 deaths per year, making suicide the tenth leading cause of death in the US. The rate of suicide in the general population has been increasing steadily over the last decade, and in 2009 reached 12 completed suicides for every 100,000 people. Older adults are overall at greater risk, with the rate reaching 14.8 per 100,000. Although in 2008 the elderly constituted 12.5% of the population, they accounted for almost 16% of all suicides. Elderly Caucasian men were at highest risk, with a rate

of 31.1 per 100,000. The spike in suicide rates is, however, the most noticeable for white men over the age of 85, for whom the rate was 45.5, almost 2.5 times the current rate for men of all ages [2]. Additional source of concern is the fact that birth cohorts carry characteristic predisposition to suicide as they age. The leading edge of the "baby boom" generation, known to have relatively higher rates of suicide, has just embarked on older adulthood raising concerns that the suicide rates and absolute suicide death numbers may increase over the next two decades.

The prevalence of attempted suicide in the elderly is much less established, however surveillance data indicate that older adults are less likely than their younger counterparts to report attempts or to present for treatment following an incomplete or aborted attempt [3]. In the general population, the ratio of suicide attempts to completed suicides ranges from 8:1 to 20:1, whereas the ratio is estimated to be 4:1 or less in the elderly. The increase in lethality of attempts in this age cohort can be explained by several factors. Older Americans are more likely than their younger counterparts to resort to violent means, such as firearms (71%), hanging (11%), jumping, and overdose (11%) [4]. Additionally, increased disease burden in this age group leads to decreased resilience and diminished capacity to withstand physical insult. Furthermore, older adults are more likely to be living alone and are more likely to take precaution against timely discovery of their act.

Risk factors

Multiple factors contribute to suicide, and never is this tragic act the consequence of a single determinant. Most of our understanding of factors that place the elderly at high risk for suicide is derived from retrospective analysis called psychological autopsy (PA). The risk factors can be categorized in various ways, but for the purpose of this text, we will review distal and proximal correlates of suicide. Distal risk factors include a wide range of contributors in sociodemographic, psychiatric, characterologic, medical, biologic, and familial domains. On the other hand, proximal risk factors are more closely associated with suicide event and represent circumstance-driven and situational correlates.

Geriatric Emergency Medicine, ed. Joseph H. Kahn, Brendan G. Magauran Jr., and Jonathan S. Olshaker. Published by Cambridge University Press.
© Cambridge University Press 2014.

Sociodemographic analysis of suicide data reveals three predominant variables impacting suicide in the geriatric population: gender, race, and marital status. The analysis concludes that male gender, white race, and unmarried status characterize the majority of suicide completers in the elderly [5].

Psychiatric illness consistently emerges as the most powerful predictor of suicide. Affective disorders, specifically major depression, are the most common disorders, present in 54–87% of cases. In comparison with younger suicide victims, the elderly seem to be more likely to suffer from single-episode unipolar depression, not complicated by substance abuse, psychosis, or medical illness, the type of depression most amenable to standard therapies. The prevalence of *substance use disorders* in elderly suicide victims varies significantly from 3 to 46%, reflecting a complex relationship between substance misuse and suicide in this age cohort, as well as indicating methodological differences among studies and diversity of populations studied. The rates of problematic drinking in the West far surpass those in the East [6]. In addition to alcohol as an independent risk factor, other postulated mechanisms of its contribution to increased risk of suicide include alcohol exacerbation of co-existing psychiatric or medical problems, and contribution to loss of social supports [7]. Primary psychotic illness, anxiety, and Axis II diagnoses appear to have less conclusive influence on elderly suicide than in younger cohorts.

Studies have identified several *characterologic constructs* as factors predisposing to suicide. Conner et al. [8] reviewed studies examining personality traits and suicide and concluded that five main psychological constructs distinguished controlled and suicide completers. These characteristics include impulsivity/aggression, depression, hopelessness, neuroticism, and self-consciousness/social disengagement, and seem to interplay with psychiatric, demographic, and medical vulnerabilities to further enhance the risk of suicide.

Numerous studies have investigated the link between *medical illness* and suicide risk. Of course, physical limitation and declining health occur commonly in the elderly making the specific association with suicide difficult to prove. There is, however, significantly increased relative risk of suicide with disorders of the central nervous system and malignant neoplasm. Additionally, visual impairment, undertreated pain, anticipatory anxiety regarding progression of physical illness, and fear of loss of autonomy or personal integrity further contribute to increased suicidality in medically compromised elders.

Abnormalities in serotoninergic, noradrenergic, and neuroendocrine systems have been implicated in the pathophysiology of suicide in the general population, underscoring *biological vulnerability* to impulsive and self-harming behaviors. Gender and age differences in suicide rates also imply a possible neurobiological process. Decreased brain concentrations of serotonin, dopamine, norepinephrine, and their metabolites, increased brain MAO-B activity, enhanced activity of the hypothalamic–pituitary–adrenal axis, and a hyperactive sympathetic system all have been implicated in depression and the normal aging process. However, the evidence of these changes being linked to suicide is inconclusive in elderly victims due to limited data [9].

Cognitive deficits in the elderly have also been linked to suicide. Elderly depressed suicide attempters exhibit poorer performance on measures of frontal executive functions, attention tests, and memory assessments [10]. Other investigations suggest evidence of brain pathology, specifically the presence of more subcortical gray matter hyperintensities on magnetic resonance imaging (MRI) in depressed elders with lifetime history of suicide attempts than in meticulously matched depressed controls without history of attempts, supporting the hypothesis that brain vascular disease may predispose to depressive disorder and suicidal behaviour [11]. Additionally, greater hippocampal neurofibrillary pathology has been identified in postmortem analysis of elderly suicides than in controls [12]. In combination, these data raise the possibility that suicide in later life is associated with disruption of neural pathways critical to regulation of cognition, mood, and behavior. Additional research, however, is needed to support and extend these findings.

A range of significant *psychosocial* circumstances is more proximally linked to suicide. Interpersonal loss through bereavement or rupture of relationships with family members, as well as alienation from other sources of support, bears important significance in late-life suicide. Psychological autopsy studies evaluated the association between specific life stressors and suicide in older adults. Beautrais found that serious relationship and financial problems distinguished suicide completers and near-fatal attempters from controls in New Zealand [13]. These findings were replicated by Rubenowitz and colleagues in Sweden [14]. Other studies have shown that older adult suicides were significantly less likely to have a confidant [15], more likely to live alone [16], and less likely to participate in community activities [17] than their peers.

Another risk factor that significantly increases the risk of suicide is *access to means*. The elderly tend to act on suicidal thoughts with greater lethality of intent and implementation, and utilize more violent means, particularly firearms. Access to lethal means increases the risk of suicide [18]: almost 75% of elderly suicide completers in the US utilized firearms as the means, and those who died by suicide were significantly more likely to have acquired a weapon within the last week of their life [19]. Among those who kept a gun, storing the weapon loaded and unlocked were also independent risk factors for suicide completion [20].

Finally, worsening of underlying depressive or anxiety disorder can be viewed as a proximal warning sign of elderly suicide. These "syndromatic clues" related to heightened risk of suicide include depression with an overlay of anxiety, dependency accompanied by guilt, rigidity alternating with impulsivity, and seemingly complete recovery from severe depression almost overnight [21] (Table 26.1).

Evaluation

The detection of suicidal elderly patients poses significant challenges to health care providers. Older adults are less likely than their younger counterparts to express suicidal ideations, yet they have a substantially higher risk of suicide, and suicidal acts orchestrated by them appear to be far more lethal in planning,

Table 26.1. Suicide risk factors

Distal factors	Demographic	Male
		Caucasian
		Unmarried
	Psychiatric	Hx MDD: unipolar, single episode
		EtOH dependence
	Personality characteristics	Impulsivity/aggression
		Depression/hopelessness
		Self-consciousness/social disengagement
		Neuroticism
	Medical	Huntington's disease
		Multiple sclerosis
		Seizure disorder
		Peptic ulcer disease
		Spinal cord injuries
		HIV/AIDS
		Malignant neoplasm
	Biological	Norepinephrine
		Serotonin
		Dopamine
		Cognitive determinants
Proximal	Psychosocial crisis	Bereavement
		Family discord
		Social isolation
		Financial stress
		Loss of independence
	Availability of means	Firearms at home
	Acute exacerbation of psychiatric illness	Depression

implementation, and outcome. Clinical intervention strategies targeting high-risk individuals based on predisposing and precipitating factors may be more effective for preventing suicide than strategies solely focused on identifying patients with suicidal thoughts or behaviors. Caregivers often fail to detect imminent suicide threat in elders as supported by the fact that about 70% of older patients who commit suicide are thought to have had contact with medical providers in the months prior to their death, 40% the week prior, and 20% on the day itself [22]. This seems to imply that suicidal older patients display certain warning signs that tend to go unnoticed by professionals. Establishing a respectful and supportive relationship with the patient, developing clinical skills, and utilizing validated and sensitive screening tools will result in improved detection and more effective prevention of suicide. Several rating scales have been developed and validated. Scales such as the Geriatric Suicide Ideation Scale or the Reasons for Living Scale–Older Adult version can help identify the presence and severity of suicidal ideations and identify resiliency/protective factors, but will not replace careful and thorough clinical inquiry. When a patient is identified as at risk, full medical and psychiatric evaluation should be conducted. First, the intensity of active suicidal thoughts should be explored, including

degrees of planning and intent as well as lethality and availability of means. Second, the patient should be asked about the mood, sleep habits, appetite, interest, motivation, and feeling of hopelessness. Additionally, previous suicide attempts, past episodes of depression, psychosis, substance abuse, impulse control, and recent stressful life events should be explored. The reliability of the report can be influenced by the patient's ability and willingness to share information, and therefore collateral sources (family members, caretakers, outpatient providers) can frequently provide critical evidence in the setting of suicidal crisis. Upon integrating the clinical data obtained during comprehensive assessment, suicidal risk is estimated and decision made regarding further interventions. In summary, clinicians should remember that suicide is the result of multiple factors and no single method of risk assessment can reliably identify who will and who will not die by suicide.

Treatment

Determination of the appropriate treatment setting is perhaps the most important decision made during the assessment. Depending on the level of risk, treatment settings can range from the most restrictive, such as involuntary hospitalization, through partial hospitalization, intensive outpatient treatment program, to the least restricting ambulatory treatment environment. Psychiatric hospitalization should be pursued for patients in immediate danger. If the patient who is deemed to be at acute risk for suicide is refusing to be admitted, the physician then becomes responsible for initiating procedures for involuntary commitment in accordance with applicable civil laws. Hospitalization protects the patient from self-harm when an adequate level of monitoring is provided. Additionally, hospitalization allows the introduction of pharmacological treatment for psychiatric conditions driving the suicidality, and yields opportunity for more thorough exploration of multiaxial problems, such as existing psychiatric and personality disorders, medical conditions as well as social stressors, vulnerabilities, and functional status. Hospitalization also allows for "step-down" referrals to treatments in day programs or ambulatory settings.

If inpatient admission is not pursued, assuring adequate monitoring at home, making prompt referral to outpatient psychiatric care, and reducing accessibility to means is considered to be necessary intervention in managing suicidal patients.

Prevention

As illustrated previously, older adults are more likely to die of suicide than are members of younger age groups because suicidal behaviors in elders are more lethal. Interventions aimed at preventing the development of suicidal state are therefore particularly critical in this age group. A wide range of approaches is needed to address this issue. *Universal* interventions involve initiatives aimed at decreasing mortality risk by affecting large groups of people. Population-based strategies of greatest relevance to late-life suicide include legislation restricting access to firearms and mandates concerning packaging and distribution of medications. In the US, the introduction of gun control through the Brady Handgun Violence Prevention Act of 1994 led to a decline in the rate of suicide by firearms among individuals older than 55 years of age [23]. In the United Kingdom, the legislated reduction in maximum package size of analgesics in 1998 was followed by a decrease in non-fatal overdoses, treatment of liver toxicity, and deaths due to analgesic self-poisoning [24].

More *selective* suicide prevention interventions target asymptomatic or pre-symptomatic individuals or groups with more distal risk factors. They may include elderly with chronic, painful, or functionally limiting conditions, or those who have become socially isolated or perceive themselves as a burden to others. Social services that provide outreach to isolated older adults in the community and care management services that address their other social needs may lower suicide risk. Work done by De Leo et al. confirms this hypothesis [25].

Finally, *indicated* suicide prevention approaches target older adults in primary care settings who have symptomatic affective illness. The Prevention of Suicide in Primary Care Elderly Collaborative Trial (PROSPECT study) compared usual care by the primary care providers with algorithm-driven treatment consisting of antidepressants, psychotherapy, education, and care management. The rates of suicidal ideations declined significantly in the intervention group [26], with greater reduction sustained over 24 months [27]. Although the Improving Mood-Promoting Access Collaborative Trial (IMPACT) did not focus explicitly on older adults with suicidal ideations or history of self-harming behaviors, it similarly revealed that a combination of problem-solving psychotherapy and antidepressant treatment reduced suicidal ideations and death wishes among depressed and dysthymic elders.

Depression

Background and epidemiology

Depression is one of the leading causes of disability worldwide [28]. Late-life depression is a common and potentially life-threatening illness. It creates enormous and far-reaching individual, family, medical, social, and economic burden. Even though late-life experiences can be associated with multiple losses and challenges, and sadness may be considered a normal response, depression is not a natural consequence of aging. Late-life depression is a heterogeneous clinical entity. Some patients have recurrent episodes beginning at a young age, and some develop depressive symptoms de novo late in life. Patients with late-onset depressive disorder tend to have less frequent family history of mood disorders, higher evidence of medical and neurological comorbidities, and higher prevalence of cognitive impairment. In turn, depression itself can exacerbate cognitive and medical limitations which then lead to social isolation. Social disruption further exacerbates both the depression and cognitive dysfunction and contributes to late-life suicide [29]. If depression is unrecognized and untreated, it is associated with significantly increased morbidity [30] and mortality from co-existing medical conditions [31] and suicide [32].

The prevalence of major depressive disorder varies from 1 to 2% in community-dwelling elders, to 5–10% of patients in medical outpatient settings, 10–15% of the medically hospitalized, and up to 14–42% of older patients residing in long-term care facilities [33]. Depression may be present in up to one-third of older ED patients [34]. It may interfere with the clinical presentation of acute medical disorders and results in a greater number of ED visits [35].

Risk factors

A wide range of predisposing and risk factors for depression has been postulated. Gender seems to play a role, as twice as many women as men are affected. Late-life depressive syndromes often emerge in the context of medical and neurological disorders. Medical illness is frequently cited as a predisposing and consequential correlate of depression, implying a bidirectional relationship between these two groups [36]. Depression is common in patients with coronary artery disease, as about one-quarter of patients who either suffered myocardial infarction (MI) or who are undergoing cardiac catheterization have major depression, and an additional 25% have minor depression [37]. Additionally, post-MI mortality is higher in depressed than non-depressed patients, implying that depression plays a contributory role in the pathogenesis of heart disease. A similar reciprocal correlation between depression and medical illness applies to a number of other conditions, including cerebrovascular diseases, Parkinson's disease, and dementia. About one-quarter to one-half of post-stroke patients suffer from depression [38], as do about one-half of those with Parkinson's disease [39].

Similarly, symptoms of depression are often present in the patients with dementia. A population study from Cache County, Utah, estimated that 20% of persons with Alzheimer's dementia (AD) suffered from dysphoria. Studies from clinical settings suggest that prevalence of major depressive disorder is 20–25%, while minor depression afflicts an additional 20–30% of AD patients.

Psychological factors of certain personality characteristics and coping styles have been linked to a higher likelihood of depression across the lifespan. High scores on personality scale measuring neuroticism are strongly related to depression in late life. Ruminative (repetitive and passive thinking about one's distress) and avoidant coping constructs have both been over-represented in individuals at higher risk of depression [40].

Social factors and life events are also associated with late-life depression (Table 26.2). These include poverty, limited social support, marital separation, and divorce, as well as recent adverse and unaccepted life events including bereavement. Functional disability is frequently cited as another factor linked to development of depression. For community-dwelling older adults, the presence of disabilities increases the risk of depression 4.2-fold per year [41]. An investigation by Penninx et al. [42] showed that depressive symptoms were in turn predictive of up to 50% greater risk of decline in physical performance, providing further evidence for bidirectional correlation between depression and functional decline.

Table 26.2. Late-life depression risk factors

Demographic	Female
Medical	Comorbid: Cardiac disease, cerebrovascular disease, diabetes, cancer
Cognitive	Mild cognitive impairment; dementia
Personality traits	Neuroticism
	Ruminations
	Avoidance
Social	Bereavement
	Deficient social support
	Poverty
	Functional disability
	Relocation

Table 26.3. ED depression screening instrument (ED-DSI)

Question	Response	
1. Do you often feel sad or depressed?	Yes	No
2. Do you often feel helpless?	Yes	No
3. Do you often feel downhearted and blue?	Yes	No

At least one positive response corresponds to a positive screening result for depression.

- depressed mood;
- anhedonia;
- anorexia;
- insomnia/hypersomnia;
- psychomotor agitation/retardation;
- fatigue/anergia;
- worthlessness/guilt;
- decreased concentration;
- death wishes/suicidal ideations/attempt or plan.

Evaluation

Older adults in North America utilize EDs at a higher rate than younger adults, and depressed elders utilize these services at a further enhanced rate, even after adjusting for chronic medical illness [43]. Depression can be particularly difficult to identify in older patients, and much of the burden of depression diagnosis falls on primary medical providers [44]. Several reasons for poor recognition of late-life depressive disorder have been identified. First, depression is often insidious and presents with vague somatic complaints or overlapping symptoms of medical illness that can mask or mimic depressive symptoms [45]. Co-existence of mild cognitive impairment or dementia may also complicate the diagnosis of depression due to either symptom overlap (anhedonia, apathy, poor concentration, and functional regression or impaired recall of symptoms) [46]. Additionally, episodes of depression can emerge as consequence of stressful life events and therefore be interpreted as "justifiable," with no need for further treatment or follow-up. The patients themselves can be reluctant to accept the diagnosis or follow up with treatment due to the stigma attached to the mental illness [47]. Lastly, the providers may lack the knowledge or awareness necessary for appropriate assessment and adequate recognition of depressive symptoms in the geriatric population [48].

The criteria delineated in the *Diagnostic and Statistical Manual of Mental Disorders IV-TR* (DSM IV-TR) should be used as diagnostic guidelines. According to DSM IV-TR, in order to meet the criteria for a major depressive episode, patients must experience at least five of the nine symptoms listed below for a period of at least two weeks. Although the prevalence of major depression appears to decrease as one becomes older [49], the incidence of clinically significant sub-syndromal or minor depression rises steadily with advancing age. Patients in this group do not meet the full diagnostic criteria because of fewer or limited duration of symptoms. They do, however, carry a similar disease burden, including poorer health and social outcomes, functional impairment, and decreased quality of life [50].

DSM IV-TR criteria for major depressive episode

Five or more of the following must be present for the same 2-week period. At least one of the symptoms must be either depressed mood or anhedonia.

Several standard tools are available to facilitate screening for depression. A simple question, "Do you often feel sad or depressed?," to which the patient is required to answer either "yes" or "no," was tested in a sample of medically ill patients in the community and had a sensitivity of 69% and specificity of 90% [51]. The Patient Health Questionaire-2 (PHQ-2) asks patients about their depressed mood: 1) "During the past weeks have you been bothered by feeling down, depressed, or hopeless?"; and 2) "During the past month have you been bothered by little interest or pleasure in doing things?" This questionnaire has a sensitivity of 100% and specificity of 77% [52]. A brief, three-question screening tool has been validated for use in the ED setting to identify individuals with depression – the Emergency Department–Depression Screening Instrument (ED-DSI) (see Table 26.3). ED-DSI has 89% sensitivity and 73% specificity in cognitively intact individuals [53].

Diagnostic depression work-up should include a thorough review of medical and neurological problems, active medications use, and questions regarding substance abuse. Additionally, assessment of psychiatric history and cognitive examination should take place. Collateral information from family members, caretakers, and friends should be sought to corroborate the history.

Treatment

As previously, mentioned, untreated depression is associated with increased mortality from co-existing medical conditions and suicide. It also increases the risk of disability and contributes to impairment in psychosocial functioning and quality of life. Failure to identify depression may also lead to overuse of resources, such as unnecessary pursuits of physical and laboratory studies, avoidable referrals to specialists, and frequent returns to EDs [54]. Adequate recognition and prompt treatment referral are therefore imperative in improving overall care of the depressed elderly [55].

Depressive disorder with severe symptomatology, particularly if accompanied by suicidal ideations, suicide intent, recent attempt, or complicated by psychotic symptoms, almost always warrants inpatient psychiatric hospitalization. Hospitalization should also be considered for individuals who have a history of poor compliance, are socially isolated or neglected, and those who suffer from complex medical comorbidities.

For less acute patients, other levels of treatment referrals should be utilized. These include referrals to partial hospitalization programs, psychiatric consultants, or primary care providers. Utilization of psychiatric consultants is appropriate when diagnostic difficulties emerge, co-existing psychiatric symptoms of anxiety or substance abuse exist, or confounding medical and neurological symptoms obscure the diagnosis. Pharmacologic interventions, psychotherapy, and electroconvulsive therapy (ECT) are effective treatments for depressed elders. Antidepressants are considered to be safe and effective in targeting depressive symptoms with clinical recommendations favoring the use of selective serotonin reuptake inhibitors (SSRIs). SSRIs are generally well tolerated, with fewer sedative and anticholinergic side effects as well as reduced risk of lethal overdose than tricyclic antidepressants [56]. The role of various forms of psychotherapy has been proposed to exercise significant benefit in suicidal patients. Psychotherapeutic interventions that enhance adherence to treatment, provide education, increase self-esteem, strengthen social supports, and diminish hopelessness are clinically recommended [57]. A large number of studies support the effectiveness of ECT in the treatment of geriatric depression [58], but side effects such as cardiac complications, cognitive decline, and delirium limit its use in some patients.

Substance abuse

Background and epidemiology

Substance use disorders in the elderly are a significant public health concern that only in recent years has begun to receive attention. As our population ages, this problem is likely to grow since the cohort of "baby boomers" grew up in an era when use of alcohol and drugs was more widespread. The majority of patients with substance abuse and dependence present in general medical settings, imposing an urgent need for medical providers to become familiar with diagnostic criteria, risk factors, consequences, and treatment options.

Alcohol remains the substance most commonly used among the elderly, however the estimates of prevalence of alcoholism vary as studies differ in their definitions of use (self-reports versus strict diagnostic criteria) and populations studied (community versus medical settings).

The lifetime prevalence of alcohol abuse and dependence in the entire sample of the Epidemiologic Catchment Area Study was 13.8% in men aged 65 or older, the lifetime prevalence was 14%, and the 1-month prevalence was 1.93%. In women aged 65 or older, the lifetime prevalence was 1.49% and the 1-month prevalence was 0.4% [59]. Rates of heavy drinking among older adults are much higher, demonstrating that 15–20% of men and 8–10% of women drink at "at risk" or "problem" drinking levels.

The rates of alcohol use disorders are higher in medical settings. Approximately 14% of ED older patients, 18% of medical inpatients, and >20% of psychiatrically hospitalized patients meet criteria for alcohol abuse or dependence [60].

DSM IV-TR describes alcohol abuse and dependence as two distinct diagnostic categories. DSM V-TR, which was published in May 2013, identifies alcohol use disorders as one separate category.

Alcohol abuse is a maladaptive pattern of drinking associated with at least one of the following: failure to fulfill obligations, drinking in hazardous situations or causing legal problems, and continued use despite social or occupational problems.

DSM IV-TR criteria for alcohol abuse

A. A maladaptive pattern of use leading to impairment or distress, as manifested by **one or more** occurring within a 12-month period:

    a. failure to fulfill role obligations at work, school, or home;

    b. recurrent use in hazardous situations;

    c. recurrent legal problems;

    d. continued use.

Alcohol dependence is described as a pattern of drinking associated with at least three of the following occurring in the same 12-month period: tolerance; withdrawal symptoms; lack of control; preoccupation with acquisition and/or use; desire or unsuccessful efforts to quit; and continued use despite adverse effects. The symptoms need to be associated with impairment in social, occupational, and recreational activities.

DSM IV-TR criteria for alcohol dependence

A. A maladaptive pattern of use leading to impairment or distress, as manifested by *three or more* occurring within a 12-month period:

    a. tolerance to alcohol;

    b. withdrawal syndrome;

    c. greater use than intended;

    d. desire to use alcohol or inability to control use;

    e. devotion of large proportion of time to getting and consuming alcohol, and recovering from alcohol use;

    f. neglect of social, work, or recreational activities;

    g. continued alcohol use despite physical or psychological problems.

The World Health Organization recognizes harmful ("evidence that use is causing adverse consequences") and hazardous drinking ("quality and pattern of use that places patients at risk of adverse consequences") as additional separate diagnostic categories.

Harmful drinking in the general population consists of alcohol intake of >14 drinks per week or more than four drinks per occasion for men and more than seven drinks per week or more than three per occasion for women, where a drink corresponds to 10–12 g of pure alcohol [61]. These quantitative guidelines are stricter for the geriatric population. The National Institute on Alcohol Abuse and Alcoholism (NIAAA) and the American

Geriatrics Society (AGS) currently define risky drinking levels for people aged 65 and older as more than seven drinks per week or more than three drinks on any single day [62,63].

About two-thirds of elderly alcoholics have developed the problem before the age of 40 ("early-onset"). Early-onset drinkers tend to have more pervasive psychiatric and medical comorbidity as well as a higher incidence of familiar pattern of use. One-third began the problematic drinking pattern later in life ("late-onset"), typically in response to stressful life events such as retirement, functional decline, and death of spouse or medical disability. Late-onset drinkers typically have fewer alcohol-related problems, have less psychiatric comorbidity, and are less likely to have family history significant for alcohol use disorders [64].

Risk factors

Problem drinking affects the elderly population differently than younger patients in that it is more likely to complicate the course of co-existing medical conditions, can adversely influence effects of commonly prescribed medications, and can exacerbate cognitive problems [65], leading to markedly increased morbidity and mortality [66]. Age-related physiologic changes make elderly patients more vulnerable to the intoxicating effects of alcohol. Volume of distribution for alcohol diminishes as the total body water decreases, leading to higher peak concentration for a given dose of alcohol. In addition, decreased activity of alcohol dehydrogenase in the stomach increases the intoxicating properties of alcohol [67].

Heavy alcohol consumption carries a significant risk of worsening co-existing medical illnesses. As such, alcohol is known to double the risk of hypertension among women consuming more than two drinks per day and men having more than four drinks per day. Alcohol impedes diabetic control and contributes to exacerbation of diabetic neuropathy and retinopathy. Additionally, it is known to contribute to gastrointestinal irritation and bleeding, and is associated with increased risk of gout and higher rates of cancer, particularly head and neck, lung, esophagus, and breast. Consuming more than two drinks per day among women and four or more among men increases the risk of liver cirrhosis. Smaller amounts can worsen the course of acute and chronic hepatitis and reduce responsiveness to interferon [68].

Chronic exposure to alcohol may lead to peripheral neuropathy, myopathy, and cerebellar damage, which in conjunction with direct impairment effects on judgment and balance, leads to increased risk of falls and injuries. Elderly alcoholics have a higher age-adjusted risk of osteoporosis and hip fractures [69].

Psychiatric comorbidities frequently implicated in chronic alcohol exposure in the elderly include affective disorders, anxiety, and cognitive impairment. Depressive symptoms are of particular concern as they are associated with increased morbidity and mortality, as well as heightened risk of suicide [70].

Evaluation

Alcohol abuse and dependence are frequently under-recognized and undertreated. Reasons why the diagnosis is missed

Table 26.4. Difficulties in applying DSM-IV Substance Abuse/Dependence criteria to elderly patients

Tolerance	Elderly drinkers may not exhibit tolerance because of increased sensitivity to intoxicating effects of alcohol
Withdrawal	Late-onset drinkers often lack physiological dependence
Loss of control (larger amounts taken than intended)	Elderly drinkers may exhibit impairment in self-monitoring due to cognitive deficits
Unsuccessful efforts to stop	Same issue across the lifespan
Large amount of time spent to obtain, use, or recover from effects of alcohol	Negative effects from alcohol can emerge even in absence of extensive time commitment
Giving up social, recreational activities	Detection may be impeded due to fewer activities
Continued use despite negative consequences	Same issue across the lifespan

Table 26.5. Physical symptoms screening triggers

- Cognitive impairment
- Depression and anxiety
- Insomnia
- Weight loss and nutritional deficiencies
- Diminished self-care
- Gait abnormalities, tremors, and frequent falls
- Refractory hypertension
- Poor glucose control
- Recurrent gastritis and esophagitis
- Recurrent seizures
- Difficulty managing warfarin dosing

appear to be multifactorial. First, applying DSM-IV TR criteria for substance abuse and dependence may be difficult in this population (Table 26.4). Second, patients, families, and providers may share ageist assumptions such as the belief that older adults' quality of life will remain poor even if they are successfully treated for their substance abuse [71]. Third, many older drinkers attribute their alcohol problems to a breakdown in moral values causing a sense of shame and stigma that ultimately prevents them from seeking help. Additionally, difficulty applying criteria to a variety of nonspecific symptoms (falls, sleep problems, confusion, irritability) [72], stereotyping (physicians are less likely to detect alcohol problems in women, the educated, and those of higher socioeconomic status) [73], and abbreviated office/ED visits [74] may further impede the clinician's ability to detect alcohol-related problems in the elderly.

Routine screening is recommended in all older patients, particularly those undergoing major life transitions or presenting with nonspecific physical symptoms. Table 26.5 summarizes physical symptoms or complaints that should increase suspicion of alcohol use disorder in the elderly [75] and trigger formal screening.

Table 26.6. CAGE questionnaire

- C (cut-down): Have you ever felt that you should cut down on your drinking?
- A (annoyed): Have people annoyed you by criticizing your drinking?
- G (guilty): Have you ever felt guilty about your drinking?
- E (eye-opener): Have you ever had a drink first thing in the morning to steady your nerves or get rid of a hangover?

Table 26.7. Short Michigan Alcoholism Screening Test: geriatric version

- Do you ever underestimate how much you drink?
- After drinking do you ever skip meals?
- Does drinking decrease shakes and tremors?
- Does drinking make you not remember parts of the day or night?
- Do you drink to relax or calm your nerves?
- Do you drink to take your mind off problems?
- Have you ever increased your drinking after a loss in your life?
- Has a doctor or nurse said they're worried about your drinking?
- Have you made rules to manage your drinking?
- When lonely, does drinking help?

Total score >2 "yes" responses points to alcohol problem.

Table 26.8. Alcohol Use Disorders Identification Test (Audit-C; figures indicate points scored)

- How often did you have a drink containing alcohol in the past year?
  Never, 0; monthly or less, 1; 2–4 per month, 2; 2–3 per week, 3; 4 or more per week, 4.
- How many drinks did you have on a typical day when you were drinking alcohol?
  1–2, 0; 3–4, 1; 5–6, 2; 7–9, 3; 10 or more, 4.
- How often did you have 6 or more drinks on one occasion in the past year?
  Never, 0; less than monthly, 1; monthly, 2; weekly, 3; daily, 4.

Several brief, practical, and well-validated screening tools for alcoholism are available. The CAGE questionnaire (Table 26.6) and SMAST-G [76] (Short Michigan Alcoholism Screening Test-Geriatric Version) (Table 26.7) are commonly used tools that can facilitate detection. SMAST-G has a sensitivity of 85% and specificity of 90% in identifying alcohol use disorders in the elderly [77], while CAGE has shown variable sensitivity (60–98%) and specificity (56–100%) in older populations [78].

There are several other validated screening methodologies that have been proven helpful in facilitating detection of alcohol use disorders in the elderly. The Alcohol Use Disorders Identification Test (AUDIT) is recommended for use in primary care settings worldwide. The Audit-C consists of three AUDIT items on consumption, frequency, and bingeing and is equivalent to the ten-item scale in identifying hazardous drinkers across a range of populations [79] (Table 26.8).

SBIRT (**S**creening, **B**rief **I**ntervention, and **R**eferral to **T**reatment) is a comprehensive, integrated, public health approach to the delivery of early intervention for individuals with risky alcohol and drug use, as well as the timely referral to more intensive substance abuse treatment for those who have

Table 26.9. Laboratory tests

- Blood count: ↑ red blood cell size; mean corpuscular volume (MCV) >100
- Liver functions tests (LFTs)
- ↑ Aspartate aminotransferase (AST) >40 u/l
- ↑ Alanine aminotransferase (ALT) >40 u/l
- AST/ALT ratio >2 → suggestive of alcoholic liver disease
- ↑ Carbohydrate-deficient transferrin (CDT): high sensitivity and specificity/good indicator of early relapse: 20 U or 2.6%
- ↑ Gamma-glutamyltransferase (GGT): levels ↑ after 70 drinks/week for several weeks >35 u/l
- Urine/serum toxicology screen: to exclude other drug use
- Electrolytes: ↓ Na, ↓Mg → ↑ risk of seizures
- Blood alcohol concentration (BAC): ~150 w/o intoxication or ~300 w/o somnolence → evidence of tolerance → ↑ risk of withdrawal

substance use disorders. It consists of brief screening aimed at quick assessment of the severity of substance use and identification of the appropriate level of treatment. The Brief Intervention focuses on increasing awareness regarding substance use and evoking motivation toward behavioral change. Finally, referral to treatment provides those identified as needing more extensive treatment with access to specialty care [80].

Complete evaluation should further include thorough physical examination aimed at identifying stigmata of chronic exposure to alcohol (palmar erythema, hepatomegaly) and assessment of medical conditions commonly associated with or exacerbated by heavy alcohol consumption. Furthermore, evaluation of risk of withdrawal syndrome is essential in determining the level of care and intensity of intervention. Laboratory findings, when combined with screening instruments, can represent an important part of improving the diagnosis of an alcohol use disorder. Indirect biomarkers illustrate the effect of alcohol on organ systems or body chemistry. Most commonly monitored biomarkers include mean corpuscular volume (MCV), gamma-glutamyltransferase (GGT), aspartate aminotransferase (AST), alanine aminotransferase (ALT), and carbohydrate-deficient transferrin (CDT) (Table 26.9).

Treatment

The treatment of the geriatric patient with an alcohol use disorder should be within a context of a comprehensive treatment plan, tailored to the patient's specific needs, readiness, and coexisting problems. The intervention needs to be provided in a nonconfrontational and supportive manner, since older adults experience a significantly greater burden of stigma and shame.

Treatment intervention needs to be stratified depending on the pattern and severity of use. The screening tools and questionnaires are helpful in identifying elders at risk. The following step in management of elder substance-abusing patients should focus on determining the risk of withdrawal syndrome. The presence of comorbid medical problems, limited reserve, susceptibility to kindling, and vulnerability to adverse effects of the medications used for treatment of withdrawal may significantly increase the risk of complicated withdrawal syndrome in this population [81]. Histories of prior complicated detoxifications, previous seizures or delirium tremens, or unstable medical comorbidities warrant inpatient detoxification [82]. The Clinical Institute Withdrawal Assessment for Alcohol (CIWA–Ar) can be useful in guiding benzodiazepine therapy for management of acute withdrawal syndrome. After medical detoxification is completed, elderly patients should be referred to residential, day treatment, or outpatient programs where psychological interventions such as psychoeducation, counseling, and motivational interviewing can be provided. The use of medications promoting abstinence has not been studied extensively in elderly subjects. Several studies have been conducted to determine the efficacy of brief interventions, either alone or in combination with medication management. Project GOAL examined the effectiveness of two 10–15-minute counseling visits that included advice, education, and contracting. Patients in the intervention arm significantly reduced weekly alcohol consumption and episodes of heavy drinking, and maintained the gains at 12-month follow-up. A more recent trial found that brief behavioral counseling within the A-FRAMES model also resulted in a significant reduction in alcohol consumption among the participants. The A-FRAMES model focuses on conducting thorough Assessment and providing objective Feedback. It subsequently stresses that Responsibility for change belongs to the patient and gives clear Advice about the benefits of change. It concludes with providing a Menu of options for treatment to facilitate change using Empathic listening and encouraging Self-efficacy.

Pharmacologic treatment with anticraving agents, such as naltrexone, has shown some efficacy (prevention of relapse) in subjects 50–74 years of age [83]. Acamprosate has been found to be safe and effective in younger populations [84].

Geriatric psychoses

Background and epidemiology

Medical dictionaries describe psychosis as gross impairment in reality testing that is manifested by delusions, hallucinations, incoherent speech, and agitated or disorganized behavior without apparent appreciation on the patient's side of the incomprehensibility of the symptoms. Psychoses in the geriatric population can be manifestations of numerous conditions and therefore pose significant diagnostic challenge for a clinician. DSM-IV TR identifies a plethora of psychotic illnesses, including schizophrenia, schizophreniform disorder, brief psychotic disorder, and psychotic disorders due to general medical conditions. In addition to primary psychotic disorders, psychotic symptoms can accompany a number of other diagnoses, such as major depressive disorder, bipolar disorder, substance intoxication, and withdrawal, as well as dementia. Onset of psychotic symptoms late in life warrants thorough diagnostic investigation, as this is frequently the first manifestation of underlying medical or neurologic conditions.

The epidemiologic data indicate that prevalence of schizophrenia and schizophreniform disorder in older adults in North America is about 1% [85], while estimates from Europe suggest prevalence rates between 1 and 2% [86]. While primary psychotic disorders remain fairly rare, approximately 16–23% of the elderly population develops psychotic symptoms related to other causes, primarily to dementia [87]. Dementia significantly increases vulnerability to psychosis, and over 50% of patients with cognitive disorders have been noted to have ideas of reference and hallucinatory experiences.

Dementia is a common neuropsychiatric syndrome associated with progressive decline in function across multiple cognitive domains. It affects 8–10% of people older than 65 and nearly 50% of those older than 85 [88]. Alzheimer's disease is the most common cause of dementia (60%), followed by vascular dementia (20%) and dementia with Lewy bodies (15%) [89]. About 80% of patients with dementia will experience some form of behavioral or psychological symptoms associated with dementia syndrome (BPSD). These symptoms include agitation and aggression, delusions, hallucination and misidentifications, screaming and repetitive vocalizations, as well as circadian rhythm dysregulation and wandering. BPSD can cause significant distress for patients and their caregivers, and are associated with poorer prognosis, rapid cognitive decline, diminished quality of life, and risk of institutionalization [90]. Successful treatment of psychiatric and behavioral problems is associated with better outcomes such as improved quality of life, decreased caregiver stress, and reduced patient suffering [91].

Primary psychotic disorders and psychotic symptoms associated with dementia must be differentiated from delirium. Delirium is a common neuropsychiatric syndrome characterized by an acute disturbance in cognition, attention, and level of consciousness, frequently accompanied by changes in sleep–wake cycle, psychomotor agitation, or retardation, as well as hallucinations and delusions. It is a common psychiatric emergency affecting an estimated 30–50% of hospitalized elders [92], yet still posing a significant diagnostic challenge for the clinicians as non-detection rates can reach up to 70% [93]. Emergence of delirium is associated with a number of adverse consequences including increased mortality [94], prolonged hospitalization, and heightened risk of institutionalization [95], as well as impeded physical and cognitive recovery at 6 and 12 months [96]. Early identification of delirium and prompt management of the underlying medical factors reduces its severity and duration, and leads to improved outcomes for the patient [97].

Risk factors

The incidence of psychosis in general increases with age, with a number of factors leading to increase in vulnerability and expression. It has been proposed that age-related deterioration of cortical areas such as the frontal and temporal lobes as well as neurochemical changes common in aging, might be implicated in the increased incidence of psychosis [98]. Because older adults who develop late-onset psychosis have high rate of decreased visual and auditory acuity, there is controversy around the relationship between the sensory deficit and predisposition to psychosis. Clinical experience indicates that improved hearing or vision has led to decreased paranoid delusions and hallucinations [99]. Furthermore, the combination of physical illnesses, social isolation, polypharmacy, and substance abuse frequently encountered in the elderly may further potentiate the vulnerability for psychosis. Geneti predisposition, certain premorbid personality constructs, primarily schizotypal and paranoid, as well as female gender have been postulated as additional risk factors for the development of psychosis in the elderly.

In patients with AD and psychosis, the presence of delusions was associated with older age, increased depression, more agitation, and worse general health. The presence of hallucinations, on the other hand, was associated with more severe dementia, being African-American, having fewer years of formal education, and struggling with gait abnormalities. Newer data indicate that psychosis in AD may have genetic determinants [100].

Evaluation

Late-life psychoses are a diverse spectrum of disorders that can present significant diagnostic and management challenges. They can be generally categorized into early- and late-onset psychoses, with the latter being further divided into psychoses without and with dementia. The most common diagnoses within the late-onset group are delirium, dementia, late-onset psychotic and mood disorders, and psychosis due to general medical conditions. The initial assessment of new-onset late-life psychosis includes a thorough medical and neurological work-up. The evaluation typically includes brain imaging and laboratory studies, such as complete blood count, comprehensive metabolic panel, B_{12} and folate levels, thyroid function tests, urinalysis, and ECG. Comprehensive review of medications, including over-the-counter and herbal agents, and substance abuse is imperative. Differentiation between delirium, dementia, and primary psychoses must occur given the variation in risk, prognosis, and management linked to these entities [101]. Table 26.10 outlines the key differences.

Delirium is a medical emergency that should not be confused with psychosis and that must be evaluated and treated urgently. Delirium is conceptualized as a multifactorial syndrome emerging from the interaction of the predisposing and precipitating factors. Its severity and likelihood increase with the number of risk factors present. Predisposing factors describe patient vulnerabilities and include age, pre-existing cognitive impairment, and sensory deficits, among others [102]. Precipitating factors, on the other hand, delineate hospital-related insults that have been linked to the onset of the syndrome [103] (Table 26.11). Elderly patients are intrinsically at risk of having a number

Table 26.10. Differential diagnosis: delirium, dementia, psychosis

	Delirium	Dementia	Psychosis
Onset	Acute	Gradual	Variable
Course	Fluctuating	Progressive	Chronic
Consciousness	Altered	Normal	Normal
Orientation	Fluctuating	Impaired	Normal
Duration	Hours–months	Months–years	Months–years
Hallucinations	Common	Rare till late	Common
Attention	Impaired	Normal till late	May be impaired

Table 26.11. Risk factors for delirium

Predisposing factors	Precipitating factors
Age (>65)	Polypharmacy
Cognitive impairment	Infection
Physical frailty	Immobility
Visual impairment	Catheters
Hearing impairment	Sleep deprivation
Male gender	Use of restraints (physical and
Dehydration on admission	pharmacological)
Infection on admission	Pain
Multiple comorbidities	High number of hospital procedures
Nutritional deficiencies	Hypoxia
Alcohol dependence	Electrolyte disturbance
Prior episodes of delirium	End organ failure
	Alcohol withdrawal

Table 26.12. Possible causes of behavioral and psychological disturbances in dementia

Medication side effects: especially anticholinergic, antimuscarinic
Delirium (infection, dehydration, acute medical illness)
Pain linked to chronic or acute medical problems
Frustration due to progressive memory/cognitive failure
Physical needs (hunger, need for toileting)
Emotional needs (separation from family)
Environmental factors (noise, overcrowding, overstimulation, understimulation)
Rigid caregiving

of predisposing factors, making them more likely to develop delirium even in response to seemingly benign triggers [104]. Iatrogenic etiology should not be overlooked, as medication use may be the sole precipitant for 12–39% of cases of delirium in the elderly [105].

Dementia that is commonly complicated by psychotic symptoms is a common neuropsychiatric syndrome associated with progressive decline in function across multiple cognitive domains. The first step in evaluating psychotic disturbance in the course of dementia is to assess and explore medical, pharmacological, and environmental variables that may precipitate the behavior. Table 26.12 gives a summary of possible factors leading to behavioral escalation in dementia patients [106].

It is essential to identify and correct all modifiable causes of behavioral distress, but the evaluation can be challenging due to the fluctuating nature of these symptoms and the patient's impeded ability to communicate the nature of the distress.

Treatment

Care of patients with behavioral symptoms and agitation typically involves a wide range of psychosocial treatments with focus on the patient's physical health, safety of the environment, and psychiatric symptoms. Behavioral complications that are primarily treated non-pharmacologically include circadian rhythm abnormalities, wandering, vocalizations, and catastrophic

Table 26.13. Non-pharmacological interventions for BPSD

Behavior	Intervention
Day–night reversal	Avoidance of nighttime fluid and diuretics
	Effective treatment of pain
	Daytime structure, socialization, exercise
	Discouragement of daytime napping
Wandering	Elimination of environmental hazards: locks, alarms on doors and windows
	Redirection techniques
	Soft nighttime illumination
Catastrophic reaction	Relaxed, supportive approach
	Avoidance of sensory overload
	Limited demands

reactions (emotional response of various intensities to an overwhelming task or situation) [107] (Table 26.13).

Other symptoms such as psychosis, agitation, and aggression have historically been described as "medication-responsive." It is important, however, to point out that at this time there is no Food and Drug Administration (FDA)-approved indication for a medication to treat these common and debilitating behavioral problems. Antipsychotic medications have been used "off-label," but FDA black-box warnings linking these medications to increased mortality (most commonly due to cardiac or infectious causes), and research findings that emphasize either modest medication efficacy or lack of it, significantly curtail prescribing practices [108]. In a recent American College of Neuropsychiatrists White Paper, a group of experts made several recommendations with regard to treatment of agitation and psychosis in patients with dementia. Identification and correction of possible reversible causative factors along with environmental, interpersonal, social, and medical interventions should be considered first. Families, patients, and caregivers should be involved in the decision-making process with full appreciation of the benefits and shortfalls of currently available strategies. Only persistent and severe symptoms should be considered for continuous pharmacological management, with the understanding that the prescribing clinician provides ongoing monitoring of effectiveness. The lowest effective medication dosages for the shortest period of time necessary to stabilize symptoms should be used [109] in this population.

Pearls and pitfalls

Pitfalls

- Older adults at are higher risk of suicide than any other segment of the population.
- There is a concern that as the "baby boom" population ages, there will be a substantial increase in the number of older adults needing treatment for substance abuse problems.
- The onset of psychotic symptoms in late life may be the first sign of a medical, neurological, or substance-induced condition.

Pearls

- Older suicide victims are more likely to have suffered from a single episode of unipolar depression, the type of depression that tends to respond well to standard therapies.
- Effective screening and intervention strategies exist, leading to improvement in substance abuse problems in the elderly.
- Primary psychotic disorders remain fairly rare in the elderly population.

References

1. World Health Organization. *World Health Report 2010*.
2. Center for Disease Control and Prevention. National Center for Injury Prevention and Control. *Web based Injury Statistics Query and Reporting System* (online, accessed September 23, 2012).
3. Moscicki EK. Identification of suicide risk factor using epidemiologic studies. *Psychiatr Clin North Am*. 1997;3:499–517.
4. Goldsmith SK, Pellmar TC, Kleinman AM, et al. (ed.) *Reducing Suicide: A National Imperative* (Washington, DC: National Academy Press, 2002).
5. Centers for Disease Control and Prevention, Atlanta, GA.
6. Conwell Y, Van Orden K, Caine E. Suicide in older adults. *Psychiatr Clin North Am*. 2011;34(2):451–68.
7. Murphy GE, Wetzel RD, Robins E, et al. Multiple risk factors predict suicide in alcoholism. *Arch Gen Psychiatr*. 1992;49(6):459–63.
8. Conner KR, Duberstein PR, Conwell Y, et al. Psychological vulnerability to completed suicide: a review of empirical studies. *Suicide Life Threat Bevah*. 2001;31(4):367–85.
9. Di Giviovann G, Di Matteo V, Esposity E (ed.). The role of dopamine and serotonin in suicidal behavior and aggression. In *Progress in Brain Research*, vol. 172, ed. Ryding E, Lindstrom M, Traskman-Bendz L (Philadelphia, PA: Elsevier, 2008).
10. Dombrovski AY, Clark L, Reynolds CF 3rd, et al. Cognitive performance in suicidal depressed elderly: preliminary report. *Am J Geriatr Psychiatr*. 2008;16(2):109–15.
11. Alexopoulos GS, Meyers BS, Young RC, et al. 'Vascular depression' hypothesis. *Arch Gen Psychiatr*. 1997;54(10):915–22.
12. Rubio A, Vestner AL, Steward JM, et al. Suicide and Alzheimer's pathology in the elderly: A case-control study. *Biol Psychiatr*. 2001;49:138–45.
13. Beautrais AL. A case control study of suicide and attempted suicide in older adults. *Suicide Life-Threat Behav*. 2002;32(1):1–9
14. Rubenowitz E, Waern M, Wilhelmson K, Allebeck P. Life events and psychosocial factors in elderly suicides- a case control study. *Psychol Med*. 2001;31(7):1193–202.
15. Miller M. A psychological autopsy of a geriatric suicide. *J. Geriatr Psychiatr*. 1977;10(2):229–42.
16. Barraclough BM. Suicide in the elderly: recent developments in psychogeriatrics. *Br J Psychiatr*. 1972;(Suppl. #6):87–97.
17. Duberstein PR, Conwell Y, Conner KR, et al. Poor social integration and suicide: fact or artifact? A case-control study. *Psychol Med*. 2004;34(7):1331–7.
18. Conwell Y, Duberstein PR, Caine ED. Risk factors for suicide in later life. *Biol Psychiatr*. 2002;52:193–204.

19. Miller M. Geriatric suicide: the Arizona study. *Gerontologist.* 1978;18:488–95.

20. Conwell Y, Duberstein PR, Connor K, et al. Access to firearms and risk for suicide behavior in middle-aged and older adults. *Am J Geriatr Psychiatr.* 2002;10(4):407–16.

21. Holkup PA, Hsiao-Chen J, Titler MG. Evidence based protocol. Elderly suicide secondary prevention. *J Gerontol Nurs.* 2003;6–17.

22. Venlaere L, Bouckaert F, Gastmans C. Care for suicidal older people: current clinical-ethical considerations. *J Med Ethics.* 2007;33:376–81.

23. Ludwig J, Cook PJ. Homicide and suicide rates associated with implementation of the Brady Handgun Violence Prevention Act. *JAMA.* 2000;284:585–91.

24. Howton K. United Kingdom legislation on pack size of analgesics: background, rationale, and effects on suicide and deliberate self-harm. *Suicide Life Threat Behav.* 2002;32(3):223–9.

25. De Leo D, Dello BM, Dwyer J. Suicide among the elderly: The long-term impact of a telephone support and assessment intervention in northern Italy. *Br J Psychiatr.* 2002;181:226–9.

26. Bruce ML, Ten Have T, Reynolds CF III, et al. Reducing suicidal ideation and depressive symptoms in depressed older primary care patients: a randomized controlled trial. *JAMA.* 2004;291(9):1081–91.

27. Alexopoulos GS, Reynolds CF III, Bruce ML, et al. Reducing suicidal ideation and depression in older primary care patients: 24 months outcomes of the PROSPECT study. *Am J Psychiatr.* 2009;166:882–90.

28. Moussavi S, Chatterji S, Verdes E, et al. Depression, chronic diseases, and decrements in health: results from the World Health Surveys. *Lancet.* 2007;370:851–8.

29. Alexopoulos GS, Buckwalter K, Olin J, et al. Comorbidity of late life depression: An opportunity for research on mechanisms and treatment. *Biol Psychiatr.* 2002;52:543–58.

30. Huang BY, Cornoni-Huntley J, Hays JC, et al. Impact of depressive symptoms on hospitalization risk in community-welling older persons. *J Am Geriatr Soc.* 2000;48(10):1279–84.

31. Schultz R, Dryer RA, Rollman BI. Depression as a risk factor for non-suicide mortality in the elderly. *Biol Psychiatr.* 2002;52(3):205–25.

32. Waern M, Runeson BS, Allebeck P, et al. Mental disorders in elderly suicides: a case control study. *Am J Psychiatr.* 2002;159(3):450–5.

33. Fiske A, Loebach Wetherell J, Gatz M. Depression in older adults. *Annu Rev Clin Psychol.* 2009;5:363–89.

34. Sanders AB. Older persons in the emergency medical care system. *J Am Geriatr Soc.* 2001;49:1390–2.

35. Meldon SW, Emerman CL, Schubert DS. Recognition of depression in geriatric ED patients by emergency physicians. *Ann Emerg Med.* 1997;30:442–7.

36. Charney DS, Reynolds CF III, Lewis L, et al. Depression and Bipolar Support Alliance Consensus statement on the unmet needs in diagnosis and treatment of mood disorders in late life. *Arch Gen Psychiatr.* 2003;60(7):664–72.

37. Carney RM, Freedland KE. Depression, mortality, and medical morbidity in patients with coronary heart disease. *Biol Psychiatr.* 2003;54:241–7.

38. Astrom M, Adolfsson R, Asplud K. Major depression in stroke patients. A 3 year longitudinal study. *Stroke.* 1993;24:976–82.

39. Cummings JL. Depression and Parkinson's disease: A review. *Am J Psychiatr.* 1992;149:443–54.

40. Fiske A, Wetherell J, Gatz M. Depression in older adults. *Annu Rev Clin Psychol.* 2009;5:363–89.

41. Prince MJ, Harwood RH, Thomas A, et al. A prospective population based cohort study of the effects of disablement and social milieu on the onset and maintenance of late life depression. The Gospel Oak Project VII. *Psychol Med.* 1998;28(2):337–50.

42. Penninx BW, Guralnik JM, Ferrucci L et al. Depressive symptoms and physical decline in community dwelling older persons. *JAMA.* 1998;279(21):1720–6.

43. Pines JM, Mullins PM, Cooper JK, et al. National trends in emergency department use, care patterns, and quality of care of older adults in the United States. *J Am Geriatr Soc.* 2013;61(1):12–17.

44. Kesser RC, Birnbaum H, Bromet E, et al. Age differences in major depression: results from the National Comorbidity Survey Replication (NCS-R). *Psycholog Med.* 2010;40(02):225–37.

45. Schwenk TL. Diagnosis of late life depression: the view from primary care. *Biol Psychiatr.* 2002;52(3):157–63.

46. Alexopoulos GS, Kiosses DN, Heo M, et al. Executive dysfunction and the course of geriatric depression. *Biol Psychiatr.* 2005;58:2004–10.

47. Thompson TL 2nd, Mitchell WD, House RM. Geriatric psychiatry patients' care by primary care physicians. *Psychosomatics.* 1989;30(1):65–72.

48. Meldon SW, Emerman CL, Schubert DS. Recognition of depression in geriatric ED patients by ED physicians. *Ann Emerg Med.* 1997;30(4):442–7.

49. Lyness JM, Kim J, Tang W, et al. The clinical significance of subsyndromal depression in older primary care patients. *Am J Geriatr Psych.* 2007;15(3):214–23.

50. Park M, Unützer J. Geriatric depression in primary care. *Psychiatr Clin North Am.* 2011;34(2):469–87, ix–x.

51. Watkins CL, Lightbody CE, Sutton CJ, et al. Evaluation of a single-item screening tool for depression after stroke: a cohort study. *Clin Rehabil.* 2007;21(9):846–52.

52. Li C, Friedman B, Conwell Y, et al. Validity of the Patient Health Questionnaire 2 (PHQ-2) in identifying major depression in older people. *J Am Geriatr Soc.* 2007;55(4):596–602.

53. Fabacher DA, Raccio-Robak N, McErlean MA, et al. Validation of a brief screening tool to detect depression in elderly ED patients. *Am J Emerg Med.* 2002;20:99–102.

54. Walsh PG, Currier G, Shah M, et al. Psychiatric emergency services for the US elderly: 2008 and beyond. *Am J Geriatr Psychiatr.* 2008;16(9):706–17.

55. DasGupta K. Treatment of depression in elderly patients: Recent advances. *Arch Fam Med.* 1998;7(3):274–80.

56. Birrer RB, Vemuri SP. Depression in late life: A diagnostic and therapeutic challenge. *Am Fam Physician.* 2004;69:2375–82.

57. Fiske A, Loebach Wetherill J, Gatz M. Depression in older adults. *Annu Rev Clin Psychol.* 2009;5:363–89.

58. Salzman C, Wong E, Wright BC. Drug and ECT treatment of depression in the elderly, 1996–2001: A literature review. *Biol Psychiatr.* 2002;52:265–84.

59. Helzer JE, Burnam A, McEvoy LT. Alcohol abuse and dependence. In *Psychiatric Disorders in America: The Epidemiologic Catchment Area Study*, ed. Robions LN, Regier DA (New York: Macmillan 1991), pp. 81–115.

60. O'Connell H, Chin A, Cunningham C, et al. The role of dopamine and serotonin in suicidal behavior and aggression. *BMJ*. 2003;327:664–7.

61. Schuckit MA. Alcohol use disorders. *Lancet*. 2009;373:492–501.

62. *Helping patients who drink too much. A Clinician's Guide, 2005 edn* (Rockville, MD: NIAAA, National Institute of Health, 2005).

63. Moore A, American Geriatrics Society Clinical Practice Committee. *Clinical Guidelines for Alcohol Use Disorders in Older Adults, November 2003*.

64. Liberto JG, Oslin DW. Early versus late onset of alcoholism in the elderly. *Int J Addict*. 1995;30(13–14):1799–818.

65. Oslin DW. Alcohol use in late life: disability and comorbidity. *J Geriatr Psychiatr Neurol*. 2000;13:134–40.

66. Friedmann PD, Karrison T, Nerney M, et al. The effect of alcohol abuse on the health status of older adults seen in the emergency department. *Am J Drug Alcohol Abuse*. 1999;25(3):529–42.

67. Ozdemir V, Fourie J, Busto U, Naranjo CA. Pharmacokinetic changes in the elderly. Do they contribute to drug abuse and dependence? *Clin Pharmacokin*. 1996;31:372–85.

68. Moore AA, Whiteman EJ, Ward KT. Risk of combined alcohol/medication use in older adults. *Am J Geriatr Pharmacother*. 2007;5(1):64–74.

69. Rigler SK. Alcoholism in the elderly. *Am Fam Physician*. 2000;61:1710–16.

70. Warren M. Alcohol dependence and misuse in elderly suicides. *Alcohol*. 2003;38(3):249–54.

71. Blow FC, Cook CA, Booth BM, et al. Age-related psychiatric comorbidities and level of functioning in alcoholic veterans seeking outpatient treatment. *Hosp Community Psychiatr*. 1992;43:990–5.

72. Finlayson RD, Hurt RE, Davis LJ, et al. Alcoholism in elderly persons: a study of the psychiatric and psychosocial features of 216 inpatients. *Mayo Clin Proc*. 1988;63:761–8.

73. Moore RD, Bone LR, Geller G, et al. Prevalence, detection and treatment of alcoholism in hospitalized patients. *JAMA*. 1989;261:403–7.

74. Keeler EB, Solomon DH, Beck JC, et al. Effects of patient age on duration of medical encounters with physicians. *Med Care*. 1982; 20:1101–8.

75. The American Geriatrics Society. *Clinical Guideliness for Alcohol Use Disorders in Older Adults* (accessed January 27, 2013 from www.americangeriatrics.org/products/positionpapers/alcoholPF, updated November 2003).

76. Blow FC, Brower KJ, Schulenberg JR, et al. The Michigan Alcoholism Screening Test–Geriatric version (MAST-G): a new elderly specific screening instrument. *Alcohol Clin Exp Res*. 1992;16:372.

77. Blow SJ, Gillespie BW, Barry KL, et al. Brief screening for alcohol problems in elderly populations using the Short Michigan Alcoholism Screening Test: geriatric version. *Alcohol Clin Exp Res*. 1998;22(Suppl.):131A.

78. Jones TV, Lindsay BA, Yount P, et al. Alcoholism screening questionnaires: Are they valid in the elderly medical outpatients? *J Gen Intern Med*. 1993;8:674–8.

79. Bradley KA, Dibenedetti AF, Volk RJ, et al. Audit-C as a brief screen for alcohol misuse in primary care. *Alcohol Clin Exp Res*. 2007;31:1208–17.

80. Center for Substance Abuse Treatment, Substance Abuse and Mental Health Administration. *Screening, Brief Intervention, and Referral to Treatment, 2008* (accessed from http://sbirt.samhsa.gov).

81. Kraemer, KL, Mayo-Smith MF, Calkins R. Impact of age on the severity, course, and complications of alcohol withdrawal. *Arch Intern Med*. 1997;157:2234–41.

82. Rigler SK. Alcoholism in the elderly. *Am Fam Physician*. 2000;61:1710–16.

83. O'Connell H, Chin AV, Cunningham C, et al. Alcohol use disorders in elderly people: redefining an age old problem in old age. *BMJ*. 2003;327(7416):664–7.

84. Rosner S, Leucht S, Lehert P, Soyka M. Acamprosate supports abstinence, naltrexone prevents excessive drinking: Evidence from a meta-analysis with unreported outcomes. *J Psychopharmacol*. 2008;22(1):11–23.

85. Cohen CI. Outcomes of schizophrenia into later life: an overview. *Gerontologist*. 1990;30(6):790–6.

86. Neugebauer R. Formulation of hypothesis about the true prevalence about the functional and organic psychiatric disorders among the elderly in the United States. In. *Mental Illness in the United States*, ed. Dohrenwend B, Dohrenwend BS, Gould MS, et al. (New York, NY: Raven Press, 1990).

87. Khouzam HR, Battista MA, Emes R, et al. Psychoses in late life: evaluation and management of disorders seen in primary care. *Geriatrics* 2005;60(3): 26–33.

88. Finkel SI. Introduction to behavioral and psychological symptoms of dementia (BPSD). *Int J Geriatr Psychiatr*. 2000;15(Suppl. 1):S2–4.

89. Overshott R, Burns A. Treatment of dementia. *J Neurol Neurosurg Psychiatr*. 2005;76(Suppl. V):v53–9.

90. Hersch EC, Falzgraf S. Management of the behavioral and psychological symptoms of dementia. *Clin Intervent Aging*. 2007;2(4):611–21.

91. Cohen-Mansfield J. Non-pharmacologic interventions for inappropriate behaviors in dementia. *Am J Geriatr Psychiatr*. 2001;9:361–81.

92. Kirshner H. Delirium: A focused review. *Curr Neurol Neurosc Rep*. 2007;7:479–82.

93. Gills AJ, McDonald HT. Unmasking delirium. *Can Nurse*. 2006;102(9);18–24.

94. McCusker J, Cole M, Abrahamowicz M, Primeau F. Delirium predicts 12-month mortality. *Arch Intern Med*. 2002;162:457–63.

95. DeFrances CJ, Hall MJ. *2002 National Hospital Discharge Survey Advanced Data from Vital and Health Statistics, 342* (Hyattsville MD: National Center for Health Statistics, 2004).

96. McCusker J, Cole M, Dendukuri N, Han L, Bedzile E. The course of delirium in older medical inpatients: a prospective study. *J Gen Intern Med*. 2003;18:696–704.

97. Sexena S, Lawley D. Delirium in the elderly: a clinical review. *Postgrad Med J*. 2009;85:405–13.

98. Lacro JP, Jeste DV. Geriatric psychosis. *Psychiatr Q.* 1997;68(3):247–60.

99. Manford M, Andemann F. Complex visual hallucinations. Clinical and neurobiological insights. *Brain.* 1998;121(10):1819–40.

100. Iglewicz A, Meeks TW, Jeste DV. New wine in old bottle: Late-life psychosis. *Psychiatr Clin North Am.* 2011;34(2):295–318.

101. Gill T, Khouzam HR, Tan DT. A mnemonic for monitoring the prescribing of atypical antipsychotics. *Geriatrics* 2004;59:41–5.

102. Burns A, Gallagley A, Byrne J. Delirium. *J Neurol Neurosurg Psychiatr.* 2004;75:362–7.

103. Meager DJ. Delirium: optimizing management. *BMJ.* 2001; 322:144–9.

104. Young J, Inouye SK. Delirium in older people. *BMJ.* 2007;334:842–6.

105. Alagiakrishnan K, Wiens CA. An approach to drug induced delirium in the elderly. *Postgrad Med J.* 2004;80:388–93.

106. Schwab W, Messinger-Rapport B, Franco K. Psychiatric symptoms of dementia: Treatable, but no silver bullet. *Cleveland Clin J Med.* 2009;76(3):167–74.

107. Tueth MJ. Dementia: diagnosis and emergency behavioral complications. *J Emerg Med.* 1995;13(4):519–25.

108. Sultzer DL, Davis SM, Tariot PN, et al. Clinical symptom responses to antipsychotic medications in Alzheimer's disease: Phase 1 outcomes from CATIE-AD Effectiveness Trial. *Am J Psychiatr.* 2008;165:844–54.

109. Jeste DV, Blazer D, Casey D, et al. ACNP White Paper: Update on use of antipsychotic drugs in elderly persons with dementia. *Neuropsychopharmacology.* 2008;33:957–70.

Chapter 27

Metabolic and endocrine emergencies in the elderly

Kristine Samson and Dany Elsayegh

Diabetic ketoacidosis and hyperosmolar hyperglycemic state

Background

Diabetic ketoacidosis (DKA) and hyperosmolar hyperglycemic state (HHS) are two of the most serious complications of diabetes. DKA is more common, occurring with an annual incidence of four to eight cases per 1000 diabetic patients [1]. It is usually seen in patients who have type I diabetes, but may occur in type II diabetics as well; HHS usually occurs in patients with type II diabetes. Exact figures for the incidence of HHS are not available but are believed to account for less than 1% of diabetic admissions to the hospital [2]. Those affected by DKA tend to present earlier for medical attention and are younger than those who present with HHS. Furthermore, the mortality rate for DKA is less than 5% while that in HHS is much higher, at 15%. Both rates are higher for the elderly [3].

Both diseases occur as a result of relative or absolute insulin deficiency with a co-existing increase in counter-regulatory hormone release (glucagon, catecholamines, cortisol, and growth hormone). In DKA, insulin deficiency together with a background of insulin resistance results in accelerated lipolysis, fatty acid production, and finally ketoacidosis [4]. As per the American Diabetes Association, DKA is defined as hyperglycemia (blood glucose >250 mg/dl), acidosis (pH <7.3, serum bicarbonate <18mmol, anion gap >10), and ketonemia [3]. The most common causes of DKA are infection, change in insulin therapy, medication noncompliance, and presentation of new onset of diabetes.

In HHS there is usually a relative insulin deficiency. Since there is some insulin secretion, ketosis is usually suppressed though there is not enough available insulin to suppress hyperglycemia. HHS is diagnosed when there is a blood glucose level >600 mg/dl and serum osmolarity is >320 mosm/kg. Some degree of ketosis may be present.

Diabetic ketoacidosis and HHS are not mutually exclusive, and patients may present on a spectrum between the two. In a retrospective study of 613 patients by Gaglia et al., 22% had DKA, 45% had HHS, and 33% had both [4]. Those who are obese or of African-American background often present with features of HHS and DKA [1]. Gaglia et al. found that almost one-third of cases showing features of both were the elderly. In HHS, the most common causes are infections and dehydration.

The most common precipitant of HHS and DKA, accounting for up to 50% of cases, are infections – pneumonia, urinary tract infection (UTI), and gastroenteritis. Medication noncompliance or inadequate diabetic treatment is the second most common precipitant, accounting for 20–40% of cases. Other less common triggers include vascular events (acute myocardial infarction [MI], stroke), pancreatitis, trauma, burns, other endocrine abnormalities (thyroid disorders, Cushing's), and medications (steroids, diuretics, antipsychotics) [4].

History

The reduced net activity of circulating insulin leads to increased glucose production and decreased glucose utilization by tissues. This results in hyperglycemia, which induces osmotic diuresis, which in turn leads to volume contraction and electrolyte loss. Patients with DKA often present earlier for medical attention because acidosis develops quickly (over a period of hours) while those with HHS present later (after several days) and thus are more dehydrated with worse electrolyte abnormalities [4].

Symptoms include those related to hyperglycemia and resulting dehydration such as polyuria, polydipsia, polyphagia, blurred vision, malaise, and weight loss. Patients in DKA may present with abdominal pain, nausea, and vomiting with a fruity odor to their breath. Those with HHS may present with altered mental status, coma, and seizures. Usually the severity of altered mental status correlates with serum osmolarity [4]. Symptoms related to the underlying cause behind the acute HHS and DKA attack may also be present (e.g., hyperthermia or hypothermia if an infection is present, chest pain if acute MI is present).

Physical

On physical examination there are usually signs of dehydration including dry mucous membranes, poor skin turgor, tachycardia, tachypnea, and Kussmaul breathing (if acidosis is present). The elderly are at increased risk for altered mental status presentation secondary to a higher risk for developing

Geriatric Emergency Medicine, ed. Joseph H. Kahn, Brendan G. Magauran Jr., and Jonathan S. Olshaker. Published by Cambridge University Press. © Cambridge University Press 2014.

hyperosmolarity (decreased glomerular filtration rate (GFR), decreased thirst sensation, and impaired ability to obtain fluids) [3].

Diagnostic testing

Blood work including complete blood count (CBC), metabolic panel, serum or urine ketones, and pH (venous blood gas [VBG] or arterial blood gas [ABG]) should be obtained. An electrocardiogram (ECG) should be performed to evaluate for underlying cardiac disease or effects of electrolyte disturbance. Furthermore, specific testing based on patient presentation and complaint and aimed at diagnosing the precipitant of the DKA or HHS episode should be obtained. For example, if infection is suspected, urinalysis, urine culture, chest radiograph, and blood cultures should be acquired. If a stroke is being considered then a computed tomography (CT) scan of the head should be obtained.

Differential diagnoses

The differential diagnoses for DKA and HHS depend on the chief complaint. If the patient presents with vomiting and abdominal pain (DKA presentation), appendicitis, gastroenteritis, gastritis, and pancreatitis may all be in the differential. If the patient presents with altered mental status and lethargy (HHS presentation), then sepsis, stroke, myxedema coma, and drug or alcohol intoxication should all be considered. If based on the findings of ketoacidosis with an elevated anion gap, then starvation ketosis, alcoholic ketoacidosis, lactic acidosis, and various alcohol poisonings (methanol, ethylene glycol) should be investigated.

Treatment

The treatment for DKA and HHS is multifold and includes replenishment of fluids to correct dehydration, control of glucose, correction of electrolyte imbalances, monitoring of acid–base status, and treatment of underlying precipitant factors.

Isotonic fluid replacement is first-line treatment. Those with DKA have an estimated fluid loss of 5–8 l, while those with HHS are even more profoundly dehydrated with estimated fluid losses of 10–12 l [1]. Underlying cardiac status should be considered when administering the recommended 5–20 ml/kg/h of intravenous (IV) fluid within the first hour [4]. Fluid repletion builds intravascular volume, improves tissue perfusion, and decreases circulating glucose levels [1]. When serum glucose levels fall below 250 mg/dl, 5% dextrose should be added to fluids. Overzealous, rapid fluid replacement may lead to cerebral edema or congestive heart failure (CHF). Cerebral edema is the most common cause of death in patients with DKA and HHS.

Insulin therapy should be initiated after the patient is hemodynamically stable and fluid resuscitation initiated. Insulin reverses ketogenesis, which corrects ketoacidosis, and decreases serum glucose levels by increasing glucose utilization and decreasing glucose production. Insulin by the IV route should be used initially because it works more rapidly and more reliably, especially if there is poor tissue perfusion.

An insulin drip of 0.1 units/kg/h titrated to decrease glucose by approximately 100 mg/dl/h is recommended [4]. The insulin infusion should not be stopped until the patient's anion gap has closed and the bicarbonate level is >18 mmol/l; at this point the patient may be transitioned to long-acting subcutaneous insulin. Again, if the serum glucose falls to below 250 mg/dl, 5% dextrose should be added to IV fluids and the insulin infusion should be continued.

Fluid resuscitation is initiated prior to insulin infusion because insulin enhances shift of intravascular fluid into cells, which may worsen pre-existing hypotension. Furthermore, if hypokalemia exists at initial presentation, potassium should be replaced before insulin is given because insulin will promote movement of potassium into the cells, worsening pre-existing hypokalemia. Severe hypokalemia may cause a malignant arrhythmia or severe muscle fatigue, leading to respiratory failure [4].

Whole-body stores of potassium are depleted in cases of DKA and HHS – potassium deficits may be 3–6 mEq/kg. However, initial serum potassium levels may be low, normal, or high. When insulin is administered, serum potassium shifts to the intracellular space so serum potassium levels often drop rapidly. Thus in cases of low or normal potassium levels, potassium supplementation should begin early [1]: 20–30 mEq/h, administered via a central line, usually keeps serum potassium within the normal range [4]. If hyperkalemia is present on initial presentation, the provider should be cautious in treating this initial abnormal lab value. Secondary to acidosis and hyperglycemia, potassium shifts from the intracellular to the extracellular space leading to an elevated initial potassium level despite the patient actually being depleted of potassium. Therapeutic interventions with fluids and insulin will usually "treat" initial hyperkalemia shifting the potassium back into cells, leading to a rapid drop in serum potassium levels and unmasking the patient's true whole-body potassium depletion.

Bicarbonate is not routinely given to treat metabolic acidosis associated with DKA because ketosis usually reverses with insulin and IV fluid therapy. In cases of severe acidemia (usually pH <6.9) with evidence of cardiovascular collapse refractory to initial fluid treatment, bicarbonate may be used [4]. Two ampules of sodium bicarbonate added to 1 l of 0.45% sodium chloride may be administered over one to two hours. After the infusion is completed, a subsequent pH should be obtained and if still <6.9, the bicarbonate infusion may be repeated. Once the pH is >6.9, no further bicarbonate infusions are necessary [4].

Serum magnesium and phosphate levels should also be monitored and replaced as necessary.

Disposition

Patients with DKA or HHS need to be admitted to a monitored setting where frequent vital signs including glucose fingersticks (which should be performed hourly) are available. When there is hemodynamic instability, such as in the setting of sepsis with DKA or HHS or acute MI with DKA or HHS, the patient may require an intensive care admission.

Thyroid disorder emergencies: myxedema coma and thyroid storm

Background

The thyroid gland produces two biologically active thyroid hormones – thyroxine (T4) and 3,5,3′ triiodothyronine (T3). T4 is produced exclusively by the thyroid gland while only 20% of T3 is produced by the thyroid gland. The majority of circulating thyroid hormone is T4, in a ratio of 20:1 with T3. T4 is converted to T3 by peripheral tissues [5]. More than 99% of T4 and T3 hormones circulate in bound form to multiple serum proteins. The less than 1% free forms of T3 and T4 are the only active form of the hormones. The hypothalamus secretes thyroid-releasing hormone (TRH) that stimulates the pituitary gland to secrete thyroid-stimulating hormone (TSH), that in turn stimulates the thyroid gland to produce T4 and T3. Elevated free T4 and T3 levels exert a negative feedback on the pituitary to decrease production of TSH.

Dysfunction of the thyroid gland is common in the elderly, with hypothyroidism occurring in over 10% of females and approximately 2% of males above the age of 60. Furthermore, 10–15% of those with hyperthyroidism are older than 60 [6]. Though common, thyroid disorders are often overlooked in the elderly because classic signs and symptoms of hypo- or hyperthyroidism may not be present and the more subtle signs of thyroid disease are often attributed to "aging" or other comorbidities.

Myxedema coma

History

Myxedema coma, a life-threatening complication of hypothyroidism, usually affects patients older than 75 years and is characterized by altered mental status and cardiovascular and respiratory collapse in the setting of severe hypothyroidism. The most common causes of primary hypothyroidism (failure of the thyroid gland to secrete thyroid hormones) include Hashimoto's thyroiditis, previous radioactive iodine ablation, dietary iodine deficiency, previous thyroidectomy, subacute thyroiditis, and medication side effects (e.g., lithium, amiodarone, and interferon-α) [5].

Clinical signs of hypothyroidism may go unrecognized because they develop slowly and are often mistaken for effects of the aging process. These include cold intolerance, weight gain, lethargy, constipation, dry skin, depression, and cognitive changes [5]. Usually there is an underlying stressor that precipitates the severe mental deterioration associated with myxedema coma. These include infection, acute MI, sedative medications, or exposure to the cold [3], which is why myxedema coma is more common during the winter months.

Physical

On examination, classic findings associated with hypothyroidism may be present and include dry skin, thinning of hair, bradycardia, hypothermia, hypoventilation, and delayed reflexes [6]. Generalized skin and soft tissue swelling, more easily seen as periorbital edema, with ptosis, macroglossia, and cool skin may also be found.

Diagnostic testing

Thyroid function tests are abnormal, with low levels of free T4 and T3 along with elevated TSH levels (primary hypothyroidism) or normal/low TSH levels (hypothalamic/pituitary failure). Additional blood work should also be requested including CBC, basic metabolic panel, creatinine phosphokinase (CPK), and ABG (if hypoventilation is present, to look for hypercarbic respiratory failure). Blood and urine cultures, urinalysis, and X-ray should be obtained to rule out infection or sepsis as the precipitating cause of myxedema coma. A head CT to rule out stroke or mass, together with ECG to rule out acute ST segment elevation MI (STEMI) and to look for bradyarrhythmias, should also be obtained. Cardiac enzymes should also be ordered.

Differential diagnoses

Any cause of altered mental status (coma, psychosis, seizure) is included in the differential. Meningitis, encephalitis, electrolyte abnormalities, sepsis (from urine, lung, abdomen), various drug overdoses (sedatives, narcotics), encephalopathic states, and strokes need to be considered. Worsening dementia is also in the differential. Hypothermia may also be found in hypoglycemic states and sepsis.

Treatment

Supportive measures, together with IV replacement of thyroid hormone, are the main components of treatment. If IV fluid administration does not correct possible severe cases of hypotension and bradycardia, vasopressor support may be necessary. Hypothermia should be treated with passive rewarming (e.g., warm blankets). Mechanical ventilation may be needed for patients with hypoventilation and hypercapnia. Thyroid hormone replacement therapy is initiated with an IV loading dose of levothyroxine of 200–500 μ, followed by 10–50 μ/day. Because severe hypothyroidism may be caused by a failure in the pituitary axis or from polyglandular autoimmune disease, consider also giving the patient stress doses of corticosteroids [1].

Thyroid storm

History

The presence of excess thyroid hormone only becomes a life-threatening emergency when thyrotoxicosis is associated with severe thermoregulatory dysfunction (elevated temperature), mental status changes, multi-organ dysfunction, and adrenergic crisis. This is known as "thyroid storm" [1]. The most common causes of thyroid storm in the elderly are Graves disease and toxic multinodular goiter [5]. Classic symptoms of hyperthyroidism including heat intolerance, diarrhea, palpitations, and tremulousness, and weight loss in spite of increased appetite may not be present in the elderly for many different reasons. For example, elderly patients usually have pre-existing constipation so "diarrhea" presents as correction of constipation with regular bowel movements. Rather than weight loss with increased appetite, many elderly patients have weight loss accompanied by loss of appetite. Furthermore, elderly patients may present with slow atrial fibrillation rather than rapid atrial fibrillation secondary to already existing medication regimens of beta blockers or calcium channel blockers. High-output heart failure may also be an initial presentation. Fatigue, lethargy, confusion, or agitation may be other presenting symptoms [6].

Patients may experience symptoms including palpitations, anxiety, cardiac failure, and excessive sweating. It is important to search for underlying insults that may trigger thyroid storm. Potential underlying entities are similar to those that may precipitate myxedema coma including acute MI, underlying infection, or cerebrovascular accident (CVA).

Physical exam

On examination, patients presenting with thyroid storm may be febrile, tachycardic, hypertensive, and have warm, moist skin and coarse tremors, muscle weakness, and hyperreflexia. If the underlying cause of thyroid storm is Graves' disease, the patient may have lid lag and exophthalmos. The patient may also have a goiter [5].

Diagnostic testing

Elevated free T4 or free T3 levels, usually in conjunction with suppressed TSH levels (primary hyperthyroidism), are found on laboratory testing. TSH levels may not be suppressed in patients whose primary dysfunction is not within the thyroid (i.e., pituitary or hypothalamic disorder), in elderly patients, or in those on chronic steroids. Abnormal liver function tests may be present and there may be signs of fluid overload on chest radiography [3].

Differential diagnoses

The differential diagnoses depend on the patient's complaints. If the patient presents with new-onset atrial fibrillation or heart failure, acute MI or acute coronary syndrome are possible etiologies. If the patient presents with anorexia and weight loss, an occult malignancy may be the source. If lethargy or confusion is the predominant symptom then an electrolyte abnormality, sepsis, infection, or brain lesion are possibilities.

Treatment

Treatment is multifold and includes stabilization of respiratory and cardiovascular systems, blocking thyroid hormone synthesis and release, blocking peripheral conversion of T4 to T3, and blocking peripheral effects of thyroid hormone.

Beta blockers, if not contraindicated, may be used to treat rapid atrial fibrillation, tachycardia, or hypertension that may be associated with thyrotoxicosis [1]. Propranolol, specifically, has the added benefit of blocking peripheral conversion of T4 to T3.

There are two medications used initially to block thyroid hormone synthesis. These are propylthiouracil (PTU) given in a loading dose of 600–1000 mg followed by 200–300 mg

administered every 4–6 hours, or methimazole given in a loading dose of 60–100 mg followed by 20–30 mg every 6–8 hours. PTU is often preferred because it also acts to decrease peripheral conversion of T4 to T3 [1].

Iodide in the form of potassium iodide (5 drops every 6 or 12 hours) or Lugol's solution (4–8 drops every 6 hours) blocks release of previously synthesized thyroid hormone [1].

High-dose steroids also block peripheral conversion of T4 to T3. The recommended dose is hydrocortisone 100 mg IV every 6–8 hours [1].

Furthermore, specific treatment of the precipitating event – acute MI, sepsis, stroke – must also be addressed.

Disposition

Patients presenting with either thyroid storm or myxedema coma often require admission to an intensive care setting.

Rhabdomyolysis

Background

Rhabdomyolysis is the breakdown of muscle fibers and release of myoglobin into the circulation, which can lead to kidney damage. There are approximately 26,000 cases of rhabdomyolysis reported annually [7]. The rate of acute renal failure occurs in 4–33% of patients afflicted with rhabdomyolysis [8]. There is a wide range of causes of rhabdomyolysis, including alcohol, drugs (cocaine, amphetamines, PCP), medication side effects (statins, antipsychotics, selective serotonin reuptake inhibitors: SSRIs), muscle injury from trauma – especially crush injuries, burns, or ischemia – prolonged immobilization, compartment syndrome, and increased muscular activity from muscle enzyme deficiencies and exercise/overexertion [8,9]. Often the causes of rhabdomyolysis are multifactorial.

When muscle injury occurs, potassium, myoglobin, creatine kinase (CK), and uric acid are released into the blood. Myoglobin as well as uric acid may cause damage directly by producing casts that obstruct renal tubules and lead to acute tubular necrosis. Dehydration and acidosis enhance development of acute renal failure that will develop within 3 to 7 days post-muscle injury if rhabdomyolysis is not treated [8].

History

The classic triad of rhabdomyolysis consists of muscle pain, weakness, and tea-colored urine [9]. Because this triad is present in only 10% of cases, a thorough history should be obtained and a high index of suspicion should be maintained. There may be an antecedent history of increased muscle use – for example, running a marathon, especially in very warm and humid conditions, or prolonged seizure activity. If the patient is a victim of high-voltage electrocution (occurs in approximately 10% of those that survive an electric shock) or trauma with crush injury, rhabdomyolysis should be considered. Prolonged immobilization may cause rhabdomyolysis. The spectrum of immobilization may range from an elderly individual who falls while alone, sustains a hip fracture, and is unable to ambulate and ends up lying on the floor for a prolonged period of time, to an alcoholic or drug overdose patient who passes out, doesn't move for a prolonged period of time, and is discovered hours to days later.

A thorough medication history is also crucial. Statins, which were prescribed 76 million times in 2000 alone, and antipsychotic medications may cause rhabdomyolysis. The FDA reported 3339 cases of rhabdomyolysis involving statins [9] in 2000 and cerivastatin was withdrawn from the market in 2001 after its association with 100 rhabdomyolysis-related deaths. A social history, including substance abuse history, should also be obtained.

The most common sites of muscle pain are in the back, thighs, and calves [8]. The patient may also complain of malaise, subjective fever, nausea, and vomiting. Darker-colored urine may be a chief complaint.

Physical exam

Findings on physical exam may be obvious in cases of trauma and may include swelling, induration, necrosis, and tenderness upon palpation, especially in cases of compartment syndrome. Those with non-traumatic causes may have very few abnormal physical findings. These patients may present with only muscle weakness, tenderness, and contractures.

In the setting of malignant hyperthermia or neuroleptic malignant syndrome the patient will be hyperthermic, with generalized muscle contraction and rigidity, together with delirium.

Diagnostic testing

Elevated levels (~fivefold) of CK, a product of muscle breakdown, are usually used to define rhabdomyolysis. Levels begin to rise approximately 2–12 hours post-muscle injury and peak in 1–3 days [8]. Myoglobin in the urine may also be present and since it is cleared so rapidly, its presence is not needed to diagnose rhabdomyolysis. A urine dipstick that shows blood but, upon microscopic examination, is devoid of RBCs suggests the presence of myoglobinuria. Urinalysis may also demonstrate proteinuria and brown casts [9].

An electrolyte panel including a blood urea nitrogen (BUN) and creatinine (CR) as well as CK should be obtained. Progression to renal failure needs to be monitored. Furthermore, life-threatening hyperkalemia caused by direct release of potassium from muscle and perhaps acute renal failure requires discovery and treatment. Coagulation studies help rule out disseminated intravascular coagulation (DIC), which is also a life-threatening complication of rhabdomyolysis. An ECG should be performed to rule out life-threatening arrhythmias. Urine toxicology studies may help rule out illicit drugs as contributing factors. Hypocalcemia should also be identified and treated rapidly.

Associated testing for traumatic injury such as radiographs to rule out fractures, or a manometer to rule out elevated pressures in compartment syndrome, should be performed if clinically indicated.

Management

Intravenous fluid (IVF) hydration is the mainstay of treatment, and should be titrated to maintain stable vital signs and a urine output of 2 ml/kg/h [8]. Mannitol and urine alkalinization have also been used to treat rhabdomyolysis, but no definitive studies have proven benefit over IVF hydration alone. Urine alkalinization with sodium bicarbonate added to D5W may help reduce crystallization of uric acid, which contributes to renal damage. Mannitol forces diuresis, which may prevent cast deposition and avoid renal damage.

In cases of acute rental failure unresponsive to IVF hydration, life-threatening hyperkalemia, or cases of fluid overload, dialysis may be indicated. Only 4% of patients with acute renal failure secondary to rhabdomyolysis will require hemodialysis [8].

Hyperkalemia, especially if ECG abnormalities are present, can be treated with IV calcium, dextrose and insulin, beta-2 agonists, and Kayexalate [8].

Disposition

Disposition will depend on the patient's stability at time of presentation and the underlying cause of rhabdomyolysis. If there is severe multi-trauma or burn injury present, a surgical intensive care unit may be necessary. Elderly patients on statins with concurrent infection and a poor ejection fraction may need closer monitoring on a telemetry or intensive care unit (ICU) setting to monitor fluid status and urine output. Patients presenting with cardiac arrhythmia, hyperkalemia, hypocalcemia, or acute renal failure and no urine output require an ICU setting.

Adrenal crisis

Background

The adrenal gland is divided into the cortex and medulla. The adrenal cortex is responsible for producing glucocorticoid and mineralocorticoid hormones while the medulla releases catecholamines. Production of glucocorticoids is regulated by the hypothalamic–pituitary axis, while the secretion of mineralocorticoids is dependent on the renin–angiotensin system [10].

Primary acute adrenal crisis is usually caused by critical illness in a patient with pre-existing chronic primary adrenal insufficiency (Addison's disease) or acute bilateral adrenal infarct or hemorrhage, which most commonly occurs in the setting of trauma or infection [11]. More common causes of adrenal insufficiency are autoimmune diseases, adrenal infections (TB, fungal infections, AIDS), and bilateral adrenal metastasis. Insufficient replacement of glucocorticoids in a steroid-dependent patient undergoing physiological stress, or abrupt withdrawal of glucocorticoids in a patient on chronic steroids, may also precipitate adrenal crisis. Secondary adrenal insufficiency usually does not precipitate adrenal crisis because mineralocorticoid function is preserved. However, in cases of acute pituitary loss or dysfunction (e.g., pituitary apoplexy), adrenal crisis may ensue.

History

Acute adrenal crisis is a life-threatening emergency. It should not be confused with Addison's disease, which is an adrenal insufficiency that occurs over a period of time. Adrenal crisis usually presents with hypotensive shock unresponsive to aggressive fluid replacement. Associated symptoms are nonspecific and may include fatigue, malaise, vomiting, abdominal pain, weight loss, lethargy, and fever [11]. In cases of primary adrenal insufficiency, the patient may also have findings of hyperpigmentation especially in non-exposed areas. Furthermore, there may be a preceding history of infectious illness that may have triggered the crisis.

Physical exam

The patient may be hypothermic or hyperthermic with hypotension. In women with primary adrenal insufficiency there may be loss of axillary and pubic hair. Again, hyperpigmentation may be seen, especially in areas that are not usually exposed to sunlight (e.g., palms). Signs of infection may be present such as rales, rashes, or nuchal rigidity.

Diagnostic tests

A CBC and electrolyte panel should be performed. In cases of acute primary adrenal crisis one may find hyponatremia and hyperkalemia. Testing to diagnose the precipitating event should be performed. An ECG should be obtained to rule out MI. Radiography, blood cultures, urine culture, and urinalysis (UA) should be obtained to rule out underlying infection. In acute illness a random cortisol level may be drawn, because in stressful situations any level <20 μg/dl is suggestive of primary adrenal insufficiency. In non-acute settings an early morning cortisol level should be drawn, and any level <10 μg/dl is suggestive of adrenal insufficiency [10].

Treatment

Isotonic fluid replacement should be started especially in cases of hypotensive shock. High-dose steroids, usually hydrocortisone 100 mg IV, should be given acutely and repeated every 6 hours. Mineralocorticoids do not need to be additionally given in acute primary adrenal crisis cases because, at high doses, supplemental hydrocortisone will have some mineralocorticoid effect. Furthermore, IV fluid resuscitation helps replace volume and electrolytes lost from lack of mineralocorticoid effect. Antibiotics in cases of underlying infection should be given. Aspirin, Plavix, heparin, beta blockers, and oxygen should be administered in cases of co-existing MI unless contraindicated. After the acute crisis has passed, the patient on chronic steroids will require a steroid taper. Those with primary adrenal insufficiency will need glucocorticoid replacement (usually hydrocortisone 10 mg twice a day) and mineralocorticoid replacement fludrocortisone 50–200 μg/day titrated to postural blood pressure and symptoms) [3].

Differential diagnosis

sepsis, meningitis, and encephalitis are included in the differential. Various causes of abdominal pain and vomiting such as gastroenteritis, appendicitis, pancreatitis, cholecystitis, and mesenteric ischemia should be considered. Cardiogenic shock from an acute MI should also be in the differential.

Disposition

A hemodynamically unstable patient, which is how a patient in adrenal crisis usually presents, requires intensive care monitoring.

Pituitary apoplexy

Background

Pituitary tumor apoplexy is a life-threatening emergency that develops when there is infarct or hemorrhage into a pre-existing pituitary adenoma. The incidence varies between 0.6 and 10%. The mean age at presentation is 50.9 years, and there is a slightly increased predominance in females (ratio 1.0:2.1) [12]. Most cases occur spontaneously in patients undiagnosed with pituitary adenoma. In 25–30%, there are predisposing factors including head trauma, radiation, cardiac surgery, anticoagulant therapy, and treatment with dopamine agonists [12].

History

Classic symptoms of pituitary apoplexy include sudden and severe headache associated with visual symptoms. Visual symptoms may include decreased visual acuity, visual field defects, or ophthalmoplegia. Patients may also present with nausea, vomiting, neck stiffness, and altered mental status [13]. Meningeal irritation is associated with leakage of blood into the subarachnoid space. Cardiovascular collapse often occurs secondary to sudden loss of adrenocorticotropic hormone (ACTH), which stimulates glucocorticoid production at a time of severe stress [12]. Thyroid deficiency secondary to loss of TSH stimulation may also be a complication.

Physical exam

Patients may present with symptoms including headache, nausea, vomiting, diplopia, and ptosis. These clinical manifestations are caused by a rapid increase in intrasellar pressure against the relatively rigid walls of the sella turcica, where the pituitary resides, causing compression of nearby cranial nerves and vascular structures. Upon cranial nerve examination, the medical provider may find visual field defects, decreased visual acuity, or disconjugate gaze. The patient may have meningeal signs secondary to leakage of blood and tissue from the pituitary causing a chemical irritation of the meninges. Findings include nuchal rigidity, altered mental status, fever, and photophobia [12]. If the internal carotid artery (ICA) spasms secondary to irritation from hemorrhage, the patient may have signs and symptoms consistent with a stroke [1]. Signs and symptoms of a cerebrospinal fluid (CSF) leak (CSF otorrhea or rhinorrhea) are a rare presentation if there is inferior extension of the hemorrhage. There may be hypertension and malignant arrhythmias if there is compression of the hypothalamus [1]. Findings of hypothyroidism and adrenal insufficiency may also be present.

Diagnostic tests

A CBC, electrolyte panel, coagulation profile, and CT scan of the brain are initial tests of choice. CT scans of the brain are easier to obtain, and in an acute presentation (within the first three days of presentation) will diagnose most hemorrhages within adenomas. An MRI or magnetic resonance angiography (MRA) may be more useful especially in subacute cases. Furthermore, an MRI or MRA delineates adjacent vessels and cranial nerves, and the effects that the adenoma with hemorrhage will have on these structures [12]. Cortisol levels and thyroid function tests should also be obtained. Lumbar puncture is not diagnostic.

Differential diagnosis

A patient presenting with severe headache, nausea, vomiting, and cranial nerve findings needs to be ruled out for subarachnoid hemorrhage, cavernous sinus thrombosis, or cerebrovascular hemorrhage. If the patient presents with headache, fever, altered mental status, and meningeal signs, then bacterial or viral meningitis needs to be considered. A differential diagnosis of stroke is included if the patient presents with hemiparesis [13]. A potential non-life-threatening diagnosis includes migraine headaches.

Treatment

If hemodynamic instability is present, the patient should be resuscitated with isotonic normal saline and given a stress dose of steroids because of acute loss of ACTH release. Neurosurgical consultation should be obtained immediately. Patients presenting with altered mental status, cranial nerve findings, and worsening hemodynamic status require emergent surgery, usually in the form of trans-sphenoidal decompression [1].

Disposition

Patients suffering from pituitary apoplexy require intensive care monitoring in an ICU setting, possibly a neurosurgical ICU.

Potassium disorders

Background

Potassium is the most abundant cation in the body. The majority of potassium stores are intracellular, with approximately 2% residing in the extracellular space. There is a large gradient between the two compartments, with approximately 150 mmol/l in the intracellular space and 3.5–5.0 mmol/l in the extracellular space. The gradient is dependent on oral potassium intake, the distribution of potassium between the two compartments, and renal excretion of potassium [14].

Patients with normal renal function excrete 90% of potassium in the urine while the rest is eliminated via the gastrointestinal (GI) tract. If the patient has renal dysfunction, the GI tract may account for up to 25% of potassium excretion [15]. Renal excretion of potassium is dependent on aldosterone stimulation, distal sodium delivery, and urine flow. Reduced urine flow (as seen in urine depletion and reduced kidney function) and increased aldosterone levels both increase renal secretion of potassium [14]. Extrarenally, potassium levels are influenced by insulin, acid–base status, catecholamines, and GI losses.

Hyperkalemia

Background

The development of hyperkalemia is usually multifactorial and includes a combination of increased potassium load, decreased renal excretion, and shifting of potassium from the intracellular to extracellular space. The most common contributing factor is renal failure, acute or chronic, which is present in 33–83% of cases. The second most important cause is medication side effects, which are implicated in 35–75% of cases [14]. Common medications that cause hyperkalemia include spironolactone (which usually causes hyperkalemia within the first ten days of starting the medication), ACE inhibitors (increase incidence of hyperkalemia in the elderly to 7%), trimethoprim (enhanced at low urine pH), and nonsteroidal anti-inflammatory drugs (NSAIDs, which cause hyporeninemic hypoaldosteronism) [14]. Increased dietary potassium only becomes a significant factor in patients with severe renal insufficiency; otherwise the renal system can handle the increased load [15]. The elderly are particularly vulnerable to the development of hyperkalemia secondary to multiple drug regimens, age-related decrease in GFR, and a blunted response to aldosterone in the face of already elevated potassium levels [16,17].

Hyperkalemia is life threatening because of the effects that elevated potassium has on cardiac muscle depolarization and the resulting development of malignant cardiac arrhythmias. ECG changes will usually begin to be seen at potassium levels of 5.5–6.0 mmol/l. ECG changes may include peaked T waves, prolonged PR interval, loss of P waves, widened QRS, sine wave pattern, bradycardia, and ventricular tachycardia. Left untreated the patient may go into cardiac arrest. The effects on the heart are not only dependent on serum potassium levels but also on their rate of increase [15].

History and physical exam

Since the causes of hyperkalemia are usually multifactorial there is a vast array of possible histories and physical findings that may be present. Patients with end-stage renal disease who have been noncompliant and have missed a hemodialysis session are frequently found to be hyperkalemic. Patients who are dehydrated or suffering from hypoperfusion secondary to sepsis, gastroenteritis, poor oral intake, or GI bleeding may be hyperkalemic secondary to acute renal failure. Trauma patients involved in severe crush injuries or who have been lying in one position for a long time after a fall may be found to have rhabdomyolysis, acute renal failure, and hyperkalemia. The combination of these aforementioned scenarios with certain medications will only exacerbate the degree of hyperkalemia.

Upon examination the patient may be found to be bradycardic, have altered mental status, paralysis, paresthesias, and respiratory distress. There may be signs and symptoms of dehydration or poor perfusion such as hypotension, dry buccal mucosa, poor capillary refill, and poor skin turgor. The patient may have physical findings consistent with end-stage renal disease such as an arteriovenous fistula or graft.

Diagnostic tests

An electrolyte panel and ECG should be obtained first. Tests to discover the underlying cause of renal failure may be obtained later.

Treatment

The treatment of life-threatening hyperkalemia is twofold. The first goal is stabilization of the cardiac membrane, especially when there is evidence of cardiac involvement on the ECG. The second goal is aimed at lowering serum potassium levels either by temporary transcellular shift or excretion from the body.

Stabilization of the cardiac membrane may be accomplished by the administration of IV calcium in the forms of calcium chloride or calcium gluconate. The effects of calcium on cardiac muscle act quickly, usually in 1–3 minutes, but are short-lived lasting only approximately 60 minutes. The dose may be repeated if the patient responds and then deteriorates again. Caution should be exercised when administering calcium in cases of digoxin toxicity associated with hyperkalemia, because new arrhythmias may develop once calcium is introduced [14,15].

Rapid decrease in serum potassium levels may be accomplished by administering medications to shift potassium from the extracellular to the intracellular space. Such medications include insulin therapy with glucose administration if serum glucose levels are not already elevated. Rebound hypoglycemia is a potential side effect especially in patients who are not diabetic and in those who have end-stage renal disease. Thus, frequent fingersticks are necessary after this intervention is performed. Insulin works quickly, usually in 15–30 minutes, and within 60 minutes serum potassium levels usually drop by 0.65–1.0 mmol/l [15]. Nebulized beta agonists, which stimulate the Na–K pump thereby increasing intracellular potassium uptake, may also be used. The dose that must be administered is higher than that used to treat reactive airway disease and usually lowers the serum potassium level by 0.53–0.98 mmol/l. Tachycardia is a side effect [15].

Definitive removal of potassium from the body requires increased excretion from the GI tract through resins such as sodium polystyrene sulfonate (Kayexalate) or via dialysis. Unfortunately, cation exchange resins work slowly, with maximal effect seen after 4–6 hours. Kayexalate should not be given in patients with bowel obstruction or the early stages of a post-renal transplant [14]. Dialysis may be limited by the arrival of a renal consult and hemodialysis nurse and availability of hemodialysis access. However, once these are in position, dialysis, especially hemodialysis, is very effective in lowering serum potassium levels. Potassium is removed at a rate of 5–50 mmol/h [14].

There is equivocal evidence to support the use of sodium bicarbonate to treat hyperkalemia, and it is best reserved to treat hyperkalemia associated with metabolic acidosis [14].

Disposition

Patients with hyperkalemia and evidence of ECG changes need admission to a cardiac monitored setting – either a telemetry unit or an ICU.

Hypokalemia

Background

Hypokalemia is one of the most common electrolyte disturbances found in hospitalized patients and is defined as a serum potassium level <3.5 mmol/l. Moderate to severe hypokalemia associated with actual symptoms such as muscle weakness, muscle cramping, and fatigue does not usually occur until serum potassium levels fall <3.0 mmol/l. In severe cases of hypokalemia, serum potassium levels fall to <2.0 mmol/l and muscle weakness can degenerate into ascending paralysis, respiratory failure or rhabdomyolysis. Furthermore, cardiac arrhythmias may develop. Patients are prone to development of ventricular tachycardia and ventricular fibrillation in cases of moderate to severe hypokalemia. A predisposition to the development of a malignant arrhythmia is enhanced in the presence of digoxin toxicity; many elderly patients take digoxin for pre-existing cardiac disease. Patients may also develop prolonged QTc syndrome, which may degenerate into torsades de pointes, a type of ventricular tachycardia that usually does not resolve until potassium and magnesium levels are adequately replaced.

Hypokalemia may develop from increased potassium loss, shift of serum potassium into cells, and decreased dietary intake. The most common causes are secondary to increased losses either from medications, most commonly diuretics, or GI losses [18]. Other less common causes may be secondary to renal tubular acidosis (RTA), laxative abuse, endocrine disorders (hyperaldosteronism or Cushing's syndrome), or co-existing hypomagnesemia. Patients with poor dietary habits, especially chronic alcoholics or nursing home residents and the elderly who are solely reliant on others for their nutrition, may often be hypokalemic and hypomagnesemic as well.

History and physical exam

The etiology of hypokalemia may be quite obvious. For example, patients may present with GI complaints of vomiting, diarrhea, and inability to tolerate oral intake. Others may complain of generalized weakness after being started on antihypertensive medications or diuretics such as hydrochlorothiazide or Lasix. Patients may appear emaciated or chronically malnourished, making the diagnosis of poor potassium intake the likely source of hypokalemia. If the source of hypokalemia is not obvious, patients with hypertension and hypokalemia may have an endocrine abnormality such as hyperaldosteronism or Cushing's disease. In normotensive patients with hypokalemia, RTA may be the cause.

Diagnostic tests

An electrolyte panel should be ordered that includes a magnesium and calcium level. A urinary potassium level may also be ordered if the cause of the hypokalemia is not obvious. An ECG should also be obtained looking for a prolonged QTc level or the presence of U waves, T-wave flattening, or ST-segment changes which usually occur in moderate to severe cases of hypokalemia [15].

Treatment

Generally, every reduction of 0.3 mmol/l in serum potassium equates to a total body potassium deficit of 100 mmol. In mild cases of hypokalemia, potassium replacement may occur via the oral route. In moderate to severe cases of hypokalemia, especially if there is evidence of ECG changes (especially a prolonged QTc), or in cases when the patient cannot tolerate PO, the IV route is preferred. The rate of IV replacement should not exceed 20 mmol/h unless the patient is in cardiac arrest [18]. However, even when the patient is in cardiac arrest, potassium should not be given as an IV push. In order to correct low potassium levels, associated low magnesium and calcium levels need to be aggressively treated as well.

Disposition

Patients with mild cases of hypokalemia who do not have any symptoms related to the potassium deficit may be discharged home with oral potassium supplementation and follow-up if they are able to tolerate oral intake. Patients with more moderate to severe cases of hypokalemia may need inpatient IV replacement of potassium. If these patients have no evidence of ECG changes, no evidence of respiratory fatigue, or evidence of ascending paralysis, they may be treated on general medical floors. Those with aforementioned findings require at least a telemetry admission or even intensive care monitoring.

Sodium disorders

Background

The normal serum sodium ranges from 135 to 145 mmol/l. Disorders of sodium and water balance increase in the elderly, and age has been found to be an independent risk factor for developing hyponatremia and hypernatremia. This is due to a number of physiological changes as the body ages. These alterations include a decrease in total body water, a decrease in GFR, decrease in urinary concentrating ability, decrease in aldosterone, decrease in thirst mechanism, and increase in antidiuretic hormone, ADH [17]. Between the ages of 30 and 85 years, renal mass, usually in the cortex, decreases in size by approximately 20–25% and GFR (excluding cases with inherent renal disease) declines by approximately 50–63% [17]. These physiological changes make it difficult for the elderly to conserve sodium in times of sodium deprivation and to excrete it in times of increased load. These changes are compounded by complex medication regimens in the elderly that may predispose to water and electrolyte abnormalities, together with poor nutritional intake especially in those with dementia, stroke (dysphagia problems), and those who are bedbound. Thus the elderly, especially in times of physiological stress, are prone to electrolyte and fluid imbalances.

Hyponatremia

Background

Hyponatremia is defined by a sodium level <135 mmol/l, with severe hyponatremia defined by a sodium level <125 mmol/l.

Hyponatremia is the most common sodium disorder and is found in approximately 11% of the outpatient elderly population and 5.3% of the inpatient population [16]. Up to 73% of hospitalized patients with hyponatremia have an iatrogenic cause (most commonly medications and IV fluid administration), and mortality rates double for the elderly when hospitalized and found to have co-existing hyponatremia.

Hyponatremia almost always occurs when sodium levels are decreased relative to total body water. This may occur when there is a loss of sodium in excess of water loss or if there is an increase in total body water so that the serum sodium becomes diluted [19]. Thus water homeostasis has a major influence on serum sodium balance. Additionally, aldosterone, which is secreted from the adrenal cortex in response to stimulation from the renin–angiotensin system, increases net sodium reabsorption. On the other hand, atrial natriuretic peptide (ANP), which is released from the atrial myocytes, inhibits sodium resorption [20].

The causes of hyponatremia may be classified by the extracellular fluid status of the patient – hypovolemic hyponatremia, euvolemic hyponatremia, and hypervolemic hyponatremia.

In cases of hypovolemic hyponatremia, sodium losses are accompanied by water losses, but hypotonic rather than isotonic solutions are used to replace losses, or inappropriate vasopressin secretion (response to hypovolemia) induces water retention. Water and sodium loss may occur via the renal system, extrarenally via the GI tract (diarrhea and vomiting) or skin (excessive sweating or burns), fluid sequestration, or medications (diuretics).

One of the most common causes of hypovolemic hyponatremia, especially in the elderly, is diuretic use. In 50–90% of cases, hyponatremia develops within the first two weeks of starting the medication [21]. Possible risk factors for thiazide-induced hyponatremia include female gender, pre-existing hypokalemia, increasing thiazide doses, and chronically high fluid intake [22].

Euvolemic hyponatremia is the most common form of hyponatremia. Causes include iatrogenic fluid administration, syndrome of inappropriate antidiuretic hormone (SIADH), hypothyroidism, adrenal insufficiency, psychogenic primary polydipsia, and medication side effects (SSRIs, tricyclic antidepressants, Ecstasy). SIADH is the most common cause of euvolemic hyponatremia and is associated with numerous disorders including malignancies such as lung cancer, infections, and central nervous system disorders. The diagnosis is typical in a patient who appears to be in normal total body water balance but is found to have hyponatremia and inappropriately dilute urine [17,20].

In patients who are extracellularly fluid overloaded but intravascularly depleted (usually secondary to poor perfusion), resulting in vasopressin secretion and water retention, hyponatremia may develop. This usually occurs in patients with CHF or those with cirrhosis. The presence of hyponatremia at time of discharge for treatment of CHF is a statistically significant predictor of mortality 60 days after discharge [23].

History and physical exam

The patient with hyponatremia may have multiple different presentations depending on the underlying cause of hyponatremia. Hyponatremia itself, especially if severe or developing rapidly over a short period of time, usually causes neurological symptoms such as dizziness, confusion, gait impairment, memory loss, lethargy, coma, and seizures [21]. If acute and rapidly evolving, the patient may develop respiratory arrest, brain stem herniation, and death [24]. Risk factors for these severe effects of hyponatremia include being a premenopausal woman or endurance athlete [25]. Other nonspecific symptoms may include weakness and vomiting.

If the underlying cause of hyponatremia is hypovolemia then signs of hypovolemia may be present such as dry mucous membranes, poor skin turgor, tachycardia, and orthostatic hypotension. If hypervolemic hyponatremia is present then signs of increased extracellular fluid may be present such as edema, ascites, rales on lung auscultation, and jugular venous distention.

Diagnostic tests

The work-up for hyponatremia includes obtaining an electrolyte panel, serum osmolality, urine osmolality, and urine sodium. A sodium level <130 mmol/l is considered significant hyponatremia.

In most cases of hyponatremia there will be a low serum osmolality (normal levels range from 275 to 290 mosm/kg) because sodium concentrations largely determine osmolality levels. However, in cases of hyperglycemia or renal failure where there is an elevated urea nitrogen level, hyponatremia may be accompanied by an elevated serum osmolality.

In cases where there is hyponatremia accompanied by a low serum osmolality, a urine osmolality will help narrow the differential. If a patient is found to be hyponatremic, ADH levels should be suppressed and the urine osmolality should be maximally diluted with levels <100 mosm/kg. If this is found to be the case, then the cause of hyponatremia is most likely primary polydipsia because ADH secretion is appropriate but intake is so high that excretion is at its maximum. Other less common causes of hyponatremia associated with low urine osmolality are reset osmostat and malnutrition. If the urine osmolality is elevated, then ADH secretion is not appropriate and the differential is narrowed to causes of inappropriate ADH secretion such as hypovolemia, heart failure, cirrhosis, and SIADH [26].

To narrow the differential further amongst cases where hyponatremia, low plasma osmolality, and high urine osmolality levels are present, one may obtain a urine sodium level. In patients that have low effective circulating volume (hypovolemic, cirrhotic, or heart failure patients), the urine sodium levels are low, usually <25 mEq/l, unless currently on diuretic therapy. If the urine sodium level is >40 mEq/l, then SIADH is the probable cause [26].

Adjunctive testing to diagnose the underlying causes of hyponatremia may include chest X-ray, B-natriuretic peptide, and ECG to aid in the diagnosis of CHF. A liver function test and coagulation panel may help diagnose cirrhosis. In cases of SIADH, a malignancy work-up or HIV testing may be appropriate.

Treatment

Treatment is based upon the underlying cause of hyponatremia as well as the presence and severity of symptoms. There is a general consensus that the rate of correction, even if symptomatic, should not exceed 8–10 mmol/l over the course of 24 hours [24], with a rate of 1 mmol/l /h as the maximum rate. If this rate is exceeded, especially in patients whose hyponatremia was chronic or occurred over a long period of time, cerebral demyelination, especially central pontine myelinolysis, may occur [19]. Risk factors for development of osmotic demyelination include the presence of alcoholic cirrhosis and hypoxia [25].

If the patient has hypovolemic hyponatremia, treatment is fluid resuscitation with isotonic fluids and discontinuation of any offending agents such as diuretics that may be contributing to the hypovolemia and hyponatremia.

If the patient's hyponatremia is secondary to hypervolemia then treatment is aimed at treating the underlying cause along with fluid restriction.

In cases of asymptomatic chronic euvolemic hyponatremia and SIADH, fluid restriction is the initial treatment. If fluid restriction does not restore normal sodium levels, then demeclocycline (300 mg four times per day for 10 days) may be used [27]. It works by inhibiting ADH effects on the kidney and induces a nephrogenic diabetes insipidus.

In cases of symptomatic severe hyponatremia (e.g., active seizures), 3% hypertonic solution may be used until symptoms have ceased or have reversed, until the sodium level reaches 120 mmol/l or the maximum of a 10 mmol/l increase has been reached [26]. As per Adrogué and Madias, hyponatremia and hypernatremia may be corrected using the following formula and characteristics [24]:

Change in Na^+ = (infusate Na^+ – serum Na^+)/(total body water + 1)

Amount of Na^+ (mmol/l) in various infusates:
3% Sodium chloride in water = 513 mmol/l
0.9% Sodium chloride in water = 154 mmol/l
Lactated Ringers = 130 mmol/l
0.45% sodium chloride in water = 77 mmol/l
5% Dextrose in water = 0 mmol/l.

To calculate estimated total body water (in liters):
0.6% and 0.5% of total body weight in nonelderly men and women, respectively
0.5% and 0.45% of total body weight in elderly men and women, respectively

Disposition

Patients with severe symptoms of hyponatremia who will require hypertonic saline infusion should be admitted to an ICU for neurological and respiratory checks, and frequent chemistry panel checks. Patients who are hyponatremic with signs and symptoms of CHF may need admission to a telemetry, cardiac care unit, or regular floor bed depending on the severity of cardiovascular and respiratory status. Asymptomatic patients may be followed closely as an outpatient to work up the underlying cause of hyponatremia.

Hypernatremia
Background

Hypernatremia is defined as a sodium level >145 mmol/l. Hypernatremia occurs less frequently than hyponatremia and is present in approximately 1% of patients older than 60 years of age admitted to the hospital, but carries an increased mortality rate of seven times that of age-matched controls [17]. The most frequent cause of hypernatremia is water loss, with less frequent causes being salt intake without water or the iatrogenic cause of hypertonic fluid administration. Risk factors for the development of hypernatremia include age greater than 80 years, female gender, dementia, and being a nursing home resident [16]. The elderly have many reasons to develop hypernatremia including an inability to maximally concentrate urine, already reduced percentage of body water, perhaps an impaired ability to get to a water source (e.g., secondary to dementia, stroke), and decreased thirst mechanisms [16,27]. Underlying triggers include febrile illness and infection, as well as surgery. Hypernatremia almost never develops in patients with intact thirst mechanisms and an ability to get to a water source.

The most common cause of hypernatremia is unreplaced water losses, which may occur via the GI and genitourinary tracts as well as via the skin. Vomiting and diarrhea with an inability to replace lost fluids may cause hypernatremia. Skin losses, both insensible and sensible, which occur in times of fever, exercise, or exposure to extreme heat, may also lead to hypernatremia. And lastly, patients with diabetes insipidus or an osmotic diuresis (hyperglycemia) may present with hypernatremia [26].

History and physical exam

A sodium level of >145 mmol/l is considered hypernatremia, while a level >158 meEq/l will cause severe symptoms. The history should include the patient's oral fluid intake and medication use (e.g., lithium). Patients with hypernatremia often appear dehydrated with decreased skin turgor, dry mucous membranes, tachycardia, orthostatic hypotension or overt hypotension, and delayed capillary refill. The physical examination should include an assessment of fluid status and mental status. The patient may present with altered mental status and seizures and, in severe cases, brain shrinkage may develop with spontaneous intracranial hemorrhage and permanent neurological damage [27]. Weakness and lethargy are common nonspecific findings. The co-existing trigger may produce signs and symptoms as well. There may be a history of vomiting and diarrhea. If fever is present there may symptoms and/or signs of infection such as cough, dysuria, frequency, flank pain, or cellulitis.

Diagnostic tests

A chemistry panel, which includes sodium, diagnoses hypernatremia. A BUN and blood glucose level will help diagnose osmotic diuresis associated with hypernatremia. Radiograph urinalysis, urine culture, and blood cultures may help diagno an infection.

Treatment

While rapid correction of hyponatremia will lead to osmot demyelination, rapid correction of hypernatremia may lead cerebral edema, especially when it occurs in patients with chron hypernatremia. Thus the rate of correction should not excee 10–12 mmol/l per 24 hours or a rate of 0.5 mmol/l/h. If the patie is initially hypotensive, then isotonic fluid resuscitation should started first. The same formulas used to correct hyponatrem may be used to reverse hypernatremia. Patients with diabet insipidus will require vasopressin treatment [25]. Targeted antib otics should be used to treat associated bacterial infections.

Disposition

Patients with obtundation, seizures, or coma will require a mo itored setting such as the ICU or stepdown unit for admissio The patient will need frequent neurological checks and freque chemistry panel checks. Patients who are in septic shock togeth with hypernatremia may also need an ICU or stepdown admi sion. Patients with less severe symptoms such as generaliz weakness may be admitted to a general medical floor.

Calcium disorders
Background

Approximately 99% of total body calcium resides in bones whi 1% resides in the extracellular fluid; 55% of extracellular ine calcium is bound to proteins and inorganic acids (the majori protein being albumin) while the rest of the extracellular ca cium is ionized and biologically active. Calcium homeostasis dependent upon parathyroid hormone (PTH) concentratio and vitamin D and calcitonin levels. In response to low calciu concentrations, PTH is secreted to increase ionized calciu levels. PTH is able to achieve this by stimulating osteoclasts increase bone resorption, stimulating the kidney to increase ca cium resorption and increasing renal production of 1,25-dih droxyvitamin D $(1,25(OH)_2D)$ [28]. $1,25(OH)_2D$ also increas calcium levels by increasing bone resorption and increasing (tract absorption of calcium and phosphate. On the other han increased calcitonin levels decrease calcium levels by inhibitir bone resorption. Normal calcium levels range from 8.5 to 10 mg/dl. Because the majority of calcium in the extracellular flu is bound to albumin, fluctuating albumin levels affect seru calcium levels such that every decrease in albumin by 1.0 m decreases actual calcium levels by 0.8 mg/dl. If accurate calciu levels are required, an ionized calcium level should be sent wi normal ranges between 4.5 and 5.0 mg/dl.

Hypercalcemia
Background

Hypercalcemia is found in approximately 1–4% of the adu population and approximately 0.5–3% of hospitalized patient

Any level >11.0 mg/dl is considered hypercalcemia, but more severe symptoms do not generally occur unless levels are >13.0 mg/dl or the levels of calcium rise rapidly [29].

The most common cause of hypercalcemia is primary hyperparathyroidism, which in 80–85% of cases is secondary to a single adenoma. Primary hyperparathyroidism is usually diagnosed in elderly women and its incidence peaks in the seventh decade [30]. Most patients are asymptomatic and are found to have hypercalcemia together with an elevated or inappropriately normal PTH level and normal renal function [30]. The levels associated with primary hyperparathyroidism are usually minimally elevated at 10.0–11.0 mg/dl.

The most common cause of hypercalcemia in hospitalized patients is malignancy. It is also the second most common cause of hypercalcemia in general, accounting for 30–40% of cases. Solid tumors such as those of the lung, head, neck, and kidney secrete PTH-related peptide, which binds to PTH receptors and acts to increase calcium levels. Multiple myeloma and breast cancer cause hypercalcemia via lytic bone metastasis. Other less common causes include sarcoidosis, immobilization, familial hypocalciuric hypercalcemia, milk-alkali syndrome, excess vitamin D ingestion, and medication side effects from drugs such as lithium and thiazide diuretics [31]. Hypercalcemia caused by malignancy is caused by osteoclastic bone activity.

History and physical exam

The most common organ systems affected by hypercalcemia are the neurological and GI tracts. Patients often present with vomiting, diarrhea, and abdominal pain. There may be some irritability, cognitive dysfunction, fatigue, lethargy, coma, and muscle weakness. Patients may complain of polyuria and polydipsia. Nephrolithiasis may develop from increased calcium excretion in the urine and the patient may complain of renal colic [28]. The patient may appear dehydrated from the vomiting, diarrhea, and polyuria with signs and symptoms including dry mucous membranes, decreased skin turgor, tachycardia, orthostatic hypotension, or overt hypotension. Patients may also present with newly diagnosed hypertension. Those with malignancies that cause lytic or blastic lesions may present with pathological fractures. That is why this disorder is known to produce "bones, stones, and abdominal groans."

Diagnostic tests

A chemistry panel including albumin, BUN, and creatinine should be obtained. Hypercalcemia may cause renal insufficiency so it is important to check the BUN and creatinine levels. PTH levels should also be drawn because elevated or normal values in the presence of hypercalcemia suggest primary hyperparathyroidism, while low levels suggest other possibilities such as malignancy. Urine calcium levels may also be procured and, if <100 mg/dl in the setting of hypercalcemia, then familial hypocalciuric hypercalcemia is a possibility. Bone mineral density scans will usually demonstrate cortical bone loss, especially at the lumbar spine, hip, and distal third of the forearm [30]. If there are signs and symptoms of renal colic, a renal ultrasound or CT abdomen/pelvis should be performed to rule out an obstructive stone and UA should be obtained to rule out co-existing urine infection. If multiple myeloma is suspected (findings of lytic lesions on radiography, elevated total protein levels with normal albumin levels together with hypercalcemia) then serum protein electrophoresis and 24-hour urine protein electrophoresis should be ordered. A work-up for other malignancies may be necessary if an unclear source of hypercalcemia is present.

Differential diagnosis

Other electrolyte disorders such as hyponatremia or hypernatremia, and endocrine disorders such as Addisonian crisis and myxedema coma, may produce symptoms of fatigue, weakness, lethargy, and coma. Hypokalemia and rhabdomyolysis may also produce muscle weakness. Polydipsia and polyuria may be seen in new-onset diabetics, DKA, and HHS patients. Nausea, vomiting, and abdominal pain may be secondary to DKA, gastroenteritis, small bowel obstruction, appendicitis, pyelonephritis, or mesenteric ischemia.

Treatment

Initial treatment for all cases of hypercalcemia is hydration. If levels are >13 mg/dl or the patient is suffering from severe symptoms, they should receive IV hydration at rates of at least 200–300 ml/h to restore intravascular volume. Loop diuretics may be added only if there is evidence of fluid overload or the patient is adequately resuscitated, to help enhance calcium secretion into the urine. Bisphosphonates, which reach maximum efficacy 24–48 hours later, are especially effective in cases of hypercalcemia secondary to malignancy. They act by inhibiting osteoclast resorption of bone. Pamidronate (60–90 mg IV over 4 hours) or zoledronate (4 mg IV over 15 minutes) may be administered. The effects of bisphosphonates on hypercalcemia may last up to one month after initial administration. Calcitonin (4 U/kg SQ), on the other hand, acts rapidly but only temporarily and tachyphylaxis tends to occur with repeat usage. Hypercalcemia secondary to sarcoidosis or lymphoma often responds to steroids. Oral prednisone may be given at 40–60 mg/day. If the patient cannot receive IV hydration (renal failure patients or those with acute congestive heart failure), or the calcium level is >18 mg/dl then hemodialysis may be required [28,31,32].

In cases of hypercalcemia secondary to malignancy, chemotherapy, surgery, or radiation therapy aimed at treating the underlying malignancy should urgently be started. In patients with symptomatic hypercalcemia from primary hyperparathyroidism, a head and neck surgeon should be consulted for potential resection.

Disposition

Patients requiring emergent hemodialysis for hypercalcemia or who are hemodynamically unstable or comatose should be admitted to a stepdown or ICU setting. Others with milder symptoms may be admitted to a general medical floor or worked up as an outpatient if asymptomatic.

Hypocalcemia

Background

Hypocalcemia is common in critically ill patients with an incidence of 15–88% [31]. Vitamin D deficiency, co-existing hypomagnesemia, severe burns, sepsis, pancreatitis, critical illness per se, and hyperphosphatemia, may cause significant hypocalcemia. Vitamin D deficiency results in less calcium absorption from the GI tract. Elevated phosphate levels, as seen in tumor lysis syndrome or rhabdomyolysis, result in calcium phosphate salt formation, which decreases ionized calcium levels [32]. Hypoparathyroidism, which is most commonly caused by previous excision of the parathyroid glands, thyroidectomy, or previous radical neck dissection, is also a common cause of hypocalcemia. Total calcium levels, 7.5 mg/dl or an ionized calcium level <2.8 mg/dl is considered significant [31]. Hypocalcemia in the severely ill has been linked to persistent hypotension and increased mortality [31]. As with hypercalcemia, the more acute the fall in calcium levels, the more severe the symptoms.

History and physical exam

Neuromuscular irritability is the main manifestation of hypocalcemia and may be as subtle as fatigue, anxiety, hyperirritability to as obvious as circumoral numbness, extremity paresthesias, and muscle cramps. In more severe cases, the hypocalcemic patient may experience mental status changes, tetany, bronchospasm, laryngospasm, and seizures. On physical exam, the patient may exhibit positive Chvostek's and Trousseau's signs. Long-standing hypocalcemia may result in papilledema, dry scaly skin, and coarse hair [33].

Diagnostic tests

An electrolyte panel including magnesium, phosphate, and albumin should be obtained. If a confirmatory test is required, an ionized calcium level may be sent. A PTH level, to rule out hypoparathyroidism, and a vitamin D level may also be procured. An ECG to rule out QT prolongation should also be obtained.

Differential diagnosis

Other electrolyte disorders and infections may produce signs and symptoms similar to those produced by hypocalcemia.

Treatment

Severe cases of hypocalcemia associated with altered mental status, seizures, or tetany require IV administration of calcium: 10 ml of 10% calcium chloride (containing 272 mg of elemental calcium) or 10 ml of 10% calcium gluconate (which has 90 mg of elemental calcium) may be given IV. Though calcium chloride contains more calcium, calcium gluconate is preferred because it causes less phlebitis and tissue necrosis if extravasation occurs. The bolus dose may be given over 20 minutes followed by a continuous infusion of 0.5–1.5 mg/kg/h of elemental calcium [33]. This should be repeated until severe symptoms resolve.

In moderate to severe cases, 4 mg of calcium gluconate should be given over 4 hours. In mild cases of hypocalcemia, oral replacement is sufficient. Calcium carbonate or calcium citrate may be administered. Co-existing hypomagnesemia should also be treated. Repeat calcium levels should be checked 6–10 hours after repletion [31].

Disposition

Patients presenting with frank tetany or seizures will require ICU or stepdown monitoring. Those with new prolonged QT intervals should be admitted to a telemetry setting. Others exhibiting milder symptoms may be admitted to a general medical floor or treated as an outpatient.

Acid–base disorders

Acid–base equilibrium is dependent on normal respiratory and renal function. Acid–base disorders commonly occur when there is a change in the normal pH that results from changes in these respiratory and renal functions. Acid–base disorders may occur as one distinct entity or in various combinations. If an acid–base disorder does develop, there is usually a compensatory reaction that attempts to correct the pH. For example, if a primarily metabolic acid–base disorder occurs, respiratory compensation attempts to correct the acidosis. However, the compensatory reaction never normalizes the pH and if this occurs then a mixed acid–base disorder should be suspected [34].

Measurements of pH, serum bicarbonate (HCO_3) and carbon dioxide (CO_2) levels help determine the type of acid–base disorder present and are calculated as follows:

$$Dissolved\ CO_2 + H_2O \leftrightarrow H_2CO_3 \leftrightarrow HCO_3 + H^+$$

$$pH = 6.10 \log ([HCO_3^-]/[0.03 \times pCO_2]).$$

There are four general types of acid–base disorder:

1. Metabolic acidosis: Decreased pH with decreased serum HCO_3; underlying disease entities that may produce metabolic acidosis include diarrhea, renal tubular acidosis, DKA, alcoholic ketoacidosis, lactic acidosis, and toxic ingestions such as methanol, ethylene glycol, and salicylate poisoning [34].
2. Metabolic alkalosis: Increased pH with increased serum HCO_3; underlying disease entities that may produce metabolic alkalosis include vomiting, continuous nasogastric suctioning, and diuretic use [34].
3. Respiratory acidosis: Decreased pH with increased pCO_2 underlying disease entities that may produce respiratory acidosis include CNS depression from drug overdoses and strokes, as well as hypercapnic respiratory failure from chronic obstructive pulmonary disease (COPD) exacerbation, severe pneumonia, CHF exacerbation, and status asthmaticus [34].
4. Respiratory alkalosis: Increased pH with decreased pCO_2; underlying disease entities such as sepsis, salicylate poisoning, and anxiety may produce acute respiratory alkalosis [34].

Metabolic acidosis

There are three underlying mechanisms for the development of metabolic acidosis – increased acid production, decreased acid excretion, and loss of bicarbonate. For every 1 mEq/l decrease in HCO_3, pCO_2 decreases by 1.2 mmHg in an attempt at respiratory compensation [35]. Compensation usually occurs rapidly.

Metabolic acidosis can be further classified into anion gap and non-anion gap. The anion gap is the difference between measured cations and measured anions, and may be calculated using the following formula: $Na - (Cl + HCO_3)$. The normal anion gap ranges from 10 to 12. Examples of disease processes that lead to an anion gap type of metabolic acidosis include lactic acidosis (from sepsis, mesenteric ischemia, metformin), DKA, various toxin ingestions (methanol, ethylene glycol, and propylene glycol), and uremia. Treatment of acidosis is aimed at the underlying process. If lactic acidosis from sepsis occurs then IVF, antibiotics, and perhaps pressors need to be used to improve tissue perfusion. If DKA is causing the metabolic acidosis then IVF and insulin are the recommended treatment modalities. As for toxic alcohol ingestions, ethanol or fomipizole are treatment agents. The difference between the measured and calculated serum osmolarity is known as the osmolal gap. Anion gap acidosis with an elevated osmolal gap is indicative of a toxic alcohol intoxication.

Examples of disease processes that lead to a non-anion gap acidosis include renal tubular acidosis type I and II, renal failure, and diarrhea. Treatment again is aimed at treating the underlying disorder. Admission to an ICU is warranted if the patient is hemodynamically unstable or altered from a toxic ingestion.

Metabolic alkalosis

Metabolic alkalosis primarily develops from excess alkali intake or increased hydrogen ion losses from the GI tract or renal system. Losses from the GI tract are usually from vomiting or persistent nasogastric suctioning. A patient may lose up to 400 mEq of acid per day from the GI tract. Acid loss is usually coupled with equivalent chloride loss. Bicarbonate losses may also occur via the renal system from diuretic use or renal tubular acidosis (Bartter's, Gitelman's, and Liddleman's syndromes). Primary mineralocorticoid excess may also lead to metabolic alkalosis [36]. Severe metabolic alkalosis, especially if the pH is >7.55, is dangerous because it may lead to cardiac arrhythmias, altered mental status, seizures, and respiratory depression [3,36].

Treatment is aimed at the underlying disorder. If GI losses are the main problem, antiemetics with IVF rehydration usually resolves metabolic alkalosis. The treatment of various renal tubular acidoses includes a combination of medications such as amiloride, triamterene, and spironolactone. Posthypercapnic metabolic alkalosis usually requires IVF and potassium administration to reverse the alkalosis [36].

Respiratory compensation occurs rapidly, and for every rise in HCO_3 by 1 mEq/l there should be a rise in pCO_2 by 0.6 mmHg [37].

Respiratory acidosis

The most common causes of respiratory acidosis are disease processes that cause hypoventilation leading to CO_2 retention and hypercarbia. Underlying central neurological disorders may lead to hypoventilation including brain trauma and CVAs. Neuromuscular disorders such as a myasthenia gravis or Guillain–Barré syndrome, drug overdoses with sedatives and narcotics, and finally, underlying cardiopulmonary disorders such as COPD exacerbation, status asthmaticus, large pulmonary emboli, and CHF exacerbation may cause respiratory acidosis. Patients may present with dyspnea, anxiety, confusion, and altered mental status or coma. Treatment is aimed at the underlying process, and in many cases adjunctive noninvasive ventilation with biphasic or continuous positive airway pressure or mechanical ventilation reverses the respiratory acidosis [38].

Metabolic compensation occurs in a slower fashion, and every 1 mmHg increase in $PaCO_2$ leads to a rise in HCO_3 of 0.4 mEq/l [37]. Patients requiring noninvasive ventilation or mechanical ventilation should be directed to the ICU or step-down monitoring.

Respiratory alkalosis

Respiratory alkalosis is usually associated with tachypnea. It may be seen in respiratory disorders such as status asthmaticus, pulmonary emboli, CHF exacerbation, and pneumonia. Anxiety and salicylate toxicity may also cause respiratory alkalosis. Symptoms include paresthesias, dizziness, muscle cramping, and tetany [38]. Treatment again is aimed at the underlying disease process. Bronchodilators and steroids are used to treat status asthmaticus, anticoagulation treats pulmonary emboli, diuretic and nitrates may treat CHF exacerbation, and antibiotics treat pneumonia.

Metabolic compensation again occurs in a slower fashion, and every 1 mmHg decrease in $PaCO_2$ leads to a fall in HCO_3 of 0.4 mEq/l [37].

Summary

The elderly are one of the most rapidly growing segments of our population. As such, the medical provider should be familiar with the unique circumstances that surround the metabolic and endocrine emergencies faced by the geriatric population. The elderly usually have comorbid conditions that make treating these emergencies more difficult and usually increase the associated morbidity and mortality. For example, strokes and dementia may make it difficult to obtain any type of history from an elderly patient, thus making a diagnosis and treatment plan more difficult. Multiple drug regimens create dangerous iatrogenic side effects. Underlying cardiovascular disease may complicate any treatment plan, thus requiring intensive monitoring if aggressive fluid hydration is warranted. The medical provider needs to be vigilant when treating the geriatric population.

Pearls and pitfalls

- Hyperosmolar hyperglycemic status usually develops over a longer period of time than DKA and, as such, these patients will need more fluid and more time for resolution of disease. Fluid status correction should be performed over a longer period of time because overzealous correction of fluid status in patients with HHS may lead to fluid overload, especially in the elderly.

- If a patient with DKA or HHS presents with initial hypokalemia, potassium should be repleted prior to insulin administration. If insulin is administered first, potassium will be driven into the intracellular space and exacerbate pre-existing hypokalemia, which may cause a malignant arrhythmia.

- Classical symptoms associated with hypothyroidism and hyperthyroidism may not be present in the elderly. For example, rapid atrial fibrillation associated with hyperthyroidism may present as atrial fibrillation with slow ventricular response if the elderly patient is already on a beta blocker or certain calcium channel blockers. Diarrhea associated with hyperthyroidism may present as a return to daily bowel movements in an elderly patient with prior constipation. Hypothyroid symptoms such as worsening constipation, cold intolerance, and cognitive decline may be mistakenly attributed to the aging process.

- In patients with myxedema coma, thyroid and glucocorticoid replacement should both be given in case thyroid deficiency is secondary to pituitary malfunction.

- Electrolyte disorders are quite common in the elderly secondary to an extensive drug regimen and thus a thorough medication list should be obtained. ACE inhibitors are common causes of hyperkalemia. Hydrochlorothiazide and other diuretics are common causes of hyponatremia. Statins may lead to rhabdomyolysis.

- Many endocrine and metabolic disorders such as DKA, HHS, rhabdomyolysis, and hypercalcemia require aggressive fluid hydration, but this must be tempered with the knowledge that many of the elderly have co-existing cardiovascular disease that may place them at risk for congestive heart failure.

- Pituitary apoplexy is classically characterized by sudden onset of severe headache associated with visual complaints including decreased visual acuity, visual field defects, or ophthalmoplegia. Unexplained shock unresponsive to aggressive fluid resuscitation should prompt a potential diagnosis of adrenal crisis.

- An inability to correct hypokalemia should prompt a check for hypomagnesemia and hypocalcemia. If calcium and magnesium levels are not replaced, potassium levels may not normalize.

- Patients with elevated potassium levels should receive an ECG. If ECG changes associated with hyperkalemia are present, the patient should receive IV calcium to stabilize the cardiac membrane.

- The rate of correction for hyponatremia, even if symptomatic, should not exceed 8–10 mmol/l over the course of 24 hours, with a maximal rate of 1 mmol/l/h. If this rate is exceeded, especially in patients whose hyponatremia is chronic or has occurred over a long period of time, cerebral demyelination, especially central pontine myelinolysis, may occur.

- Initial treatment for all cases of hypercalcemia is hydration.

- The compensatory reaction to an acid–base disorder never normalizes the pH. If this occurs then a mixed acid–base disorder should be suspected.

References

1. Goldberg PA, Inzucchi SE. Critical issues in endocrinology. *Clin Chest Med*. 2003;24(4):583–606.
2. Kitabachi AE. *Online Epidemiology and Pathogenesis of Diabetic Ketoacidosis and Hyperosmolar Hyperglycemic State* [online]. UptoDate; 2012 (accessed from www.uptodate.com).
3. Kearney T, Dang C. Diabetic and endocrine emergencies. *Postgrad Med J*. 2007;83(976):79–86.
4. Gaglia JL, Wyckoff J, Abrahamson MJ. Acute hyperglycemic crisis in the elderly. *Med Clin North Am*. 2004;88(4):1063–84.
5. Wallace K, Hoffman MT. Thyroid dysfunction: how to manage overt and subclinical disease in older patients. *Geriatrics*. 1998;53(4):32–8, 41.
6. Rehman SU, Cope DW, Senseney AD, Brzezinski W. Thyroid disorders in elderly patients. *South Med J*. 2005;98(5):543–9.
7. Melli G, Chaudhry V, Cornblath DR. Rhabdomyolysis: an evaluation of 475 hospitalized patients. *Medicine (Baltimore)*. 2005;84(6):377–85.
8. Bagley WH, Yang H, Shah KH. Rhabdomyolysis. *Intern Emerg Med*. 2007;2(3):210–18.
9. Huerta-Alardin AL, Varon J, Mark PE. Bench-to-bedside review: Rhabdomyolysis – an overview for clinicians. *Crit Care*. 2005;9(2):158–69.
10. Bouillon R. Acute adrenal insufficiency. *Endocrinol Metab Clin North Am*. 2006;35(4):767–75.
11. de Herder WW, van der Lely AJ. Addisonian crisis and relative adrenal failure. *Rev Endocr Metab Disord*. 2003;4(2):143–7.
12. Nawar RN, AbdelMannan D, Selman WR, Arafah B. Pituitary tumor apoplexy: a review. *J Intensive Care Med*. 2008;23(2):75–90.
13. Shields LBE, Balko MG, Hunsaker JC. Sudden and unexpected death from pituitary tumor apoplexy. *J Forensic Sci*. 2012;57(1):262–6.
14. Evans KJ, Greenberg A. Hyperkalemia: A Review. *J Intensive Care Med*. 2005;20(5):272–90.
15. Alfonzo AVM, Isles C, Geddes C, Deighan C. Potassium disorders – clinical spectrum and emergency management. *Resuscitation*. 2006;70(1):10–25.
16. Schlanger LE, Bailey JL, Sands JM. Electrolytes in the aging. *Ad Chronic Kidney Dis*. 2010;17(4):308–19.
17. Luckey AE, Parsa CJ. Fluid and electrolytes in the elderly. *Arch Surg*. 2003;138(10):1055–60.
18. Rastergar A, Soleimani M. Hypokalemia and hyperkalemia. *Postgrad Med J*. 2001;77(914):759–64.
19. Smith DM, McKenna K, Thompson CJ. Hyponatremia. *Clin Endocrinol (Oxf)*. 2000;52(6):667–78.
20. Patel GP, Balk RA. Recognition and treatment of hyponatremia in acutely ill hospitalized patients. *Clin Ther*. 2007;29(2):211–29.

21. Egom EEA, Chirico D, Clark AL. A review of thiazide-induced hyponatremia. *Clin Med*. 2011;11(5):448–51.

22. Hix JK, Silver S, Sterns RH. Diuretic-associated hyponatremia. *Semin Nephrol*. 2011;31(6):553–66.

23. Upadhyay A, Jaber BL, Madias NE. Incidence and prevalence of hyponatremia. *Am J Med*. 2006;119(7 Suppl. 1):S30–5.

24. Adrogué, HJ, Madias NE. Hyponatremia. *N Engl J Med*. 2000;342(21):1581–9.

25. Wakil A, Atkin SL. Serum sodium disorders: safe management. *Clin Med*. 2010;10(1):79–82.

26. Sterns RH. *Online Causes of Hypernatremia* [online]. UptoDate; 2012 (accessed from www.uptodate.com).

27. Tareen N, Martins D, Nagami G, Levine B, Norris KC. Sodium disorders in the elderly. *J Natl Med Assoc*. 2005;97(2):217–24.

28. Ariyan CE, Sosa JA. Assessment and management of patients with abnormal calcium. *Crit Care Med*. 2004;32(4 Suppl.):S146–54.

29. Pellitteri PK. Evaluation of hypercalcemia in relation to hyperparathyroidism. *Otolaryngol Clin North Am*. 2010;43(2):389–97.

30. Marcocci C, Cetani F. Clinical practice. Primary hyperparathyroidism. *N Engl J Med*. 2011;365(25):2389–97.

31. French S, Subauste J, Geraci S. Calcium abnormalities in hospitalized patients. *South Med J*. 2012;105(4):231–7.

32. Moe SM. Disorders involving calcium, phosphorus, and magnesium. *Prim Care*. 2008;35(2):251–37.

33. Kelly A, Levine MA. Hypocalcemia in the critically ill patients. *J Intensive Care Med*. 2013;28(3):166–77.

34. Haber RJ. A practical approach to acid–base disorders. *West J Med*. 1991;155(2):146–51.

35 Emmet M. *Online Simple and Mixed Acid–Base Disorders* [online]. UptoDate; 2012 (accessed from www.uptodate.com).

36. Laski ME, Sabatini S. Metabolic alkalosis, bedside and bench. *Semin Nephrol*. 2006;26(6):404–21.

37. Herd AM. An approach to complex acid–base problems: keeping it simple. *Can Fam Physician*. 2005;51:226–32.

38. Ayers P, Warrington L. Diagnosis and treatment of simple acid–base disorders. *Nutr Clin Pract*. 2008;23(2):122–7.

Alternative geriatric care and quality metrics

Mary E. Tanski and Jesse M. Pines

This chapter will discuss alternatives to traditional geriatric care, including home care, transitional care, mobile acute care units for the elderly (MACE), hospital at home, and other alternatives. Methods of measuring quality of care in the hospital and other settings will be discussed in this chapter.

Introduction

With the growing number of older adults in society, the need for medical care has expanded tremendously [1]. A recent study found that the use of hospital-based emergency departments (EDs) in older adults outpaced population growth, with the largest growth coming in the oldest old (85+ years) [2]. According to data from the National Hospital Ambulatory Medical Care Survey (NHAMCS) in 2008, patients aged 65–74 years account for 14% of ED visits and approximately 31% were admitted. Patients 75 years and older accounted for 29% of visits and had an admission rate of 41%. These rates are both considerably higher than the admission rate for patients less than 65 years, which was only 13% [3–5].

Older adults use EDs for a variety of reasons. While most visits are for real or potential emergencies, many older adults – similar to younger patients – use EDs as an around-the-clock provider of primary medical care and as a safety net. Compared with the rest of the adult population, older adults have a higher ED utilization rate and have higher rates of adverse health outcomes after ED visits [6,7]. The average three-month mortality rate for an older adult after an ED visit has been estimated at 10% [1]. Older adults also have a 72-hour ED return rate of 24%, and as many as a quarter of these patients who return to the ED are subsequently hospitalized [1]. Despite the large number of older adults visiting EDs, emergency physicians report feeling less confident in caring for their unique needs and report lower job satisfaction taking care of older adults [8]. Many providers think that training, research, and continuing education in the specialty of geriatric medicine is lacking. In a survey of practicing emergency physicians, 45% reported increased difficulty caring for older patients compared with younger patients, and 75% anticipated a greater problem with ED and intensive care unit (ICU) crowding as the population ages [9]. Also, many providers are unfamiliar with protocols to screen for the presence of cognitive dysfunction and elder abuse in their older patients, and are unaware of how to access and utilize resources available to them such as transportation, home nursing care, and financial programs [7,8].

There are various reasons for higher rates of admissions and adverse events in older adults. First, older adults present to the ED more acutely ill than other populations and they have a higher inherent risk of adverse outcomes due to higher prevalence of disease. They more frequently have atypical presentations with multiple comorbid conditions, putting them at risk for missed or delayed diagnoses and subsequent decline [7]. Reasons for higher admission rates also come from physicians who fear that older adults may not be able to return to the ED or seek medical care if their condition worsens [3,8]. Many physicians are unaware of outpatient resources for older adults. Some feel uneasy sending older adults back home into an environment that may not have sufficient support. Emergency physicians also perceive that they do not have enough time to screen older patients for their needs and seek out resources for them. As a result, the decision is often to simply admit the patient and allow issues to be sorted out by an inpatient team. Finally, family and caregiver demands often influence admission decisions. Families or caregivers may feel overwhelmed with changes in the patient's health and functional status, and may feel uncomfortable taking care of their new needs during an acute problem.

However, some research demonstrates that patients and their family members prefer medical care in their familiar home environment [10], and this may improve patient satisfaction. As research continues in this area, providers will be charged with searching for alternative means to traditional inpatient hospital geriatric care including admission avoidance home care, transitional care, and mobile acute care units. Avoiding hospital admission is desirable beyond cost implications because hospital admission itself can have real risks, including higher rates of infections and deconditioning, leaving patients with lower functional status. Over the past several decades, other resources outside of hospitals have become available to older adults. This chapter aims to discuss alternatives to traditional inpatient geriatric hospital care and to reveal methods of measuring quality of care in the ED and in alternative care environments. In this chapter, we use Brent Asplin's Input–Throughput–Output model as a way to frame where interventions for older adults

Geriatric Emergency Medicine, ed. Joseph H. Kahn, Brendan G. Magauran Jr., and Jonathan S. Olshaker. Published by Cambridge University Press. Cambridge University Press 2014.

Table 28.1. Asplin's Input–Throughput–Output model

Intervention	Description	Impact
Hospital at Home after early discharge	Continuation of hospital-level treatment in the home environment	6% improvement in ADL, no impact on Barthel score [16]
Admission Avoidance Hospital at Home	Substitution for inpatient care using multi-faceted team approach, providing hospital-level care in the home environment [26]	Decreased hospital readmission, need for inpatient rehabilitation, and hospital-acquired complications with reduced overall health care costs. Improved quality of life (QoL). Longer average length of stay (LoS). No change in morbidity, mortality, or overall neurologic function [27,29]
Identification of seniors at risk	Brief survey to identify risk factors in early re-presenters, to provide an intervention that may prevent return [34]	Improved follow-up, home visits, and psychiatric service interventions instituted. Further study required to clarify impact
Intervention-dedicated geriatrician	Geriatrician provided chronic medication review, education on self-management of disease, and detailed communication with outpatient providers. Systematic screening evaluation	Decreased readmission to the hospital at 3 months [14]
Telemedicine	Use of technology to bring patients and physicians together without limitation of transportation to a common location, frequent "check-ins" to monitor health status regularly [37]	Decreased depressive symptoms and ED return visits. Improved self-reported QoL. More studies needed to determine the best way to utilize this technology [38,39]
Geriatric-focused ED	Alternative area of the ED dedicated to geriatric care, or focused geriatric protocols initiated in the ED	Improved physical location including decreased stimulation and more comfortable facilities, dedicated pharmacists to evaluate medication interactions, specific call-back protocol to provide opportunity for reassessment after discharge
Geriatric consult service	Comprehensive evaluation by a geriatric team in the ED to determine the need for inpatient treatment, outpatient follow-up, or transfer to a convalescent facility for care [41]	Decreased admission to the hospital with low rate of hospital readmission and morbidity [41]
Case-based liaison service	Brief screening visit during ED visit to assess for delirium, malnutrition, vision, hearing, and dental needs, transportation issues, and ability to perform activities of daily living [43]	Trend towards lower ED revisits but not statistically significant, low rate of compliance with referrals initiated [43]
Transitional Care	Establish line of communication between sending and receiving facilities and patient's care management teams, assess for unmet needs and make appropriate referrals [45,46]	Increased follow-up with referrals, but not effective in reducing overall service use. Reduced nursing home admissions among high-risk, and improved patient satisfaction. No effect on health care costs or QoL [48]
Geri-FiTT	Geriatricians educate staff members and caregivers in geriatric care principles, contact primary care physician to establish continuity of care, and ensure follow-up after discharge [47]	Greater patient satisfaction, improved primary physician knowledge of care course, improved communication. No significant change in overall care transition. More study is required to assess impact [47]
Acute Care Elderly Unit (ACE Unit)	Specific area in the hospital dedicated to older patients, utilizing multidisciplinary rounds directed by a geriatrician. Focus on early mobilization and rehabilitation, medication management, treatment of specific disease, and comprehensive discharge planning	Decreased length of service by 1 day, reduced cost by 21%. Lower one-year readmission rates [49]
Mobile Acute Care Elderly Unit (MACE Unit)	Similar to ACE Unit, but without the constraints of a physical location dedicated to geriatric patients [50]	Shorter LoS, lower cost, no change in in-hospital mortality or readmission rates

can safely reduce the rates of ED use and hospitalization in this high-risk population [11]. Broadly, this includes input or entry into the hospital itself, comprehensive care of the patient in the ED or inpatient side if they are admitted to the hospital, and robust discharge planning with assistance, resources, and care at home. See Table 28.1.

Input (reducing ED and hospital use)

For the purposes of this chapter, we define input as the demand for ED and hospital-based services by older adults. One of the

goals of geriatric care is to reduce the requirement for ED and hospital-based care. This goal aims to keep community-dwelling older adults in their home settings being cared for by outpatient providers who are familiar with their medical and social issues. However, the population of older adults presenting to the ED for medical care is complex, and patient characteristics and illness severity dictate the most appropriate location for medical care. Some geriatric research has focused on reducing the number of patients seeking hospital care. But since many older adults have critical illness and require resource-intensive care, reducing these visits is unlikely to have a large impact on overall utilization of the hospital and resources [12]. The top three complaints for older adults in hospital EDs between 2001 and 2009 were chest pain, abdominal pain, and fever, all three of which are high-risk. Many physicians may be uncomfortable managing these issues [2]. Older patients make up 36% of the acute care setting in hospitals [13]. The acutely ill subset of the geriatric population who require a resource-intensive approach and immediate interventions, where aggressive management is desired, is undoubtedly best cared for in hospital-based settings.

There are other groups, however, that call for medical attention that is less resource-intensive and could potentially be managed in clinic-based settings. These patients may require assessment and treatment but may not benefit from inpatient hospital care, and could potentially be harmed by it. With proper alternatives outside of the hospital, it may be possible for these patients to avoid hospital care altogether. Given the cost of inpatient hospitalization, admission avoidance has become a focus of health systems as well as national health plans [14]. From a public health perspective, avoiding hospital admission is an attractive proposition considering the research showing the risks of even a few days of inpatient admission on functioning in older adults [15]. Many hospitalized older adult patients are discharged in a worse health state than when they were originally admitted, and 20–30% die within a year of hospital discharge [13]. One study showed that 35% of older adults who were hospitalized demonstrated a functional decline in activities of daily living (ADL) from admission to discharge, and this rate was greater than 50% in patients older than 85 years [15]. While some of this decline may be attributable to acute illness, hospitalization itself plays a role as well [16]. Some risk factors for this decline are thought to be those such as sleep deprivation, as well as the noisy, stimulating hospital environment and excessive bed rest with insufficient physical or occupational therapy to maintain mobility. Polypharmacy and iatrogenic issues can also be detrimental [17]. The loss of the ability to perform ADL is a significant problem for older adults, considering that the ability to dress, bathe, and use the commode independently may be the difference between a patient being able to be discharged home with assistance and requiring skilled nursing care. From an emergency physician perspective, utilizing alternatives to traditional inpatient geriatric care may be feasible and beneficial to the older adult population and could prevent morbidity and functional decline experienced in the hospital.

Avoiding ED presentation with primary care

One group of older adults who use the ED has low-acuity complaints or illnesses that could be addressed acutely and immediately with referral back to a primary care physician. This group of patients usually presents with urgent but non-emergent needs, and has effectively substituted the ED for a clinic-based setting. This can occur for several reasons.

The first is that many patients may be unable to make an appointment to see their primary physician in a timely manner because of the relative shortage of primary care physicians and geriatricians. In 2009, there were only 7345 geriatricians in the US – approximately half of what was required based on the population of elderly patients. As the older adult population continues to grow, the projected shortfall of geriatricians by the year 2030 is 24,047 [18]. Some patients have to wait for weeks to obtain an appointment with their doctor. With packed primary physician schedules, there are ever fewer urgent ambulatory appointments available. Because of this, patients are sometimes referred to the ED for care, crowding the department with issues that could potentially be managed in an outpatient clinic setting [18]. The Institute of Medicine (IOM) Report *Retooling for an Aging America: Building the Health Care Workforce* highlights that, in addition to the lack of geriatric primary care providers, there are also deficiencies in other geriatric health care personnel including nurses, pharmacists, and physical therapists. The report stated that the current workforce is poorly prepared in geriatrics, and insufficient to meet the needs of the growing elderly population. The IOM created a committee to address these concerns in 2007, focusing on increasing recruitment and retention of health care workers specializing in geriatrics, as well as improving how care is provided [19]. Some proposals have been set forth to increase graduate medical education (GME) payments to increase the number of geriatricians, and that all institutions that receive Medicare or Medicaid funding may be required to train their health professionals in geriatric care principles [19]. Other proposals have suggested that family physicians and internists can partner with geriatricians for patients whose cases are more complex, thus providing the patients with the service of complementary skill sets and geriatric expertise. This partnership may allow generalists to care for the majority of needs of their older population, but would be able to provide education for when it is appropriate to involve a geriatrician. This would allow the limited supply of geriatricians to care for the most vulnerable or at-risk older population [20]. By making geriatric care a national health priority, it may be possible to increase the proportion of the geriatric population that has an accessible medical home and reduce lower-acuity ED use.

Second, many acute medical issues arise during off-hours when physician offices are not open. The ED serves as a convenient alternative to awaiting evaluation in a clinic. Many medical providers have advice lines available, although many do not have any after-hours care available. In some cases, patients are advised to go to the ED for all complaints regardless of actual or perceived acuity, as providers are unable to evaluate the patient face-to-face and may have malpractice or other clinical concerns. Solutions to this could include nurse lines that could make rapid appointments with primary physicians, physician house calls, or extended after-hour clinics to reduce low-acuity ED visits. While these may seem like reasonable alternatives to sending patients to the ED, in many models there is little incentive for primary providers to open up their schedules for these urgent appointments. However, as more practices move to becoming medical homes in the coming years, it is possible that open-scheduling and improved off-hours communication may reduce some low-acuity visits for older adults that currently take place in the ED [21].

Third, recent trends for insurance providers toward cost sharing have driven up co-payments for many outpatient visits. As the co-pay for each appointment increases, elderly patients may be less enticed to use their medical home for maintenance visits, which may lead to greater utilization of hospital care [22]. In the year after office-based co-payments increased, patients with plans that increased cost sharing had fewer outpatient visits, as well as an increased number of hospital admissions and inpatient hospital days than plans that did not increase co-payments [22]. The effect was even greater for patients of lower socioeconomic status and those with chronic medical conditions. Lower use of ambulatory care can lead to poorer monitoring and missed opportunities to catch subtle declines in health status early so that an ED visit and hospitalization may not be required. For example, well-managed congestive heart failure patients depend on regular visits with their cardiologist for weight management and medication adjustment. Without these regular visits, the potential exists for unrecognized decompensation and need for an ED visit.

"Hospital at Home"

"Hospital at Home" is an increasingly studied care model which allows the patient to receive inpatient care in their own home environment. Patients may be more comfortable in a home environment, may be less likely to become confused, and may have more help from family. There are two approaches to using Hospital at Home.

The first type of Hospital at Home occurs after early discharge from an inpatient setting and attempts to continue the course of treatment the patient was receiving in the setting of their own home. This type of care is often recommended by a hospitalist or treating physician, and can provide a vast array of services such as intravenous (IV) antibiotics, blood transfusions, care after minor strokes, or care for heart failure. One study evaluated the effect of Hospital in the Home in a group of patients who were deemed to still require inpatient care by the treating team. The study required that patients be discharged early to receive their care in their home within 24 hours of diagnosis. These patients had a statistically significant change in their instrumental ADL (IADL) of 6% compared with the in-hospital control group, but did not show improvement in their Barthel scores or Mental Status Questionnaire (MSQ) [16]. The Barthel score measures a patient's functional disability by evaluating their performance of ADL related to mobility and self-care [23]. It is suggested that this more apparent improvement in IADL could be related to the fact that IADL are more sensitive to change in acute illness. Patients in the hospital are less able to continue to perform IADL and hence they are prone to decline more quickly, whereas they continue to do basic ADL even as inpatients. The MSQ is a tool used to discover and determine the severity of mental impairment in older patients [24]. In that study, both patients in hospital and those treated with Hospital at Home showed improvement in their MSQ, but no significant difference between the groups was discovered [16]. Caplan et al. also previously reported improvement in iatrogenic complications such as bladder and bowel function, as well as decreased confusion in patients discharged early with treatment at home [25].

The second type of Hospital at Home is more relevant to emergency physicians, and is called Admission Avoidance Hospital at Home. This model aims to avoid entering into the ED or hospital system altogether by providing all hospital-level care in the home environment [26]. It can be initiated by a primary care physician after an office visit [27] or after evaluation by an emergency physician who determines the patient may not benefit from direct hospital care, specialty emergency diagnostic procedures, or diagnostic investigation. Given the trend toward early hospital discharge especially in Medicare and Medicaid patients [28], Admission Avoidance Hospital at Home is based on the finding that there may be limited health benefit for patients in short hospital stays and that much care provided in the hospital can actually be done at home. From a cost perspective, Admission Avoidance Hospital at Home has potential to create less of a financial burden than inpatient hospital care without sacrificing important quality measures [27,29]. However, research reviewing the cost-saving possibilities of the program is mixed, with some studies reporting costs savings that were not recognized in other studies. The reason for this is unclear, but could be related to the particular medical condition being examined [30].

In order for Admission Avoidance Hospital at Home to substitute for an inpatient stay, it is important that it is able to provide physician and nursing care similar to that found in a hospital environment, and this care must be different than that provided by usual community-based home care services. This model provides active medical care and treatment for a condition that would have otherwise required inpatient hospital management, and has been found to be efficacious and on-par with quality standards [31]. It is built on a multi-faceted team approach involving physicians, nurses, and other health professionals and has a strong focus on assessment and education. Models are very heterogeneous, and have been studied in the context of specific diseases such as chronic obstructive pulmonary disease (COPD) exacerbations, pneumonia, cellulitis, heart failure, and first-time ischemic stroke. In one study of elderly patients experiencing an acute exacerbation of COPD who were treated in the Hospital at Home environment, patients were found to have a significantly reduced risk of hospital readmission and better patient outcome at 6 months with increased quality of life. Although these patients had a mean treatment length that was longer than patients admitted to the hospital, they incurred lower health care costs overall and none was admitted to a long-term care facility, compared with 11.5% of those treated in the hospital [32]. They also had the opportunity to participate in rehabilitation in the home setting, and reported increased scores on patient satisfaction surveys. Another example looks at first-time occurrence of ischemic stroke. In one study, patients with first-time ischemic stroke were randomized to treatment in the hospital compared with treatment at home after initial evaluation in the ED with a computed tomography (CT) scan, lab work, and neurologic evaluation. The patients treated at home had a longer treatment course, but had decreased need for inpatient rehabilitation after care was complete, had better scores on depression screens, and had no change in morbidity, mortality, or overall neurologic function [33].

When patients were offered Hospital at Home care compared with traditional inpatient care, 69% opted to receive their treatment at home [31]. While it has not been shown to improve cognition, daily functioning, or quality of life, Hospital at Home has been associated with greater patient satisfaction with care overall, and patients have a decreased risk of death at 6 months. Some studies of patients who avoided hospital admission and underwent Hospital at Home care showed fewer hospital-related complications such as urinary tract infections, bowel complications, and falls, and that these patients underwent a lower number of invasive procedures [16,27]. In studies looking at patients with dementia, fewer problems with behavior, aggression, and sleep were reported in those utilizing Admission Avoidance Hospital at Home, even in those experiencing functional decline [27]. Despite its positive impact on patient satisfaction and its trend toward decreased hospital-associated complications, a systematic review in the Cochrane database showed that patients treated in Admission Avoidance Hospital at Home settings found no difference in actual health outcome than those treated with traditional inpatient hospital care [27], and another systematic review showed no statistically significant difference in patient or caregiver health [30]. More studies are clearly needed to evaluate its overall impact.

As noted, the array of provisions offered by Admission Avoidance Hospital at Home providers is vast, and the jury is still out about cost savings, effectiveness, and practicality. Some of the conflicting results may be related to the particular health condition focused on in the various studies [30]. In addition, it may be difficult for providers to determine the type of patient who would benefit from utilization of Hospital at Home care. In general, patients who are unstable would likely benefit from an inpatient hospital setting where they have direct access to specialists and diagnostics. It is important to note that Admission Avoidance Hospital at Home and inpatient hospital care are not mutually exclusive, and patients whose condition deteriorates at home would be able to be admitted to the hospital if necessary.

Preventing hospital returns

One way to reduce ED use is to identify patients at high risk for hospital return and intervene early before their repeat ED visit. Older adults who are discharged from the ED often re-present after a short time period, and some come back frequently. In one study, 44% made at least one return visit to the ED, with 19% returning within 30 days. Additionally, 8% of these patients returned three or more times during the next six months [34]. Another study found that about 24% of elderly patients who were discharged home from the ED returned over the next three months [35]. ED returns can expose patients to duplicate testing and additional prescription medications, and increase their likelihood of hospital admission. Of patients who re-presented to the ED in one study, about 1 in 4 was hospitalized [35]. The high rate of ED recidivism and hospital readmission is costly and currently makes up more than $17

billion of Medicare spending. Soon, Medicare and other payers will not reimburse hospitals for readmissions within 30 days of discharge, in an attempt to incentivize health care systems to provide quality inpatient care and enhance discharge planning. Patients who are ultimately readmitted will create a large financial burden on hospitals, so when patients re-present to the ED, there may be pressure on ED physicians to discharge rather than readmit them [21].

Patients who re-present do so for various reasons including exacerbations or progression of chronic disease, inadequate initial quality of care, lack of follow-up or monitoring, or absence of social support. Research has been focused on identifying common risk factors in early re-presenters to attempt to provide an intervention that may prevent the return. One study focused on the development of a self-assessment questionnaire entitled "Identification of Seniors At Risk (ISAR)," which patients and their families completed [34]. Questions focused on evaluating adverse outcomes at 6 months such as mortality, admission to a nursing home, and decrease in functional status. The study found that continued symptoms or exacerbations of chronic conditions contributed most to early returns. A follow-up study to evaluate the use of ISAR was undertaken a few years later, which showed good to excellent validity for detecting functional impairment and depression in the ED setting [36]. Depression, lack of social support, and functional impairment are risks for patient return to the ED, so it follows that early returns could possibly be mitigated by improving the initial quality of care and ensuring better outpatient follow-up, when available. It is also possible that intervention by psychiatric services or home visits could potentially mollify frequent visits and lead to better health. Clearly, further study is required in this area, but it appears that surveys such as this, looking at pertinent risk factors and identifying areas of need, may identify older adults who might require further services or referrals to prevent re-presentation to the ED.

Similarly, immediately after discharge from an inpatient hospital facility, older adult patients are at risk for short-term re-presentation to health care settings such as the ED and often need to be readmitted to the hospital. This may be due to inability to comply with instructions suggested by their physicians, side effects of new medications, or misunderstanding of their care plans by themselves or caregivers [14]. A method to prevent these immediate readmissions was studied in Paris. In the study, an intervention-dedicated geriatrician targeted three areas in the care of elderly hospitalized patients: chronic medication review according to geriatric prescribing principles, education on self-management of disease, and detailed transition-of-care communication with outpatient health care professionals. They also provided systematic screening evaluations [14]. The intervention-dedicated geriatricians made recommendations to the patient's primary geriatrician in each of the three areas during the patient's stay. Changes included at least one major drug change for 70% of patients. Screening identified depression in more than 43%, and malnutrition or risk of malnutrition in 78.5%. With these interventions, patients in the study group demonstrated significantly decreased readmission to the hospital at 3 months [14].

In 1994, Caplan et al. attempted to predict which groups of patients with specific disease entities would present to the hospital for admission in the Discharge of Elderly from the Emergency Department (DEED) I Study. He followed 468 patients aged 75 and older living in the community for 4 weeks and found that 17% were admitted to the hospitals during this time. Of these patients who were admitted, there was no disease or disease category that was predictive of admission to the hospital during the month [4]. However, admitted patients shared several pre-existing risk factors including dependency in ADL, inability to independently manage transportation, medications, and finances, cognitive impairment, and living alone. The study concluded that if these at-risk patients could be identified and interventions performed, perhaps admission to the hospital could be avoided by addressing the social issues and barriers to care. This hypothesis became the basis for the DEED II trial. This was a randomized controlled trial of more than 700 patients aged 75 and older who were discharged from the ED. Patients were randomized to an immediate assessment and intervention group, which took place in their homes, by a team of geriatricians, nurses, and other service providers who were tasked with identifying specific patient needs for one month and coordinating their care plan. The control group received regular care. They then received follow-up at 1, 3, 6, 12, and 18 months. During the screening assessment, an average of 1.65 problems per patient were discovered and an action was taken, be it a referral to a primary physician, a specialist or physical therapist, nursing, or allied health professional. This study showed that after the referral, patients had lower one-month rates of admission to the hospital (both elective and emergent) but there was no statistically significant difference in emergent hospital admission. The intervention group had increased visits to primary care and less decline in cognitive function at 1 and 3 months as measured by their Barthel index. However, this difference disappeared at 18 months. These studies show that identification, intervention, and referral during the ED or hospital stay can reduce re-presentation to the health care setting and may positively affect health, at least in the short term.

Telemedicine

Another proposed intervention to prevent re-presentation to the hospital and to encourage health maintenance in vulnerable populations is the concept of telemedicine. Telemedicine, defined by the American Telemedicine Association as the "use of medical information exchanged from one site to another via electronic communications to improve patients' health status," provides a unique opportunity for evaluation of older adults in their home environment [37]. It brings patients in front of physicians, bypassing the need for a common physical location and the barrier of transportation issues. This allows the patient and the doctor to communicate with each other and for the physician to make an assessment.

Telemedicine has the potential to bring in-home care to those who may otherwise have been managing their disease on their own and has the potential to positively impact patients. One randomized controlled trial evaluated the use of telemedicine in older adults with chronic illness. Nurses coached patients with functional limitations in areas such as medication adherence, symptom monitoring, and increasing physical activity. The telemedicine group was a central part of the patients' care plan, and helped manage efficient communication with the care team as well as timely patient referrals. This group of patients showed a favorable effect in terms of reduced depressive symptoms and improvement in self-reported overall quality of life. They also had a significantly decreased number of return ED visits [38]. Another study involving veterans with multiple chronic medical problems utilized nurse practitioners and telemedicine technology to educate patients, monitor their health status at home, and coordinate their care in a rural community. The study found decreased ED visits and hospitalizations as well as better perceived health overall [39].

However, while proposed as a way to save at-risk older adults from avoidable hospital admissions and ED visits, results of trials evaluating telemedicine have not all been positive [40]. In a randomized controlled trial that used telemedicine to monitor blood pressure, weight, and symptoms of high-risk older adults at home, no reductions in hospital admissions or ED visits were found compared with usual care [40]. However, this trial was aimed at patients with congestive heart failure, and outcome measures were compared against standard care, which was defined as in-office visits. The authors surmised the control patients participating in the study already were receiving high-quality care, which could have contributed to it being a negative study. Additional studies examining whether telemedicine might have a positive impact on patients who would otherwise not have transportation or resources to attend clinic or have other barriers to standard health care can be undertaken to help counteract this potential bias. Interest in telemedicine as a way to overcome obstacles of decentralized health care and service provision to the older adult population is growing, yet challenges remain in how to best utilize this system in a way to feasibly benefit the geriatric population.

Throughput (care of patients within the ED)

In our current system of emergency care, EDs evaluate and treat all-comers from infants to older adults. However, this busy, sometimes chaotic environment may not be suitable for all patients [41]. As the number of Americans aged 65 and over is projected to increase from 35 million in 2000 to about 72 million by 2030, we can expect to continue to see more elderly patients in the ED [2,42]. When evaluating this group of patients, it is recognized that traditionally used rapid-triage diagnosis may be impossible in the older patient with multiple comorbidities, polypharmacy, and functional and cognitive impairments who often presents with subtle clinical signs and symptoms of acute illness [42].

The concept of geriatric-focused EDs has begun to evolve, recognizing that the geriatric ED is a separate subsection of a ED where elderly patients are taken care of by medical personnel specifically trained in geriatric medicine, in a space away from the stressful busy environment of the ED. Alternatively geriatric EDs don't necessarily need to be in a different physical location and can be implemented through changing protocols for older adults, focusing on their unique need. Some changes to the physical location include extra-thick bed mattresses to prevent pressure injuries, walls that are painted in soothing colors, and wooden floors without the usual glare or slick polished look to prevent falls. These departments have dedicated pharmacists to review a patient's medications to assess for interactions. In addition, there is a call-back system where staff contact discharged patients to see how they are doing at home and how they are managing their medications. This allows for reassessment of the patient and is an opportunity to bring the patient in for re-evaluation if necessary. For a more detailed discussion of geriatric EDs, please refer to Chapter 2, The geriatric emergency department.

Emergency departments are also recognizing that it is important to take a more holistic approach to dealing with geriatric patients. When it comes to providing comprehensive quality care, there are many benefits to a geriatric consult service. In Hong Kong, a comprehensive geriatric assessment took place in the ED in an attempt to avoid admissions [41]. During this study, patients were referred from the ED to a geriatrics team of a geriatrician and a nurse. They were comprehensively assessed by the team and then admitted if they required acute hospital care, discharged to home, or transitioned to a convalescent facility for further geriatric care. Only 15% of patients were admitted to the hospital, there was only a 1.6% adverse event rate defined as death in 14 days, and only 1.6% re-presented to the hospital in the same 14-day period. This represented a significant reduction in geriatric hospital admission rates [41]. However, this type of intervention has its challenges. For this type of intervention to be effective, the comprehensive geriatric care team must be available 24–7. They must have the resources to provide patients with the services they need, and must be able ensure continuity of care.

Emergency departments may provide an opportunity to address unmet geriatric needs regardless of patients' chief complaints. While waiting in the ED, geriatric patients can be screened for previously undetected medical, dental, social, or cognitive need. One study by Miller et al. assessed geriatric patients in the ED for their ability to perform activities of daily living, presence of delirium, nutritional status, vision evaluation, hearing evaluation, need for dental intervention, and transportation issues in a case-finding and liaison service fashion [43]. All information was gathered over 30 minutes on average, and recommendations were made to the ED physicians regarding additional testing and referrals to specialists. Additionally, if discharged, patients were contacted by phone in 7–10 days for assistance with setting up the recommended appointments. This study found that the aforementioned problems were common in elderly patients visiting the ED and that most were relatively inexpensive to identify and initiate referral. However, patients and their caregivers often did not comply with the ED's recommendations and improvements in functional health status were not realized. The failure of this approach may have been due to difficulties with ensuring outpatient follow-up for the referrals. At follow-up the authors found trends toward fewer subsequent visits to EDs by intervention patients, although these results were not statistically significant. This study concluded that identification of patients with overlooked needs can be done at relatively low cost, and that referrals can easily be made. However, many EDs are not equipped to provide these services directly and may not have adequate influence on ensuring recommendations are followed through in a way to influence post-ED outcomes [43].

It is recognized that increasing the breadth and scope of services provided to geriatric patients in the ED could potentially benefit overall health but can also lead to delays in disposition and increased length of stays as patients await the consultants and recommendations. More research is needed to determine what effect the delay in disposition has on ED crowding and to determine whether the benefit of being able to discharge a proportion of elderly patients awaiting geriatric assessment in the ED is worth this delay.

Output (safely transitioning patients out of the ED)

Once a patient has been evaluated and treated in the ED and their acute medical issue has been assessed, many barriers still exist to discharging the patient. Issues with transportation, home safety, and caregiver familiarity with treatment plans are common. Furthermore, it is known that older adults discharged from the ED have high rates of poor health outcomes. Nearly a quarter who are discharged re-present to the ED in the following 3 months [35], and many are admitted to the hospital [1,44]. Older adults can become disoriented by frequent changes in their surroundings, and new caregivers may be unfamiliar with patients' medications and medical problems due to poor communication and lack of standardization in patient hand-offs [28].

"Transitional Care"

One way to enhance discharge home and to ensure that care plans are understood and implemented is the model of "Transitional Care." The goal of Transitional Care is to establish a link between the sending and receiving ends of a patient's care team through coordination, comprehensive communication, and continuity as the patient transitions from one health care setting to another [45]. This includes careful education of all health care providers, involving patients and their families in care plan decisions, ensuring medication and treatment accuracy, and anticipating difficulties patients may face outside of the hospital setting to allow for early intervention and prevention of readmission to the hospital [45]. The transition from the hospital to home or inpatient facilities can be a difficult time for older adults and their caregivers [46]. Transitions from one health care setting to another frequently happen after hours or on weekends. There is poor communication between multiple specialists leading to fragmented health care plans, medical errors, difficulty addressing patient values and family preferences, and failure to establish goals of care [47]. Transitional Care models seek to identify the unique needs of each patient, and to facilitate a collaborative effort between all team members to ensure safety and satisfaction.

One randomized controlled trial evaluated the effectiveness of comprehensive Transitional Care in older adults in the ED and its effect on subsequent service utilization. This study examined rates of service utilization including repeat ED visits, hospitalizations, nursing home admissions, and health care costs at 30 and 120 days. An advanced nurse practitioner in the ED assessed each patient, evaluated unmet needs, and made appropriate primary care or community service referrals. This study showed an increase in follow-up with referrals among intervention patients but was not effective in reducing overall service use. However, it also reduced nursing home admissions among patients deemed to be high-risk, but quality of life and health care costs were unaffected. Patients also reported more satisfaction with the process of ED discharge [48].

Another program called the Geriatric Floating Interdisciplinary Transition Team, or Geri-FITT, sought to improve the quality of geriatric care and facilitate movement from one setting to another while improving patient satisfaction. It did so by combining inpatient geriatric evaluation and transitional care into one model. Here, patients were evaluated by a geriatrician or nurse practitioner with geriatric training while in the hospital. The geriatricians helped educate hospital staff members and other caregivers in geriatric care principles, contact the patient's primary care physician to establish continuity of care, and ensure follow-up soon after discharge from the hospital [47]. Fourteen days after discharge, patients responded to a survey including a three-question Care Transition Measure (CTM-3) rating their satisfaction with their transition from hospital to home, and four questions evaluating their inpatient hospital course. The relationship between hospital service and their CTM-3 score was evaluated in a multivariable linear regression model. Although patients exposed to the model reported slightly greater satisfaction both while in the hospital and with their primary physician's knowledge of their hospital course, the Geri-FITT model did not appreciably alter care transition with statistical significance. Despite this, the Geri-FITT model was able to bring geriatric-specific focused care to patients and to coordinate evaluation of the geriatric patient with the Transitional Care service [47]. Emergency physicians may be able to play a valuable role in this model of care by initiating the referral to a geriatric specialist, involving the patient's providers early in the course, and becoming a valuable component of the patient's care team. Enhanced communication among providers helps to more seamlessly facilitate care transition, which could reduce rates of ED use and hospital readmission. Thus, this concept may be an attractive area for future research.

Acute Care Elderly Unit/Mobile Acute Care Elderly Unit

Another model which may help with safe and comfortable transition is the Acute Care Elderly Unit, or ACE Unit. This is an expanded multidimensional model of care designed to address all aspects of the geriatric patient's needs while admitted in the hospital. A physician with specialized geriatric training typically coordinates the patient's care team [12]. The goals are to address the individual needs of a hospitalized older adult with a focus on early mobilization and rehabilitation, pharmaceutical management, level of functioning, treatment of specific disease, and comprehensive discharge planning. It aims to incorporate multidisciplinary rounds into the care plan, including nutrition and dietary planning, physical and occupational therapy, physician or geriatrician, social work, and nursing. In one study, the use of ACE Units was shown to decrease the length of service by 1 day, reduce costs by 21%, and was associated with lower readmission rates within one year [49].

Another study took the concept of the ACE Unit further and developed a Mobile ACE Unit. Similar to the ACE Unit, geriatric patients admitted to the hospital received geriatric-based comprehensive medical care including outpatient care coordination, family meetings, caregiver education, and post-discharge follow-up phone calls. However, rather than caring for patients solely located in the geographic area of the ACE Unit, the study investigators carried ACE Unit principles to admitted patients throughout the hospital in various locations and medical units. This study found shorter length of service and lower costs, with no change in in-hospital mortality or readmission rates [50]. Therefore, it may be possible to provide similar benefits obtained by an ACE Unit to a larger population of admitted elderly patients without the limitations of geographical space.

Quality indicators of care

Some older adult patients present with vague complaints and atypical presentations of illness, and often have a more profound medical history and list of prescription medications than the general population [41,51,52]. Because of this, their care often is more time intensive for emergency providers. Some of the attributes of emergency medicine, including high stress of physicians, high acuity of patients, immediate decision making with incomplete data, and an inability to control patient volume make older people uniquely susceptible to error in the ED [53]. Recognizing this, much effort has been applied to research and develop quality indicators to ensure that older adults are receiving safe appropriate care, and to target areas that need improvement.

One organization that has worked extensively to develop quality indicators for geriatric care is the Society of Academic Emergency Medicine (SAEM) Geriatric Task Force. This group was formed in 2005 by the SAEM with input from the Academic College of Emergency Physicians (ACEP), and has focused on three areas of potential improvement, namely cognitive assessment, pain management, and transitional care [51,54]. For each topic, a content expert was tasked with developing quality indicators using an If–Then format and the Assessing Care of Vulnerable Elders (ACOVE) quality indicator approach. These indicators were designed to help focus quality improvement efforts.

It has been shown that the presence of cognitive impairment including both delirium and cognitive impairment without delirium, is highly prevalent in patients over the age of 65 years old presenting to ED. It is thought that at least one-quarter of these elderly patients in the ED have some form of cognitive dysfunction, and the prevalence increases with age [55,56]. The etiologies of this mental impairment are numerous, including medication use, systemic disease, central nervous system (CNS) disease, infection, and withdrawal [56]. Delirium alone affects around 10% of patients (57) and may signify critically unresolved underlying medical issues. Patients with delirium that is not diagnosed in the ED have three times the mortality rate than those whose condition is recognized [51]. Patients with cognitive dysfunction without delirium may also suffer, as their mental condition may affect their ability to comprehend medical information, follow up instructions, and return precautions if discharged from the ED. The impact of this condition on health is real, and affected patients have an increased rate of morbidity and mortality after discharge [55]. Unfortunately, most of these patients are not recognized by emergency physicians [56,58]. The possibility for intervention is great, as nearly 70% of these patients have no underlying diagnosis of dementia or cognitive impairment and could benefit from identification and intervention or referral in the ED [55].

Because of the magnitude of this potential impact of identifying cognitive dysfunction in the ED, the Geriatrics Task Force recommends that emergency providers should conduct an evaluation of mental status for all elderly patients presenting to the ED [51]. A standardized, general approach that meets quality standards and is not time consuming has been suggested by Wilber et al. First, the provider may determine the patient's level of consciousness, with normal being alert and interactive. Then, the provider can use a validated cognitive scale such as the Six-Item Screener (SIS) which is very simple, takes approximately one minute to perform, and assesses both short-term memory and orientation. If abnormal mental status is elicited, the provider should document whether this is a change from baseline. If it is found to be a change from baseline, strong consideration should be given to hospitalizing the patient for further care and evaluation. If the patient is to be discharged, the provider should document adequate support in the home and a follow-up or referral plan [51].

The next quality indicator targeted was adequate pain management for geriatric patients in the ED. Despite the fact that pain is now considered the "fifth vital sign" and many patients present to the ED with complaints of acute pain, pain is often ineffectively and inadequately treated [59,60]. It has been shown that geriatric patients with untreated pain have poorer outcomes overall due to missed rehabilitation sessions, longer hospital stays, and pain-induced induction of delirium, yet advanced age is a strong predictor of oligoanalgesia in the ED [52]. There are multiple reasons why pain is poorly addressed in older adults. First, emergency physicians may believe that older adults experience less pain than younger adults [60] when, in reality, cognitive and sensory impairments in elderly patients may make them less able to advocate for their own care in a busy ED setting. In one study, only 64% of older adult patients who experienced hip fracture received pain medications despite complaining of pain, and of those, just more than half received an opioid. When pain medication was provided, there was often a delay greater than 2 hours from patient presentation to administration [59]. A study by Terrell et al. showed

that patients 80 years of age or older received opioid analgesic pain medications significantly less than younger patients for both fracture and non-fracture diagnoses [52].

In a survey regarding pain control in the elderly, many emergency physicians stated that they felt their emergency medicine training or continuing education was inadequate to prepare them for pain management in the elderly population. Nearly half stated that they felt uncomfortable treating pain in the elderly because of concerns of drug interactions, side effects, or fear of oversedation [9,61]. Their hesitancy to provide adequate pain medication leads to patient and caregiver dissatisfaction as well as repeat ED visits. In an attempt to improve the management of acute pain in the ED, the Geriatrics Task Force established quality indicators based on the amount of time patients have been in the ED. For example, patients need to have a formal assessment of pain documented within 1 hour of their arrival to the ED. If they are in the department for 6 hours they need to have a second evaluation of their pain, and if they are to be discharged they need to have a follow-up assessment to address any ongoing pain before they are sent home. Additionally, if patients are to be sent home on narcotic pain medications, they should also have a bowel regimen prescribed to prevent constipation [52].

Other medication prescriptions are cause for concern as well. Providers are often concerned about medication interactions when prescribing or administering drugs, as elderly patients are more likely to be on multiple medications and are susceptible to polypharmacy. A survey of ED patients showed that only half could give their physician information about what medications they take and their dosing schedule [61]. Providers may be wary of prescribing medications with incomplete knowledge of home medication regimens and fear of medication interactions or concern for the effect medications may have on vital signs [60].

In general, older adults use a larger proportion of prescription medications compared with the general population, and as adults age and research expands the number of drugs used for medical care, prescription use is steadily increasing. In 1968 a US Task Force reported that 10% of the population was older than 65 and used 25% of all prescription medications. Currently, approximately 13% of the population is aged 65 and older, and use 31% of prescriptions. And in 2040, it is projected that 20% of the population will be 65 or older and using 50% of medications. A recent survey of ambulatory adults found that 12% of respondents 65 years and older reported taking 10 or more medications, and 50% took five or more medications [62]. The larger the number of medications used, the higher the likelihood of medication reactions and interactions. Patients who see multiple providers or who use multiple pharmacies to obtain their medication are at greater risk of polypharmacy. When patients are seen and treated in the ED, they often leave with additional prescriptions which may or may not be communicated to their primary physicians. Providers sometimes do not cross-check for medication interactions and as a result patients may suffer morbidity. Evaluation in the ED may present an opportunity to review and identify potential complications of polypharmacy and prevent untoward effects of drug interactions.

In addition to the aforementioned quality indicators, Carpenter et al. attempted to expand on these initiatives to include medication management, screening and prevention, and functional assessment. They found evidence to be lacking to make conclusions about minimum care standards for the ED care of older adults. They did, however, highlight the importance of providing high-quality care, and highlighted these as areas of potential further quality research [54].

Summary

In summary, the older adult population is growing larger and will be requiring geriatric-specific medical care on multiple levels. From admission-avoidance Hospital at Home, to telemedicine, to focused geriatric care units, there are several potential areas of intervention to make caring for this vulnerable population more cost effective, more rewarding for physicians, and safer for patients overall. More research and study is required to recognize the potential of these interventions and to ensure high-quality effective care is provided.

It is apparent that our traditional view of emergency medical care, treatment, and disposition may not be fit for the complicated medical and social issues of the geriatric patient. Holistic management with coordination between patients and families, as well as between providers and specialist services, may be the most beneficial to ensure appropriate care [1,53].

Pearls and pitfalls

- Admitting older adult patients to the hospital is a decision that requires a thorough understanding of the potential risks and benefits. Older adult patients who are admitted to the hospital often suffer adverse consequences such as delirium, falls, and hospital-acquired infections, and sometimes experience functional decline in activities of daily living after discharge.

- Transitions of care between providers are a period of increased vulnerability for older patients. Ensuring patients have a clear discharge plan, reliable home support, and dependable follow-up can help prevent unanticipated return to the ED.

- Simple screening tools can be utilized in the ED and may help identify unmet medical and social needs for older adult patients.

- Quality improvement indicators for older adults in the ED center on mental status assessment, pain control, and polypharmacy, and emphasize a comprehensive holistic approach to care of the older patient.

References

1. Aminzadeh F, Dalziel WB. Older adults in the emergency department: a systematic review of patterns of use, adverse outcomes, and effectiveness of interventions. *Ann Emerg Med*. 2002;39(3):238.

2. Pines JM, Mullins PM, Cooper JK, Feng LB, Roth KE. Trends in emergency department use, care patterns, and quality for older adults in the United States. *J Am Geriatr Soc*. 2013;61(1):12–17.

3. US Department of Health and Human Services. *Ambulatory Care Visits to Physician Offices, Hospital Outpatient Departments, and Emergency Departments: United States, 2001–02. Series 13, No 159* (accessed from www.cdc.gov/nchs/products/series.htm).

4. Caplan GA, Williams A, Daly B, Abraham K. A randomized, controlled trial of comprehensive geriatric assessment and multidisciplinary intervention after discharge of elderly from the emergency department – the DEED II study. *J Am Geriatr Soc*. 2004;52(9):1417.

5. Kozak LJ, Hall MJ, Owings MF. National Hospital Discharge Survey: 2000 annual summary with detailed diagnosis and procedure data. Vital and health statistics. Series 13. *Data from the National Health Survey*. 2002;153:1.

6. Hastings S, Heflin MT. A systematic review of interventions to improve outcomes for elders discharged from the emergency department. *Acad Emerg Med*. 2005;12(10):978.

7. Hogan T, Losman E, Carpenter C, et al. Development of geriatric competencies for emergency medicine residents using an expert consensus process. *Acad Emerg Med*. 2010;17(3);316.

8. Schumacher, JG. Emergency medicine and older adults: continuing challenges and opportunities. *Am J Emerg Med*. 2005;23(4):556.

9. McNamara R, Rousseau E, Sanders A. Geriatric emergency medicine: a survey of practicing emergency physicians. *Ann Emerg Med*. 1992;21(7):796.

10. Leff B, Burton L, Mader S, et al. Satisfaction with hospital at home care. *J Am Geriatr Soc*. 2006;54(9):1355.

11. Asplin B, Magid D, Rhodes K, Solberg L, Camargo C. A conceptual model of emergency department crowding. *Ann Emerg Med*. 2003;42(2):173–80.

12. Cassel CK. *Geriatrics: A Vital Core of Hospital Medicine. Caring for the Hospitalized Elderly: Current Best Practice and New Horizons: a Special Supplement to the Hospitalist: the Official Publication of the Society of Hospital Medicine*, 2005 (2–3) (accessed from http://books.google.com/books?id=VB1fNwAACAAJ).

13. Lanfield CS. Improving health care for older persons. *Ann Intern Med*. 2003;139(5):421.

14. Legrain S, Tubach F, Bonnet-Zamponi D, et al. A new multimodal geriatric discharge-planning intervention to prevent emergency visits and rehospitalizations of older adults: the optimization of medication in AGEd multicenter randomized controlled trial. *J Am Geriatr Soc*. 2011;59(11):2017.

15. Covinsky KE, Palmer RM, Fortinsky RH, et al. Loss of independence in activities of daily living in older adults hospitalized with medical illnesses: increased vulnerability with age. *J Am Geriatr Soc*. 2003;51(4):451.

16. Caplan GA, Coconis J, Woods J. Effect of hospital in the home treatment on physical and cognitive function: A randomized controlled trial. *J Gerontol A Biol Sci Med Sci*. 2005;60(8):1035.

17. Leff B, Burton L, Madder S, et al. Comparison of functional outcomes associated with hospital at home care and traditional acute hospital care. *J Am Geriatr Soc*. 2009;57(2):273.

18. Committee on the Future Health Care Workforce for Older Americans, Institute of Medicine. *Retooling for an Aging America: Building the Health Care Workforce*. (Washington, DC: The National Academies Press, 2008), accessed from www.nap.edu/openbook.php?record_id=12089&page=15), 46 pp.

19. Institute of Medicine. *Retooling for an Aging America: Building the Health Care Workforce*. Washington, DC: The National Academies Press, 2008.

20. Fried LP, Hall WJ. Editorial: Leading on behalf of an aging society. *J Am Geriatr Soc*. 2008;56(10):1791.

21. NCQA.org [Internet]. Washington, DC: National Committee for Quality Assurance; c2011 (cited July 12, 2012; accessed from www.ncqa.org/tabid/631/Default.aspx).

22. Trivedi AN, Moloo H, Mor V. Increased ambulatory care copayments and hospitalizations among the elderly. *N Engl J Med*. 2012;362(4):320.

23. Mahoney FI, Barthel D. Functional evaluation: the Barthel Index. *Maryland State Med J*. 1965;14:61.

24. Pfeiffer E. A short portable mental status questionnaire for the assessment of organic brain deficit in elderly patients. *J Am Geriatr Soc*. 1975;23(10):433.

25. Caplan GA, Ward JA, Brennan NJ, et al. Hospital in the home: a randomised controlled trial. *Med J Australia*. 1999;170(4):156.

26. Montalto M. *Hospital in the Home: Principles and Practice* (Melbourne: ArtWords Publishing, 2002).

27. Shepperd S, Doll H, Angus RM, et al. Hospital at home admission avoidance. *Cochrane Database Syst Rev*. 2008;(4):CD007491.

28. Murtaugh CM, Litke A. Transitions through postacute and long-term care settings: patterns of use and outcomes for a national cohort of elders. *Med Care*. 2002;40(3):227.

29. Brennan TA, Leape LL, Laird NM, et al. Incidence of adverse events and negligence in hospitalized patients: results of the Harvard Medical Practice Study I. 1991. *Qual Safety Health Care*. 2004;13(2):145.

30. Leff B. Acute? care at home. The health and cost effects of substituting home care for inpatient acute care: a review of the evidence. *J Am Geriatr Soc*. 2001;49(8):1123.

31. Leff B, Burton L, Mader S, et al. Hospital at home: feasibility and outcomes of a program to provide hospital-level care at home for acutely ill older patients. *Ann Intern Med*. 2005;143(11):798.

32. Aimonino Ricauda N, Tibaldi V, Leff B, et al. Substitutive "hospital at home" versus inpatient care for elderly patients with exacerbations of chronic obstructive pulmonary disease: a prospective randomized, controlled trial. *J Am Geriatr Soc*. 2008;56(3):493.

33. Aimonino Ricauda NA, Bo M, Molaschi M, et al. Home hospitalization service for acute uncomplicated first ischemic stroke in elderly patients: a randomized trial. *J Am Geriatr Soc*. 2004;52(2):278.

34. McCusker J, Cardin S, Bellavance F, Belzile E. Return to the emergency department among elders: patterns and predictors. *Acad Emerg Med*. 2000;7(3):249.

35. Hastings SN, Heflin M. A systematic review of interventions to improve outcomes for elders discharged from the emergency department. *Acad Emerg Med*. 2005;12(10):978.

36. Dendukuri N, McCusker J, Belzile E. The identification of seniors at risk screening tool: further evidence of concurrent and predictive validity. *J Am Geriatr Soc*. 2004;52(2):290.

37. Chae YM, Heon Lee J, Hee Ho S, et al. Patient satisfaction with telemedicine in home health services for the elderly. *Int J Med Informatics*. 2001;61(2–3):167.

38. Gellis ZD, Kenaley B, McGinty J, et al. Outcomes of a telehealth intervention for homebound older adults with heart or chronic respiratory failure: a randomized controlled trial. *Gerontologist*. 2012;52(4):541.

39. Kobb R, Hoffman N, Lodge R, Kline S. Enhancing elder chronic care through technology and care coordination: report from a pilot. *Telemedicine J E-health*. 2003;9(2):189.

40. Takahashi PY, Pecina JL, Upatising B, et al. A randomized controlled trial of telemonitoring in older adults with multiple health issues to prevent hospitalizations and emergency department visits. *Arch Intern Med*. 2012;1960:1.

41. Yuen TMY, Lee LLY, Or ILC, et al. Geriatric consultation service in emergency department: how does it work? *Emerg Med J*. 2013;30(3):180–5.

42. Hwang U, Morrison RS. The geriatric emergency department. *J Am Geriatr Soc*. 2007;55(11):1873.

43. Miller DK, Lewis LM, Nork MJ, Morley JE. Controlled trial of a geriatric case-finding and liaison service in an emergency department. *J Am Geriatr Soc*. 1996;44(5):513.

44. McCusker J, Jacobs P, Dendukuri N, et al. Cost-effectiveness of a brief two-stage emergency department intervention for high-risk elders: results of a quasi-randomized controlled trial. *Ann Emerg Med*. 2003;41(1):45.

45. Coleman EA, Berenson RA. Lost in transition: challenges and opportunities for improving the quality of transitional care. *Ann Intern Med*. 2004;141(7):533.

46. Coleman, EA. Falling through the cracks: challenges and opportunities for improving transitional care for persons with continuous complex care need. *J Am Geriatr Soc*. 2003;51(4):549.

47. Arbaje AI, Maron DD, Yu Q, et al. The geriatric floating interdisciplinary transition team. *J Am Geriatr Soc*. 2010;58(2):364.

48. Mion LC, Palmer RM, Meldon SW, et al. Case finding and referral model for emergency department elders: a randomized clinical trial. *Ann Emerg Med*. 2003;41(1):57.

49. Jayadevappa R, Chhatre S, Weiner M, Raziano D. Health resource utilization and medical care cost of acute care elderly unit patients. *Value Health*. 2006;9(3):186.

50. Farber JI, Korc-Grodzicki B, Du Q, Leipzig R, Siu AL. Operational and quality outcomes of a mobile acute care for the elderly service. *J Hosp Med*. 2001;6(6):358.

51. Terrell KM, Hustey FM, Hwang U, et al. Quality indicators for geriatric emergency care. *Acad Emerg Med*. 2009;16(5):441.

52. Terrell KM, Heard K, Miller DK. Prescribing to older ED patients. *Am J Emerg Med*. 2006;24(4):468.

53. Sanders AB. Quality in emergency medicine: an introduction. *Acad Emerg Med*. 2002;9(11):1064.

54. Carpenter CR, Heard K, Wilber S, et al. Research priorities for high-quality geriatric emergency care: medication management, screening, and prevention and functional assessment. *Acad Emerg Med*. 2011;18(6):644.

55. Hustey FM, Meldon SW. The effect of mental status screening on the care of elderly emergency department patients. *Ann Emerg Med*. 2003;41(5):678.

56. Wilber ST. Altered mental status in older emergency department patients. *Emerg Med Clin North Am*. 2006;24(2):299.

57. Hustey FM, Meldon SW. The prevalence and documentation of impaired mental status in elderly emergency department patients. *Ann Emerg Med*. 2002;39(3):248.

58. Sanders AB. Missed delirium in older emergency department patients: a quality-of-care problem. *Ann Emerg Med*. 2002;39(3):338.

59. Hwang U, Richardson LD, Sonuyi TO, Morrison RS. The effect of emergency department crowding on the management of pain in older adults with hip fracture. *J Am Geriatr Soc*. 2006;54(2):270.

60. Neighbor ML, Honner S, Kohn MA. Factors affecting emergency department opioid administration to severely injured patients. *Acad Emerg Med*. 2004;11(12):1290.

61. Rupp T, Delaney KA. Inadequate analgesia in emergency medicine. *Ann Emerg Med*. 2004;43(4):494.

62. Kaufman DW, Kelly JP, Rosenberg L, Anderson TE, Mitchell AA. Recent patterns of medication use in the ambulatory adult population of the United States: the Slone survey. *JAMA*. 2002;287(3):337.

Chapter

29

Functional assessment of the elderly

Kirk A. Stiffler

Physical function can be seen as the person's ability to perform the tasks of everyday living, and it has been recognized that the assessment of such function is a key factor in the health care of elderly patients. Higher levels of functioning are associated with an increase in number of healthy and independent years of life. Measures of physical function are associated with modifications of those life years, and are associated with future health care events, disability, institutionalization, and even mortality. Loss of physical function, or functional decline, can be described as the loss of independent living skills and can be a result of any number of factors that impact patients such as medical illnesses, cognitive declines, affective disorders, environmental issues (including social support), economic stability, and even spirituality issues. As the population in the US continues to age, more and more elderly patients will present to the emergency department (ED) with issues that are a direct result of, or will directly impact, their subsequent functional status. Understanding how to reliably assess functional status and identify patients at high risk for subsequent decline thus becomes imperative for the practicing emergency medicine health care provider.

This chapter will review the common tools available which may be feasibly used to assess the physical function status of elderly patients in the ED, as well as the prediction tools used to help identify patients at risk for functional decline after an ED visit or during and after inpatient hospitalization. Additionally, screening tools for other common issues encountered in the elderly such as vision loss, hearing impairment, alcohol use disorders, malnutrition, and falls will be reviewed.

Comprehensive geriatric assessment

Functional assessment of elderly patients is an integral part of a comprehensive geriatric assessment (CGA). CGA typically involves an in-depth evaluation of an elderly person's medical (including comorbidities and polypharmacy), psychosocial (including mood, social support, and nutrition), functional (including activities of daily living and risk of falls), and environmental resources and problems, and then attempts to link that person with an overall plan (including resources) for the treatment and follow-up of those issues identified [1,2]. It is a method of case finding, or identifying

Table 29.1. Risk factors identified for functional decline

Increasing age
Pre-existing functional impairment
Recent ED visit or hospitalization
Visual impairment
Pre-existing cognitive impairment
Polypharmacy
Social isolation/lack of social support
Recent falls
Decubitus ulcer
Poor self-rated health status

health and wellness issues which currently exist, but do so without detection by health care providers. While CGA may be of benefit when used in settings other than the ED, its benefit is less definitive when ED-based CGA and intervention is reviewed [1,3]. Outcomes evaluated in various ED CGA studies include repeat ED visits, subsequent hospitalization or nursing home placement, functional status measures such as activities of daily living (ADL) and instrumental ADL (IADL), patient and caregiver satisfaction, quality of life, and mortality (Table 29.1).

Early reviews of ED CGA showed inconclusive results overall; however, functional status stands out as one area in which these trials demonstrated a benefit, with three out of the four trials measuring functional decline demonstrating a reduction in the decline for the intervention group [3,4]. A more recent systematic review of CGA concludes that a two-step process of screening patients with validated tools such as the Identification of Seniors at Risk (ISAR), the Triage Risk Screening Tool (TRST), or others as discussed below, to identify patients at high risk of functional decline is more efficient than age-based screening, and that CGA performed in the ED, followed by appropriate interventions, improves outcomes such as functional decline, ED readmissions, and possibly nursing home admissions [5]. CGA may be feasible if additional ED resources are available. However, the time required for such an assessment is often prohibitive without dedicated staff and resources.

Geriatric Emergency Medicine, ed. Joseph H. Kahn, Brendan G. Magauran Jr., and Jonathan S. Olshaker. Published by Cambridge University Press. © Cambridge University Press 2014.

Assessment tools for functional status

Activities of daily living and IADL measures are commonly used by health care providers to assess the function of people with possible disability in carrying out daily tasks of living. Original activities were proposed by Lawton and Brody in an attempt to standardize the functional assessment of geriatric patients [6]. ADL scales, adapted from the original Lawton and Brody proposals, encompass both basic biologic (or life-sustaining activities) (BADL) and instrumental (or higher functional competence) activities (IADL). The Older American Resources and Service (OARS) functional measure incorporates these ADL into a standardized questionnaire which can be administered either face to face or via a telephone interview, and have been validated for use in the ED [7,8].

The basic ADL include seven items: eating, dressing/undressing, grooming, walking, transfers to/from bed or chair, bathing, and continence. The IADL consist of an additional seven items reflecting the person's ability to maintain an independent household: using the telephone, travel, shopping, meal preparation, housework, taking medication, and management of finances. Each of the 14 items are scored on a scale of 0–2: 2 meaning the patient can perform the activity without any help, 1 meaning the activity requires some help, and 0 meaning the patient is completely unable to perform the activity. Self-reported responses are recorded. Higher scores therefore indicate greater independence and any loss of points on subsequent measures of ADL indicates a decline in function. Measurement of ADL in some form or another has become routine in many national surveys of older people, and these have been shown to be predictors of nursing home admissions, paid home care, hospital services, living arrangements, physician services, insurance coverage, and mortality [9].

Performance testing of function

In contrast to ADL scales which are scored on self- or proxy-reported responses, physical function performance testing requires the patient to attempt certain physical tests while under direct observation. Objective measurements and/or scores are compiled, many of which have been shown to be predictive of mortality, disability, hospitalization, and even nursing home admission. These tests include items such as hand grip strength, walking speed, balance testing, "up and go" testing, and chair rising.

Brief screening tools (each usually performed in <2–3 minutes) for gait, balance, and lower extremity strength have been proposed which may be feasible in the ED for selected cases. The timed "up and go" test has a high sensitivity for detecting functional mobility issues, and is considered abnormal if the patient takes longer than 20 seconds to rise from an armchair, walk 3 meters, turn, walk back, and sit down again [10]. Slow gait speed (13 seconds to walk 10 meters) has also been shown to be predictive of recurrent falls and poor overall survival. This can be rapidly assessed in most EDs [11,12]. Regarding balance, the inability to stand on one leg for more than 5 seconds is indicative of being frail and at risk for injurious falls [13]. More common balance testing includes assessing the ability of patients to maintain side-by-side, semi-tandem, and tandem standing for 10 seconds [14]. The measurement of hand grip strength requires the use of a hand-held dynamometer, while the strength of the lower extremities themselves is often tested by having the patient rise from a straight-backed chair (with their arms folded across their chest) to a standing position 5 times in succession, with a time requirement of greater than about 15 seconds being considered abnormal [15]. Several of these tests (balance, walking speed, chair rising) were combined into a Short Performance Physical Battery assessing lower extremity function, and this was shown to be predictive of mortality and nursing home admission, and correlated well with self-rated health status [16].

Other more in-depth evaluations of balance and mobility include the Gait Assessment Rating Scale, the Berg Functional Balance Scale, and the Tinetti Balance and Mobility Scale. While these scales provide a more in-depth picture of any given patient's mobility and balance, they may be prohibitively lengthy to be performed in the emergency setting.

Prediction tools for post-ED functional decline

ISAR

The ISAR tool was developed in an attempt to predict adverse health outcomes during the initial 6 months after an ED visit by patients 65 years and older [17]. The tool itself was derived as the best subset of screening questions which were developed from a literature review of general factors and specific questions that might predict functional decline. These questions assessed aspects of functional status both prior to the acute problem which prompted the ED visit, as well as the change in function since the onset of the problem. Topics queried included those pertaining to physical, social, functional, and cognitive risk factors, as well as medical history (including medications), medical resource usage, and alcohol use or abuse.

From these initial questions studied, the best subset of items was derived and tested in a prospective 6-month follow-up study of geriatric ED patients (admitted or discharged from the ED) [17]. This study validated the tool (40% of the cohort) for detection of adverse health outcomes in older ED patients. Adverse health outcomes were defined as death during 6 months after ED visit, institutionalization, or clinically significant decline in physical function (defined as a 3-point or greater decline on the OARS ADL scale) within 6 months of the ED visit. The 6 items on the ISAR tool are: 1) Before the illness or injury that brought you to Emergency, did you need someone to help you on a regular basis? 2) Since the illness or injury that brought you to Emergency, have you needed more help than usual to take care of yourself? 3) Have you been hospitalized for one or more nights during the past 6 months? 4) In general, do you see well? 5) In general, do you have serious problems with your memory? 6) Do you take more than three different medications every day?

Various cutoff points can be used with the ISAR tool, depending on available resources of the ED or associated hospital system, with a positive score of 2 or more demonstrating a sensitivity/specificity of 72/58%, a score of 3 or more 44/80%, and a score of 4 or more 23/92% in detecting older patients at risk for adverse health outcome within the immediate 6 months following an ED visit. The ISAR tool performs well in both admitted and discharged ED patients. Subsequent studies demonstrated its ability to help identify elderly patients who are more likely to return to the ED and/or be admitted to an acute care hospital within the next 6 months, in addition to the detection of adverse health outcomes. Used in conjunction with disclosure of the results, notification of primary care and home providers, and other referrals such as home care services, the ISAR tool has been shown to reduce the rate of functional decline after an ED visit for patients over the age of 65 [18].

BRIGHT

Boyd et al. evaluated the Brief Risk Identification for Geriatric Health Tool (BRIGHT) in a cross-sectional study of elderly ED patients from New Zealand [19]. Items addressed in the tool include yes or no questions regarding help with bathing, personal hygiene, dressing the lower body, getting around indoors, difficulty making decisions about everyday activity, shortness of breath, recent falls, perception of general health, memory problems, ability to do ordinary housework, and depression. The BRIGHT questionnaire was conceptualized as a means to identify older people with disabilities living in a community who might have unmet social, functional, and health care needs (community case finding).

The 11-item BRIGHT tool, which can be either self-administered or administered with assistance from untrained personnel, successfully identifies older adults in the ED who have decreased function at baseline when they present to the ED for a medical complaint. It therefore may be useful to identify older ED patients who need a more comprehensive geriatric assessment (ED case finding) [19]. A cutoff value of 3 or more positive answers to any of the 11 BRIGHT questions has similar discriminatory ability as the ISAR tool for ED case finding, though it may be slightly better at detecting IADL deficits than other tools. The tool does not predict outcomes such as repeat ED use, institutionalization, functional decline over time, morbidity, or mortality, and it has not been studied in a controlled manner in conjunction with interventions to assess its utility in reducing such adverse outcomes.

SIGNET/TRST

The Systematic Intervention for a Geriatric Network of Evaluation and Treatment (SIGNET) model was developed as a means of case finding at-risk community-dwelling older people and linking them to pre-existing medical and community agencies or resources [20]. TRST consists of 6 relatively easy historical factors: the presence of cognitive impairment, living alone or no caregiver willing or able to provide assistance, difficulty walking or transferring from/to chair, ED visit within the previous 30 days or hospitalization within the last 90 days, five or more prescription medications, and professional recommendation (reflecting the ED nurse's clinical judgment). Potential at-risk patients are defined as having cognitive impairment or two or more of the remaining five risk factors. The TRST screening tool has been shown to be useful in identifying elderly patients who are most likely to have repeat ED visits, hospitalizations, or nursing home placement within 30 days and 120 days after an initial ED visit. TRST typically takes only 1–2 minutes to complete. A simple cutoff of 2 or more positive answers on the TRST screen identifies those at risk.

More germane to the understanding of functional assessment of elderly ED patients is the ability of TRST to identify baseline functional impairment in older ED patients and to predict subsequent functional decline after an initial ED visit, similar to the ISAR tool discussed above [21]. TRST scores correlated with baseline ADL and IADL impairments, as well as with self-perceived physical health. A score of 2 or more was also moderately predictive of ADL or IADL decline at 30 and 120 days after an index ED visit. Advantages of TRST include the ease of use and completion without additional resources beyond normal questioning of the patient during the ED visit, whereas several of the ISAR items require inquiries regarding pre-morbid or acute functional dependence and impaired vision and hearing issues, which may not be a part of routine ED triage processes at many institutions.

HARP

The Hospital Admission Risk Profile (HARP) was developed to assess the risk of functional decline in those patients aged 70 and older who are admitted to the hospital as opposed to being discharged from the ED [22]. HARP consists of a total 29 questions; age, cognitive function (as measured by a 21-item abbreviated mini-mental status exam), and the 7 IADLs. High-risk patients identified by HARP were three times more likely to show a loss in ADL function at hospital discharge, some of which persisted at up to 3 months post-hospital discharge. HARP may be best used to identify those admitted elderly patients who could most benefit from comprehensive hospital discharge planning, specialized geriatric inpatient care, and inpatient/outpatient post-hospital rehabilitation.

SHERPA

Pascale Cornette and others developed a similar tool attempting to predict the functional decline of hospitalized patients over the age of 70 [23]. SHERPA (Score Hospitalier d'Evaluation du Risque de Perte d'Autonomie) consists of five variables: age, premorbid IADL score, abbreviated mini-mental status exam, a history of fall in the previous year, and poor self-perceived health. Scores on SHERPA categorize patients into low-, mild-, moderate-, and high-risk profiles. Functional decline was again defined as a loss of at least one point on the ADL scale. The SHERPA score showed moderate discrimination for predicting functional decline at 3 months post-hospital discharge. With each category increase, there is an approximate twofold increase in the risk of functional decline. The score has yet to be validated on an independent population, but as with the HARP, the authors suggest it could be used as an initial screening tool to help guide either the placement of elderly patients into more appropriate inpatient units and/or the early initiation of additional rehabilitation services.

Inouye et al.

Another predictive index for in-hospital functional decline was developed by Inyoue et al. for patients aged 70 and older admitted to a general medical floor [24]. Data were collected regarding self-reported physical function and IADL, a mini-mental status exam, pre-illness social activity level, depression scale, social networks and supports, vision and hearing tests, delirium screening, and a standardized skin check. Four factors were incorporated into the predictive tool: decubitus ulcer, cognitive dysfunction, low social activity, and existing functional impairment. This skin check for decubiti is unique to functional decline instruments. Each categorical advancement in this scale represents an approximate fourfold increase in the prevalence of functional decline at hospital discharge. It is of particular note that the existence of skin breakdown has the highest independent risk for in-hospital functional decline for this population.

Screening for common issues in elderly ED patients

Visual impairment screening

Visual impairment, typically defined as worse than 20/40 corrected vision on a standard eye chart, is a common problem in the US and increases dramatically with advancing age [25]. Some of the most common causes of visual loss are age related, and include macular degeneration, diabetic retinopathy, presbyopia, cataracts, and glaucoma. These diseases can lead to a variety of ill effects on vision such as overall reduced visual acuity, loss of contrast sensitivity, scattered scotomas, light scatter, altered color perception, glare sensitivity, myopia, loss of depth perception, and loss of central or peripheral visual fields [26].

Visual loss adversely affects several aspects of everyday function for many geriatric patients. Impairment of function is seen with and can be predicted by increasing levels of visual loss. It is also associated with lower leisure time physical activity, difficulty driving an automobile, depression, and hip fractures. Remediation of visual loss through a variety of techniques such as medical management, surgical intervention, assistive devices (corrective eyewear, magnifiers, monoculars, or binoculars) or environmental alteration (large print, high contrast usage, alternative lighting techniques) can help mitigate some of these adverse effects. This visual rehabilitation can be performed by the patient's health care team outside of the ED, and guided by such questionnaires as the Activities of Daily Vision Scale which evaluates visual disability not captured by routine visual acuity testing [27]. Such in-depth assessment of visual disability screening as that obtained by these types of questionnaires is typically considered impractical in the everyday practice of emergency medicine, though many aspects of

the questionnaire may be typically covered in a comprehensive geriatric assessment.

Rapid methods of visual impairment assessment available in the ED include self-reporting of visual impairment upon direct query and traditional visual acuity testing. Self reporting of visual impairment with a question such as, "How would you rate your distant and near vision?" is thought to be a fairly reliable measure of visual function [28]. This type of self-reporting may capture more disability than simple acuity testing, since it addresses the functional aspects of vision in the patient's daily life, rather than simple visual acuity. Additionally, corrective eyewear is not always readily available in the ED for visual acuity testing. Nonetheless, visual acuity testing is a simple, familiar, and rapid means by which to categorize patients as vision impaired. Those patients testing worse than 20/40 are considered vision impaired, and those testing 20/200 or worse are considered legally blind [29]. The US Preventive Services Task Force concluded that current evidence is insufficient to assess the benefit/harm balance for visual acuity screening in older adults [30]. Nonetheless, if significant functional visual impairment is detected in the ED, patients and/or families should be referred to the appropriate resources within the community to further assess and maximally remediate the impairment in an attempt to avoid the associated morbidities.

Hearing impairment

Age-related hearing loss, or presbycusis, affects a significant portion of the geriatric population and increases with age [31]. Although age-related conductive hearing losses such as collapse of the cartilaginous auditory canal, stiffening of the tympanic membrane and ossicular chain, otitis media, cholesteatomas, tumors, and cerumen impaction do occur, the most significant age-related hearing losses are sensorineural in origin. With aging, there is a general alteration of the size, number, and neurochemical makeup of the entire central auditory system, as well as the cumulative aggregation of environmental and iatrogenic damage such as prolonged exposure to loud noises, exposure to ototoxic substances, and local and systemic diseases [32]. These changes lead to a hearing loss which is typically gradual, progressive, bilateral, and characterized by high frequency loss which makes understanding speech and hearing or localizing high-frequency sounds (such as beepers, turn signals, escaping steam) particularly difficult at first. These losses progress to involve lower frequencies, making even the simple detection of speech difficult.

As with visual impairment, presbycusis can have significant adverse effects. Hearing loss not only leads to difficult with speech recognition and detection, but with localization of sounds, enjoyment of music, and participation in social activities [33]. Decreased levels of physical, social, and cognitive function, depression, and diminished quality of life have all been shown to be associated with hearing impairment. Hearing impairment is also thought to be predictive of future functional impairment [34].

Screening for such losses can be accomplished in a variety of manners, including a single question for self-reporting, the whisper test, the Hearing Handicap Inventory for the

Elderly–Screening Version (HHIE-S), and audiometry. Each of these tests is estimated to take less than 1–2 minutes. Self-reported hearing loss is felt to be an acceptably sensitive and specific method for detection, with a positive or equivocal response to questions such as, "Would you say you have any difficulty hearing?" or "Do you feel you have hearing loss?" showing adequate detection rates in the geriatric population, especially given the high pretest probability [35,36]. The whisper test is performed by whispering random numbers and letters behind the patient at arm's length, while occluding the non-tested ear. Failure to repeat at least 3 out of 6 letters or numbers indicates significant hearing loss [37]. HHIE-S is a self-administered questionnaire measuring social, emotional, and functional aspects of hearing loss which do not always correlate well with objective hearing losses [38]. Audiometry has the highest accuracy in detecting hearing loss in the elderly [39]. Given that audiometric devices may not be readily available in most EDs, current reviews suggest initial screening with either a single direct hearing question or the whispered voice test, followed by audiometry in those failing either initial test [32]. Although the data on the efficacy of hearing impairment treatment in restoring hearing-related quality of life and overall quality of life are questionable, screening may still be of value, particularly for those patients willing and able to comply with treatments [40,41].

Malnutrition

Malnutrition, including over- and underweight conditions, is common in the elderly population, with estimates ranging from 5–10% for community-dwelling elderly to as high as 30–60% of hospitalized elderly and can adversely affect health and well-being [42]. A number of factors influence dietary patterns and therefore overall nutrition, including physical activity levels which may decrease with aging, overall diminished physical functioning, health issues which limit intake such as medical comorbidities, age-associated loss of taste and smell, poor dentition, poor cognitive function, social factors such as loss of a spouse and isolation, and financial concerns. Although there are a multitude of assessments that can be performed to thoroughly understand the nutritional status of any given patient, the goal of nutritional screening is to rapidly and easily identify those at risk for the adverse outcomes associated with malnutrition such as increased mortality, increased susceptibility to infection, and reduced quality of life.

Self-reporting of weight and height may be adequately sensitive, and therefore simply asking the elderly patient about unintentional weight loss could indeed be the simplest manner in which to screen for malnutrition [43]. Height and weight are often collected routinely on ED patients, and from these two data points the anthropometric body mass index (BMI) can be calculated as kilograms/meters^2. Those with a BMI <18.5 (underweight) or >25 (overweight) are at risk for malnutrition. Additional screening measures include the Mini Nutritional Assessment (MNA) and the Nutrition Screening Initiative. These screening tools allow for the detection of malnutrition despite normal anthropometric or biochemical parameters, since they inquire about issues such as quantity and quality of

food intake, as well as physical and social issues surrounding dietary intake [42,44,45]. The United States Preventive Services Task Force (USPSTF) recommends that clinicians screen all adult patients for obesity and offer counseling and behavioral interventions [46]. As with vision and hearing screening, if time allows, brief screening by either simple query regarding nutrition or by the MNA-short form may be of value, particularly in the setting of a comprehensive geriatric assessment for appropriately selected geriatric ED patients at high risk.

Alcohol abuse

Estimates of alcohol-related problems for those over 65 years of age range from 2 to 22% [47]. These problems include heavy drinking, driving after drinking, and alcohol-related adverse health, social, legal, or behavioral issues [48]. Alcohol consumption is one of the leading causes of death in the US, and those elderly who use alcohol may present with symptoms of use at lower levels than younger counterparts because of age-related physiological changes and the interaction between the alcohol and overall declining health and comorbidities, medication use, and diminished physical functioning. Though not specific to the geriatric population, the USPSTF recommends screening and behavioral counseling interventions to reduce alcohol misuse by all adults in primary care settings [49]. Others agree, extending the recommendation for screening and brief intervention to those in the ED [50].

Several relatively brief screens exist to help identify alcohol use and misuse [51]. The most widely used and studied instrument is the CAGE questionnaire, which asks about feeling the need to "Cut" down on drinking, being "Annoyed" by others criticizing the level of alcohol use, feeling "Guilty" about drinking, and the need for an "Eye-opener" in the morning [52]. A positive response to two or more of the questions is used as the cutoff for probable alcohol misuse. The TWEAK questionnaire is also brief and easy to administer, asking about five aspects of alcohol use (Tolerance, Worry, Eye-openers, Amnesia, and the need to "Kut" down) [53]. The Short Michigan Alcoholism Screening Test–Geriatric Version (SMAST-G) was one of the first screens which addressed the unique aspects of alcohol use problems in the elderly, which include lowering the sensible limits and de-emphasizing social and occupational complications which do not impact the geriatric population as profoundly [54]. Two or more yes answers on the SMAST-G is considered a positive screen. The Alcohol Use Disorder Identification Test (AUDIT) questionnaire was shown likely to be advantageous in those with confounding psychiatric issues [55,56]. Cyr and Wartman propose a simple two-question screen, asking, "Have you ever had alcohol problems?" and "Was your last drink within 24 hours?" If either is answered positively, then alcohol misuse is probable [57]. The Alcohol-Related Problems Survey (ARPS) has been shown to have good sensitivities in detecting alcohol issues resulting from the interaction of alcohol use and medical comorbidities, but can take up to ten minutes to complete, thereby limiting its utility in the ED [58,59]. No ideal screening tool for the ED has been identified; the familiarity, brevity, and ease of use suggest that the CAGE questions be used (taking less than 30 seconds) as an initial screen in the ED for possible alcohol use disorders [60].

Extending the role of the ED beyond simple screening for alcohol misuse, the concept of screening, brief intervention, and referral to treatment for alcohol misuse while patients are in the ED (ED-SBIRT) has been shown to reduce unhealthy drinking, at least in the short term, and is endorsed by a multitude of national health care organizations as strategy to improve the health of ED patients [61,62]. After initial screening, those people identified as misusing alcohol undergo a brief intervention. This brief intervention typically consists of a brief negotiated interview where introspective questioning eventually leads to an assessment of the patient's willingness to alter their alcohol use, followed by the development of specific alcohol use reduction goals and referral to appropriate outpatient treatment resources [63]. The use of ED-SBIRT for substances other than alcohol and for its use in the elderly population in particular has been less well studied.

Balance, gait, falls

Falls are a common occurrence in the elderly population, with up to one-third of community-dwelling individuals 65 or older falling each year [64,65]. The incidence of elderly patients falling within hospitals and nursing homes is estimated to be even higher [66]. These falls precipitate a significant number of injuries and ED visits. They also produce a large psychological burden on the individual and an enormous financial burden on the health care system [67–69]. Fall prevention programs or exercise programs are effective in reducing the fall rate in both populations [70–72]. The USPSTF recommends exercise or physical therapy and vitamin D supplementation in community-dwelling elderly who are at risk of falls, but not routine in-depth risk assessment [73]. Screening for falls can be done by asking the patient about falls within the last 12 months (2 or more) and whether they have any difficulty with gait or balance issues. If patients answer positive to any of those screening questions, they should likely undergo a multifactorial fall assessment to evaluate the modifiable risk factors for falling, which include acute illness, urinary incontinence, visual and sensory loss, medication side effects, home hazards, and improper foot wear. This assessment should include orthostatic vital signs and visual testing, along with medication, ADL, and cognitive and home environment assessments. In addition, further assessment of gait, balance, and lower extremity strength should be performed [74,75].

Summary and recommendations

The functional status of elderly ED patients is an important aspect of their well-being. It not only affects their day-to-day quality of life, but is also clearly predictive of a variety of issues including the future use of health care services, disability, and even mortality. Comprehensive geriatric assessments are an ideal means by which to assess this issue, but are in reality too time and resource intensive to be completed for all elderly ED patients. Validated tools such as TRST, ISAR, and possibly BRIGHT could be used as the initial step in case-finding elderly ED patients who are at risk of adverse outcomes after their ED visit and discharged back into the community setting, while tools such as HARP, SHERPA, and that of Inouye et al. could

Table 29.2. Suggested optimal timing of effective screening tools for common elderly issues

Vision	Self-reporting
	Visual acuity testing
Hearing	Self-reporting
	Whispered voice test
Malnutrition	Self-reporting
	BMI calculation
Alcohol misuse	CAGE questionnaire
	Cyr and Wartman 2-part questionnaire
Gait, balance, falls	Self-reporting

be performed on those patients requiring acute hospitalization after their ED evaluation in order to identify those in need of more advanced hospital discharge planning, intervention, and care.

Screening for the multitude of common problems seen in elderly ED patients such as vision loss, hearing loss, substance abuse, etc. can be time consuming. Many tools exist as previously discussed, but these tools, when used in aggregate, are too cumbersome for the day-to-day practice of emergency medicine. Practicing physicians should maintain a high index of suspicion, understanding the profound impact any one of these problems can have on the well-being of their patients. Screening for most of these issues can be as simple as a direct query to the patient or proxy while in the ED. If a positive response is found, further formal assessments as detailed above may be performed either in the ED, or during appropriate and timely follow-up health care encounters outside the ED (Table 29.2).

Pearls and pitfalls
Pearls

- The functional status of elderly ED patients should always be considered, especially for those being considered for discharge to an environment lacking health care and/or social support.
- Physical performance tests assessing parameters such as gait speed, strength, and balance are useful predictors of disability, future health care needs, and even mortality.
- Validated brief screening tools exist which, if performed, can help predict future adverse health outcomes.
- Many elderly patients have unrecognized sensory or substance abuse issues which may be amenable to remediation.

Pitfalls

- Never discharge an elderly patient home from the ED without considering and/or assessing their ability to fulfill their basic activities of daily living.
- Ignoring the reason for a fall in an elderly person misses the opportunity to offer or refer the patient to appropriate interventions which may prevent a repeat ED visit or other future adverse health outcome.

- Giving important medical information such as discharge instructions to someone with visual or hearing impairment without addressing those limitations essentially guarantees noncompliance with the information.
- Underestimating the extent of substance abuse in elderly patients leads to many missed opportunities for brief interventions or counseling.

References

1. Stuck AE, Siu AL, Wieland GD, et al. Comprehensive geriatric assessment: a meta-analysis of controlled trials. *Lancet*. 1993;342:1032–6.

2. Rubenstein LZ, Stuck AE, Siu AL, et al. Impacts of geriatric evaluation and management programs on defined outcomes: overview of the evidence. *J Am Geriatr Soc*. 1991;39:8–16S; discussion, 17–18S.

3. Hastings SN, Heflin MT. A systematic review of interventions to improve outcomes for elders discharged from the emergency department. *Acad Emerg Med*. 2005;12:978–86.

4. Aminzadeh F, Dalziel WB. Older adults in the emergency department: a systematic review of patterns of use, adverse outcomes, and effectiveness of interventions. *Ann Emerg Med*. 2002;39:238–47.

5. Graf CE, Zekry D, Giannelli S, et al. Efficiency and applicability of comprehensive geriatric assessment in the emergency department: a systematic review. *Aging Clin Exp Res*. 2011;23:244–54.

6. Lawton MP, Brody EM. Assessment of older people: self-maintaining and instrumental activities of daily living. *Gerontologist*. 1969;9:179–86.

7. George LK, Fillenbaum GG. OARS methodology. A decade of experience in geriatric assessment. *J Am Geriatr Soc*. 1985;33:607–15.

8. Fillenbaum GG. *Multidimensional Functional Assessment of Older Adults: The Duke Older Americans Resources and Services Procedures* (Dallas, TX: Erlbaum, 1988).

9. Wiener JM, Hanley RJ, Clark R, et al. Measuring the activities of daily living: comparisons across national surveys. *J Gerontol*. 1990;45:S229–37.

10. Podsiadlo D, Richardson S. The timed "Up & Go": a test of basic functional mobility for frail elderly persons. *J Am Geriatr Soc*. 1991;39:142–8.

11. Fritz S, Lusardi M. White paper: "Walking speed: the sixth vital sign." *J Geriatr Phys Ther (2001)*. 2009;32: 46–9.

12. Hardy SE, Perera S, Roumani YF, et al. Improvement in usual gait speed predicts better survival in older adults. *J Am Geriatr Soc*. 2007;55: 1727–34.

13. Michikawa T, Nishiwaki Y, Takebayashi T, et al. One-leg standing test for elderly populations. *J Ortho Sci*. 2009;14:675–85.

14. Cesari M, Onder G, Zamboni V, et al. Physical function and self-rated health status as predictors of mortality: results from longitudinal analysis in the ilSIRENTE study. *BMC Geriatr*. 2008;8:34.

15. Cesari M, Kritchevsky SB, Newman AB, et al. Added value of physical performance measures in predicting adverse health-related events: results from the Health, Aging and Body Composition Study. *J Am Geriatr Soc*. 2009;57:251–9.

16. Guralnik JM, Simonsick EM, Ferrucci L, et al. A short physical performance battery assessing lower extremity function: association with self-reported disability and prediction of mortality and nursing home admission. *J Gerontol*. 1994;49:M85–94.

17. McCusker J, Bellavance F, Cardin S, et al. Detection of older people at increased risk of adverse health outcomes after an emergency visit: the ISAR screening tool. *J Am Geriatr Soc*. 1999;47: 1229–37.

18. McCusker J, Verdon J, Tousignant P, et al. Rapid emergency department intervention for older people reduces risk of functional decline: results of a multicenter randomized trial. *J Am Geriatr Soc*. 2001;49: 1272–81.

19. Boyd M, Koziol-McLain J, Yates K, et al. Emergency department case-finding for high-risk older adults: the Brief Risk Identification for Geriatric Health Tool (BRIGHT). *Acad Emerg Med*. 2008;15:598–606.

20. Meldon SW, Mion L, Palmer R, et al. Case finding of at-risk elders in the emergency department (ED): A multicenter study. *Acad Emerg Med*. 2000;7:1166.

21. Hustey FM, Mion LC, Connor JT, et al. A brief risk stratification tool to predict functional decline in older adults discharged from emergency departments. *J Am Geriatr Soc*. 2007;55:1269–74.

22. Sager MA, Rudberg MA, Jalaluddin M, et al. Hospital admission risk profile (HARP): identifying older patients at risk for functional decline following acute medical illness and hospitalization. *J Am Greiatr Soc*. 1996;44:251–7.

23. Cornette P, Swine C, Malhomme B, et al. Early evaluation of the risk of functional decline following hospitalization of older patients: development of a predictive tool. *Eur J Public Health*. 2006;16:203–8.

24. Inouye SK, Wagner DR, Acampora D, et al. A predictive index for functional decline in hospitalized elderly medical patients. *J Gen Intern Med*. 1993;8:645–52.

25. Nelson KAD. Statistical Brief #36: Severe visual impairment in the United States and in each state, 1990. *J Vis Imp Blind*. 1993;87:80–5.

26. Watson GR. Low vision in the geriatric population: rehabilitation and management. *J Am Geriatr Soc*. 2001;49:317–30.

27. Mangione CM, Phillips RS, Seddon JM, et al. Development of the 'Activities of Daily Vision Scale'. A measure of visual functional status. *Med Care*. 1992;30:1111–26.

28. Lee PP, Smith JP, Kington RS. The associations between self-rated vision and hearing and functional status in middle age. *Ophthalmology*. 1999;106:401–5.

29. Rubin GS, West SK, Munoz B, et al. A comprehensive assessment of visual impairment in a population of older Americans. The SEE Study. Salisbury Eye Evaluation Project. *Invest Ophthalmol Visual Sci*. 1997;38:557–68.

30. US Preventive Services Task Force. Screening for impaired visual acuity in older adults: US Preventive Services Task Force recommendation statement. *Ann Intern Med*. 2009;151:37–43.

31. Cruickshanks KJ, Tweed TS, Wiley TL, et al. The 5-year incidence and progression of hearing loss: the epidemiology of hearing loss study. *Arch Otolaryngol Head Neck Surg*. 2003;129:1041–6.

32. Bagai A, Thavendiranathan P, Detsky AS. Does this patient have hearing impairment? *JAMA*. 2006;295:416–28.

33. Gates GA, Mills JH. Presbycusis. *Lancet.* 2005;366:1111–20.

34. Reuben DB, Mui S, Damesyn M, et al. The prognostic value of sensory impairment in older persons. *J Am Geriatr Soc.* 1999;47:930–5.

35. Clark K, Sowers M, Wallace RB, et al. The accuracy of self-reported hearing loss in women aged 60–85 years. *Am J Epidemiol.* 1991;134:704–8.

36. Nondahl DM, Cruickshanks KJ, Wiley TL, et al. Accuracy of self-reported hearing loss. *Audiology.* 1998;37:295–301.

37. Pirozzo S, Papinczak T, Glasziou P. Whispered voice test for screening for hearing impairment in adults and children: systematic review. *BMJ (Clinical Research edn).* 2003;327:967.

38. Ventry IM, Weinstein BE. The hearing handicap inventory for the elderly: a new tool. *Ear Hearing.* 1982;3:128–34.

39. McBride WS, Mulrow CD, Aguilar C, Tuley MR. Methods for screening for hearing loss in older adults. *Am J Med Sci.* 1994;307:40–2.

40. Chou R, Dana T, Bougatsos C, et al. Screening adults aged 50 years or older for hearing loss: a review of the evidence for the US preventive services task force. *Ann Intern Med.* 2011;154:347–55.

41. Pacala JT, Yueh B. Hearing deficits in the older patient: "I didn't notice anything." *JAMA.* 2012;307:1185–94.

42. Guigoz Y, Vellas B, Garry PJ. Assessing the nutritional status of the elderly: The Mini Nutritional Assessment as part of the geriatric evaluation. *Nutrition Rev.* 1996;54:S59–65.

43. Sahyoun NR, Maynard LM, Zhang XL, et al. Factors associated with errors in self-reported height and weight in older adults. *J Nutrition Health Aging.* 2008;12:108–15.

44. Salva A, Pera G. Screening for malnutrition in dwelling elderly. *Public Health Nutr.* 2001;4:1375–8.

45. Posner BM, Jette AM, Smith KW, et al. Nutrition and health risks in the elderly: the nutrition screening initiative. *Am J Public Health.* 1993;83:972–8.

46. US Preventive Services Task Force. Screening for obesity in adults: recommendations and rationale. *Ann Intern Med.* 2003;139:930–2.

47. Adams WL, Cox NS. Epidemiology of problem drinking among elderly people. *Int J Addictions.* 1995;30:1693–716.

48. Reid MC, Anderson PA. Geriatric substance use disorders. *Med Clin North Am.* 1997;81:999–1016.

49. US Preventive Services Task Force. Screening and behavioral counseling interventions in primary care to reduce alcohol misuse: recommendation statement. *Ann Intern Med.* 2004;140:554–6.

50. D'Onofrio G, Degutis LC. Preventive care in the emergency department: screening and brief intervention for alcohol problems in the emergency department: a systematic review. *Acad Emerg Med.* 2002;9:627–38.

51. O'Connell H, Chin AV, Hamilton F, et al. A systematic review of the utility of self-report alcohol screening instruments in the elderly. *Int J Geriatr Psychiatr.* 2004;19:1074–86.

52. Ewing JA. Detecting alcoholism. The CAGE questionnaire. *JAMA.* 1984;252:1905–7.

53. Cherpitel CJ. Screening for alcohol problems in the emergency department. *Ann Emerg Med.* 1995;26:158–66.

54. Conigliaro J, Kraemer K, McNeil M. Screening and identification of older adults with alcohol problems in primary care. *J Geriatr Psychiatr Neurol.* 2000;13:106–14.

55. Saunders JB, Aasland OG, Babor TF, et al. Development of the Alcohol Use Disorders Identification Test (AUDIT): WHO Collaborative Project on Early Detection of Persons with Harmful Alcohol Consumption – II. *Addiction (Abingdon, England).* 1993;88:791–804.

56. Philpot M, Pearson N, Petratou V, et al. Screening for problem drinking in older people referred to a mental health service: a comparison of CAGE and AUDIT. *Aging Mental Health.* 2003;7:171–5.

57. Cyr MG, Wartman SA. The effectiveness of routine screening questions in the detection of alcoholism. *JAMA.* 1988;259:51–4.

58. Fink A, Morton SC, Beck JC, et al. The alcohol-related problems survey: identifying hazardous and harmful drinking in older primary care patients. *J Am Geriatr Soc.* 2002;50:1717–22.

59. Fink A, Tsai MC, Hays RD, et al. Comparing the alcohol-related problems survey (ARPS) to traditional alcohol screening measures in elderly outpatients. *Arch Gerontol Geriatr.* 2002;34:55–78.

60. D'Onofrio G, Bernstein E, Bernstein J, et al. Patients with alcohol problems in the emergency department, part 1: improving detection. SAEM Substance Abuse Task Force. Society for Academic Emergency Medicine. *Acad Emerg Med.* 1998;5:1200–9.

61. Academic ED SBIRT Research Collaborative. The impact of screening, brief intervention and referral for treatment in emergency department patients' alcohol use: a 3-, 6- and 12-month follow-up. *Alcohol Alcoholism (Oxford, Oxfordshire).* 2010;45:51419.

62. Bernstein E, Topp D, Shaw E, et al. A preliminary report of knowledge translation: lessons from taking screening and brief intervention techniques from the research setting into regional systems of care. *Acad Emerg Med.* 2009;16:1225–33.

63. Vaca FE, Winn D. The basics of alcohol screening, brief intervention and referral to treatment in the emergency department. *West J Emerg Med.* 2007;8:88–92.

64. Tinetti ME. Clinical practice. Preventing falls in elderly persons. *N Engl J Med.* 2003;348:42–9.

65. Rubenstein LZ, Josephson KR. The epidemiology of falls and syncope. *Clinics Geriatr Med.* 2002;18:141–58.

66. Nurmi I, Luthje P. Incidence and costs of falls and fall injuries among elderly in institutional care. *Scand J Prim Health Care.* 2002;20:118–22.

67. Tinetti ME. Prevention of falls and fall injuries in elderly persons: a research agenda. *Preventive Med.* 1994;23:756–62.

68. Li F, Fisher KJ, Harmer P, et al. Fear of falling in elderly persons association with falls, functional ability, and quality of life. *J Gerontol B, Psycholog Social Sci.* 2003;58:P283–90.

69. Stevens JA, Corso PS, Finkelstein EA, et al. The costs of fatal and non-fatal falls among older adults. *Injury Prevention.* 2006;12:290–5.

70. Chang JT, Morton SC, Rubenstein LZ, et al. Interventions for the prevention of falls in older adults: systematic review and meta-analysis of randomised clinical trials. *BMJ (Clin Res edn).* 2004;328:680.

71. Cameron ID, Murray GR, Gillespie LD, et al. Interventions for preventing falls in older people in nursing care facilities and hospitals. *Cochrane Database Syst Rev.* 2010:CD005465.

72. Gillespie LD, Robertson MC, Gillespie WJ, et al. Interventions for preventing falls in older people living in the community. *Cochrane Database Syst Rev.* 2009:CD007146.

73. Moyer VA. Prevention of Falls in Community-Dwelling Older Adults: US Preventive Services Task Force Recommendation Statement. *Ann Intern Med.* 2012;157:197–204.

74. Ganz DA, Bao Y, Shekelle PG, et al. Will my patient fall? *JAMA.* 2007;297:77–86.

75. American Geriatrics Society/British Geriatrics Society. Summary of the Updated American Geriatrics Society/British Geriatrics Society clinical practice guideline for prevention of falls in older persons. *J Am Geriatr Soc.* 2011;59:148–57.

Chapter 30

Palliative and end-of-life care in the emergency department

Paul L. DeSandre and Karen M. May

Introduction

Most chronic incurable illness occurs in the elderly and the proportion of elderly is rising. In the US, the median age of death is over 75 years and is rising. By 2030, the proportion of people over 85 years old will have doubled, with almost one-quarter having dementia [1]. Excluding infants, people over the age of 75 use the emergency department (ED) more often than any other age group [2]. The quality of care at the end of life is often poor, with patients suffering in their last days [3,4]. Although most patients prefer to die at home, they most often die in hospitals or nursing homes [5].

Palliative care is intended to "prevent and relieve suffering" and "support the best possible quality of life for patient and their families, regardless of their stage of disease or the need for other therapies, and in accordance with their values and preferences" [6]. Intensive care unit (ICU)-based studies have demonstrated that earlier involvement of palliative care decreases length of stay, results in fewer non-beneficial interventions, and creates better concordance between patients and families for the goals of medical interventions [7]. At the end of life, earlier palliative care involvement improves symptom management and family satisfaction [8,9].

In our daily practice in emergency medicine, we already assess and communicate prognoses for certain situations, relieve pain and other symptoms, articulate goals of care to determine appropriate interventions and dispositions, utilize understanding of ethical and legal concerns in the care of our patients, and provide culturally sensitive care and communication in the last hours of living and after death. Therefore, we already perform many aspects of general palliative care in our everyday practice. What is needed is an improvement in comfort and skills in managing the many patients and families facing these life-changing events in our EDs [10]. This chapter will focus on recognizing patients on a trajectory of dying and provide a structure to rapidly identify, intervene, and establish appropriate disposition on patients with immediate palliative care need.

Trajectories of illness and prognosis

With aging, progressive functional decline usually develops from the cumulative effects of multiple chronic illnesses.

Exacerbations of individual diseases, compounded by other comorbid conditions, can lead to more rapid functional decline. Death may occur with a particularly aggressive and unexpected exacerbation, or through the relentless accumulation of illnesses which eventually overwhelm the body's physiologic defenses irretrievably. For the emergency clinician to quickly navigate critical medical decision making with a patient or family, it is essential to first understand where a patient may be on their trajectory of illness, and their immediate risks for mortality, with and without intervention.

Functional trajectories have been developed to assist clinicians in recognizing decline in patients with advanced progressive illness. Functional trajectories measure decline in the activities of daily living such as eating, bathing, toileting, and ambulating to assess a patient's functional status. A decreasing functional status generally correlates to a higher risk of death over time [11] (Figure 30.1).

Typically, when patients with serious progressive disease survive an acute illness or exacerbation, they may recover but not return to their prior level of function. A relatively straightforward process of combining functional assessment with disease-specific estimations of prognoses can give a clearer sense of risks and benefits of immediate interventions in the ED relative to the goals of the patient and family. In patients with dementia presenting with complex severe illness, the context of recent functional ability over the past weeks and months can facilitate critical communications with family on a mutually acceptable approach to care. In an effort to objectify the relatively unpredictable process of decline in dementia, functional scales specific to dementia have been created. Although validated and commonly used, the Functional Assessment Staging (FAST) scale is less predictive of 6-month mortality in patients entering nursing homes than the Mortality Risk Index Score (MRIS) [12]. The most reliable predictor of 6-month mortality was "not awake most of the day." This simple indicator may provide an emergency clinician the opportunity to quickly contextualize the presenting illness, and allow a useful dialogue with family on how to best proceed with either life-sustaining or palliative interventions, including referral to hospice from the ED.

When patients are at risk of dying in the ED, intensive resources are required from the point of arrival until the person is either transferred out of the ED, or death occurs and the

---

Geriatric Emergency Medicine, ed. Joseph H. Kahn, Brendan G. Magauran Jr., and Jonathan S. Olshaker. Published by Cambridge University Press.
© Cambridge University Press 2014.

Proposed Trajectories of Dying

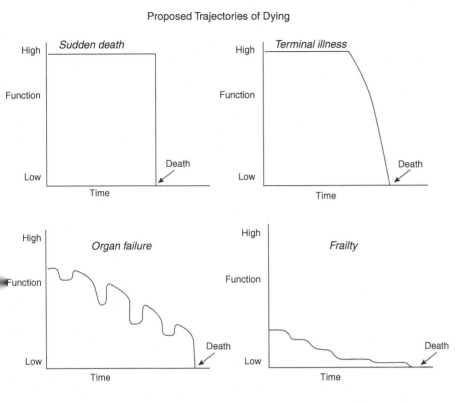

Figure 30.1. Trajectories of dying. Reproduced with permission from Lunney et al. [11].

family has left the ED. If death is inevitable, the patient must be rapidly assessed, goals determined, and interventions performed immediately. Seven trajectories have been identified to describe these different scenarios, along with recommended palliative interventions [13]. When the goals of the patient are unclear, the necessary default is to perform life-sustaining interventions. When the goals of the patient are clear, the clinician must carefully weigh the relative benefits and burdens of each intervention while protecting the patient from outcomes that would be inconsistent with their goals (Table 30.1).

Cardiopulmonary resuscitation and prognosis in advanced illness

With a clear understanding of the trajectories of illness and outcomes of cardiopulmonary resuscitation (CPR), emergency clinicians can effectively guide decision making that best aligns with the patient's goals for medical care. Patients and their families may lack understanding of the patient's disease trajectory as well as the outcomes of CPR, which can profoundly influence decision making. There are several factors that likely contribute to the disparity of the perceptions of clinicians and patients. Physicians and patients often have different perspectives on the need to share prognostic information, so prognosis may not be discussed at all [14]. In approximately one-third of cases, concordance is poor between physician and patient estimation of prognosis [15]. Prognosis is often overestimated by oncologists and potentially more so by patients [16–19]; and an overestimation of prognosis may significantly influence treatment preferences for CPR and life-sustaining interventions [20]. Paradoxically, longer patient–physician relationships may result in less accurate prognostic

communications, favoring the presumed objectivity of clinicians such as hospitalists (or emergency clinicians), which may be preferred by patients [16,21].

The original use of CPR was an attempt to intervene in otherwise healthy patients with witnessed and unexpected cardiac arrest [22]. Currently in the US, CPR is applied to all patients with cardiac arrest, regardless of medical condition, unless an order to not attempt resuscitation is in place. The known outcomes of CPR are poor.

In hospital, cardiac arrest survival to discharge is approximately 17% [13]. Of survivors of in-hospital cardiac arrest, 51% are discharged home and 47% are discharged to institutions, with the best functioning patients pre-arrest sustaining a 25% decline. Of patients who achieve return of spontaneous circulation, 63% are subsequently given orders to not attempt resuscitation and 44% have life-sustaining interventions withdrawn [23]. Factors associated with higher likelihood of survival to discharge with in-hospital cardiac arrest include coronary artery disease and ICU as location of cardiac arrest. Negative predictors of survival to discharge include sepsis, metastatic cancer, dementia, serum creatinine >1.5mg/dl, African-American race, and dependent status [24].

Out-of-hospital cardiac arrest has significantly worse outcomes than in-hospital cardiac arrest, with only 7.6% survival to discharge, and this has been essentially unchanged for the past 30 years [14]. Return of spontaneous circulation is achieved in approximately 22% of out-of-hospital cardiac arrests. Of those, if the initial arrhythmia is ventricular fibrillation or ventricular tachycardia, 14–25% survive to discharge. If the initial arrhythmia is asystole, only 0.2–5% survive to discharge. The strongest predictor of survival to discharge in out-of-hospital cardiac

Table 30.1. A) Example symptoms and signs of mortality and factors that contribute to the perception of approaching death

Category of symptoms/signs	Examples
Mechanism of injury	• Penetrating trauma/gunshot wound to the head • Auto vs. pedestrian at high speed • Stab wound to the heart or multiple stab wounds
Chief complaint	• Chest pain • Dyspnea • Abdominal pain • Altered level of consciousness
Physiological indicators and diagnostic findings	• Vital signs (temp, BP, pulse, RR, SaO$_2$) • Cardiac rhythm (e.g., ventricular fibrillation, asystole) • Massive intracranial hemorrhage on head CT with midline shift and uncal herniation
Physical examination findings	• Cranial vault disruption • Brain parenchyma outside the cranial vault • Evidence of disseminated intravascular coagulation • Lab/radiographic findings suggestive of severe or advanced stage of pathology (e.g., urosepsis, aspiration pneumonia, high-grade subdural hematoma) • Abnormal neurological findings (e.g., pupils fixed and dilated)
Demographic factors	Developmental indicators (e.g., age, height disproportionate to expected weight)
Patient's sense of impending doom or approaching death	• Patient stating they are "going to die" or "don't let me die" • Clinicians listen to patients when the patient perceives that he/she is going to die in the absence of a psychiatric problem
Required procedures	• Cardiopulmonary resuscitation: chest compression, intubation, cardiac pacing • Rapid, massive transfusions • Subdural hematoma evacuation

RR = respiratory rate; BP = blood pressure
Reproduced with permission from Chan [13].

B) Observed ED death trajectories, trajectory characteristics, and example palliative care interventions

Trajectory	Characteristics	Palliative care interventions for the patient or family
1. Dead on arrival	• Patient has injuries/medical condition incompatible with life • EMTs provided resuscitative efforts in the field • Consensus among ED clinicians regarding the finality of death • Patient declared dead within minutes of arrival to the ED	*Physical/symptoms* - No intervention *Psychological and social* - Family witnessed resuscitation - Skillful death notification *Spiritual* - Chaplain, social worker, or any clinician - Cultural considerations for postmortem care
2. Prehospital resuscitation with subsequent ED death	• Physical examination findings and physiological indicators help to determine that the patient is likely to die • ED clinicians use all resources that are available and at their disposal in an effort to resuscitate the patient • Clinicians have concerns about neurological outcome if the patient is resuscitated • Clinicians and/or family members may have differing opinions that death is imminent • ED clinicians may, however, continue resuscitation efforts despite obvious signs of death because of other factors (e.g., SIDS, pediatric trauma)	*Physical/symptoms* - Consider withholding/withdrawing life-sustaining therapies and medicate for distressing symptoms *Psychological and social* - Clarification of goals of care and match interventions to these goals - Assess for advance directives - Family witnessed resuscitation - Skillful delivery of serious news and/or death notification *Spiritual* - Chaplain, social worker, or any clinician - Cultural considerations for postmortem care
3. Pre-hospital resuscitation with survival until admission	• EMTs and ED clinicians use various signs of mortality to achieve perceptions of approaching death	

Trajectory	Characteristics	Palliative care interventions for the patient or family
3a. Resuscitative efforts are likely to be effective	• ED clinicians strive to save a life because of their perception that the patient is likely to survive • ED clinicians use aggressive/invasive/heroic efforts in attempt to resuscitate the patient • Clinicians do not perceive that death is a probability because they fully engage in resuscitative interventions	*Physical/symptoms* - Consider pain and symptom medications that will not interfere with hemodynamics (e.g., fentanyl) *Psychological and social* - Clarification of goals of care and match interventions to these goals - Assess for advance directives - Determine how decisions are made within the family (patient autonomy vs. shared decision making) - Family witnessed resuscitation - Skillful delivery of serious news *Spiritual* - Chaplain, social worker, or any clinician
3b. Resuscitative efforts are unlikely to be effective	• Uncertainty as to the ending of a patient's life • Resuscitation interventions may have a temporary effect to maintain signs of life • Clinical actions: - are designed to prove to the family and sometimes to themselves that death is the only possible outcome; - are in agreement with the patient's previously stated wishes in an advance directive; - are congruent with patient/family wishes or expectations to protect the clinician and hospital from litigation; - are congruent with the clinician's own moral values; - are congruent with acceptable standards of practice to protect the clinicians' and hospital's reputation and to avoid litigation	*Physical/symptoms* - Consider pain and symptom medications that will not interfere with hemodynamics (e.g., fentanyl) - Consider withholding/withdrawing life-sustaining therapies and medicate for distressing symptoms *Psychological and social* - Clarification of goals of care and match interventions to these goals - Assess for advance directives - Determine how decisions are made within the family (patient autonomy vs. shared decision making) - Family witnessed resuscitation - Skillful delivery of serious news *Spiritual* - Chaplain, social worker, or any clinician
4. Terminally ill and comes to the ED	• Patient, family, and primary provider achieve informal recognition and establish formal prognostication/certification that death is near (e.g., prognosis <6 months enabling hospice enrolment) • Family nonetheless activates emergency medical system (e.g., calls 911) to bring patient to the ED because of: - misunderstanding of role of hospice - lack of experiential knowledge of signs of impending death - cultural/spiritual considerations	*Physical/symptoms* - Pain and symptom medications - Consider withholding/withdrawing life-sustaining therapies and medicate for distressing symptoms *Psychological and social* - Assess the reasons for coming to the ED - Clarification of goals of care and match interventions to these goals - Assess for advance directives - Determine how decisions are made within the family (patient autonomy vs. shared decision making) - Assess caregiver coping - Assess caregiver resource network and support - Family witnessed resuscitation - Skillful delivery of serious news *Spiritual* - Chaplain, social worker, or any clinician
5. Frail and hovering near death	• Patients are frail and critically ill and share many aspects with the terminally ill patient population (e.g., poor health/functional status) • ED clinicians, although uncertain, anticipate that the patient will die during this hospitalization • No informal recognition or formal prognostication/certification that death is near (e.g., no prognosis <6 months) • Absence of this recognition or certification process causes ED clinicians to question the hopes and goals of the therapies that they initiate for the patient	*Physical/symptoms* - Pain and symptom medications - Consider withholding/withdrawing life-sustaining therapies and medicate for distressing symptoms *Psychological and social* - Assess the reasons for coming to the ED - Clarification of goals of care and match interventions to these goals - Assess for advance directives - Determine how decisions are made within the family (patient autonomy vs. shared decision making)

Table 30.1 B) *(cont.)*

Trajectory	Characteristics	Palliative care interventions for the patient or family
		- Assess caregiver coping
		- Assess caregiver resource network and support
		- Skillful delivery of serious news
		Spiritual
		- Chaplain, social worker, or any clinician
6. Alive and interactive on arrival, but arrests in the ED	• Death unexpected for both the clinicians and the family • ED clinicians are surprised by the sudden death or arrest of the patient while they are in the process of trying to rule in or rule out life-threatening pathology or are actively trying to treat life-threatening pathology • ED clinicians use all appropriate resources in an attempt to resuscitate the patient	*Physical/symptoms* - Pain and symptom medications *Psychological and social* - Clarification of goals of care and match interventions to these goals - Assess for advance directives - Determine how decisions are made within the family (patient autonomy vs. shared decision making) - Family witnessed resuscitation - Skillful delivery of serious news *Spiritual* - Chaplain, social worker, or any clinician
7. Potentially preventable death by omission or commission	• The patient is approaching death and is dying but this is not recognized until it is potentially too late • Can occur in both routine and unfamiliar situations • Index of suspicion of death or adverse event is not high and mistakes may be made • ED clinicians' perceptions and what they choose to focus their attention on may lead them down the wrong evaluation or treatment pathway • The clinicians either forget guidelines for care, prioritize care for different patients differently, become desensitized to the care needs of the patient, or lack knowledge about how to deliver the best possible care	*Physical/symptoms* - Consider pain and symptom medications that will not interfere with hemodynamics (e.g., fentanyl) - Consider withholding/withdrawing life-sustaining therapies and medicate for distressing symptoms *Psychological and social* - Clarification of goals of care and match interventions to these goals - Assess for advance directives - Determine how decisions are made within the family (patient autonomy vs. shared decision making) - Family witnessed resuscitation - Skillful delivery of serious news and death notification *Spiritual* - Chaplain, social worker, or any clinician

EMT = Emergency medical technician
Reproduced with permission from reference [13].

arrest is the return of spontaneous circulation prior to arrival in the ED [25].

Patients with cancer have worse outcomes overall, with 6.2% survival to discharge from in-hospital cardiac arrest [26]. One well-performed retrospective review of 243 cancer patients over a 5-year period in a single tertiary care cancer hospital demonstrated that when cardiac arrest occurred as a result of a gradual medical decline including sepsis, progressive cardiogenic shock, acidosis, or multiple organ dysfunction syndrome, survival to discharge was zero [27].

Patients and families are generally uninformed of the likely outcomes of CPR [28]. When given information regarding outcomes of CPR, patients with advanced illness often change their preferences in favor of avoiding CPR [29,30].

Pre-hospital

Attitudes surrounding end-of-life care and interventions are improving with pre-hospital providers. There is strong support for honoring advance directives, but additional experience, training, and protocol-based support is needed to improve comfort in appropriately withholding life-sustaining interventions [31]. Specific rules for termination of care, policy implementation, and coordinated systems of palliative and emergency care have all been effective interventions to limit non-beneficial attempts at CPR in the pre-hospital setting [32–34].

Family presence in resuscitation

Given the poor prognosis associated with CPR, it is important to anticipate the grieving process of the family while attempting to effect return of spontaneous circulation. A direct approach to supporting families is to allow their presence while performing CPR in the ED. Family presence during resuscitation is gaining acceptance, particularly in pediatric EDs [35,36]. In addition, family presence has not been shown to cause disruption during CPR, and families reflect positively on the ability to be present during these

Table 30.2. Nine steps of family presence in resuscitation

Step	Process	Example phrases
1: Introduction	Family support person introduces family members to clinicians performing resuscitation Resuscitation team leader introduces self to family	"This is George Smith, the son of our patient" "I am Dr. Jones and I am providing the medical care to your mother"
2: Status	Review current condition in concrete terms	"Your mother's heart is not pumping, and we are trying to make the heart start pumping again"
3: Prognosis	Provide a warning statement	"We are worried that your mother may not survive this very serious situation"
4: Plan	State what will be done next	"We will continue to provide all possible medical interventions to try to get your mother's heart to start pumping again"
5: Provide	Continue resuscitation efforts	
6: Review	ROSC* a. Review: Summarize events b. Plan: Explain process of moving to the intensive care unit or other next level of care No ROSC a. Overview: State the event b. Review: Paint the picture c. Recommendations: Ask for team input for concordance d. Transition: Prepare the family for the discontinuation e. Pronouncement of death f. Condolence: provide empathic communication, establish silence by turning off all alarms and medical equipment, and provide space for family to be present with their loved one	a. "Ms. Smith has sustained an unwitnessed cardiac arrest with no return of spontaneous circulation" b. "We have assured adequate ventilation and chest compressions for 20 minutes and have not achieved spontaneous circulation with a persistent non-perfusing rhythm of pulseless electrical activity on the monitor" c. "Are there any additional recommendations from the resuscitation team at this time?" d. "I'm afraid your mother is not going to survive. Would you like to come closer to say 'good bye'? Are there other family members outside the room who may need to say 'goodbye'?" e. "The patient is pronounced dead at 02:36 am" f. "I'm so sorry for your loss. I would like to inform the rest of your family if that is alright. Would you like to come with me or remain here with your mother?"
7: Acknowledge	Communicate recognition of the effort of the medical team	"Thank you team for your skill and commitment in this extremely difficult situation"
8: Inform	Resuscitation team leader offers to communicate outcome and provide formal death disclosure to remaining family in a quiet room	See Table 30.3, "Death disclosure"
9: Self and staff care	Resuscitation leader debriefs team and provides time for self-reflection prior to returning to patient care	"Let's take a moment to reflect on the process of the case, and how we are doing personally" "Any thoughts on what went well or what could have been improved?" "Let's please take a moment to honor the life of this patient and the grief of their loved ones. Please also take a moment to regroup alone or with the support of one another"

*Return of spontaneous circulation.

aggressive attempts at preventing death, possibly as an aspect of pre-grieving. Despite this support, practice patterns are variable and no universal guidelines yet exist to assist in the process of including families during resuscitative efforts. Protocols are generally recommended to assist in assuring a smooth process [37–39]. While encouraged, family presence should be agreed upon among the involved providers prior to allowing family members into the room. A support person without clinical duties should be assigned to stay with a predetermined and limited number of family members at any given time to assure understanding, psychosocial support, and a controlled environment [40]. A useful structure based on the Education in Palliative and End of Life-Emergency Medicine (EPEC-EM) curriculum breaks the process down into nine steps (see Tables 30.2 and 30.3) [41].

Rapid identification and assessment in the ED

SPEED

In addition to life-threatening circumstances, patients with palliative care needs often enter the hospital through the ED [42]. Several outcomes of patient and family satisfaction as well as costs of care can be improved with early palliative care involvement [43,44]. The usual emergency focus on identifying or ruling out the life-threat, intervening, and establishing disposition may not recognize the needs of patients with advanced progressive illness. Efforts to identify stable patients with unmet palliative care needs in the ED have generally relied on trained practitioners placed there

Table 30.3. Death disclosure [41,49]

1: Preparation	• Family arrival
	• Available information is clear, including full name of patient
	• Prepared interdisciplinary team enters room together with cell phones and pagers given to colleagues
	• Environment
	• Quiet and respectful
	• Seating and facial tissues
2: Engagement	• Introductions with appropriately serious demeanor
	• Introduce the team
	• Verify the identity of the patient by full name
	• Identify the person closest to the patient (the primary survivor) and their relationship to the patient
	• Children
	• Recommend, based on age and maturity, whether children should be present initially
	• Sit down
	• Closest to primary survivor, whether or not they choose to sit
	• Maintain culturally sensitive body language with position and touch
3: Transition	• Relate information about events immediately preceding death
	• Example: "I'm not sure what you know about what has happened, but I'm afraid I have some bad news about (your father, Mr. Jones) …"
4: "Dead" or "Died"	• Avoid euphemisms
	• Example: "I'm afraid (your father, John Jones) has died"
5: Reaction tolerance	• Time and presence
	• Empathic communication
	• Acknowledge
	• "This is not what you were expecting"
	• "You seem angry"
	• Legitimize
	• "Many people in this situation would feel angry"
	• Explore
	• "Can you tell me what your are most concerned about right now?"
	• Empathize
	• "I wish the news were better"
	• Commit
	• "I will make sure we have a good plan in place before you leave today" [80]
6: Information	• Speak on lack of suffering and unconsciousness prior to death
	• Request needed information to report on cause of death
	• Example: "To better understand what happened to (deceased patient's name), may I ask you some questions about his/her medical history? I can also tell you what we know and answer any questions you may have"
7: Viewing	• Offer viewing with staff guidance
8: Conclusion	• Offer condolences and contact information for any additional questions
	• If the deceased is a child, offer something tangible such as a lock of the child's hair
9: Self and staff care	• Debrief
	• Check-in

[45,46]. In an effort to simplify the identification of these patients, a consensus panel of experts designed the Screen for Palliative and End of Life Care Needs in the Emergency Department (SPEED). It is a brief multidimensional assessment tool that has been tested for reliability and validity in cancer patients presenting to the ED, and can be rapidly administered as early as triage [47]. Five major domains of palliative care needs are addressed with the SPEED tool: physical, therapeutic, psychological, social, and spiritual. In a recent assessment of this tool, nearly half of patients screened had pain in the moderate to severe range at the time of presentation. One-quarter of patients had rated at least moderate difficulty on several functional parameters such as medication problems, care needs at home, acquiring medical care consistent with their goals, and feeling generally overwhelmed [48].

ABCD

In both trauma and non-trauma patients in critical condition, initial assessment and intervention involves a standard "ABCD" sequence of "Airway," then "Breathing," then "Circulation," then "Disability." For patients in critical condition who are in functional trajectory near the end of life, a similar approach can provide a structure for active intervention while simultaneously addressing the goals of the patient and family. The following section is an adaptation of the ABCD structured approach to rapid palliative care assessment from EPEC-EM [49].

Advance directive

The presence of an advance directive can change the course of emergency decision making. It is tangible evidence of the autonomous perspective of the patient, which is one of the most important guiding principles in bioethics, whether in the ED or elsewhere. When physicians act in good faith, based on reasonable evidence, and exercise good professional judgment, the application of an order to not attempt resuscitation is legally and ethically supportable [50,51]. The reverse must be considered as well. If there is ample evidence in an available advance directive to withhold life-sustaining interventions, and the evidence is willfully ignored, then a physician may be exposed to liability [52]. When applied systematically, standardized forms such as the Physician Orders for Life Sustaining Treatments (POLST) assure that life-sustaining interventions are easily recognized and applied consistent with the patient's expressed goals [53].

If the patient's critical condition is the natural consequence of the progression of disease, then the advance directive is often useful in guiding decision making. Despite this general durability, it should be noted that there are times when acting on an advance directive does not support an ethically sound decision. The context of an advance directive must always be considered prior to deciding to withhold life-sustaining interventions. A particularly challenging example would be a patient with severe progressive illness and an advance directive who presents to the ED for attempted suicide. If the patient were acting in a state of suicidal depression, then like any other suicide attempt, the principles of autonomy would no longer apply [54,55]. In these difficult situations, the four basic principles of bioethics best help to guide our decision making by balancing questions of autonomy, beneficence, non-malfeasance, and justice.

Better symptom control

Symptoms can be addressed simultaneously while gathering additional information to guide more invasive interventions. Initially, less invasive interventions may be tried, such as biphasic positive airway pressure (BiPAP) or intravenous (IV) fluid resuscitation, until the goals for medical interventions are clear. During this time a social worker may be helpful in identifying and locating an appropriate surrogate decision maker to allow a brief review of goals for medical intervention. Pain, dyspnea, and delirium are disturbingly common symptoms that can be managed quickly in most patients, even as goals are evolving.

When a patient enters the ED near the end of life, acute severe pain must be addressed immediately. This remains true even if the patient is hypotensive with poor renal function. In such a case, fentanyl would be a reasonable choice. It has the least effect on blood pressure among opioids and is not dependent on renal function for excretion. Doses as low as 0.25–0.50 μg/kg may be administered every 5 minutes until pain is controlled or unacceptable side effects ensue limiting continuation, such as lethargy or vomiting. In other situations, morphine or hydromorphone would be acceptable considerations in appropriate equivalent doses. If the patient is opioid tolerant and in acute severe pain, the recommended initial intravenous dose is 10–20% of the total equivalent opioid taken in the prior 24 hours. After a 15-minute reassessment (a reasonable estimate of the concentration maximum for parenteral dosing), if the patient remains alert and pain is unaffected, the recommendation is to increase the dose by 50–100%. If the pain score is improved at all, and the patient remains alert, but the pain is persistent and moderate to severe, the recommendation is to repeat the initial calculated dose. The National Comprehensive Cancer Network provides comprehensive guidelines for the management of cancer pain, including acute situations. The guidelines are based on best evidence and expert consensus, and provide an excellent basis for safe general pain management in patients at the end of life [56]. The recommendations reflect similar guidelines from the American Pain Society [57].

Dyspnea may be the most distressing symptom experienced at the end of life [58]. Attempts at treating the underlying cause of dyspnea are certainly the most effective intervention when possible. Symptom control may begin with commonly used ED interventions such as oxygen, nebulized beta agonist therapy, or diuretics depending on the situation. Other simple mechanical and environmental interventions may also be effective, such as providing a fan, open space, a quiet environment, and upright positioning to alleviate the diaphragmatic work of breathing. When the underlying condition is no longer treatable, or when other interventions are inadequate, adjunctive opioid treatment should be considered. While there is ample evidence to support the safe use of opioids for intractable dyspnea, they remain underutilized [59]. Their mechanism is complex, but in part involves a reduction in brain stimulation at a small area of the periaqueductal gray matter, which is more broadly stimulated by pain experiences [60,61]. Doses for opioid-naïve patients may be as low as one-tenth to one-third the usual calculated doses for severe pain, whereas doses of opioid-tolerant patients may involve a 25% increase in usual breakthrough pain dose equivalent. When repeated doses of opioids appear inadequate or if there is a significant anxiety component to the dyspnea, midazolam may be added at low incremental doses such as 1–2 mg every 5 minutes until effective [62].

In addition to pain and dyspnea, delirium is also a disturbing and common symptom at the end of life. Delirium can be defined as an acute (hours to days) waxing and waning alteration of consciousness with a change in cognitive function. The focus of treatment is on identifying and reversing the cause of delirium whenever possible. Of dying cancer patients, delirium is present in up to 88%, but a reversible cause for delirium may be discovered in only 50% of these cases [63]. With acutely agitated delirium, immediate intervention is warranted. Haloperidol is considered an effective initial intervention for delirium, with the advantage of having the least sedating effects.

Table 30.4. C-U-R-V-E-S

Step 1 Determine capacity for medical decision making	**C**ommunicate and choose?	Is the patient able to communicate an objective choice among alternatives?
	Understand?	Can the patient recognize the "risks, benefits, alternatives, and consequences" in their choices?
	Reason?	Does the patient rationally explain why they are making the choice among other choices?
	Value?	Is the decision consistent with the patient's known system of values?
Step 2 Determine need to immediately intervene	**E**mergency?	Is there an immediate risk to life or limb?
	Surrogate?	Is there a need for, and reasonably available, surrogate decision maker?*

*Order of surrogates for medical decision making is based on applicable state law, and decisions should always consider the terms of a legitimate advance directive.

Initial doses of 0.5–1.0 mg subcutaneously (SC) may be given every 30–60 minutes until effective and then scheduled every 6 hours. In severe agitation with inadequate response to halo-peridol or other neuroleptic, benzodiazepines such as loraze-pam (0.5–1.0 mg IV or SC) may be added every 1–2 hours until effective. If rapid onset or if sedation is required, midazolam may be titrated in 1–2 mg increments IV every 5 minutes until effective, then repeated at the effective dose every 6 hours [64].

Capacity

Decisions for all medical care should be based on the patient's own statements, with autonomy being the guiding and primary bioethical principle. If the patient is lacking decisional capacity, then surrogate decision makers must be sought to represent the patient's perspective whenever possible. If there is an advance directive, then the surrogate would hopefully support the patient's statements in the advance directive to guide medical recommendations.

Advance directives are often a reliable guide for medical interventions. In addition, they offer information directly from the patient, thereby supporting the patient's autonomous decision making. Occasionally, the advance directive may be medically inconsistent or difficult to apply to the particular circumstance. In these situations, which may not be uncommon, the most important designation on any advance directive is that of a surrogate or health care decision maker, sometimes referred to as the "durable power of attorney for health care." If that individual or the highest-level legal surrogate (which is state specific) is reasonably available at the time of presentation and understands the patient's previously expressed goals of care, then immediate decision making can be negotiated quickly. Multiple and equally important issues regarding the involvement of the patient or the surrogate need to be addressed simultaneously prior to medical intervention, even with the threat to life and limb. A useful mnemonic, CURVES, uses a series of inquiries in a two-step process to rapidly assess the situation, and to determine when to intervene (see Table 30.4) [65].

Is there a reasonably available surrogate decision maker? This inquiry must consider the order of surrogates for medical decision making based on applicable state law. This inquiry also assumes that any available advance directive is considered.

If an immediate life or limb threat exists, the patient does not have the capacity for medical decision making, and a legal surrogate cannot reasonably be accessed, then intervention must be guided by available advance directives. If there is no advance directive in such situations, intervention must proceed based on the best interest of the patient with the goal being the immediate preservation of life and limb. If the patient has capacity, or the surrogate decision maker is present, goals of medical interventions must then be determined immediately. For example, a medical goal of intubation might be to prevent immediate or short-term progression to death. If the goal of the patient is to not die on mechanical ventilation in an ICU and this is a predictable outcome of the intubation due to the patient's premorbid and comorbid conditions, then intubation would not be consistent with the patient's autonomously expressed goals. Therefore, attempts should be made to understand the patient's perspective prior to intervention, including an immediate life threat. The EPEC-EM curriculum provides an excellent structure for applying a rapid approach to establishing these goals in patients with advanced illness [49]. The following is an adaptation of that structure, which is rooted in the "ask-tell-ask" model for effective communication.

Goals of care: the six steps

1. Prepare

   In order to initiate a reasonable and expedient discussion of goals of care, gather as much information as possible including the advance directive if available. Next, if the patient lacks capacity for medical decision making, make reasonable efforts to communicate with the most appropriate surrogate decision maker in order of legal designation.

2. Inquire

   (i) Known information
   - The first and most important step is asking what is already known about the patient's condition. This establishes whether the clinicians and the patient and family have the same or different understandings of the situation.

   (ii) Expectations/hopes
   - The next and crucial step is to establish the patient's and family's expectations for the overall outcomes of medical interventions. This helps the emergency clinician assess whether those goals are realistically achievable. If the patient is clearly dying, and the family

states, "I know dad is going to die, I just don't want to see him suffer," then subsequent communications can guide medical interventions to assure as comfortable and peaceful a death as possible. On the other hand, if the same patient's family were to communicate their hope is to see the patient leave the hospital in a functional condition, then a different communication would need to happen prior to agreeing to medical interventions that would not be expected to achieve those goals.

3. Present options

When attempting to present possible or available approaches to the patient's care, it is often useful to speak in more general but related terms to help create a more objective dialogue. The initial communication should help to identify the current condition of the patient such as, "When we see patients who are close to dying …" or "when we see patients who appear to only have days or weeks left to live …" The second part of the communication offers options and should be related to what interventions are possible and what the expected outcomes would be. The basis of this approach is essentially providing informed consent prior to intervention. It is important to keep in mind that in the case of a dying patient, the likely outcome with or without aggressive interventions is still death. The death may occur at a later point with life-sustaining interventions such as intubation, but the outcome would be death in the ICU as opposed to other possibilities such as an inpatient hospice unit or at home with hospice. If questions remain about likely outcomes of initiating life-sustaining interventions in a particular situation, consultation from the critical care team may be helpful.

4. Recommend

Once the perspective of the patient is presented, the options for intervention provided, then as with most clinical communications with patients and families, a recommendation should be given. Emergency clinicians are in a profoundly important position to assist in medical decision making by recommending interventions most consistent with the goals of the patient and family.

5. Agree

With the patient or surrogate decision maker, the clinician can now establish agreement to proceed and with appropriate interventions. If outcomes are unclear and goals remain uncertain, then the default is always toward life-sustaining interventions to allow the family more time. In such situations, the communications prior to the interventions will resonate and promote ongoing dialogue that is likely to continue in the ICU.

6. Plan

The final plan of care is driven by agreed goals for interventions. If the patient is actively dying, and the agreement is to limit immediate suffering, then perhaps aggressive symptom management is the plan. In such situations, the patient may not be reasonably moved from the environment of the ED. The primary plan may be to control the environment and create as much privacy as possible while remaining in the ED. For example, the patient may need to be moved to a closed room, monitors turned off, phlebotomy avoided, and vital signs checks discontinued. With the frequent assessments and aggressive treatments involved, such situations may require a nurse-staffing adjustment. If the family is hopeful for an unrealistic outcome with life-sustaining interventions under way, final communications should strive to share in the hope for the same outcome while preparing the family for the likelihood of deterioration. In common parlance: "hope for the best, and prepare for the worst."

Decision and disposition

Once the goals of care are clear in a critical situation, final decisions may be made about proceeding, avoiding, or discontinuing critical interventions.

Ventilator discontinuation

There are times when patients are already undergoing life-sustaining interventions that are clearly inconsistent with previously communicated goals of care. An important example is the patient who is placed on a ventilator prior to the availability of an advance directive or reliable surrogate decision maker that would unequivocally challenge the intervention. Once concordance is established that the ventilator is inconsistent with the patient's goals of care, intervention must now involve the removal of the ventilator. With the focus having shifted away from life-sustaining interventions, it may not be possible to transfer such a patient to an ICU. However, if there are available beds, and the critical care team is comfortable with the process, ICU transfer may still be possible. Some hospitals may have access to an inpatient hospice or palliative care unit that may consider receiving the patient and performing the ventilator withdrawal after the patient has left the ED. There may be advantages to this arrangement if available and if acceptable to the family. The environment would likely be more peaceful, the patient would be supported by expert symptom management, and the family would be given expert communications and sustained bereavement support. Most other situations require the emergency clinician to perform this procedure independently and skillfully. A structured approach assures that the process is safe, comfortable, and efficient.

The first and most important step is to establish consensus on whether or not to proceed with ventilator discontinuation. An existing advance directive or the statements from a reliable surrogate decision maker should guide a perspective from the patient's point of view given the medical circumstances. If the goals of the patient are clearly inconsistent with being maintained on a ventilator, then interdisciplinary professionals available to the ED should be brought together to assess and confer opinions. Available interdisciplinary team members may include nurses, physicians, social workers, chaplains, or other professionals. The intent is to verify as objectively as possible that the goals of the patient are incompatible with maintaining the ventilator, and thus requiring expedient removal [66].

Documentation of the purpose of performing the procedure in the ED should be the next step. This should be treated like an informed consent and should be documented in a similar manner. Like any other procedure, the risks, benefits, and alternatives must be communicated and understood by the surrogate decision makers. The concordance of the family and the interdisciplinary team should also be documented, along with a clear statement about how the intervention of removal of the ventilator is expected to provide benefit for the patient.

Once consensus to proceed is established and documented, the family must then be informed of the process and given explicit preparation for what to expect. For example, given the noise, lack of privacy, and lack of space common to many EDs, the patient may need to be moved to a different area. It would be prudent to inform the family and encourage the removal of monitors and alarms to limit distraction away from the patient's comfort as the focus of care. Another consideration is whether to maintain endotracheal intubation when discontinuing the ventilator. If airway obstruction is a concern, then maintaining the endotracheal intubation may be preferable to extubation when discontinuing the ventilator. It is important in these situations that other medical interventions to assure comfort are emphasized, such as judicious use of opioids or benzodiazepines. It is important to note that there is increasing evidence that appropriate dosing of opioids for dyspnea and benzodiazepines for anxiety at the end of life would not be expected to hasten death [67,68].

In preparing the family for what to expect, it is crucial to describe the predictable transition from ventilator homeostasis to ventilator independence. It is important to distinguish between normal expected reflex responses (such as apneic pauses and gasp reflexes) and signs of distress (such as accessory muscle use, nasal flaring, grunting, or facial grimacing). Family engagement with the patient should be encouraged with gentle touch or verbal reassurances. Finally, the family must be prepared for the possibility that the patient may continue breathing. Depending on the circumstances, this may continue for several days. In this case, the patient would need to be admitted to the hospital or to an inpatient hospice or palliative care unit. If the patient is likely to die in the ED, symptoms must be managed aggressively with as much interdisciplinary support as possible for the family throughout the dying process.

End of life

The actively dying patient

When patients who are actively dying present to the ED, the focus of care shifts away from life-sustaining interventions and toward comfort for the patient and the family. The clinician must first identify these situations, then intervene with care and compassion [69]. Family members may be unable to physically or psychologically care for the patient who is actively dying at home, even when hospice has been involved. Respiratory distress or an acute neurologic change is the most common reason patients present to the ED at the end of life [70].

A recent history of events at home may help recognize the actively dying patient prior to obvious signs that the patient is physiologically dying. Over several days or weeks, patients become increasingly weak and socially withdrawn while losing the interest and capacity to maintain nutrition and hydration. As physiologic death becomes more apparent, vital signs become abnormal, skin becomes clammy and mottled, respirations become irregular with apneic periods, and loss of swallowing reflexes leads to pooling of secretions in the oropharynx that may bubble in the glottis. This is sometimes referred to as a "death rattle," and although not usually distressing to patients, may be distressing to family. Since the etiology is loss of swallowing reflexes, suctioning is generally ineffective and more likely to induce discomfort. The fastest and most effective intervention is glycopyrrolate (0.2–0.4 mg) or atropine (1 mg) IV or SC every 2 hours as needed [71,72].

Once the patient is identified as actively dying, concurrent interventions to optimize the dying process need to be initiated, such as accessing support staff, optimizing the environment of care, and actively managing physical symptoms. When a patient is dying, interdisciplinary support staff can be invaluable in addressing their complex psychological, social, and spiritual needs. Chaplaincy, social work, and other available support staff can provide reassurance to family and even alert clinicians to signs of distress, while assuring a comfortable milieu. If death is imminent, the patient should remain in the ED to minimize chaos for the family, and every attempt should be made to place patient and family in a quiet area with privacy [73]. Monitors and alarms should be turned off, phlebotomy discontinued, and vital sign assessments limited. Even if death is hours to days away, the patient may stay in the ED for a significant period of time given the long holding times in EDs. Emergency physicians should therefore be comfortable managing distressing symptoms [74]. For specific recommendations, see B (Better symptom control) above under ABCD.

Hospice patients in the ED

Hospice is a multidisciplinary care system that aims to provide supportive care to patients in the last phase of a terminal disease. The focus is on improving the quality of life by effectively managing pain and other symptoms, addressing emotional, psychosocial, and spiritual patient needs, while providing support and bereavement care to families. Patients are eligible for hospice care if they have a prognosis of 6 months or less if their disease runs its usual course and they desire medical treatment aimed at alleviating symptoms and maintaining quality of life, not life prolongation. Patients may have any diagnosis to qualify for hospice, with non-cancer diagnoses now representing over half of all patients admitted to hospice. Common non-cancer diagnoses include end-stage chronic obstructive pulmonary disease, congestive heart failure, dementia, failure to thrive, and progressive neuromuscular diseases. While enrollment in hospice decreases ED visits, it does not eliminate them [75].

Hospice patients presenting to the ED

Hospice patients may present to the ED for a variety of reasons. It is paramount not to assume the patient is in search of aggressive treatments, but to first clearly identify the trigger for the visit. Common triggers include poor symptom control (uncontrolled pain or terminal dyspnea), fever, malfunction of support devices (PEG tube), inability to cope with impending death, and caregiver fatigue. When early in the hospice relationship, these stressors may quickly become overwhelming before the hospice program has had sufficient opportunity to intervene. Recognize also that psychological, social, or spiritual issues may be contributing to the patient's distress in addition to their physical symptoms.

When a hospice patient presents to the ED, early communication with the hospice program is essential. This can help provide information on the patient's advance directives as well as help clarify their overall goals of care [76]. The emergency physician should treat any distressing physical symptoms the patient has and tailor further treatments based on their goals. Further discussion may be needed with the patient and the family, but generally this involves low-burden, noninvasive testing, and interventions to improve comfort or relieve burdensome symptoms. If consistent with goals, make every attempt to discharge the patient back home or to an inpatient hospice unit when appropriate.

Hospice referrals from the ED

Emergency physicians routinely manage patients with terminal illness. Early identification and referral of appropriate patients to hospice improves patient and family satisfaction with care at the end of life.

The Centers for Medicare and Medicaid Services provide general guidelines, which are available online to assist in recognizing the likelihood of a patient dying within 6 months [77]. If a patient is deemed eligible for hospice and their goals are aligned with a hospice approach to their care at the end of life, the emergency physician should introduce the concept of hospice to the patient and family. Whenever possible, the primary care physician should be involved prior to this discussion. It is often helpful to frame the discussion about hospice in accomplishing previously established goals of living with optimal comfort and support at this important time. Using this approach may help assuage a person's fears that hospice means "giving up" or is "a place where people die." If the patient is agreeable, the emergency clinician may initiate the referral with local hospice resources. A social worker can be very helpful in assisting this process [78,79].

Summary

With our increasingly elderly population, crises related to advanced progressive illness are expected to propel a greater need for emergency care that is sensitive to palliative care concerns. Using available interdisciplinary resources and a structured approach to palliative care principles, emergency specialists can quickly and skillfully guide patients and families through optimal medical care that best aligns with their goals.

References

1. Kung HC, Hoyert DL, Xu J, Murphy SL. Deaths: final data for 2005. *National vital statistics reports: from the Centers for Disease Control and Prevention, National Center for Health Statistics, National Vital Statistics System.* 2008;56:1–120.

2. NHAMCS 2008. *National Hospital Ambulatory Medical Care Survey: 2008 Emergency Department Summary Tables.*

3. Shugarman, LR, Lorenz, K, Lynn, J. SUPPORT study; End-of-life care: An agenda for policy improvement. *Clin Geriatr Med.* 2005;21(1):255–72.

4. Morden NE, Chang CH, Jacobson JO, et al. End-of-life care for Medicare beneficiaries with cancer is highly intensive overall and varies widely. *Health Aff (Millwood).* 2012;31(4):786–96.

5. Barnato AE, Herndon MB, Anthony DL, et al. Are regional variations in end-of-life care intensity explained by patient preferences? *Med Care.* 2007;45(5):86–393.

6. AAHPM, American Academy of Hospice and Palliative Medicine. *Statement on Clinical Practice Guidelines for Quality Palliative Care* (2006, online, accessed August 15, 2012).

7. Campbell ML, Guzman JA. Impact of a proactive approach to improve end-of-life care in a medical ICU. *Chest.* 2003;123:266–71.

8. Delgado-Guay MO, Parsons HA, Li Z, Palmer LJ, Bruera E. Symptom distress, interventions, and outcomes of intensive care unit cancer patients referred to a palliative care consult team. *Cancer.* 2009;115:437–45.

9. Gelfman LP, Meier DE, Morrison RS. Does palliative care improve quality? A survey of bereaved family members. *J Pain Symptom Management.* 2008;36:22–8.

10. Smith AK, Fisher J, Schonberg MA, et al. Am I doing the right thing? Provider perspectives on improving palliative care in the emergency department. *Ann Emerg Med.* 2009;54(1):86–93.

11. Lunney JR, Lynn J, Hogan C. Profiles of older medicare decedents. *J Am Geriatr Soc.* 2002;50:1108–12.

12. Mitchell SL, Kiely DK, Hamel MB, et al. Estimating prognosis for nursing home residents with advanced dementia. *JAMA.* 2004;291(22):2734–40.

13. Chan GK. Trajectories of approaching death in the emergency department: clinician narratives of patient transitions to the end of life. *J Pain Symptom Manage.* 2011;42(6):864–81.

14. Hancock K, Clayton JM, Parker SM, et al. Discrepant perceptions about end-of-life communication: a systematic review. *J Pain Symptom Manage.* 2007;34(2):190–200.

15. Fried TR, Bradley EH, O'leary J. Prognosis communication in serious illness: perceptions of older patients, caregivers, and clinicians. *J Am Geriatr Soc.* 2003;51:1398–403.

16. Christakis NA, Lamont EB. Extent and determinants of error in doctors' prognoses in terminally ill patients: prospective cohort study. *BMJ (Clin Res ed.).* 2000;320(7233):469–72.

17. Glare P, Virik K, Jones M, et al. A systematic review of physicians' survival predictions in terminally ill cancer patients. *BMJ (Clin Res ed.).* 2003;327:195–8.

18. Meropol NJ, Weinfurt KP, Burnett CB, et al. Perceptions of patients and physicians regarding phase I cancer clinical trials: implications for physician-patient communication. *J Clin Oncol.* 2003;21(13):2589–96.

19. Weeks JC, Cook EF, O'day SJ, et al. Relationship between cancer patients' predictions of prognosis and their treatment preferences. *JAMA.* 1998;279(21):1709–14.

20. Haidet P, Hamel MB, Davis RB, et al. Outcomes, preferences for resuscitation, and physician-patient communication among patients with metastatic colorectal cancer. SUPPORT Investigators. Study to Understand Prognoses and Preferences for Outcomes and Risks of Treatments. *Am J Med.* 1998;105(103):222–9.

21. Lamont EB, Siegler M. Paradoxes in cancer patients' advance care planning. *J Palliat Med.* 2000;3(1):27–35.

22. Kouwenhoven WB, Jude JR, Knickerbocker GG. Closed-chest cardiac massage. *JAMA.* 1960;173:1064–7.

23. Peberdy MA, Kaye W, Ornato JP, et al. Cardiopulmonary resuscitation of adults in the hospital: a report of 14720 cardiac arrests from the National Registry of Cardiopulmonary Resuscitation. *Resuscitation.* 2003;58(3):297–308.

24. Ebell MH, Becker LA, Barry HC, Hagen M. Survival after in-hospital cardiopulmonary resuscitation. A meta-analysis. *J General Intern Med.* 1998;13(12):805–16.

25. Sasson C, Rogers MA, Dahl, J, Kellermann AL. Predictors of survival from out-of-hospital cardiac arrest: a systematic review and meta-analysis. *Circulation Cardiovascular Qual Outcomes.* 2010;3(1):63–81.

26. Reisfield GM, Wallace SK, Munsell MF, et al. Survival in cancer patients undergoing in-hospital cardiopulmonary resuscitation: a meta-analysis. *Resuscitation.* 2006;71(2):152–60.

27. Ewer MS, Kish SK, Martin CG, Price KJ, Feeley TW. Characteristics of cardiac arrest in cancer patients as a predictor of survival after cardiopulmonary resuscitation. *Cancer.* 2001;92(7):1905–12.

28. Heyland DK, Frank C, Groll D, et al. Understanding cardiopulmonary resuscitation decision making: perspectives of seriously ill hospitalized patients and family members. *Chest.* 2006;130(2):419–28.

29. Murphy DJ, Burrows D, Santilli S, et al. The influence of the probability of survival on patients' preferences regarding cardiopulmonary resuscitation. *N Engl J Med.* 1994;330(8):545–9.

30. El-Jawahri A, Podgurski LM, Eichler AF, et al. Use of video to facilitate end-of-life discussions with patients with cancer: a randomized controlled trial. *J Clin Oncol.* 2010;28(2):305–10.

31. Stone SC, Abbott J, Mcclung CD, et al. Paramedic knowledge, attitudes, and training in end-of-life care. *Prehosp Disaster Med.* 2009;24(6):529–34.

32. Sherbino J, Keim SM, Davis DP. Clinical decision rules for termination of resuscitation in out-of-hospital cardiac arrest. *J Emerg Med.* 2010;38(1):80–6.

33. Grudzen CR, Hoffman JR, Koenig WJ, et al. The LA story: what happened after a new policy allowing paramedics to forgo resuscitation attempts in pre-hospital cardiac arrest. *Resuscitation.* 2010;81(6):685–90.

34. Burnod A, Lenclud G, Ricard-Hibon A, et al. Collaboration between pre-hospital emergency medical teams and palliative care networks allows a better respect of a patient's will. *Eur J Emerg Med.* 2012;19(1):46–7.

35. Morrison LJ, Kierzk G, Diekema, DS, et al. Part 3: Ethics: 2010 American Heart Association Guidelines for Cardiopulmonary Resuscitation and Emergency Cardiovascular Care. *Circulation.* 2010;122(18 Suppl. 3):S665–75.

36. Kleinman MD, deCaen AR, Chameides L, et al. Part 10: Pediatric Basic and Advanced Life Support: 2010 International Consensus on Cardiopulmonary Resuscitation and Emergency Cardiovascular Care Science With Treatment Recommendations. *Circulation.* 2010;122(16 Suppl. 2):S466–515.

37. Dingerman RS, Mitchell EA, Meyer EC, Curley, MA. Parent presence during complex invasive procedures and cardiopulmonary resuscitation: a systematic review of the literature. *Pediatrics.* 2007;120(4):842–54.

38. Dudley NC, Hansen KW, Furnival RA, et al. The effect of family presence on the efficiency of pediatric trauma resuscitations. *Ann Emerg Med.* 2009;53(6):777–84.

39. Tinsley C, Hill JB, Shah J, et al. Experience of families during cardiopulmonary resuscitation in a pediatric intensive care unit. *Pediatrics.* 2008;122(4):e799–804.

40. Farah MM, Thomas CA, Shaw, KN. Evidence-based guidelines for family presence in the resuscitation room. A step-by-step approach. *Pediatr Emerg Care.* 2007;23(8):587–91.

41. Desandre PL, May K. Palliative care in the emergency department. In *Oxford Textbook of Palliative Medicine*, 5th edn, ed. Cherny N, Fallon M, Kaasa S, Portenoy R, Currow D [To be published by Oxford University Press in 2014].

42. Institute of Medicine. *Hospital Based Emergency Care: At the Breaking Point* (Washington, DC: Institute of Medicine, 2006).

43. Casarett D, Pickard A, Bailey FA, et al. Do palliative consultations improve patient outcomes? *J Am Geriatr Soc.* 2008;56(4):593–9.

44. Morrison RS, Penrod JD, Cassel JB, et al. Cost savings associated with US hospital palliative care consultation programs. *Arch Intern Med.* 2008;168(16):1783–90.

45. Mahony SO, Blank A, Simpson J, et al. Preliminary report of a palliative care and case management project in an emergency department for chronically ill elderly patients. *J Urban Health.* 2008;85(3):443–51.

46. Glajchen M, Lawson R, Homel P, Desandre P, Todd KH. A rapid two-stage screening protocol for palliative care in the emergency department: a quality improvement initiative. *J Pain Symptom Manage.* 2011;42(5):657–62.

47. Richards CT, Gisondi MA, Chang CH, et al. Palliative care symptom assessment for patients with cancer in the emergency department: validation of the Screen for Palliative and End-of-life care needs in the Emergency Department instrument. *J Palliat Med.* 2011;14(6):757–64.

48. Quest T, Gisondi M, Engle K, et al. *Implementation of the Screening for Palliative Care Needs in the Emergency Department (SPEED) Instrument in Two Emergency Departments* (Boston, MA: Society for Academic Emergency Medicine Annual Meeting, 2011).

49. Emanuel L, Quest T. ed. *Education in Palliative and End-of-life Care of Emergency Medicine (EPEC-EM)* (Chicago, IL: EPEC Project, Buehler Center on Aging, Health & Society, Northwestern University, 2008).

50. In re Dinnerstein, 6 Mass. App. Ct. 466, 380 N. E. 2d, 134 (1978).

51. Cruzan v. Director of Missouri Department of Health, 109 S. C 3240 (1990).

52. Scheible v. Joseph Morse Geriatric Center Inc., District Court o Appeal of Florida, Fourth District, No. 4D07–3064 (2008).

53. Hickman SE, Nelson CA, Moss AH, et al. The consistency between treatments provided to nursing facility residents and orders on the physician orders for life-sustaining treatment form. *J Am Geriatr Soc.* 2011;59(11):2091–9.

54. Leeman C. Distinguishing among irrational suicide and other forms of hastened death: implications for clinical practice. *Psychosomatics.* 2009;50(3):185–91.

55. Entwistle V, Carter SM, Cribb A, Mccaffery K. Supporting patient autonomy: the importance of clinician-patient relationships. *J Gen Intern Med.* 2010;25(7):741–45.

56. National Comprehensive Cancer Network (2012). Adult Cancer Pain, v. 1.2012. NCCN Clinical Practice Guidelines in Oncology (NCCN Guidelines).

57. American Pain Society. *Principles of Analgesic Use in the Treatment of Acute Pain and Cancer Pain*, 6th edn (Glenview, IL: American Pain Society, 2008).

58. Campbell ML. Dyspnea prevalence, trajectories, and measurement in critical care and at life's end. *Curr Opin Support Palliative Care.* 2012;6(2):168–71.

59. Jennings AL, Davies AN, Higgins JP, Gibbs JS, Broadley KE. A systematic review of the use of opioids in the management of dyspnoea. *Thorax.* 2002;57(11):939–44.

60. Mahler DA. Understanding mechanisms and documenting plausibility of palliative interventions for dyspnea. *Curr Opin Support Palliative Care.* 2011;5(2):71–6.

61. Von Leupoldt A, Sommer T, Kegat S, et al. Down-regulation of insular cortex responses to dyspnea and pain in asthma. *Am J Resp Crit Care Med.* 2009;180(3):232–8.

62. Ben-Aharon I, Gafter-Gvili A, Paul M, Leibovici L, Stemmer SM. Interventions for alleviating cancer-related dyspnea: a systematic review. *J Clin Oncol.* 2008;26(14):2396–404.

63. Lawlor PG, Gagnon B, Mancini IL, et al. Occurrence, causes, and outcome of delirium in patients with advanced cancer: a prospective study. *Arch Intern Med.* 2000;160(6):786–94.

64. Centeno C, Sanz A, Bruera E. Delirium in advanced cancer patients. *Palliative Med.* 2004;18(3):184–94.

65. Chow GV, Czarny MJ, Hughes MT, Carrese JA. CURVES: a mnemonic for determining medical decision-making capacity and providing emergency treatment in the acute setting. *Chest.* 2010;137(2):421–7.

66. Curtis, J. Interventions to improve care during withdrawal of life-sustaining treatments. *J Palliat Med.* 2005;8(Suppl. 1):16–31.

67. Chan JT, Treece PD, Engleberg RA, et al. Association between narcotic and benzodiazepine use after withdrawal of life support and time to death. *Chest.* 2004;126(1):286–93.

68. Campbell MB, Bizeck KS, Thill M. Patient responses during rapid terminal weaning from mechanical ventilation: A prospective study. *Crit Care Med.* 1999;27(1):73–7.

69. Savory E, Marco CA. End-of-life issues in the acute and critically ill patient. *Scand J Trauma Resusc Emerg Med.* 2009;17(21):doi: 10.1186/1757-7241-17-21.

70. Lamba S, Nagurka R, Murano T, Zalenski RJ, Compton S. Early identification of dying trajectories in emergency department patients: Potential impact on hospital care. *J Palliat Med.* 2012;15(4):392–5.

71. Ferris FD. Last hours of living. *Clin Geriatr Med.* 2004;20(6):641–67.

72. Abraham JL. *The Last Days…and the Bereaved. A Physician's Guide to Pain and Symptom Management in Cancer Patients* (Baltimore, MD: The Johns Hopkins University Press, 2005), pp. 397–435.

73. Bookman K, Abbott J. Ethics Seminars: Withdrawal of treatment in the emergency department. When and how? *Soc Acad Emerg Med.* 2006;13(12):1328–32.

74. Chan GK. End-of-life models and emergency department care. *Acad Med.* 2004;11(1):79–86.

75. Zieske M, Abbott J. Ethics Seminars: The hospice patient in the ED: An ethical approach to understanding barriers and improving care. *Soc Acad Emerg Med.* 2011;18(11):1201–7.

76. Olsen ML, Bartlett AL, Moynihan TJ. Characterizing care of hospice patients in the hospital setting. *J Palliat Med.* 2011;12(2):185–9.

77. Centers for Medicare & Medicaid Services, Medicare Coverage Database [online]. Updated May 25, 2012. Local Coverage Determination (LCD) for Hospice: Determining Terminal Status (L32015). [Accessed September 6, 2012].

78. Lamba S, Mosenthal AC. Hospice and palliative medicine: A novel subspecialty of emergency medicine. *J Emerg Med.* 2010;43(5):1–5.

79. Lamba S, Quest TE. Hospice care and the emergency department: Rules, regulations, and referrals. *Ann Emerg Med.* 2011;57(3):282–90.

80. Fogarty LA, Curbow BA, Wingard JR, McDonnell K, Somerfield MR. Can 40 seconds of compassion reduce patient anxiety? *J Clin Oncol* 1999;17(1):371–9.

Chapter

31

Social services and case management

Ravi K. Murthy and Morsal R. Tahouni

Introduction

The gradual aging of the US population has led to a significant rise in emergency department visits by geriatric patients
[1,2]. Moreover, the "graying" of the "baby boomer" generation
is expected to lead to a further increase in the number of emergency department (ED) visits. An unforeseen consequence of
this rise is the risk posed to elderly patients in the days and
weeks that follow the ED visit. Multiple studies show that this
patient group suffers from increased recidivism, health care
utilization, adverse outcomes, and even mortality [1–5]. It is
only relatively recently that emergency medicine (EM) practitioners have become aware of the many issues facing these
patients.

Furthermore, this gradual aging of the population has led
to a concomitant increase in health care costs [6,7]. Health
care expenditures currently make up 17.6% of gross domestic
product, with an expected increase to 26% by 2035 [8], a percentage that is deemed incompatible with continued economic
growth by most economic analysts. A significant portion of
these expenditures comes from those 65 years and older [6–8],
either through Medicare, private insurance, or other sources.
With the impending rise of pay-for-performance and global
reimbursement, and greater focus on appropriate health care
utilization [9–11], there will be increased pressure on providers to minimize unnecessary costs while optimizing utilization
among the geriatric population.

This chapter aims to further delineate the issues facing
geriatric patients after an initial ED visit, and then to discuss
various methods aimed at reducing the risk of these issues.
Furthermore, this chapter will outline how an ED should
integrate its care with other providers involved with geriatric
patients. Finally, we discuss screening tools used to evaluate
whether elderly patients are safe to operate motor vehicles, and
the responsibility of the EM practitioner to discuss this issue
with their patients.

Issues facing geriatric patients in the ED

Over the last three decades, EDs have seen a significant increase
in the number of visits [12]. No group has experienced this more
than the geriatric patient population. Between 1993 and 2003,

patients aged 65 years and older experienced a 34% increase in
ED visits [1,12]. Moreover, if this trend continues, the number of geriatric ED visits could have increased to 11.7 million
by 2013, up from 6.4 million visits annually two decades prior
[1]. With this sharp increase in visits, EM providers should be
aware of some of the unique factors facing geriatric patients
both in the ED and in the time period that follows.

As a consequence of these increased visits, research into
the patterns and after-effects of a geriatric patient's ED visit has
grown significantly. Several factors have been found to differentiate the geriatric ED visit from those of other patients. When
they arrive at the ED, these patients tend to have longer length
of stay (LoS), require more resources than other patients, and
have more diagnostic tests performed [2,3]. Further, elderly
patients face higher levels of urgency and rates of admission
[2,3].

In addition, geriatric patients face higher rates of adverse
health outcomes in the time period following their visit. In
the first six months after discharge, ED recidivism tends to be
higher among geriatric patients than among other groups – as
high as 25% in one study [2–4,13]. This recidivism, coupled
with more frequent primary care physician (PCP) visits in
patients with frequent ED visits, leads to higher overall health
care utilization [4]. Geriatric patients are also more likely to
suffer from polypharmacy, and therefore are at increased risk
of suffering a medication-related complication when prescribed a new medication during a visit [13]. Moreover, after
discharge from the ED these patients have a higher risk of mortality and functional decline [2]. Finally, geriatric patients have
more difficulty understanding discharge instructions [3,14],
have higher levels of dissatisfaction with their visit, and are
more likely to leave with their initial problem unresolved [3].
These combined issues may make understanding the full clinical picture more difficult for providers. Overall, the geriatric
ED visit tends to be significantly more complex than those of
other patients (Table 31.1).

Adding to this complexity is the integration of ED care with
the multiple other sources of care a geriatric patient may be
receiving. Health care experts have long been advocating the
model of the medical home in the US to manage the multiple
medical issues faced by patients. This is especially important

Geriatric Emergency Medicine, ed. Joseph H. Kahn, Brendan G. Magauran Jr., and Jonathan S. Olshaker. Published by Cambridge University Press.
© Cambridge University Press 2014.

Table 31.1. Summary of trends of ED use by elderly patients

- More likely to be admitted
- Appropriate use of ED
- Overrepresented in the ED population
- More likely to arrive in daytime
- More likely to arrive via ambulance
- More medical diagnoses
- Serious illness
- More diagnostic tests
- Longer length of stay
- Do not understand instructions
- Not asked about ability for self-care
- Have worse functional outcomes
- Higher rate of recidivism
- Higher level of noncompliance
- More incorrect diagnoses
- Problem not resolved
- Higher ED charges

Adapted from Greif [3].

in geriatric patients, as they tend to have many complex medical issues and require more care providers (specialist, visiting nurses, home-health aides) than other patients. Failure to properly communicate with a patient's medical home may lead to difficulties in follow-up and establishment of appropriate services after a recent ED visit [15]. Furthermore, it may lead to increased ED recidivism [15].

It is for these reasons that EM providers should view an ED visit by a geriatric patient as a sentinel event in their health care. Once the provider begins to assess such a patient, they should be acutely aware of the various issues the patient faces both while in the ED and after discharge home. Awareness of these issues should prompt the provider to screen these patients more thoroughly, and engage services intended to avoid potential adverse outcomes.

Case management

One major difficulty in assessing the ever-increasing needs of the geriatric population is determining who will require further assistance after leaving the ED. It is well recognized that the initial visit to the ED can often be seen as a sentinel event, marking the functional decline of an elderly patient [16,17]. While many screening tools have been developed and studied, there still remains some debate as to what key factors are most important when implementing geriatric case management in the ED. Furthermore, where and when these interventions are to be implemented, and by whom, remains a further significant area of discussion.

First and foremost, ED providers should determine what model of case management would best suit their patient population. Multiple evidence-based models have been proposed and studied; however, further research has shown several key factors as important in developing a geriatrics case management program for the ED (see Figure 31.1) [18]. Having a keen understanding of these factors will help providers choose and develop a more effective program [18].

One of the most essential of these factors is determining the ideal place to implement case management. In the busy ED, adding additional tasks to the jobs of the already overworked staff runs the risk of making a challenging job nearly impossible [17]. As daunting as this may seem, there are several key reasons that make initiation of geriatric case management in the ED important. As noted earlier, the rate of visits from the elderly population is growing rapidly, and soon this age range will become the highest represented age group of ED visits [1,2]. Combined with the high rate of post-ED visit complications, rapid assessment of a geriatric patient will become important not just in minimizing post-visit complications, but also necessary in continuing the flow and throughput of a busy ED [1].

Additionally, the limited access to primary care providers continues to be an issue. As long as access to care is limited, the ED will act as the safety net to which patients will turn in times of illness [19,20]. Furthermore, with the institution of the Patient Protection and Affordable Care Act and a shift toward global payments as a reimbursement model, there will be increased pressure on EM practitioners to minimize health care costs. Screening from the ED can help avoid potentially unnecessary admissions and repeated ED visits, while making sure that those who do need admission are not overlooked. The above facts, combined with the convenience of the ED and the fact that a majority of hospital admissions continue to come via the ED [21], make it clear why this is an ideal place to begin the case management process.

Although we have established the importance of screening geriatric patients in the ED, the question remains as to who should conduct this screening. In most studies that evaluated geriatric screening in the ED, a specialized nurse was used to perform the screening [16,22–24]. This nurse, ancillary to the ED staff, was in charge of either screening the patient or, in some studies, assisting in the management of the patient. Because they are removed from the primary team providing care for the patient, these specialists are better equipped to evaluate for issues that may have been missed during the initial emergency evaluation [18]. This specialized staff may be charged with screening all geriatric patients, or focusing on those who present with special issues such as medication compliance, recent discharge from an inpatient service, repeated ED visits, a fall at home, or caregiver stress. Multiple studies have shown that these "aged care" specialists were successful in identifying those at risk, creating an active treatment plan for those being admitted, or creating a plan for follow-up for those being discharged [16,23–26].

It is important to note that that the people performing case management are specialized and trained for this role. The task of assessing and evaluating the geriatric patient is no simple matter. The role of a case manager necessitates a deeper look at the patient past their chief complaint into their functional status and other non-clinical issues [18]. This aspect can often be overlooked or bypassed by the staff treating their initial complaint. It is for this very important reason that both the medical and social evaluations be done in close connection, but by different and separately trained staff.

1. Evidence-based Practice Model

Practice models will continue to evolve around the identified and perceived needs of older patients and their caregivers that are associated with an index ED visit. Model effectiveness can be improved through using documented evidence around specific components (high-risk screening tools) or practices (post-discharge follow-up) to inform overall model development.

2. Nursing Clinical Delivery Involvement or Leadership

The involvement of nurses and mid-level clinicians to lead or be involved in the delivery of a broader multidisciplinary intervention allows them to address both the health and often interrelated social concerns of older patients, more so than social workers and other allied health professionals working in isolation rather than as part of an interdisciplinary team.

3. High-risk Screening

Given the clinical heterogeneity of the older population, high-risks screening with a validated risk-screening tool allows the most vulnerable patients to be identified and for their needs to be prioritized and addressed, especially within interventions challenged with limited staffing and resources. Furthermore, universal screening mechanisms ensure that vulnerable patients are not overlooked, especially if a patient could not be treated during an index ED visit, and give the case manager a basis on which to establish follow-up for these patients.

4. Focused Geriatric Assessment

Performing more focused as opposed to the more time-intensive and detailed comprehensive geriatric assessments that outpatient or hospital inpatient-based geriatricians usually perform allows for the more appropriate examination of a patient's problems that may otherwise be overlooked in general ED assessments. Identification of additional clinical and nonclinical issues such as an individual's functional status or social supports allows for care planning to look beyond the presenting complaint, which may more significantly affect the probability of revisitation.

5. Initiation of Care and Disposition Planning in the ED

Allowing for the initiation of care and disposition planning early during a patient's ED visit can help avoid inappropriate admissions and identify and facilitate necessary admissions. Ensuring that continuity of care is established before a patient is discharged can occur through the initiation of external communications and linkages with outside care providers during the visit.

6. Interprofessional and Capacity-building Work Practices

Having geriatric nurses and mid-level clinicians working in partnership with other ED, hospital, and primary care and community care providers, within and beyond the hospital, allows their unique expertise to be better understood and leveraged by others, enhancing the overall delivery of care within a system.

7. Post-ED Discharge Follow-up with Patients

The provision of follow-up with patients allows the integrity of earlier care and disposition planning efforts to be maintained or adapted in using these additional encounters to identify new or ongoing issues, solve problems, or further facilitate care as necessary.

8. Establishment of Evaluation and Monitoring Processes

All interventions should establish routine evaluation and monitoring processes to measure outcomes of interest and to improve on quality and effectiveness measures to continuously improve an organization's approach.

Adapted from Sinha et al. [18].

Figure 31.1. Key factors in developing a geriatrics case management program for the ED.

Given the scope of their work, case managers often need assistance in their job, and for this reason the ED social worker also plays a vital role in geriatric case management. While the case managers, with the physicians, are involved in the screening and building of a treatment plan, the social worker can be looked at as the glue that brings it together. They are generally charged with investigating family support, living conditions, and transportation for follow-up appointments, essentially ensuring that a treatment plan is realistic and feasible. Without this integral part of the team, successful interventions by case management would be significantly more difficult.

Another key factor to geriatric case management noted by several studies is the need for a multidisciplinary approach, no matter where the process begins [18,27], in order to ensure the success of that system. No one person or ED is equipped to deal with all aspects of the coordinated care needed for the complex needs of the geriatric patient [18]. Studies have shown that screening in the ED has been successful in identifying those that would require specialized care [23]. However, despite care management interventions in the ED, without a team equipped to handle the specific needs of the geriatric patient, there were no benefits to the patient regarding need for admission, length of stay, or functional decline [23]. It is at this point in care where the idea of a "medical home" becomes especially important. By ensuring proper communication with the gatekeeper of

a patient's care, the ED staff can help ensure proper implementation of a care plan.

Finally, any implemented case management program should have a mechanism for tracking and evaluating its intervention [18]. With any new system, monitoring outcomes is essential in making sure that the desired effect is being achieved. This process would also allow for continuous improvement of a program to reach its desired goals [18]. As an example, some studies used patient satisfaction of their care [24]. There is no clearly defined model of the best way to evaluate such a program, but it remains a key mechanism for allowing these programs to succeed.

Discharge planning

A significant problem when dealing with the geriatric population revolves around discharge, whether from the ED or the inpatient team. Studies have evaluated how well patients understood their discharge instructions, and furthermore, looking at four main areas regarding discharge: diagnosis of illness, course of illness, self-care, and return precautions [14]. They noted that over half the patients discharged did not understand the course of illness or the return precautions and 21% did not even understand the diagnosis itself [14]. Correlating with these statistics and demonstrating the importance of the issue there was a noted increase in adverse events in the groups that did not understand their diagnosis or course of illness [14].

Many studies have looked at how to improve the current discharge systems and noted key factors that seem to be more beneficial in preventing negative outcomes for patients and reducing ED recidivism. Nevertheless, a recurring factor in all the above studies is the use of a separate provider whose sole focus is discharge planning, their role often coinciding with that of the case management team. The role of this specialized discharge planner is one that extends over many fields and can have a great impact on outcomes. This provider has many roles in the ED. For example, they may give more education to patients at time of discharge, coordinate follow-up appointments, make follow-up calls to the patients, and are accessible to the patients after discharge. It was noted that the use of the planner in this setting reduced return visits and patients had higher rates of satisfaction at time of discharge [24].

Another critical factor is the need for coordinated care at time of discharge, not only with the ED and PCP, but with ancillary services as well. While extensive planning for discharge and outpatient management can be made from the ED, without the support of other services, there is little benefit to the geriatric patient [23]. Although discharge planning has been used to get better access to primary care or local health centers, the single most important factor in preventing of functional decline after an ED visit was found to be access to home care [16,22].

To further elucidate this factor, one study evaluated the effect of a multidisciplinary approach to discharge planning. The study found that when an ED geriatric assessment, an ED discharge planner, and a hospital-based multidisciplinary team were combined to create a 28-day post-discharge plan for geriatric patients, the results were remarkable. When compared with the standard discharge group at one month, the group that had coordinated care had significantly less use of resources (ED visits and hospital admissions) and a greater degree of normal mental and physical function [27]. Unfortunately, despite the positive effects, the overall mortality was not significantly different and the authors noted that even with these interventions, at 1 year, the same amount of functional decline was noted in patients admitted to the hospital [27]. Conversely, several other studies with similar interventions found that there was no significant decrease in ED utilization [4,25]. Unfortunately, the question as to what exact interventions will truly benefit the elderly remains unanswered.

Effectiveness of case management

There is an enormous amount of research into the area of geriatrics and case management due to the reasons highlighted above: increasing age of the population [1,2], increasing health care costs [6–8], and the increasing usage of the ED by the geriatric population [3]. The studies have shown that intervention in the ED is not only appropriate, but feasible [17,18]. Furthermore, these studies have identified a population at risk [23,24], by the use of ED case managers specialized in the field of geriatrics, in conjunction with ED staff and social workers. The identification of those at risk has led to interventions to prevent ED recidivism, functional decline in patients, and mortality. From this work, we have found that a multidisciplinary approach is required to address the needs of the geriatric patient, both in and out of the hospital [18,27,28]. However, despite multiple types of interventions, no combination has been found to decrease mortality after a hospital presentation or have a significant effect on functional decline and recidivism [4,23,25,27,29].

Of special note is the increased research into the concept of the geriatric ED. Often times, geriatric patients are cared for by staff and teams not ready to handle their needs [2,3]. In the geriatric ED, everything from its layout to types of beds and flooring, and even lighting could be tailored for the needs of the geriatric patient [30]. In this setting, practitioners would have the multidisciplinary approach and the specialists needed for their intricate care [28,30]. The importance of case management is emphasized even more in these models [28–30].

The future of geriatric case management will need to resolve what interventions have the greatest impact on patient care, along with what system is most effective in implementing these interventions. Current literature is equivocal about how best to implement a case management program, and has yet to clarify precisely which interventions will decrease mortality and recidivism. For the practicing EM physician, there are multiple models to choose from, based on the specific volume and need of their patient population. Further research will hopefully aid practitioners in developing and refining their case management programs.

Assessing older driver safety

One aspect of geriatric screening that is new to the ED is that of driving assessment. Over the last decade, the number of drivers 65 years and older has increased 20%, compared with 11% for all other driver groups [31]. This subgroup of drivers is at increased risk for being involved in a motor vehicle collision compared with all other groups aside from teenagers [32]. Recent reports in both the academic literature and the popular media have brought this issue into increased focus. Complicating matters is the fact that there are multiple issues at the core of driver assessment that have a great impact not only for the geriatric patient, but on public safety as well. With the significant increase in the number of older drivers [31], EM practitioners may have to be responsible for screening and assessing transportation mobility in their geriatric patients.

Various factors affect the ability of the geriatric patient to safely operate a motor vehicle. Decreases in visual acuity, cognitive ability, and functional ability make driving increasingly difficult [32–35]. Further, medical issues such as heart disease, dementia, and diabetes, and the medications used to treat these issues, may further affect driving ability [34,35]. Coupled with the increase in frailty that comes with aging, geriatric patients are not only at increased risk of being involved in a motor vehicle accident, but also of having more significant injuries when involved [36]. Moreover, individual mobility has a significant impact on the quality of life for older patients. Multiple studies show that driving cessation negatively impacts mental health, social involvement, independence and even health status and mortality [37,38]. This is the context in which EM practitioners should consider geriatric driver assessment.

There are currently multiple driver screening tools available for the geriatric patient, but a full review of all screening and assessment methods would be beyond the scope of this chapter. The vast majority were developed for use in the primary care setting, elderly driver programs, or state-run motor vehicle departments [39,40]. Unfortunately, none of these tools has been well validated in the literature [35, 39–41] and few have been evaluated for use in the ED setting. However, by reviewing the most recent literature, certain factors that have significant bearing upon the ability of geriatric patients to drive become clear.

The American Medical Association (AMA) has published one screening tool meant to serve as a foundation for provider screening of driving ability. The Assessment of Driving-Related Skills (ADReS), a part of the *Physician's Guide to Assessing and Counseling Older Drivers* published in conjunction with the AMA, evaluates three key areas related to the operation of a motor vehicle: vision, cognition, and motor/somatosensory function [35]. Participants are evaluated in multiple skills within each area, and then an assessment as to driving ability is made by the provider. The authors go on to note that evaluation of these skills serves as an indirect assessment of driving skill, and does not represent an individual's crash risk [35]. The evaluation is used to guide the provider's decision regarding whether or not the patient should be recommended to drive. Unfortunately, the full ADReS may be too unwieldy to be routinely performed in the ED. It better serves to illustrate to EM providers the various factors affecting driving performance, and when older patients may require further screening.

Other assessment tools involve the use of neuropsychologic testing, the Trail-Making Test B (TMT-B) being one such example. This short test may be predictive of difficulty in operating a motor vehicle [42]. One study has found this test is easily conducted within the ED setting, and may aid in screening older drivers for further assessment [39]. Furthermore, a CAGE-based screening tool, the 4C, is in development to also aid EM providers in screening older drivers. The 4C test evaluates patients in four areas: crash/citation, concern, clinical status, and cognition [43]. A score is assigned from one to four based on the patient's status in each category, with a higher score correlating with a higher driving risk. Those who failed the assessment were found to be more likely to fail a road test [43] (Figure 31.2).

Although these tools serve as an example of older driver screening, unfortunately there is currently little research validating the use of any of these tools in the ED. What is likely more important for the EM practitioner is to be aware of the multiple factors that affect an older patient's ability to operate a motor vehicle. These include patients with significant visual impairment, multiple severe medical conditions, significant neurocognitive dysfunction, history of recent motor vehicle crashes, or physical disability. These patients should be counseled to refrain from driving until further driving assessments can be made. Once counseled, these patients can be referred to

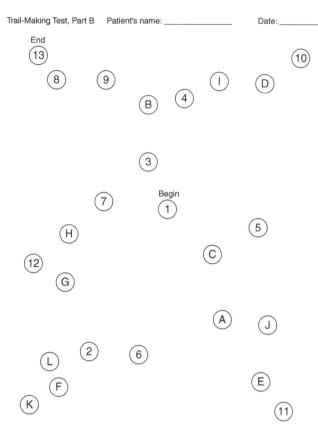

Figure 31.2. Trail-Making Test B, from ADReS (www.nhtsa.gov). Patients are instructed to connect the circles in ascending order, alternating between numerical and alphabetical values.

Reproduced from American Medical Association/National Highway Traffic Administration. *Physicians' Guide to Assessing and Counseling Older Drivers*, 2nd edn (Washington, DC: Dept of Transportation, 2003), 30 pp.

their primary medical doctor, an elderly driver program, or the state motor vehicle department to complete their assessment.

As the scope of case management expands within the ED, older driver screening may become a further responsibility. However, the question remains as to which patients should be screened within the ED. Screening every geriatric patient who drives may prove to be unfeasible with most ED resources, while screening those only recently involved in a motor vehicle crash has the potential to miss many patients with impaired driving ability. At this time, further research is required to delineate which patients should undergo screening.

Summary

The geriatric patient population faces many specific issues during and after an ED visit. These issues will only become more apparent as the number of emergency geriatric visits rises and places an increased burden on the already strained health care system. Adding to the vast responsibilities of the EM practitioner will be a thorough understanding of these issues and how to best address them.

Many appropriate screening tools have been discussed in this prior chapter. However, these must be implemented appropriately to have the best possible effect. Ideally, EDs with a significant geriatric population will use an integrated team approach to caring for geriatric patients, supplementing the existing staff with an on-site nurse, case managers, and social workers. This team will aid in identifying issues facing the patient both in the ED and after their disposition. They will also help in communicating with the patient's medical home, as well as with the patient's other care providers.

Discharge planning plays another vital role during the geriatric emergency visit. Studies have shown increased dissatisfaction and adverse medication reactions with poor discharge planning. Compounding this are higher rates of confusion about diagnosis and return, and improper follow-up. A coordinated health care team similar to those described above can help subvert these issues by carefully discussing instructions with patients and care providers, and reviewing medication changes and their possible interactions. Inclusion of a clinical pharmacist may aid further in discharge planning by reviewing new medications, checking for interactions with current medications, and helping in medication reconciliation. This team can also help coordinate follow-up with the patients' medical home, and set up post-discharge care such as a visiting nurse, physical/occupational therapy evaluation, or placement in a skilled nursing facility for further rehabilitation.

Furthermore, the EM provider must be aware of the special risk posed by driving to the geriatric population. Multiple factors contribute to the difficulty faced by geriatric patients when operating a motor vehicle. While no well-validated screening tool exists for use in the ED, providers may need to inquire about the driving habits of their older patients, and when appropriate, refer them for further evaluation, either through their primary medical doctor or through state-sponsored driving assessment programs. Simple tests such as the TMT-B may soon come into use for screening older drivers in the ED.

While the issues facing this patient population may be better defined, more research is required regarding which interventions reduce negative outcomes, and how to best implement them in the ED. As practitioners gain more experience evaluating and caring for this population with an integrated, multidisciplinary team, further evidence will help refine the advances already in progress. The onus is on the practitioner to be aware of this new research in the future.

Pearls and pitfalls

Geriatric ED visits are increasing annually, and are expected to increase over the next two decades.

These visits have been shown to be a significant marker for negative outcomes in the future, and practitioners ignore them at their own, or the patient's, risk.

An effective case management program uses a separate registered nurse, case manager, and social worker who work separately from the primary team in assessing patient need. These individuals should be specifically trained to evaluate for the issues facing geriatric patients.

Regardless of disposition, communication with the patient's medical home as well as other care providers is key to continuity of care and minimizing negative outcomes.

- Case management from the ED is not only feasible but necessary for the overall care of the geriatric patient, but success requires a coordinated multidisciplinary approach both in and outside the hospital.

- The use of an aged care specialist at time of discharge improves patient satisfaction, patient understanding of their care, and lowers ED recidivism.

- Multiple factors affect the geriatric patient's ability to safely operate a motor vehicle. ED physicians should be aware of these factors, and be prepared to refer patients for further evaluation if needed.

References

1. Roberts DC, McKay MP, Shaffer A. Increasing rates of emergency department visits for elderly patients in the United States, 1993 to 2003. *Ann Emerg Med.* 2008;51(6):769–74.

2. Aminzadeh F, Dalziel WB. Older adults in the emergency department: A systematic review of patterns of use, adverse outcomes, and effectiveness of interventions. *Ann Emerg Med.* 2002;39(3):238–47.

3. Grief CL. Patterns of ED use and perceptions of the elderly regarding their emergency care: A synthesis of recent research. *J Emerg Nurs.* 2003;29(2):122–6.

4. Horney C, Schmader K, Sanders LL, et al. Health care utilization before and after an outpatient ED visit in older people. *Am J Emerg Med.* 2012;30(1):135–42.

5. McCusker J, Healey E, Bellavance F, Connolly B. Predictors of repeat emergency department visits by elders. *Acad Emerg Med.* 1997;4(6):581–8.

6. Fuchs VR. Provide, provide: The economics of aging. NBER Working Paper 6642; 1998.

7. Spillman BC, Lubitz J. The effect of longevity on spending for acute and long-term care. *N Engl J Med.* 2000;342(19):1409–15.

8. Baicker K, Skinner JS. Health care spending growth and the future of US tax rates. NBER Working Paper 16772; 2011.

9. Institute of Medicine. Report Brief: Rewarding Provider Performance: Aligning Incentives in Medicare. National Academy of Sciences; 2006.

10. Rosenthal MB, Dudley RA. Pay-for-performance: Will the latest payment trend improve care? *JAMA.* 2007;297(7):740–4.

11. Rosenthal MB, Landon BE, Normand SL, Frank RG, Epstein AM. Pay for performance in commercial HMOs. *N Engl J Med.* 2006;355(18):1895–902.

12. National Hospital Ambulatory Medical Care Survey. 2008 Emergency Department Summary Tables; 2008.

13. McCusker J, Roberge D, Vadeboncoeur A, Verdon J. Safety of discharge of seniors from the emergency department to the community. *Healthc Q.* 2009;12:24–32.

14. Hastings SN, Barrett A, Weinberger M, et al. Older patients' understanding of emergency department discharge information and its relationship with adverse outcomes. *J Patient Saf.* 2011;7(1):19–25.

15. Rosenthal TC. The medical home: Growing evidence to support a new approach to primary care. *J Am Board Fam Med [online].* 2008;21(5):427–40.

16. McCusker J, Dendukuri N, Tousignant P, et al. Rapid two-stage emergency department intervention for seniors: Impact on continuity of care. *Acad Emerg Med.* 2003;10(3):233–43.

17. Hustey FM, Mion LC, Connor JT, et al. A brief risk stratification tool to predict functional decline in older adults discharged from emergency departments. *J Am Geriatr Soc.* 2007;55(8):1269–74.

18. Sinha SK, Bessman ES, Flomenbaum N, Leff B. A systematic review and qualitative analysis to inform the development of a new emergency department-based geriatric case management model. *Ann Emerg Med.* 2011;57(6):672–82.

19. Lowthian JA, Smith C, Stoelwinder JU, et al. Why older patients of lower clinical urgency choose to attend the emergency department. *Intern Med J.* 2013;43(1):59–65.

20. Naughton C, Drennan J, Treacy P, et al. The role of health and non-health-related factors in repeat emergency department visits in an elderly urban population. *Emerg Med J.* 2010;27(9):683–7.

21. Studnicki J, Platonova EA, Fisher JW. Hospital-level variation in the percentage of admissions originating in the emergency department. *Am J Emerg Med.* 2012;30(8):1441–6.

22. McCusker J, Jacobs P, Dendukuri N, et al. Cost-effectiveness of a brief two-stage emergency department intervention for high-risk elders: Results of a quasi-randomized controlled trial. *Ann Emerg Med.* 2003;41(1):45–56.

23. Basic D, Conforti DA. A prospective, randomised controlled trial of an aged care nurse intervention within the emergency department. *Aust Health Rev.* 2005;29(1):51–9.

24. Guttman A, Afilalo M, Guttman R, et al. An emergency department-based nurse discharge coordinator for elder patients: Does it make a difference? *Acad Emerg Med.* 2004;11(12):1318–27.

25. McCusker J, Verdon J. Do geriatric interventions reduce emergency department visits? A systematic review. *J Gerontol A Biol Sci Med Sci.* 2006;61(1):53–62.

26. Hastings SN, Heflin MT. A systematic review of interventions to improve outcomes for elders discharged from the emergency department. *Acad Emerg Med.* 2005;12(10):978–86.

27. Caplan GA, Williams AJ, Daly B, Abraham K. A randomized, controlled trial of comprehensive geriatric assessment and multidisciplinary intervention after discharge of elderly from the emergency department – the DEED II study. *J Am Geriatr Soc.* 2004;52(9):1417–23.

28. Hickman L, Newton P, Halcomb EJ, Chang E, Davidson P. Best practice interventions to improve the management of older people in acute care settings: A literature review. *J Adv Nurs.* 2007;60(2):113–26.

29. Mion LC, Palmer RM, Meldon SW, et al. Case finding and referral model for emergency department elders: A randomized clinical trial. *Ann Emerg Med.* 2003;41(1):57–68.

30. Hwang U, Morrison RS. The geriatric emergency department. *J Am Geriatr Soc.* 2007;55(11):1873–6.

31. US Department of Transportation: National Highway Traffic Safety Administration. Traffic Saftey Facts 2009 Data – Older Population; 2009.

32. Bayam E, Liebowitz J, Agresti W. Older drivers and accidents: A meta analysis and data mining application on traffic accident data. *Expert Syst App.* 2005;29(3):598–629.

33. Stiffler KA, Wilber ST. Older emergency department drivers: Patterns, behaviors, and willingness to enroll in a safe driver program. *West J Emerg Med.* 2011;12(1):51–5.

34. Eby DW, Trombley DA, Molnar LJ, Shope JT. *The Assessment of Older Drivers' Capabilities: A Review of the Literature* (Ann Arbor, MI: The University of Michigan Transportation Research Institute, 1998).

35. Carr DB, Schwartzenberg JG, Manning L, Sempek J. Assessing functional ability. In *Physician's Guide to Assessing and Counseling Older Drivers*, 2nd edn (Chicago, IL: American Medical Association, 2010), p. 17.

36. Li G, Braver ER, Chen LH. Fragility versus excessive crash involvement as determinants of high death rates per vehicle-mile of travel among older drivers. *Accid Anal Prev.* 2003;35(2):227–35.

37. Edwards JD, Lunsman M, Perkins M, Rebok GW, Roth DL. Driving cessation and health trajectories in older adults. *J Gerontol A Biol Sci Med Sci.* 2009;64(12):1290–5.

38. Ragland DR, Satariano WA, MacLeod KE. Driving cessation and increased depressive symptoms. *J Gerontol A Biol Sci Med Sci.* 2005;60(3):399–403.

39. Betz ME, Fisher J. The trail-making test B and driver screening in the emergency department. *Traffic Inj Prev.* 2009;10(5):415–20.

40. Shepperd S, McClaran J, Phillips CO et al. Discharge planning from hospital to home. *Cochrane Database Syst Rev.* 2010(1):CD000313.

41. Martin AJ, Marottoli R, O'Neill D. Driving assessment for maintaining mobility and safety in drivers with dementia. *Cochrane Database Syst Rev.* 2009(1):CD006222.

42. Classen S, Horgas A, Awadzi K, et al. Clinical predictors of older driver performance on a standardized road test. *Traffic Inj Prev.* 2008;9(5):456–62.

43. O'Connor MG, Kapust LR, Lin B, Hollis AM, Jones RN. The 4C (crash history, family concerns, clinical condition, and cognitive functions): A screening tool for the evaluation of the at-risk driver. *J Am Geriatr Soc.* 2010;58(6):1104–8.

Chapter

32

Falls and fall prevention in the elderly

Christopher Carpenter

Epidemiology

A fall is an unintentional, sudden descent to a lower level. Most geriatric falls that result in an emergency department (ED) evaluation occur from a standing level of less than six feet (2 m), and these are the falls referred to in this chapter. Falls and fall-related injuries are frequently encountered conditions in geriatric ED patients. In fact, 27% of community-residing geriatric adults will fall each year and the rates of injurious falls continue to increase faster than that expected by the "baby boomer" population surge alone [1,2]. The incidence of falls increases with age and as many as 50% of those over age 80 years will fall each year [1]. Over half of falls in community-residing older adults occur in and around the home and as many as 20% of falls result in serious injury [3]. Fall-related hospitalizations increased 50% from 373,128 to 559,335 cases in the US between 2001 and 2008 [4]. In response, the Centers for Medicare and Medicaid Services identified eight preventable conditions called "never events" in 2007. Falls in hospitals were one of those "never events," now known as preventable serious adverse events, which would restrict or reduce future hospital reimbursements [5].

Morbidity and mortality

Standing-level falls produce injuries that are disproportionate to the mechanism and are the leading cause of traumatic geriatric mortality, at a cost of $19 billion (2000, $US) annually in the US alone [6,7]. Falls frequently precede a downward spiral of fear of falling, social isolation, functional decline, and institutionalization [8]. The term "long lies" are used to describe an inability to arise following a fall, a phenomenon that may leave a fall victim on the ground for over three hours after a standing-level fall [9,10]. Injurious falls are defined by the occurrence of severe lacerations or fractures from a standing-level fall. In the period between 2000 and 2004, the National Hospital Ambulatory Care Survey reported 21 million injury-related ED visits in the US in those over age 65, and falls represent 38% of all injury-related ED encounters at a rate of 5.9 patient visits per 100 patient-years [11]. With a total of 48 million geriatric patient visits to US EDs between 2000 and 2002, trauma represents over 20% of these ED encounters [12]. In the United

Kingdom, injuries are the root cause of 33% of geriatric ED visits [13].

Fall-related injuries include intracranial hemorrhage, fractures, lacerations, and contusions. The determinants of injury from a fall include the kinetic energy of the fall impact, the direction of the fall, as well as the absorptive capacity of the bodily tissue and floor material. Fall-related fracture type also depends upon the fall mechanism and gender. In descending frequency, men fracture their hip, ribs, spine, humerus, or pelvis, whereas women fracture their hip, humerus, wrist, pelvis, or ankle. A sideways fall increases the risk of a hip fracture whereas a backwards fall increases the risk of wrist fracture [14,15].

Hip fractures are the most common fractures in men and women, with 300,000 occurring each year in the US, a number projected to double by 2040 [16]. Following a standing-level fall, hip fractures may not be immediately obvious on X-rays so magnetic resonance imaging can be cost-effective by diagnosing the bony injury days earlier than would otherwise occur [17]. Vertebral and wrist fractures are the next most common fracture injuries [18]. Wrist or distal radius fractures are the second most common fall-related fracture, found in 12–29% of all fall fractures, including Colles' fracture from a backwards fall on an outstretched hand [19]. Proximal humeral fractures represent 8–11% of fall fractures. Hand fractures are more common in long-term care facilities [20].

Falls are the most common cause of acute spinal fractures, with 90% of odontoid fractures in geriatric adults being the result of a fall [21,22]. Falls are an independent predictor of spinal cord injury, and the incidence of fall-related spinal cord injuries is increasing [23,24]. Central cord syndrome, defined by bilateral and usually distal upper extremity motor weakness, is the most common spinal cord syndrome in geriatric adults.

Rib fractures comprise 6% of fall-related fractures in institutionalized geriatric adults [20]. Pelvic fractures comprise 4–8% of community-dwelling geriatric fall fractures, but 85% of pelvic fractures in the elderly are the result of a fall [20,25,26]. The most common pelvic fracture is a pubic ramus injury. The management of fall-related injuries in geriatric patients generally requires a multidisciplinary approach that involves emergency medicine, orthopedic surgery, geriatrics, physical and occupational therapy, and pharmacy [17].

Geriatric Emergency Medicine, ed. Joseph H. Kahn, Brendan G. Magauran Jr., and Jonathan S. Olshaker. Published by Cambridge University Press.
© Cambridge University Press 2014.

Head injuries, like subdural hematoma, account for 46% of fall-related deaths. When falls occur in individuals using warfarin anticoagulation, deaths are more common (48 versus 16%). In general, more severe intracranial injuries occur with less blunt force when a patient is on warfarin [27]. Acute subdural hematoma is associated with 85% of fatal ground-level falls and is much more common in those over age 70 [28]. Since subdural hematoma can manifest with vague symptoms, clinicians must be vigilant to these intracranial hemorrhages following a fall and use family to gauge the current cognitive status compared to the patient's expected baseline for that time of day [29].

Risk factors (identifying high-risk fallers)

Fall risk factors are labeled as either intrinsic (an attribute of the individual) or extrinsic (environmental hazards) [30]. Figure 32.1 illustrates numerous examples of fall risk factors and common fall injuries. Most ED personnel do not have the opportunity to review the patient's home, but pre-hospital personnel are investigating methods to survey the home and rapidly assess fall risk to convey to ED staff [31,32]. A number of fall risk-stratification instruments are described in both inpatient and outpatient settings, but they lack validation in the ED [33–37].

One falls prevention screening tool was validated in ED settings, called the CAREFALL Triage Instrument (CTI). The CTI is based on eight modifiable fall risk factors: medication, balance and mobility, fear of falling, orthostatic hypotension, mood, osteoporosis risk, impaired vision, and urinary incontinence. The CTI is a secondary prevention instrument and derivation occurred in one academic ED in the Netherlands. Validation of the CTI in EDs other than the original derivation/validation site has yet to occur [38]. In addition, the 44-item CTI self-administered survey is probably too long for practical ED application.

The Prevention of Falls in the Elderly Trial (PROFET) was another secondary falls prevention study based in the United Kingdom. The PROFET investigators identified three predictors of falls and three factors which reduced the risk of falls (Table 32.1) [39]. One prospective single-center observational cohort assessed risk factors for falls within 6 months in ED patients who had been evaluated for any condition other than a fall. They identified three fall risk factors [40].

A systematic review of non-ED-based studies reported significant likelihood ratios for numerous risk factors (Tables 32.2 and 32.3) [41]. Past falls are consistently associated with future falls, but medications, foot problems, abnormal bedside functional tests, and cognitive dysfunction have not always increased the risk of falls in older adults in ED settings. Furthermore, in fall-risk stratification studies functional tests such as the "Get up and go" test are often poorly tolerated by geriatric ED patients [40]. For example, in one ED study of primary falls prevention, 50% of enrolled patients either refused or were incapable of performing the "Get up and go," chair stand, or tandem gait walk tests [40]. These tests of ambulatory strength and stability may be challenging in ED settings for a variety

of reasons. ED patients are acutely ill and their performance status probably does not reflect their baseline capabilities. With diminished physiological reserve, illness reduces the vigor and willingness to comply. In addition, most EDs are not geriatric friendly in either infrastructure design or personnel training [42,43]. Therefore, ED physicians rarely screen for fall risk, though nurses often do [44]. Normally ambulatory geriatric ED patients at risk for falls who cannot or will not perform ambulatory tests and who live in the community should raise concerns regarding the appropriateness of discharge. If admitted, inpatient teams should be alerted to the risk of falls to prevent inpatient injury and to prompt appropriate referrals and interventions.

Validating instruments that will accurately and reliably estimate short-term fall risk is an essential step for any interventional efforts to succeed. There will likely be more than one such instrument, since various subsets of geriatric adults are not homogeneous for fall risk. For example, the young-old (age 65–74) have different fall risk than the old-old (age 75 and older) patients, as do community-dwelling versus long-term care facility patients and physiologically frail patients. The location in which a fall occurs is also an important determinant of future fall risk and affects subsequent management strategies [45]. In addition, valid instruments to detect cognitive dysfunction in the ED have only recently been described and dementia has usually been an exclusion criterion in interventional falls trials, so extrapolation of most preventative effort to the cognitively impaired is not possible [46].

Pearls and pitfalls for fall prevention

Emergency department personnel who evaluate geriatric fall patients have two essential objectives. The first is to identify the cause of the fall and the second is to delineate any fall-related injuries. The cause of the fall is not always obvious and may be multifactorial, as depicted in Figure 32.1. Both British and American Geriatric Societies have jointly published fall prevention guidelines (Figure 32.2) [47]. Although these guidelines target primary care or the ED, as previously noted most of these fall risk factors have not been consistently associated with falls or injurious falls in ED settings. In addition, the optimal personnel to perform fall screening, and its timing within the time-deprived ED, remains elusive [44]. Nonetheless, ED's have an essential role to play in reducing fall risk, even if the most effective interventions to reduce injurious falls will be multidisciplinary and occur outside the traditional scope of practice for emergency medicine [17,48].

Any fall prevention strategy requires a willing, able, and compliant patient to be effective. Providing high-risk fall patients with exercise prescriptions or referrals to "fall teams" often fails due to patient-related factors of transportation problems, social isolation, or divergent patient values [49–51]. Similarly, providing nurses and physicians with evidence-based guidelines to reduce falls does not change practice patterns nor reduce injurious falls [52]. The PROFET trial provides one example of an effective and rigorously integrated multidisciplinary secondary falls prevention program. In this trial

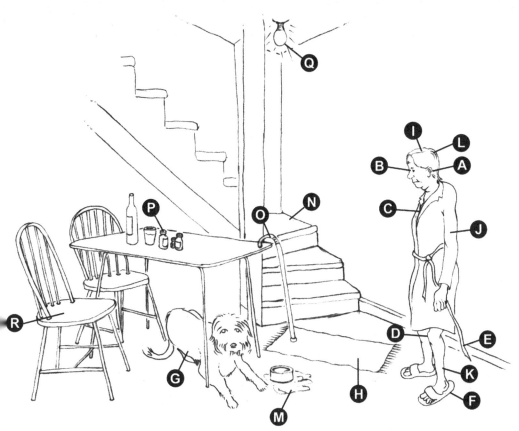

(a) **Pre-fall factors** A. Disequilibrium; B. Visual deficits; C. Dysrhythmia, Orthostatic hypotension; D. Degenerative joint disease; E. Loose fitting clothing; F. Poorly fitting footwear or foot sores; G. Pets; H. Rugs or loose mats; I. Dementia, Parkinson's Disease; J. Malnutrition; K. Deconditioning, frailty, muscle wasting; L. Pre-existing stroke or other motor deficit; M. Slippery surface; N. Stairs; O. Walker or crutches; P. Medications, alcohol; Q. Inadequate lighting; R. Transfers from sitting to standing.

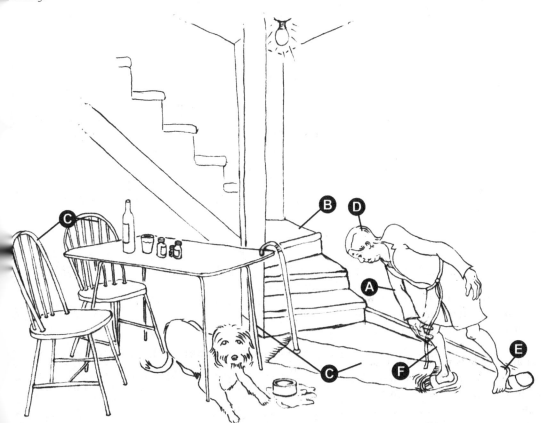

(b) **Intra-fall factors** A. Impaired reflexes to ease fall; B. Lack of handrails; C. Cluttered furniture; D. Diminished awareness of falling; E. Impaired proprioception; F. Diminished core body strength.

Figure 32.1 Standing level falls in the geriatric patient – risk factors in the home and common injuries. (Reproduced with permission of John Wiley & Sons Publishing Company.)

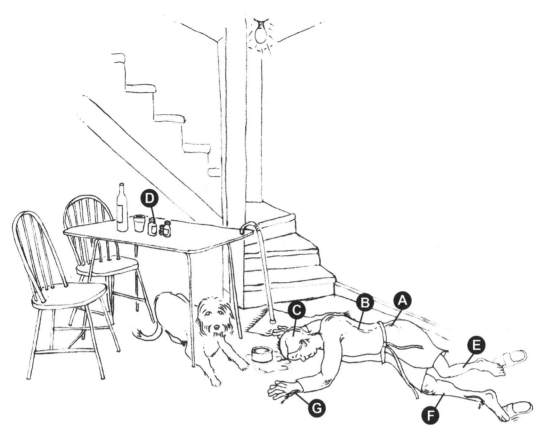

(c) **Post-fall factors and injuries** A. Osteoporosis = fractures with minor trauma; B. Spinal cord stenosis and cervical spine degenerative disc disease = spinal cord contusion (anterior cord syndrome); C. Cerebral wasting = subdural hematoma; D. Medications (anticoagulants, antiplatelet agents) = increased risk of intracranial (and other) bleeding; E. Muscle wasting = inability to rise and "long lies"; F. Diminished body fat/padding = more force to brittle bones; G. Frail skin = tears and lacerations.

Figure 32.1 (*cont.*)

Table 32.1. Predictors and protective factors for falls in ED elderly following a fall

Variable	Odds ratio (95% CI)*
Falls in last 12 months	1.5 (1.1–1.9)
Indoors fall	2.4 (1.1–5.2)
Inability to rise after fall	5.5 (2.3–13.0)
Moderate alcohol use	0.55 (0.28–1.1)
Reduced mental test score	0.70 (0.53–0.93)
Hospital admission due to fall	0.26 (0.11–0.61)

* Odds ratio >1 = increased risk of fall whereas odds ratio <1 = decreased risk of fall.

Table 32.2. Most significant risk factors for one or more falls in 12 months

Risk factor	Positive likelihood ratio (95% CI)	Negative likelihood ratio (95% CI)
Benzodiazepine, phenothiazine, or antidepressant use	27 (3.6–270)	0.88 (0.82–0.95)
Dementia	17 (1.9–149)	0.99 (0.97–1.0)
Previous stroke findings on exam[a]	15 (3.6–67)	0.91 (0.86–0.96)
Parkinson's disease	5.0 (1.5–16)	0.98 (0.97–1.0)
Unable to rise from chair without using arms[b]	4.3 (2.3–7.9)	0.77 (0.66–0.90)
≥5 errors on the Short Portable Mental Status Questionnaire	4.2 (1.9–9.6)	0.88 (0.81–0.96)
Fall in the previous month	3.8 (2.2–6.4)	0.84 (0.77–0.92)
≥4 days in bed during month prior to baseline	3.7 (1.6–8.6)	0.94 (0.89–0.99)
≥1 fall during previous year	2.8 (2.1–3.8)	0.86 (0.81–0.92)

[a] Women; [b] Men.

patients who had presented to one ED after a fall were followed by a team consisting of a general practitioner and an occupational therapist. This multidisciplinary intervention reduced falls by 20% [53].

Davison et al. conducted another falls prevention trial in the United Kingdom randomizing community-dwelling fallers after they had presented to the ED for a recurrent fall to a multidisciplinary intervention versus standard care. These investigators noted no differences in the fall risk, number of falls, or hospital admissions at one year, though the duration of subsequent hospitalizations was reduced by 3.6 days and overall confidence in balance was also improved [54]. The PROFET

Table 32.3. Significant risk factors for two or more falls in 12 months

Signs	Positive likelihood ratio (95% CI)	Negative likelihood ratio (95% CI)
Dementia	13 (2.3–79)	0.97 (0.94–1.0)
Stroke	3.2 (1.9–5.4)	0.87 (0.78–0.97)
Frequent fear of falling	2.6 (1.9–3.5)	0.70 (0.59–0.84)
Unable to complete tandem walk test[a]	2.4 (2.0–2.9)	0.51 (0.38–0.68)
≥1 fall during previous year	2.3 (1.8–2.9) to 2.4 (1.9–3.0)	0.60 (0.47–0.76) to 0.61 (0.49–0.76)
Needs >10 seconds to do 3 chair stands[b]	2.3 (1.8–2.9)	0.66 (0.54–0.80)
Self-perceived mobility problem	2.0 (1.7–2.4)	0.48 (0.34–0.68)

[a] Tandem walk test involves walking with the heel of one foot touching the toe of the other over 2 m.

[b] Get up from and sit down in a chair 3 times in a row.

and Davison trials probably yielded inconsistent estimates of one-year fall prevention effectiveness for a number of reasons. Davison et al. excluded patients with only one fall, as well as those with a medical etiology for their fall, while PROFET included those lower-risk patients. PROFET lost more patients to follow-up (23 versus 10%). Fall incidence over the one-year follow-up was measured using diaries and monthly postcards in the Davison study, while PROFET used postcard queries every 4 months. The PROFET patients reported fewer falls than the Davison patients (42.8 versus 62.6%). The multidisciplinary interventions in the PROFET and Davison trials were of similar intensity, complexity, and duration. Therefore, the most obvious explanations for the diverging effectiveness estimates between the two trials are the baseline fall risk of the populations studied (higher in the Davison trial) and the method used to identify falls during the one-year follow-up (more detailed and more frequent in the Davison trial). Of note, neither trial conducted their intervention in the ED. Instead, both screened ED patient registration logs and contacted fall patients by letter or telephone in the days after their episode of emergency care.

One systematic review analyzed 111 trials involving over 55,000 community-dwelling participants in 15 countries, but only 6 were ED-based. The fall-prevention interventions tested included exercise, vitamin D supplementation, pacemaker placement, cataract surgery, and environmental interventions. Ten studies assessed multiple interventions simultaneously, while 31 tested multifactorial interventions in which the therapy was dependent upon unique patient characteristics. Home-based exercises and tai chi reduced fall rates while overall exercise interventions reduced fracture rates (relative risk 0.36; 95% CI 0.19–0.70). In patients with cardioinhibitory carotid sinus hypersensitivity, cardiac pacing reduced the rate of falls without reducing the number of fractures. Providing new glasses paradoxically increased the rate of falls and fracture risk, but home safety interventions appear particularly effective

in patients with impaired visual acuity. Yaktrax walkers reduced outdoor falls in slippery winter conditions. Interventions that did not reduce fall rates or fall-related fractures included medication modification, vitamin D supplementation, patient education, and cognitive-behavioral modifications [55]. However, a more recent meta-analysis of 26 trials suggests that vitamin D combined with calcium reduces the risks of falls [56]. Exercise-based interventions also improved other important aspects of well-being [57]. Hip protectors did not reduce hip fracture rates in nursing home or community-dwelling patients [58]. Multifactorial interventions were ineffective for frail community-dwelling fallers [59]. Cost-effectiveness of multifactorial interventions has not yet been demonstrated because clinical effectiveness is inconsistent [60].

Recommendations and future directions

Geriatric fall patients often fail to receive guideline-directed care when they present to the ED [61]. Worldwide, clinicians of all specialties struggle to implement falls prevention research into routine care [62–64]. One ED-based implementation approach in Australia used a referral pathway, audit and feedback, and additional falls-specialty staff to improve clinician compliance with guidelines, resulting in improvement in fall-risk screening from 62.7 to 89.0% and enhanced referrals from 3.4 to 20.6% [65]. Emergency physicians often fail to screen for fall risk, though nurses do so more reliably [44]. ED case managers and social services serve as a vital link to community-based falls prevention resources for patients and families. Websites can be used to direct fall prevention advocates to low-cost local or regional resources [66–68].

High-yield opportunities for geriatricians and emergency medicine physicians to collaboratively improve the identification and efficient management of higher-risk geriatric fallers in the ED have been proposed [69]. These priorities include:

1. Validation of instruments in the ED that will accurately risk-stratify higher-risk fallers requiring admission or expedited outpatient evaluation.
2. Development of pragmatic ED-based interventions to reduce injurious fall rates.
3. Evaluation of mobile acute care for elderly unit in the ED prior to admission or discharge, to increase the efficiency with which risk of patient fall matches available inpatient or outpatient resources within a community.
4. Evaluation of hospital-at-home models to care for high-risk fallers in lieu of routine admissions.
5. Facilitation of reliable and accurate point-of-care fall-risk stratification using electronic medical records.

In the past, fall research has intentionally excluded patients with cognitive dysfunction and indirectly excluded frail and economically disadvantaged populations [70]. On average, only half of community-dwelling adults adhere to falls prevention interventions in clinical trials [71]. Future fall-risk assessment and interventional researchers will need to include these populations. Additionally, various fall-risk stratification methods have yet to be tested for feasibility, accuracy, and reliability

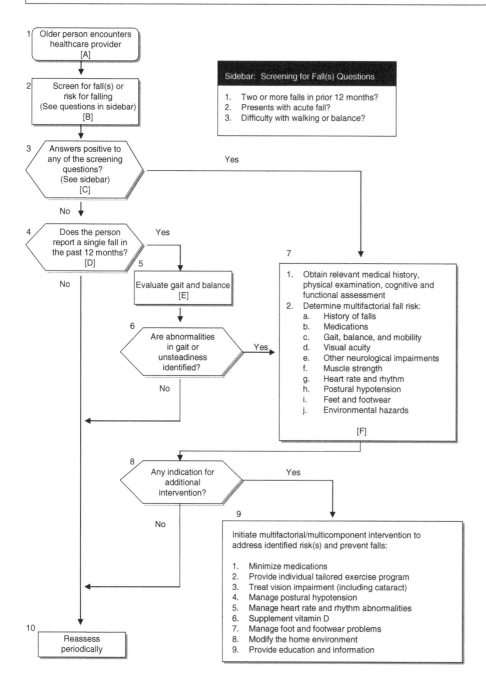

Figure 32.2. Joint fall prevention guidelines published by the British and American Geriatric Societies.

in ED settings, including balance assessments [72], functional mobility tests like the alternate-step test or stair ascent [73], and gait speed [74]. New management strategies such as vitamin D supplementation also need to be evaluated in ED settings [56]. Observation units offer one avenue for EDs to further evaluate geriatric patients at risk for post-discharge falls [75].

Summary

Geriatric falls represent an increasingly prevalent presenting complaint in the ED worldwide. The cause of falls in older adults is rarely one amenable problem, but multifactorial with intrinsic and extrinsic risk factors which are not always easily modified. Fall-risk stratification instruments for inpatient and outpatient populations are not always accurate predictors of

future falls in ED patients, and the results of "ED-based" trials have not been consistent. Nonetheless, the scope of fall-related morbidity in geriatric adults necessitates continued efforts to streamline the identification and appropriate management of high-risk fallers. Emergency providers will fill an essential role in reducing fall risk as part of a multidisciplinary care team, even if the most effective interventions to reduce injuries occur outside the traditional site and scope of practice for emergency medicine.

References

1. Stalenhoef PA, Crebolder HFJM, Knottnerus JA, et al. Incidence, risk factors, and consequences of falls among elderly subjects living in the community: a criteria-based analysis. *Eur Pub Health*. 1997;7:328–34.

2. Kannus P, Parkkari J, Koskinen S. Fall-induced injuries and deaths among older adults. *JAMA*. 1999;281:1895–9.

3. Masud T, Morris RO. Epidemiology of falls. *Age Aging*. 2001;30:3–7.

4. Hartholt KA, Stevens JA, Polinder S, et al. Increase in fall-related hospitalizations in the United States, 2001–2008. *J Trauma*. 2011;71:255–8.

5. Mattie AS, Webster BL. Centers for Medicare and Medicaid Services' "never events": An analysis and recommendations to hospitals. *Health Care Manag*. 2008;27:338–49.

6. Stevens JA, Corso PS, Finkelstein EA, et al. The costs of fatal and non-fatal falls among older adults. *Inj Prev*. 2006;12:290–5.

7. Sterling DA, Bonadies J. Geriatric falls: injury severity is high and disproportionate to mechanism. *J Trauma*. 2001;50:116–19.

8. Russell MA, Hill KD, Blackberry I, et al. Falls risk and functional decline in older fallers discharged directly from emergency departments. *J Gerontol A Biol Sci Med Sci*. 2006;61:1090–5.

9. Tinetti ME, Liu WL, Claus EB. Predictors and prognosis of inability to get up after falls among elderly persons. *JAMA*. 1993;269:65–70.

10. Grisso JA, Schwarz DF, Wolfson V, et al. The impact of falls in an inner-city elderly African-American population. *J Am Geriatr Soc*. 1992;40:673–8.

11. Carter MW, Gupta S. Characteristics and outcomes of injury-related ED visits among older adults. *Am J Emerg Med*. 2008;26:296–303.

12. Carter MW, Datti B, Winters JM. ED visits by older adults for ambulatory care-sensitive and supply-sensitive conditions. *Am J Emerg Med*. 2006;24:428–34.

13. Downing A, Wilson R. Older people's use of accident and emergency services. *Age Aging*. 2005;34:24–30.

14. Nevitt MC, Cummings SR. Type of fall and risk of hip and wrist fractures: The study of osteoporotic fractures. The Study of Osteoporotic Fractures Research Group. *J Am Geriatr Soc*. 1993;41:1226–34.

15. Norton R, Campbell AJ, Lee-Joe T, et al. Circumstances of falls resulting in hip fractures among older people. *J Am Geriatr Soc*. 1997;45:1108–12.

16. Cummings SR, Rubin SM, Black D. The future of hip fractures in the United States. Numbers, costs, and potential effects of postmenopausal estrogen. *Clin Orthop Relat Res*. 1990:163–6.

17. Carpenter CR, Stern ME. Emergency orthogeriatrics: concepts and therapeutic alternatives. *Emerg Med Clin North Am*. 2010;28:927–49.

18. Lips P. Epidemiology and predictors of fractures associated with osteoporosis. *Am J Med*. 1997;103:3–8S.

19. Tromp AM, Smit JH, Deeg DJ, et al. Predictors for falls and fractures in the Longitudinal Aging Study, Amsterdam. *J Bone Miner Res*. 1998;13:1932–9.

20. Cali CM, Kiel DP. An epidemiologic study of fall-related fractures among institutionalized older people. *J Am Geriatr Soc*. 1995;43:1336–40.

21. Lovasik D. The older patient with a spinal cord injury. *Crit Care Nurs Q*. 1999;22:20–30.

22. Müller EJ, Wick M, Russe O, et al. Management of odontoid fractures in the elderly. *Eur Spine J*. 1999;8:360–5.

23. Pirouzmand F. Epidemiological trends of spine and spinal cord injuries in the largest Canadian adult trauma center from 1986 to 2006. *J Neurosurg Spine*. 2010;12:131–40.

24. Clayton JL, Harris MB, Weintraub SL, et al. Risk factors for cervical spine injury. *Injury*. 2012;43:431–5.

25. Tinetti ME, Doucette JT, Claus E, et al. Risk factors for serious injury during falls by older persons in the community. *J Am Geriatr Soc*. 1995;43:1214–21.

26. Alost T, Waldrop RD. Profile of geriatric pelvic fractures presenting to the emergency department. *Am J Emerg Med*. 1997;15:576–8.

27. Chisholm KM, Harruff RC. Elderly deaths due to ground-level falls. *Am J Forensic Med Pathol*. 2010;31:350–4.

28. Hartshorne NJ, Harruff RC, Alvord EC. Fatal head injuries in ground-level falls. *Am J Forensic Med Pathol*. 1997;18:258–64.

29. Velasco J, Head M, Farlin E, et al. Unsuspected subdural hematoma as a differential diagnosis in elderly patients. *South Med J*. 1995;88:977–99.

30. Tinetti ME. Clinical practice. Preventing falls in elderly persons. *N Engl J Med*. 2003;348:42–9.

31. Snooks H, Cheung WY, Close J, et al. Support and Assessment for Fall Emergency Referrals (SAFER 1) trial protocol. Computerised on-scene decision support for emergency ambulance staff to assess and plan care for older people who have fallen: Evaluation of costs and benefits using a pragmatic cluster randomised trial. *BMC Emerg Med*. 2010;10:2.

32. Comans TA, Currin ML, Quinn J, et al. Problems with a great idea: Referral by pre-hospital emergency services to a community-based falls-prevention service. *Inj Prev*. 2013;19:134–8.

33. Nandy S, Parsons S, Cryer C, et al. Development and preliminary examination of the predictive validity of the Falls Risk Assessment Tool (FRAT) for use in primary care. *J Public Health*. 2004;26:138–43.

34. Oliver D, Papaioannou A, Giangregorio L, et al. A systematic review and meta-analysis of studies using the STRATIFY tool for prediction of falls in hospital patients: how well does it work? *Age Aging*. 2008;37:621–7.

35. Russell MA, Hill KD, Day LM, et al. Development of the falls risk for older people in the community (FROP-Com) screening tool. *Age Aging*. 2009;38:40–6.

36. Gates S, Lamb SE, Fisher JD, et al. Multifactorial assessment and targeted intervention for preventing falls and injuries among older people in community and emergency care settings: a systematic review and meta-analysis. *Brit Med J*. 2008;336:130–3.

37. Bongue B, Dupré C, Beauchet O, et al. A screening tool with five risk factors was developed for fall-risk prediction in community-dwelling elderly. *J Clin Epidemiol*. 2011;64:1152–60.

38. van Hensbroek PB, van Dijk N, van Breda GF, et al. The CAREFALL Triage instrument identifying risk factors for recurrent falls in elderly patients. *Am J Emerg Med*. 2009;27:23–36.

39. Close JC, Hooper R, Glucksman E, et al. Predictors of falls in a high risk population: results from the prevention of falls in the elderly trial (PROFET). *Emerg Med J*. 2003;20:421–5.

40. Carpenter CR, Scheatzle MD, D'Antonio JA, et al. Identification of fall risk factors in older adult emergency department patients. *Acad Emerg Med*. 2009;16:211–19.

41. Ganz DA, Bao Y, Shekelle PG, et al. Will my patient fall? *JAMA*. 2007;297:77–86.

42. Hwang U, Morrison RS. The geriatric emergency department. *J Am Geriatr Soc.* 2007;55:1873–6.

43. Hogan TM, Losman ED, Carpenter CR, et al. Development of geriatric competencies for emergency medicine residents using an expert consensus process. *Acad Emerg Med.* 2010;17:316–24.

44. Carpenter CR, Griffey RT, Stark S, et al. Physician and nurse acceptance of geriatric technicians to screen for geriatric syndromes in the emergency department. *West J Emerg Med.* 2011;12:489–95.

45. Kelsey JL, Procter-Gray E, Berry SD, et al. Re-evaluating the implications of recurrent falls in older adults: location changes the inference. *J Am Geriatr Soc.* 2012;60:517–24.

46. Shaw FE, Bond J, Richardson DA, et al. Multifactorial intervention after a fall in older people with cognitive impairment and dementia presenting to the accident and emergency department: A randomized controlled trial. *Brit Med J.* 2003;326:73–8.

47. Kenny RAM, Rubenstein LZ, Tinetti ME, et al. Summary of the Updated American Geriatrics Society/British Geriatrics Society clinical practice guideline for prevention of falls in older persons. *J Am Geriatr Soc.* 2011;59:148–57.

48. Bloch F, Jegou D, Dhainaut JF, et al. Do ED staffs have a role to play in the prevention of repeat falls in elderly patients? *Am J Emerg Med.* 2009;27:303–7.

49. Bleijlevens MHC, Hendriks MRC, van Haastregt JCM, et al. Process factors explaining the ineffectiveness of a multidisciplinary fall prevention programme: A process evaluation. *BMC Public Health.* 2008;8:332.

50. Hughes K, van Beurden E, Eakin EG, et al. Older persons' perception of risk of falling: implications for fall-prevention campaigns. *Am J Public Health.* 2008;98:351–7.

51. Horne M, Speed S, Skeleton D, et al. What do community-dwelling Caucasian and South Asian 60–70 year olds think about exercise for fall prevention? *Age Aging.* 2009;83:68–73.

52. Baraff LJ, Lee TJ, Kader S, et al. Effect of practice guidelines for Emergency Department care of falls in elder patients on subsequent falls and hospitalizations for injuries. *Acad Emerg Med.* 1999;6:1224–31.

53. Close J, Ellis M, Hooper R, et al. Prevention of falls in the elderly trial (PROFET): A randomised controlled trial. *Lancet.* 1999;353:93–7.

54. Davison J, Bond J, Dawson P, et al. Patients with recurrent falls attending Accident and Emergency benefit from multifactorial intervention – a randomised controlled trial. *Age Aging.* 2005;34:162–8.

55. Gillespie LD, Robertson MC, Gillespie WJ, et al. Interventions for preventing falls in older people living in the community. *Cochrane Database Syst Rev.* 2009;2: CD007146.

56. Murad MH, Elamin KB, Abu Elnour NO, et al. Clinical review. The effect of vitamin D on falls: A systematic review and meta-analysis. *J Clin Endocrinol Metab.* 2011;96:2997–3006.

57. Fairhall N, Sherrington C, Clemson L, et al. Do exercise interventions designed to prevent falls affect participation in life roles? A systematic review and meta-analysis. *Age Aging.* 2011;40:666–74.

58. Parker MJ, Gillespie LD, Gillespie WJ. Hip protectors for preventing hip fractures in the elderly. *Cochrane Database Syst Rev.* 2004;3:CD001255.

59. Faes MC, Reelick MF, Melis RJ, et al. Multifactorial fall prevention for pairs of frail community-dwelling older fallers and their informal caregivers: A dead end for complex interventions in the frailest fallers. *J Am Med Dir Assoc.* 2011;12:451–8.

60. Peeters GM, Heymans MW, de Vries OJ, et al. Multifactorial evaluation and treatment of persons with a high risk of recurrent falling was not cost-effective. *Osteoporos Int.* 2011;22:2187–96.

61. Salter AE, Khan KM, Donaldson MG, et al. Community-dwelling seniors who present to the emergency department with a fall do not receive Guideline care and their fall risk profile worsens significantly: a 6-month prospective study. *Osteoporos Int.* 2006;17:672–83.

62. Tinetti ME, Baker DI, King M, et al. Effect of dissemination of evidence in reducing injuries from falls. *N Engl J Med.* 2008;359:252–61.

63. Lord SR, Sherrington C, Cameron ID, et al. Implementing falls prevention research into policy and practice in Australia: Past, present and future. *J Safety Res.* 2011;42:517–20.

64. Speechley M. Knowledge translation for falls prevention: the view from Canada. *J Safety Res.* 2011;42:453–9.

65. Waldron N, Dey I, Nagree Y, et al. A multi-faceted intervention to implement guideline care and improve quality of care for older people who present to the emergency department with falls. *BMC Geriatr.* 2011;11:6.

66. Stopping Falls One Step at a Time. Fall Prevention Center of Excellence website. Available at www.stopfalls.org/ (accessed July 9, 2012).

67. Think Tall, Prevent a Fall Arizona Fall. Prevention Coalition website. Available at www.azstopfalls.org/ (accessed July 9, 2012).

68. Falls – Older Adults Centers for Disease Control website. Available at www.cdc.gov/HomeandRecreationalSafety/Falls/index.html (accessed July 5, 2012).

69. Carpenter CR, Shah MN, Hustey FM, et al. High yield research opportunities in geriatric emergency medicine research: pre-hospital care, delirium, adverse drug events, and falls. *J Gerontol Med Sci.* 2011;66:775–83.

70. Stineman MG, Strumpf N, Kurichi JE, et al. Attempts to reach the oldest and frailest: Recruitment, adherence, and retention of urban elderly persons to a falls reduction exercise program. *Gerontologist.* 2011;51:S59–72.

71. Nyman SR, Victor CR. Older people's participation in and engagement with falls prevention interventions in community settings: An augment to the Cochrane systematic review. *Age Aging.* 2012;41:16–23.

72. Muir SW, Berg K, Chesworth B, et al. Quantifying the magnitude of risk for balance impairment on falls in community-dwelling older adults: A systematic review and meta-analysis. *J Clin Epidemiol.* 2010;63:389–406.

73. Tiedemann A, Shimada H, Sherrington C, et al. The comparative ability of eight functional mobility tests for predicting falls in community-dwelling older people. *Age Aging.* 2008;37:430–5.

74. Quach L, Galica AM, Jones RN, et al. The nonlinear relationship between gait speed and falls: The Maintenance of Balance, Independent Living, Intellect, and Zest in the Elderly of Boston Study. *J Am Geriatr Soc.* 2011;59:1069–73.

75. Ganz DA, Alkema GE, Wu S. It takes a village to prevent falls: reconceptualizing fall prevention and management for older adults. *Inj Prev.* 2008;14:266–71.

Chapter
33
Financial issues in geriatric emergency care

Brendan G. Magauran Jr.

Background

The business side of medicine is enough to make most emergency physicians' eyes glaze over and tune out. The practice of emergency medicine is what drew most physicians to this field. However, in an environment where health care is consuming an ever-increasing share of the Gross Domestic Product (GDP) and the US is spending close to double the amount of money per capita than the next industrialized nation without substantial improvement in health care outcomes [1], the emergency physician must understand the impact health care reform efforts will have on emergency medicine practice. This chapter will focus on the financial issues particular to geriatric emergency medicine: how geriatric care is financed, the many parts of Medicare, US and geriatric population demographics, EMTALA and the Affordable Care Act.

The majority of industrialized nations pay for health care through a government-financed system based on tax collections. The US finances health care through a market-based system of charging employers and employees for private health care coverage. As is the case with all markets, government has a role in insuring "market failures" (i.e., patients too young, the disabled, and the elderly).

With the impending implementation of provisions of the Patient Protection and Affordable Care Act (PPACA) or the Affordable Care Act (ACA), there is renewed focus on providing increased insurance access and restructuring payments to providers and facilities in government-sponsored health plans. With respect to paying for emergency medicine services, the emergency department (ED) has traditionally been viewed as the most expensive place to receive care. This statement is generally accepted as true on a cost-per-visit basis [2] and has led many to health care reforms premised on reducing ED utilization. Insufficient research has been undertaken to determine the value received both medically and financially from an expedited ED work-up with regard to patient outcomes.

Demographics

Americans are living longer and the geriatric population in the US is rapidly increasing. Life expectancy increased nearly 30 years in the 20th century, from 47.3 to 76.8 years [3]. As life expectancy continues to increase, so does the geriatric population. It is estimated that by 2050, the geriatric population in the US will exceed 88.5 million, more than double the number from 2000 [4]. The geriatric population by 2050 will represent 20.2% of the US population as compared with 4.1% in 1900 and 12.4% in 2000 [5].

The ED has long been considered an expensive site for care, particularly for non-urgent patients. A non-urgent ED visit is defined as a patient who could safely be seen by a health care provider more than 24 hours later without any adverse effects to health. In a 1993 report focusing on ED access and usage, the US General Accounting Office (GAO) found that a majority of patients came to the ED with non-urgent conditions [6].

The GAO (now known as the Government Accountability Office) is an independent, non-partisan agency that audits spending of taxpayer dollars by government programs. The report entitled "Emergency Departments: Unevenly affected by growth and change in patient use" concluded that "43% of ED patients had illnesses or injuries that could have been treated in a less expensive setting, if available, but most patients went to the ED even when there were alternative sources of non-urgent care" [7].

EMTALA

The 1986 Emergency Medical Treatment and Active Labor Act (EMTALA) also limited the ED's ability to redirect non-urgent patients to less costly sites of care. EMTALA mandates that all patients who come to the ED requesting care must receive a medical screening exam to determine whether an emergency medical condition truly exists. In addition, all patients presenting to the ED requesting to be seen for any medical complaint had to be seen regardless of ability to pay and ED staff could not delay the evaluation while registration staff obtained insurance status.

Since this time, there have been numerous efforts to reduce non-urgent ED visits without a clear understanding of the reasons why patients choose the ED. Difficulty accessing primary care due to a limited infrastructure and individual perception of an emergency condition are the main drivers of ED visits. Young et al. reported in 1996 that in addition to 45% of walk-in patients presenting to an ED believing a medical emergency

Geriatric Emergency Medicine, ed. Joseph H. Kahn, Brendan G. Magauran Jr., and Jonathan S. Olshaker. Published by Cambridge University Press. © Cambridge University Press 2014.

existed, another 19% of patients reported being told to go to the ED by their health care provider representative [8]. Despite over 20 years of efforts to have patients select less costly sites of care, ED usage is still increasing annually.

Given that the US population is increasing and the "baby boom" generation is aging, ED usage by the geriatric population insured by Medicare will increase as well. Controlling Medicare costs will continue to be a major policy issue in health care reform. Reducing costs associated with ED usage does deserve a second look as perhaps the trend towards increased admissions through the ED actually reflects a cost-effective, streamlined care process that contributes to decreased hospitalizations, reduced hospital length of stays, and less cost overall.

Medicare

The financing of health care in the US is a mix of public and private financing, as well as out-of-pocket spending. Health care spending in the US for 2010 approached 2.6 trillion dollars, or 17.6% of GDP. On a per capita basis, health care spending in 2011 amounted to approximately $8608 dollars [9]. Public financing through the government is primarily through entitlement programs such as Medicaid and Medicare (there are other federal, state, and local programs). Private financing is primarily through an employer-based health insurance system in addition to individual out-of-pocket spending.

Medicare is a social insurance program that offers enrollees aged 65 years and older defined health care benefits. There are essentially four parts to Medicare: Part A for hospital coverage, Part B for outpatient services, Part C which is now private Medicare Advantage Programs, and Part D which is for drug coverage (again provided by private companies) [10]. All benefits are subject to "medical necessity." Medical necessity doctrine determines eligibility for medical items and services and the Social Security Act.

Medicare part A covers inpatient hospital services provided in a hospital. A hospital is considered to include inpatient rehabilitation facilities and long-term care facilities. Part A also covers skilled nursing facilities, hospice care services, and home health care services [11]. Medicare part B will pay for outpatient services that are medically necessary. Medically necessary is defined by accepted standards of medical care, and is generally thought of as "medical insurance." Such outpatient services include doctors' services, diagnostic testing including lab and radiology tests, vaccinations for flu and pneumonia, ambulance services, chemotherapy, clinical research, durable medical equipment (wheelchairs, walkers, commodes, hospital beds), some home health services, mental health services (inpatient and outpatient), and some preventive screening services such as mammography and pap smears [12]. Medicare part B is premium based according to income. Participants must first meet the Medicare deductible and then pay 20% of what Medicare determines to be a reasonable charge; Medicare will pay the remaining 80% [12].

Medicare part C is represented by Medicare Advantage plans. Private companies approved by Medicare offer plans that combine the part A and B benefits and may include drug coverage as well. The different types of plans include health maintenance organizations (HMO), preferred provider organizations (PPO), private fee for service plans (PFFS), and special needs plans (SNP). Medicare part C health plans also include demonstration and pilot programs as well as Programs of All-inclusive Care for the Elderly (PACE) [13]. Medicare part D is a drug prescription plan. Patients have a choice of joining a Medicare advantage plan with drug coverage or staying with original Medicare and receiving parts A and B benefits with the addition of part D. There is a coverage gap ("the donut hole") with most Medicare drug plans. Once in the coverage gap, enrollees pay 47.5% of plan cost for brand name prescriptions and 79% of plan cost for generic prescriptions.

Examples of situations paid for by Medicare parts A and B are outlined in Table 33.1 [14].

When a Medicare patient is admitted to the hospital, the physician must write an order to admit the patient to either an inpatient or observation level of services, but there is general confusion on the part of physicians and patients as to what these levels of service represent. The hospital payment for each level of services differs substantially, as an observation level of service is intended to require no more than two days in the hospital for the patient. Medicare enrollees also see quite a difference in terms of their bill, dependent upon their status as an outpatient or an inpatient.

Once the Medicare deductible is paid, an inpatient admission is covered under part A, with Medicare part A paying for both the hospital and the physician services. If the Medicare enrollee is admitted to observation-level services, then they must meet the Medicare deductible and part B will pay a significantly lower payment for the hospital and for 80% of the doctor's services. Part B will not pay for the drugs received in the outpatient setting.

Another important distinction for Medicare beneficiaries admitted under observation-level status is eligibility for a Skilled Nursing Facility (SNF) upon discharge. Medicare requires a prior inpatient-level hospital admission for at least 3 consecutive days (not including day of discharge) within 30 days of hospital discharge. An outpatient-level admission will not qualify the Medicare beneficiary for payment of SNF placement. Hospitals may change the status from inpatient to observation level, but it must conform to the requirements of "Condition Code 44" which requires the status to be changed prior to patient discharge. The Utilization Review (UR) committee must make the decision (or designee) and the patient attending physician must agree as documented in the medical record. The patient must also be informed of this change in writing. An order for observation-level status must also be placed in the medical record and the hospital must not have already billed Medicare for an inpatient-level status admission [15].

Affordable Care Act

President Barack Obama signed the Affordable Care Act into law on March 23, 2010, to be incrementally implemented over

Table 33.1. Examples of situations for which Medicare parts A and B will pay [14]

Situation	Inpatient or outpatient	Part A pays	Part B pays
You're in the Emergency Department (ED) (also known as the Emergency Room or "ER") and then you're formally admitted to the hospital with a doctor's order	Inpatient	Your hospital stay	Your doctor services
You visit the ED for a broken arm, get X-rays and a splint, and go home	Outpatient	Nothing	Doctor services and hospital outpatient services (e.g., ED visit, X-rays, splint)
You come to the ED with chest pain and the hospital keeps you for 2 nights for observation services	Outpatient	Nothing	Doctor services and hospital outpatient services (e.g., ED visit, observation services, lab tests, ECGs)
You come to the hospital for outpatient surgery, but they keep you overnight for high blood pressure. Your doctor doesn't write an order to admit you as an inpatient. You go home the next day	Outpatient	Nothing	Doctor services and hospital outpatient services (e.g., surgery, lab tests, intravenous medicines)
Your doctor writes an order for you to be admitted as an inpatient and the hospital later tells you they're changing your hospital status to outpatient. Your doctor must agree, and the hospital must tell you in writing – while you're still a hospital patient – that your hospital status changed	Outpatient	Nothing	Doctor services and hospital outpatient services

an 8-year period. The key features of the ACA include: expanding insurance coverage; eliminating pre-existing conditions discrimination; tying quality to performance with bundled payments; provisions to recruit and train geriatric health care providers as well as primary care providers; an individual mandate requiring all citizens to obtain health insurance; health insurance policies with minimum standards and no annual or lifetime caps; and importantly for seniors, elimination of the Medicare coverage gap for the "donut" hole in prescription drug coverage [16].

Emergency medicine physicians will need to be cognizant of these differences, as Medicare beneficiaries will be financially incentivized to ask about their status given the greater financial impact of outpatient admission status. Hospitals are similarly incentivized for emergency medicine physicians to understand the need for documentation that supports inpatient level of care. A Medicare denial for inpatient level of care carries a heavy penalty. Hospitals are not allowed to rebill the services as an outpatient status: they can only bill outpatient-level status on a Medicare patient initially leveled as inpatient if Condition Code 44 is met.

Criteria for determining inpatient hospital admission verses observation status are not clear-cut. Screening tools employed to aid in determining status level include McKesson's Interqual criteria and Milliman care guidelines (MCG). New updated versions are published on an annual basis and sometimes updated during the year. It is a daunting task to ask emergency medicine physicians to familiarize themselves with these tools on an annual basis, and hospitals are hiring care managers to fulfill this role and thereby aid the emergency and admitting physicians in this complex process. Increasingly, hospitals will require emergency physicians to document sufficient medical necessity to ensure an inpatient admission destination that will survive review by fiscal intermediary and scrutiny from Medicare area contractors (MAC). These are the companies hired by Medicare to process Medicare claims.

This is critical to hospital performance in two ways: avoiding Medicare inpatient level of care denials of payment (loss of all revenue for that visit) and avoiding recovery audit contractor (RAC) audits.

The impact of the ACA on emergency medicine overall appears to be significant. The Congressional Budget Office (CBO) estimates that by 2019, 32 million more Americans will have insurance coverage, but 23 million will remain uninsured [17]. In estimating the impact of this increase in access to insurance on utilization of emergency services, the experience in Massachusetts after the 2006 passage of comprehensive health care reform suggests that ED visits will increase [18]. The primary care infrastructure did not increase relative to the number of newly insured, so timely access to primary care physicians remained a problem. EMTALA provides that the ED remains the only guaranteed access to health care as the true safety net in the health care system, but does not guarantee payment for these services.

The majority of newly insured will not be elderly, but geriatric patients will be greatly affected nonetheless. ED crowding and patient boarding remain critical problems that will be exacerbated by more insured patients seeking emergency care. This impacts all ED patients. The National Ambulatory Medical Care Survey (NAMCS) from 2008 demonstrated that 15.4% of patients triaged as immediate/emergent had to wait over one hour to be seen by a physician. Another 2.7% of patients left without being seen, although the time that patients waited is not clearly documented. Efforts are under way at hospitals to redirect non-urgent patients to less expensive care sites and to improve ED throughput by reducing ED patient boarding. Redirecting non-urgent patients from the ED carries its own risks in terms of mistaken triage.

Summary

Health care reform aimed at increasing insurance access is primarily aimed at non-geriatric patients. Geriatric patient demographics suggest a continued increase in number of patients and an increasing overall percentage of patients accessing emergency services. Given the greater medical complexity of geriatric patients and increasing ED utilization trends, geriatric patients will continue to be resource intense in terms of ED evaluation and necessity of hospital admission. ED crowding and patient boarding will be further impacted without more significant efforts to address these critical problems facing emergency medicine.

Pearls and pitfalls

Pearls

- The geriatric population by 2050 will represent 20.2% of the US population as compared with 4.1% in 1900 and 12.4% in 2000.
- There is a substantial difference between admission and observation status in terms of Medicare's payment to hospitals and billing of enrollees.
- Under the Affordable Care Act, 32 million more Americans will have medical insurance coverage by 2019, but 23 million will remain uninsured.

Pitfalls

- If Medicare denies payment for an inpatient level of care, hospitals cannot re-bill Medicare as an observation (outpatient) status.
- Medicare part B will not pay for medications administered during observation status.
- Medicare requires at least 3 days of inpatient level of care in order to cover the cost of a skilled nursing facility (SNF) upon discharge. Observation status does not qualify the patient for SNF coverage.

References

1. Squires D. Explaining High Health Care Spending in the United States: An International Comparison of Supply, Utilization, Prices, and Quality, The Commonwealth Fund, May 2012 (accessed January 31, 2013 from www.commonwealthfund.org/Publications/Issue-Briefs/2012/May/High-Health-Care-Spending.aspx#citation).

2. Lopez S. The emergency room bill is enough to make you sick (accessed January 31, 2013 from http://articles.latimes.com/2009/nov/22/local/la-me-lopez22–2009nov22).

3. *National Vital Statistics Reports*, Vol. 61, No. 3, September 24, 2012, Table 19 (accessed January 31, 2013 from www.cdc.gov/nchs/data/nvsr/nvsr61/nvsr61_03.pdf).

4. The Next Four Decades – The Older Population in the United States: 2010 to 2050 Population Estimates and Projections (accessed January 31, 2013, from www.aoa.gov/AoARoot/Aging_Statistics/future_growth/DOCS/p25–1138.pdf).

5. Older Population as a Percentage of the Total Population: 1900 to 2050 (accessed February 4, 2013 from www.aoa.gov/Aging_Statistics/future_growth/future_growth.aspx#age).

6. US General Accounting Office: Emergency Departments unevenly affected by growth and change in patient use. Washington, DC GAO, 1993 (accessed February 21, 2013 from www.gao.gov/assets/160/152912.pdf).

7. Emergency Departments: Unevenly Affected by Growth and Change in Patient Use, HRD-93–4, 1993 (accessed February 21, 2013 from www.gao.gov/products/HRD-93–4).

8. Young GP, Wagner MB, Kellerman AL, Ellis J, Bouley D. Ambulatory visits to hospital emergency departments: patterns and reason for use. *JAMA*. 1996;276:460–5.

9. World Health Organization (accessed March 12, 2013 from www.who.int/countries/usa/en/).

10. What Medicare covers (accessed March 12, 2013 from www.medicare.gov/what-medicare-covers/index.html).

11. What does Medicare Part A cover? (accessed March 12, 2013 from www.medicare.gov/what-medicare-covers/part-a/what-part-a-covers.html).

12. What does Medicare Part B cover? (accessed March 12, 2013 from www.medicare.gov/what-medicare-covers/part-b/what-medicare-part-b-covers.html).

13. Medicare Advantage Plans cover all Medicare services (accessed March 12, 2013 from www.medicare.gov/what-medicare-covers/medicare-health-plans/what-medicare-advantage-plans-cover.html).

14. Centers for Medicare and Medicaid Services. Are You a Hospital Inpatient or Outpatient? (accessed March 12, 2013 from www.medicare.gov/pubs/pdf/11435.pdf).

15. CMS Manual System, Pub. 100–04 Medicare claims processing, transmittal 299. Subject: Use of Condition Code 44 (accessed May 25, 2013 from www.cms.gov/Regulations-and-Guidance/Guidance/Transmittals/downloads/r299cp.pdf).

16. Key Features of the Affordable Care Act, By Year (accessed February 21, 2013 from www.health care.gov/law/timeline/full.html).

17. Preliminary Estimate of the Effects of the Insurance Coverage Provisions of the Reconciliation Legislation Combined with H.R. 3590 as Passed by the Senate (www.cbo.gov/sites/default/files/cbofiles/attachments/hr4872_0.pdf, accessed April 28, 2013).

18. Massachusetts Division of Health Care Finance and Policy, Outpatient Emergency Department Visit Data (accessed May 24, 2013 from www.mass.gov/chia/docs/g/chia-regs/114-1-17-ed-data-specs.pdf).

Elder mistreatment

Judith A. Linden and Jonathan S. Olshaker

Elder mistreatment affects approximately 10–20% of the geriatric population in the US [1–3]. Many experts prefer use of the term elder mistreatment to elder abuse, because mistreatment encompasses both the intentional behaviors of abuse and unintentional behaviors which may also constitute abuse or neglect. While elder mistreatment shares many of the same considerations and risks as other types of family violence, certain unique aspects (such as cognitive impairment, isolation, poor health, and potentially decreased decisional capacity) make elder abuse a more complex and difficult situation, both in terms of identification and intervention. Elder mistreatment is often seen as a private affair, and therefore elders may be hesitant to report mistreatment to authorities. Older patients visit emergency departments (EDs) with increased frequency, and therefore ED staff may be the first to recognize and intervene on behalf of the abused elder. Presentations of elder abuse/neglect in the ED may vary from a patient with dementia who presents with intentional injuries, to an elder patient with severe dehydration, to a patient who presents after a fall with a hip fracture from a cluttered apartment. The emergency physician must have a high level of suspicion and be familiar with social service supports within the hospital, local resources, and local mandated reporting requirements.

History

Descriptions of elder abuse and intentional neglect/suicide can be found as far back as in ancient Greek literature. The first modern descriptions of elder abuse can be found in the British medical literature in the 1970s, with two reports (1975 and 1977) describing a phenomenon termed "granny battering" [4,5]. While intimate partner violence and child abuse have received wide attention and federal funding, elder abuse has received less public recognition, and funding has lagged. Older individuals are the fastest-growing population in the US due to better medical treatments and care that have extended life expectancy. The US Census Bureau reports that people aged 65 and older comprised 13% of the US population in 2010. It is estimated that by the year 2030 this group will comprise 19.3% and by the year 2050, 20.2% [6]. Once a person reaches 65 years, they can expect to live an average of 17 more years [7]. The longer one lives the greater the chances of the need for

some form of assistance, increasing vulnerability to abuse and neglect.

The issue of elder abuse came to the attention of the national government in the late 1970s and early 1980s, as it held congressional hearings which heralded the development and expansion of agencies and resources to combat elder mistreatment. The first federal government measures to address elder abuse came in Title XX of the Social Security Act of 1974. This act authorized individual states to use social service block grant funds to protect both elderly persons and children. In 1985, Congress passed the Elder Abuse Prevention, Identification, and Treatment Act, which clarified terminology by defining elder abuse. This act also directed the secretary for Health and Human Services to create the National Resource Center for Elder Abuse (NCEA), a division of the United States Administration on Aging (AoA), as a resource for combating elder abuse. The NCEA provides funding for research investigating the incidence and causes of elder abuse, a clearinghouse for summary of research findings, and compiles and distributes resources for elder abuse education and prevention. The Elder Abuse Task Force, a part of the Department of Health and Human Services, was created in 1990. Shortly after, the Joint Commission on Accreditation of Healthcare Organizations also began to specifically include elder mistreatment as a form of domestic violence. Most recently in 2011, the Elder Justice Act (EJA), a part of the Affordable Care Act, authorized a crucial increase in funding for studies evaluating elder abuse, as well as for training, services, and intervention programs to prevent and respond to elder abuse [8].

Definitions

The definition of "elder," as related to abuse, varies between 60 and 65, by individual state, and in the literature. Furthermore, many studies subdivide elder into "old" (aged 65–74), older (75–84), and oldest old (≥85). As mentioned earlier, many experts prefer the term elder mistreatment to elder abuse, because this includes passive abuse or neglect, as well as active or intentional abuse. Elder mistreatment encompasses many forms of elder abuse, including physical, emotional/psychological, sexual, and financial abuse, as well as neglect and abandonment. Self-neglect may also be included.

Geriatric Emergency Medicine, ed. Joseph H. Kahn, Brendan G. Magauran Jr., and Jonathan S. Olshaker. Published by Cambridge University Press. Cambridge University Press 2014.

Table 34.1. Elder abuse categories (NCEA) [24]

Physical abuse	Inflicting, or threatening to inflict physical pain or injury in a vulnerable elder, or depriving them of a basic need
Emotional abuse	Inflicting mental pain, anguish, or distress on an elder person through verbal or non-verbal acts
Sexual abuse	Non-consensual sexual contact of any kind
Financial exploitation/abuse	Illegal taking, misuse, or concealment of funds, property, or assets of a vulnerable adult
Neglect	Refusal or failure by those responsible to provide food, shelter, health care, or protection for a vulnerable adult
Abandonment	The desertion of a vulnerable elder by anyone who has assumed responsibility for care or custody of that person
Self-neglect	Behaviors of a vulnerable elder that threatens his or her own safety. Manifests by refusal or failure to provide him-/herself with adequate food, water, clothing, shelter, personal hygiene, medication (when indicated), and safety precautions

Physical abuse is the most visible form of abuse, and includes any form of physical violence against the elder. This may include behaviors such as pushing, hitting, punching, kicking, scratching, inappropriately restraining, or otherwise injuring the elder. Emotional or psychological abuse is defined as inflicting anguish or distress through verbal aggression, threats, intimidation, or other forms of verbal harassment. Sexual abuse is defined as non-consensual sexual contact of any kind. This may include not only penetration, but also non-consensual fondling, forced viewing of pornography, or forced performance of an act by the elder on another person. This type of abuse is likely very underreported due to the shame of the elder to report, and lack of the provider to consider elders as beings who could be subjected to this behavior. Financial abuse may be difficult to identify in the ED, and includes misappropriation of funds, theft of cash or social security checks, and coercion into signing over assets.

Neglect is the most common form of elder abuse, and can include intentional or unintentional withholding of food, medication, or other necessities, such as glasses, hearing aids, walkers, or wheelchairs. It can also include social isolation from human contact. Self-neglect, while not mistreatment by another, is sometimes included in the spectrum of mistreatment. Self-neglect is defined as the "behavior of an elderly that threatens his/her own health and safety." This may include refusal or failure to provide oneself with adequate food, water, clothing, shelter, personal hygiene, medication (when indicated), and safety precautions. Specific behaviors can include hoarding, poor self-hygiene, and other environmental hazards such as filthy living conditions, spoiled food, and lack of medications. Note that this excludes a situation in which a mentally competent older person, who understands the consequences of decisions, makes a conscious and voluntary decision to engage in acts that threaten his/her health or safety as a matter of personal choice. The prevalence of self-neglect increases with lower health status and poor physical and cognitive function [1,9].

Epidemiology

Elder abuse has been defined by NCEA, who further divided it into seven different types of behavior (Table 34.1). Elder abuse can be further separated into community and institutional elder abuse.

Recent studies reveal a prevalence of any type of elder mistreatment in the past year of approximately 10% of community-dwelling elders. When divided by type of abuse, emotional mistreatment (4.6–12.9%), financial mistreatment (3.5–6.6%), and potential neglect (5.1–5.4%) are the most commonly reported, with physical mistreatment (0.2–2.1%) less commonly reported and sexual mistreatment (0.3–0.6%) the least commonly reported. It should be noted that many of these studies, although they have the strength of being population based and asking behaviorally specific questions (both shown to increase identification), include only elders who are cognitively intact and have a phone. Thus the actual prevalence of mistreatment of community-dwelling elders is likely higher.

Elders who suffer from mistreatment of any type have a threefold increased risk of 1-year mortality. Those who suffer from self-neglect also have an increased risk of mortality [10,11].

Risk factors for abuse

Risk factors for elder mistreatment are controversial, and are related to both elder and caregiver factors. Some studies report that those aged >80 are at greatest risk, with others finding that those aged <70 are also at increased risk [1,2].

While any dependent elder person is at risk for mistreatment, low social support and prior traumatic experiences were found to be risk factors for elder abuse [1]. Possible risk factors related to the elder include the following [3,12,13].

- Functional or cognitive impairment;
- social isolation;
- poor health status;
- low socioeconomic status;
- lack of access to resources;
- previous psychological problems;
- previous history of family violence;
- substance abuse.

Caregiver factors include the following [14,15]:

- substance abuse;
- caregiver stress;
- previous family violence;
- financial dependence on the elder.

The contributions of race and gender are controversial, and are probably more related to confounding variables. It should be noted that many of these studies included only cognitive intact, community-dwelling elders and therefore the effect of cognitive impairment on risk is difficult to determine.

Suspicious presentations

Physical abuse

While falls and injuries occur with increasing frequency in the elderly, particularly among those with mobility issues, gait instability, or on anticoagulants, the practitioner should always evaluate these injuries for possible indicators of physical abuse. Some examples of suspicious injuries include: bruises on areas of the body that are not over bony prominences; injuries in pattern marks (i.e., a hand, a belt, a shoe); burns; multiple fractures or bruises of different ages; bruises/abrasions around the wrists or ankles from restraining; and delayed presentation to the ED.

Sexual abuse

Signs of sexual abuse may include new incontinence or soiling of clothes; unexplained anal or genital bleeding or genital injuries; unexplained genital infections; and bruises on the breasts, genitals, or anus.

Neglect

Neglect can present as bedsores; soiled or dirty clothing; severe dehydration; poor hygiene; and medical problems that are out of control due to lack of medications (e.g., diabetes or hypertension).

Historical indicators

Repeated visits to the ED;
unexplained delay in seeking treatment;
medical problems that are out of control due to lack of medications;
unexplained past injuries;
conflicting accounts of the injury;
new incontinence or soiling of clothes. [16–18]

Physical indicators

Bruises on areas of the body that are not over bony prominences;
bruises/abrasions around the wrists or ankles from restraint;
injuries in pattern marks (i.e., a hand, a belt, a shoe);
burns (especially cigarette);
multiple fractures or bruises of different ages;
fractures in places other than hip, wrist, vertebral compression;
unexplained anal or genital bleeding or genital injuries;
unexplained genital infections;
injuries to or bruises on the breasts, genitals, or anus;
malnutrition, severe dehydration;
absence of hearing aids, eyeglasses, or other aids;
bedsores.

Behavioral indicators

- Being extremely withdrawn;
- being emotionally upset or agitated;
- sudden change in behavior (as reported by caregiver);
- fear or hesitancy to talk;
- desertion of the elder at the hospital;
- caregiver who will not allow the patient to be interviewed in private;
- an elder's report of being mistreated.

Screening for elder abuse

While it is not feasible for the emergency physician to screen all geriatric patients for abuse and neglect, the practitioner should consider screening, or involving a social worker to screen, when there is a high index of suspicion. As in cases of domestic violence, patients should be interviewed privately. While many screens for elder abuse exist, some are too time intensive for the emergency physician and are meant to be used by highly trained individuals, and many have not been validated [19–21]. Yaffe et al. developed the Elder Abuse Suspicion Index (EASI) screen, and validated it in a group of family practitioners [22]. The EASI screen demonstrated a sensitivity of 0.47 and specificity of 0.75 when compared with a detailed social work evaluation. Most importantly, the screen took less than 2 minutes to administer. See Tables 34.2 and 34.3 for possible screening questions.

Documentation

Presentations that are suspicious for elder mistreatment should be carefully documented in the medical record. The same principles that apply to documentation in cases of intimate partner violence and child abuse pertain to elder abuse. Statements made by the patient should be documented in quotes, or preceded by "patient states" whenever possible. Observations about the behavior of the patient should be recorded in the chart in objective terms (e.g., withdrawing when provider approaches, very tearful, poor eye contact) rather than in subjective terms (e.g., afraid of provider, upset or sad). Concerns about caregiver interactions may also be recorded (e.g., caregiver speaking for patient or handling them in a rough manner). Injuries should be recorded, including size, description using a body map, and photography if available. Any provider concerns and referrals to social services, or reporting to adult protective services, should also be documented.

Legal/ethical considerations

Elders are protected by laws in all 50 states, but elder abuse reporting status varies by state. Mandatory reporting is required in many, but not all states. The presence of mandatory reporting may at times put the provider in conflict with the cognitively intact patient if the patient does not want the provider to report. The provider can address this concern by framing the report as an opportunity to find additional services that may be available to the patient, rather than a "report" or "investigation."

Table 34.2. AMA suggested routine screening for elder abuse [25]

Has anyone ever hurt you?

Has anyone ever touched you without your consent?

Has anyone ever made you do things you didn't want to do?

Has anyone ever taken anything that was yours without asking?

Has anyone ever scolded or threatened you?

Have you ever signed documents that you didn't understand?

Are you afraid of anyone at home?

Are you alone a lot?

Has anyone ever failed to help you take care of yourself when you needed help?

Table 34.3. Elder Abuse Suspicion Index (EASI) [22]

Within the last 12 months:

Patient answers these questions

1) Have you relied on people for any of the following: dressing, bathing, shopping, banking, meals?

2) Has anyone prevented you from getting food, clothes, medication, glasses, hearing aids, or medical care, or from being with people that you wanted to be with?

3) Have you been upset because someone talked to you in a way that made you feel ashamed or threatened?

4) Has anyone tried to force you to sign papers or to use your money against your will?

5) Has anyone made you afraid, touched you in ways that you did not want, or hurt you physically?

Doctor answers the final question

6) Elder abuse may be associated with findings such as: poor eye contact, withdrawn nature, malnourishment, hygiene issues, cuts, bruises, inappropriate clothing, or medical compliance issues. Did you notice any of these today or in the past 12 months?

Regardless of the presence of mandatory reporting laws, providers have an ethical and moral obligation to report any consideration of abuse. Most states offer the provider who reports in good conscience immunity from civil and criminal liability, and many states have penalties for not reporting suspected abuse. When questioning whether to report, the provider should err on the side of reporting, as this may bring much-needed resources and assistance to the elder [23]. It is then the responsibility of Adult Protective Services (APS) to investigate these cases. Abuse of community dwelling elders is reported to, and investigated by, Adult Protective Services (APS). Abuse of institutional dwelling elders is reported to, and investigated by, the Long Term Care Ombudsman program (LTCOP). Ombudsman is a Swedish term for "trusted intermediary." The LTCOP provides assistance and advocacy to long-term care residents. The LTCOP may investigate and intervene, or may then involve the APS. Adult protective services can inform the physician on how to locate the local LTCOP.

Once the report is made, adult protective services will then investigate. Investigation may lead to increased services, support, and resources for the senior and their family. Individual state resources and laws can be found on the NCEA website at www.ncea.aoa.gov/NCEAroot/Main_Site/Find_Help/State_Resources.aspx. If the provider believes that the patient is in imminent danger, the patient should be admitted to the hospital, since APS may not investigate immediately.

Preventive services

The physician can often face the dilemma of suspecting abuse but the patient is a competent elder who wants no report made. Another challenging situation is when there is no suspicion of intentional abuse or neglect but there are concerns that the patient and/or caregiver have insufficient support or resources. Certainly the suspicion of abuse should lead to formal reporting, but there are many other options to improve patient well-being. Case managers and social workers are excellent resources to connect patients and caregivers to social support services, visiting nurses, community programs, affordable transportation, mental health services, and other types of support that may make a significant difference. In addition, involving primary care physicians in these plans will be an important part of the handoff of ED care.

National and state emphasis on controlling costs and preventing ED revisits and hospital admissions will likely increase funding for resources such as ED case management. As mentioned earlier, ED case managers can be of tremendous assistance in connecting elderly patients to crucial resources, thus improving their quality of life and likely decreasing their risk of future abuse and neglect.

Conclusion

Since elders comprise a large proportion of ED visits and previous literature has shown that victims of elder abuse have significant interactions with the ED, all emergency physicians should have a high level of suspicion and be able to think critically about the possibility of abuse and neglect in elders presenting to the ED. The provider should be empowered to report potential abuse and neglect to the appropriate adult protective services, so that the case can be investigated and additional resources or services offered.

Pearls and pitfalls

Pearls

- Low social support is significant risk factor for elder abuse
- Substance abuse in elder or caregiver is risk factor.
- Suspicious injuries include bruises on areas of the body not over bony prominences, injuries in pattern marks, restraining injuries, and delayed presentation to the ED.
- ED case managers are outstanding resources.

Pitfalls

- Providers often do not consider elders as being subjected to sexual abuse.
- Failure to consider medical problems out of control as sign of neglect (especially due to lack of medications).

- Failure to consider behavior changes as a potential sign of abuse or neglect.

References

1. Acierno R, Hernandez MA, Amstadter AB, et al. Prevalence and correlates of emotional, physical, sexual, and financial abuse and potential neglect in the United States: the National Elder Mistreatment Study. *Am J Public Health*. 2010;100(2):292–7.

2. Laumann EO, Leitsch SA, Waite LJ. Elder mistreatment in the United States: prevalence estimates from a nationally representative study. *J Gerontol B Psychol Sci Soc Sci*. 2008;63(4):S248–54.

3. Amstadter AB, Zajac K, Strachan M, et al. Prevalence and correlates of elder mistreatment in South Carolina: the South Carolina elder mistreatment study. *J Interpers Violence*. 2011;26(15):2947–72.

4. Baker AA. Granny battering. *Nurs Mirror Midwives J*. 1977;144(8):65–6.

5. Burston GR. Letter: Granny-battering. *Br Med J*. 1975;3(5983):592.

6. Vincent GK, Velkoff VA. *The Next Four Decades, The Older Population in the United States; 2010 to 2050* (Washington, DC: US Census Bureau, 2010), pp. 25–1138.

7. Anon. *Sixty-five Plus in America* (Washington, DC: US Bureau of the Census, 1992), pp. 1023–178.

8. Dong X, Simon MA. Enhancing national policy and programs to address elder abuse. *JAMA*. 2011;305(23):2460–1.

9. Dong X-Q, Simon M, Evans D. Cross-sectional study of the characteristics of reported elder self-neglect in a community-dwelling population: findings from a population-based cohort. *Gerontology*. 2010;56(3):325–334.

10. Dong X, Simon M, Mendes de Leon C, et al. Elder self-neglect and abuse and mortality risk in a community-dwelling population. *JAMA*. 2009;302(5):517–526.

11. Lachs MS, Williams CS, O'Brien S, Pillemer KA, Charlson ME. The mortality of elder mistreatment. *JAMA*. 1998;280(5):428–32.

12. Dong X, Simon M, Rajan K, Evans DA. Association of cognitive function and risk for elder abuse in a community-dwelling population. *Dement Geriatr Cogn Disord*. 2011;32(3):209–15.

13. Mitka M. Elder abuse. *JAMA*. 2011;305(14):1402.

14. Homer AC, Gilleard C. Abuse of elderly people by their carers. *BMJ*. 1990;301(6765):1359–62.

15. Wiglesworth A, Mosqueda L, Mulnard R, et al. Screening for abuse and neglect of people with dementia. *J Am Geriatr Soc*. 2010;58(3):493–500.

16. Gorbien MJ, Eisenstein AR. Elder abuse and neglect: an overview. *Clin Geriatr Med*. 2005;21(2):279–92.

17. Kleinschmidt KC. Elder abuse: a review. *Ann Emerg Med*. 1997;30(4):463–72.

18. Lachs MS, Pillemer K. Abuse and neglect of elderly persons. *N Engl J Med*. 1995;332(7):437–43.

19. Moody LE, Voss A, Lengacher CA. Assessing abuse among the elderly living in public housing. *J Nurs Meas*. 2000;8(1):61–70.

20. Nelson HD, Nygren P, McInerney Y, Klein J. Screening women and elderly adults for family and intimate partner violence: a review of the evidence for the U.S. Preventive Services Task Force. *Ann Intern Med*. 2004;140(5):387–96.

21. Reis M, Nahmiash D. Validation of the indicators of abuse (IOA) screen. *Gerontologist*. 1998;38(4):471–80.

22. Yaffe MJ, Wolfson C, Lithwick M, Weiss D. Development and validation of a tool to improve physician identification of elder abuse: the Elder Abuse Suspicion Index (EASI). *J Elder Abuse Negl*. 2008;20(3):276–300.

23. Heath JM, Kobylarz FA, Brown M, Castaño S. Interventions from home-based geriatric assessments of adult protective service clients suffering elder mistreatment. *J Am Geriatr Soc*. 2005;53(9):1538–42.

24. Anon. *Major Types of Elder Abuse* (Orange, CA: National Center on Elder Abuse, 2011, available at www.ncea.aoa.gov/FAQ/Type_Abuse/index.aspx).

25. Levine JM. Elder neglect and abuse. A primer for primary care physicians. *Geriatrics*. 2003;58(10):37–40, 42–4.

Index